MEDICAL EDUCATION IN OKLAHOMA
VOLUME II

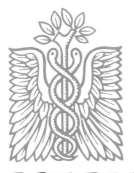

MEDICAL EDUCATION IN OKLAHOMA VOLUME II

The University of Oklahoma
School of Medicine and
Medical Center 1932–1964

Mark R. Everett and
Alice Allen Everett

Norman · University of Oklahoma Press

Library of Congress Cataloging in Publication Data

Everett, Mark Reuben, 1899-
    Medical education in Oklahoma.

    Includes bibliographical references and index.
        1. Oklahoma. University. School of Medicine—
History. 2. Oklahoma. University. Medical Center,
Oklahoma City—History. I. Everett, Alice Allen,
joint author. II. Title.
R747.067E82   610'.7'1176638   70-177333

This book is inscribed to
President Emeritus George Lynn Cross and
Director of Public Welfare Lloyd Edwin Rader
for reasons they best know

Preface

 The second volume on the history of medical education in Oklahoma requires fewer citations of original sources than the previous volume inasmuch as applicable references and documentations are available in various complicated university files, which have been arduously culled over a period of 33 years.

Starting on the presumption that the Board of Regents of the University of Oklahoma constituted the official core of medical center affairs, it became apparent from the start that no history of any facet of the university could be complete without a thorough examination of the regents' minutes which are on file in Norman. Other voluminous records, accessible in Oklahoma City, were in approximately three dozen filing cabinets in the office of the dean of the School of Medicine, some gradually becoming obscured through age and others almost too fragile to handle. Copies of certain pertinent records from faculty minutes, University Hospital records, Oklahoma legislative sessions laws, and correspondence have been placed in the library of the Medical Center.

The second half of the present volume is less concerned with the perennial struggle for survival than previously, its distinguishing feature being the changes in medical education which were occurring in a rapidly evolving medical center.

The appendices contain complete lists of faculty members and graduates of the Schools of Medicine and Nursing to July 1, 1964, as well as tabulations relative to administrators, hospital management personnel, preceptors, and other pertinent officials.

Alice Allen Everett, my wife and coauthor of this volume, contributed her industry and determination to assessing and editing the complex and sometimes taxing data assembled for this manuscript, a service which forwarded the completion of our task immeasurably. The reader is referred to Volume I, page vi, for acknowledgments of assistance from other individuals who made the preparation of a history of medical education in Oklahoma possible.

We are also indebted to Emil P. Kraettli and Mrs. Barbara James of the university regents' staff in Norman and to courteous staff members of libraries who freely contributed to our efforts.

Here in Oklahoma City I was helped by three part-time secretaries, Mrs. G. Kay McClanahan, Mrs. Nila Foreman, and Mrs. Betty Collier. Mrs. Collier, one of my secretaries during my term as dean, handled with patience and perfection the typing of the manuscript and associated tasks.

We owe our thanks to three deans who rendered important guidance, financial assistance, and encouragement during the study, James L. Dennis, the late Robert M. Bird, Tom Lynn, presently dean of the University of Oklahoma School of Medicine, and to Edward A. Shaw, director of the University Press.

Finally, we are indebted to our son, Mark Allen Everett, professor of dermatology, who encouraged us in our project and who made available to us excellent office space and other facilities in the dermatology clinic building during the years we have devoted to putting together the history of medical education in Oklahoma.

Mark R. Everett
Alice Allen Everett

Contents

Illustrations

MEDICAL EDUCATION IN OKLAHOMA
VOLUME II

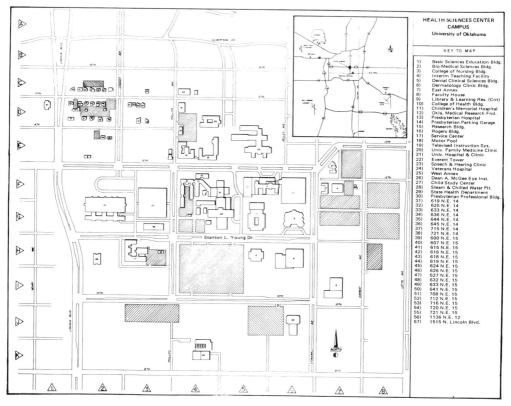

Present Health Sciences Center campus of the University of Oklahoma in Oklahoma City.

Chapter I.
Political Doldrums
and Divided Authority:
1932–35

 William H. Murray was in his second year as governor of Oklahoma in 1932, and, while he did not immediately raise new obstacles for the University Hospitals, considerable uneasiness continued to persist in the medical center as a result of rumors. For instance, a rumor came to the attention of Dean Lewis J. Moorman that the governor desired the discharge of Harry C. Smith, business manager of the University Hospitals, because of his political attitudes. As a matter of fact, there is a copy of a letter in the dean's office files from a councillor of the Oklahoma State Medical Association to Governor Murray, in which the councillor spoke of this rumor and stated that he believed matters had been grossly misrepresented to the governor; and he informed him that the A rating of the School of Medicine was very heavily dependent upon admissible evidence that the school was in no manner dominated by political influences such as those dictated by his gubernatorial actions in the previous year.[1]

The councillor further stated that the alumni of the school, as well as other representative members of the medical profession in Oklahoma, were vitally interested in the School of Medicine and its teaching hospitals, and that they were requesting the governor to join them in helping to keep the present management of the University Hospitals from being disrupted. Actually, Harry C. Smith had served the hospitals faithfully for several years and had made definite economies in the administrative expenses, while increasing the average number of patients from 330 to 408 per day.

Governor Murray's ideas of economy were really not economy at all, and one of his methods of inflicting annoying torment was his insistence that the business affairs of the University of Oklahoma and its School of Medicine were improperly managed. Within the year, he requested the dismissal of Harry Smith, eventually forcing his resignation because of purported disloyalty to and discourteous remarks about the chief executive; all of which was rather paradoxical in the light of the state examiner and inspector's audit of financial

---

[1] Mark R. Everett, *Medical Education in Oklahoma*, (Norman, University of Oklahoma Press, 1972), I, 243–48.

affairs at the two hospitals of the School of Medicine, as reported to the university regents on March 30. The audit showed that all accounts were in good order and commended the institution's officers for their efficiency in keeping records.

When the question of forced collection of the costs for charity patients from the various counties was introduced at the regents' March meeting, Judge Claude C. Hatchett stated that, under existing laws, any money spent in such an attempt would be wholly wasted. The $15 per week which counties were supposed to pay for the care of indigent patients would not have begun to reimburse even the basic hospital costs, to say nothing about the enormous amount of gratuitous service and diagnostic treatment—medical and surgical—contributed by members of the faculty and the hospital staff. Moreover, there are no words adequate to describe the fine constructive work which was conducted by the clinical staff members of the Crippled Children's Hospital. Such an institution was describable only ''as a blessing to the state.''[2]

The fact of the matter was that, since many of the counties claimed inability to pay even the small charge of $15 per week, the University Hospitals were forced to carry unpaid accounts in excess of $300,000 yearly. This produced such an acute financial problem that the university regents at their December meeting instructed President William B. Bizzell to provide for the collection of the county accounts. This directive corresponded with a decline in the health of the superintendent of University Hospitals, J. B. Smith, who became superintendent on August 1, 1931. All of these events only compounded the fiasco created by the eleventh legislature on March 9, 1927, in setting up financing of the care of the charity patients in Crippled Children's Hospital by payments from the counties, when the Supreme Court had previously ruled, on February 15, that such a contract was unconstitutional.[3] The year was one of disappointment, representing as it did an ill-advised retreat in financial support of medical education in the state of Oklahoma.

Wann Langston was clinical head of the outpatient department in 1932, and Harry Wilkins was named head of a neurosurgery service which, in time, developed into a nationally recognized specialty department that contributed a long line of neurosurgeons to American medicine. Walter W. Wells was appointed acting chairman of the Department of Obstetrics when John A. Hatchett, former chairman and professor of obstetrics and gynecology since 1911, could no longer serve because of poor health.

Charles S. Bobo, a former dean of the School of Medicine, was appointed director of the Student Health Service on the main campus of the university at Norman, following the death of Gayfree Ellison who had recently served in that capacity. Dr. Ellison, a kindly and beloved physician, had been a faculty member of the School of Medicine since 1910, voluntarily caring for faculty members and students often without monetary remuneration. Small wonder that the new infirmary on the Norman campus was named in his honor.

[2] *Journal of the Oklahoma State Medical Association*, Vol. XXV (1932), 212, 213.
[3] As cited in Everett, *Medical Education in Oklahoma*, I, 204, footnote 4.

There were 155 faculty members in the School of Medicine during the academic year 1932–33. Those newly appointed included:

Joseph Macglashan Hill, M.D.
  assistant professor of pathology
Fay Maxey Cooper, M.D.
  instructor in ophthalmology
Herman Fagin, M.D.
  instructor in medicine
Euel Park Hathaway, M.D.
  instructor in genitourinary diseases
Nesbitt Ludson Miller, M.D.
  instructor in medicine
Ben Hamilton Nicholson, M.D.
  instructor in pediatrics

John Copeland Pickard, M.D.
  instructor in otorhinolaryngology
Herbert John Rinkel, M.D.
  instructor in medicine
William Ward Rucks, Jr., M.D.
  instructor in medicine
Gladys Taylor, B.S.
  instructor in dietotherapy
Marion Weber, B.S.
  instructor in dietetics
Oscar Rogers White, M.D.
  instructor in surgery

In March, Fred C. Zapffe, secretary of the Association of American Medical Colleges, inspected our institution and proposed recommendations for guidance of the School of Medicine. These included reduction of hours in the regular schedule for medical students to approximately eighteen hundred, the discontinuance of operative teaching clinics in surgery, provision of half-day periods of experience for the clinical clerkships in the hospitals, reduction of didactic clinical lectures to a minimum, and more direct contact of the preclinical faculty with clinical cases for the purpose of instruction. Dr. Zapffe also suggested that the pathology department should reduce the required amount of microscopic work for medical students, with more emphasis on clinical pathology; and it was his opinion that the head of the department should be a physician who would have charge of all autopsies, and that the autopsy findings should be used more actively in the teaching program. Dr. Zapffe's advice was that the school should reconstitute and develop its graduate courses which had been curtailed by recent budgetary restrictions.

In regard to clinical experience for students on clerkships in the hospitals, two associate supervisors were appointed to help R. Q. Goodwin in the management of clinical clerkships, each devoting approximately six hours daily to this service.[4]

The establishment of cancer clinics around the country was part of a national trend which was endorsed by the clinical departmental heads and, subsequently, initiated by the faculty under the direction of M. N. Newquist of the American College of Surgeons, who assisted in the organization of the new clinic in the University Hospitals. John F. Kuhn, professor of gynecology, was designated executive director of the first cancer clinic.

The practice of appointing hospital residents, which began with the opening of the University Hospital in 1919, was a great step forward in postgraduate clinical education in Oklahoma. The first two residents, Raymond L. Murdoch in surgery and gynecology and Basil Hayes in medicine and obstetrics, were enthusiastically praised for their services by members of the hospital staff at the

[4] *Journal of the Association of American Medical Colleges*, Vol. IX (1934), 229.

time. The significance of the residency program which developed throughout America, particularly in the teaching hospitals, cannot be overstressed because it led to a diversity of instruction as the system of residencies expanded and progressed. This was by no means a detrimental step, because concentration on specific areas of medicine made it possible for the physician to become more expert in a special field.

The funds appropriated by the thirteenth legislature for the School of Medicine were $94,053; for the University Hospital, $308,521; and for Crippled Children's Hospital, $179,187, making a total of $581,761 in revenue for the medical unit of the University of Oklahoma. However, the regents reduced these provisions during the year to $84,649, $280,169 and $171,468, respectively, a reduction of $45,475 in the total amount appropriated for medical education by the legislature.

The Oklahoma State Medical Association again budgeted $700 for support of a postgraduate program in 1933, affirming that the extension department of the School of Medicine was doing excellent work in providing medical clinics in short-time graduate courses for physicians throughout the state.[5]

The School of Medicine granted 47 M.D. degrees in June, 1932, and the School of Nursing awarded 40 certificates of Graduate Nurse. The total number of students enrolled in medicine for the year 1932–33 was 259, and the tuition for nonresident students was $200. The medical curriculum offered 16 hours of electives in the second year, 48 hours in the third year, and 96 hours in the fourth year. At the same time, the School of Nursing had an enrollment of 95 students and a three-year curriculum.

There is a letter in the dean's office files from Floyd Bolend, associate professor of medicine, listing the names of members of the medical classes of 1932 and 1933 who volunteered emergency services during the 1932 flood in Oklahoma City. Cited particularly for prolonged service and assistance in alleviating suffering during the flood were Charles E. Leonard, Herman W. Roth, and Clifford A. Traverse.

There were 425 teaching hospital beds available during the period 1932–33, 225 in the main hospital and 200 in the Crippled Children's Hospital. There were 2,471 admissions to the Crippled Children's Hospital, 69 per cent of whom were county patients, 23 per cent pay clinical, and 8 per cent private patients. The outpatient department cared for 150 to 200 patients daily. St. Anthony Hospital had 375 beds and Central State Hospital 1,800 beds. The Holmes Home of Redeeming Love continued to be used in obstetrical teaching, as was the case for the ensuing five years.

Lewis J. Moorman, a gentleman of considerable professional honor and high ideals, entered upon his administrative duties as dean of the School of Medicine in a period of discouragement, resulting from sustained harassment and interference by Governor Murray. In fact, Dr. Moorman displayed remarkable

---

[5.] As cited in Everett, *Medical Education in Oklahoma*, I, 240.

courage in undertaking the dean's duties at all on September 1, 1931, in the face of such inadequate support at the state level.

The necessary expansion of the faculty and various operational services was limited by financial difficulties and by pressure from the governor and the regents to reduce expenditures, while the very real and great charity of the medical profession continued.[6] Meanwhile, criticism of the governor himself increased justifiably, and he lost appreciable strength in the house of representatives even before the fourteenth legislature convened in January, 1933. As a result of his so-called economy drive, state financial aid to the postgraduate program was diminished. The Oklahoma State Medical Association provided half of the financial support for the two postgraduate courses given in eleven counties of the state in 1932, making at least a reduced program possible.[7] A total of 749 physicians attended the sessions on gynecology, obstetrics, and surgical diagnosis in five centers of the state; other courses included a series in the northeast part of the state and one course in ear, nose, and throat in Oklahoma City.[8]

The only stimuli to the School of Medicine's educational program were Dr. Zapffe's favorable report on the progress of the School of Medicine in the past year and his helpful suggestions regarding modernization of the medical curriculum. These recommendations the administration attempted to carry through even without additional funds.

While there was a movement in a number of medical schools in the country to require a fifth year as an intern in an approved hospital in order to receive an M.D. degree, the faculty of the University of Oklahoma set aside this requirement on December 6, since the stipulation had been voted without publication prior to admission of the present student body. This action proved to be for the best since the various state licensing laws eventually resolved the matter.

During 1933, the third year of executive interference in medical education from the governor's office, new punitive attempts at economizing occurred. On February 23 the university regents were requested, in a letter from the governor, to lower faculty salaries *in order to buttress the funds of the state treasury*; and on June 27 the president of the university reported that he had received an executive order from Governor Murray, issued to the State Board of Affairs, which directed that board to transfer the property of the Union Soldiers Home in Oklahoma City to the regents of the University of Oklahoma as an annex to the University Hospitals, for the exclusive use of crippled children. The double surprise for President Bizzell was that the university regents, without a whimper, not only instructed him to take over the Union Soldiers Home, in

[6] Two faithful early supporters of the University of Oklahoma School of Medicine, Dr. Fred S. Clinton and Dr. Francis Fite of Muskogee, were inducted into the Oklahoma Hall of Fame in 1932.

[7] Editorial, *Journal of the Oklahoma State Medical Association*, Vol. XXVI (1933), 450–53.

[8] As cited in note 2.

accordance with the governor's order, but to provide facilities for the patients in residence in the home until such time as they could be accommodated elsewhere.

Under additional pressure from the governor, the ax fell again when the regents succeeded in dividing the administration of University Hospitals by appointing Lewis J. Moorman superintendent of the hospitals, in charge of all medical and laboratory divisions, as of July 1, 1933, and P. B. Bostic of Muskogee as business manager of the University and Crippled Children's Hospitals, replacing Harry C. Smith, as of the same date. Mr. Bostic was given control of the nonmedical personnel, subject only to approval by the president of the university and the regents. His salary was fixed at $4,500 annually.

Dr. Moorman's salary was fixed at $6,000 per annum, of which $3,500 was to be procured from the School of Medicine's budget and the remainder from University Hospital funds. All professional appointments were made subject to the approval of the superintendent of the hospitals and the president of the university.

This official action by the regents eliminated the services of Wann Langston as an administrator by forcing his resignation, which was part of the governor's strategy in the first place. There is a pertinent letter in the office files of the dean of the School of Medicine, addressed to Dean Moorman, May 20, 1933, in which Dr. Langston wrote,

> In regard to our conference of a day or two ago concerning relieving me as a half-time employee of the medical school, I want you to know that I appreciate fully the circumstances that compel this decision. I want to assure you that I accept this decision in the same spirit that I have accepted others, and assure you of my continued loyalty to you and to the medical school . . . . I think you will appreciate the fact that members of the clinical staff have largely built their reputations and practices by virtue of their connection with the School of Medicine, whereas, by virtue of my capacity I have lost the opportunity of building an adequate practice, having given the best years of my professional life to the building of this institution and placing it upon a sound financial basis. . . . Since I must now devote myself energetically to the practice of medicine, I should like to be relieved of those time-consuming and grief-laden assignments that I have carried for the last two years, namely the direction of the Outpatient Department and the supervision of the interns. . . . Thanking you for your many consider-ations, . . . and assuring you again of my personal and institutional loyalty.

These troubled words epitomize the allegiance and despair of a man devoted to medical education, who became a victim of political machinations. That Dr. Langston's many services and contributions should have been ignored by the governor and inconsiderately cast aside by authorities of the university is almost unbelievable.

Meanwhile, less traumatic changes took place, for better or for worse, in the ranks of the staff of the medical center. J. B. Smith retired on July 1 as superintendent of University Hospitals, commended for his faithful services by the regents, and Hiram D. Moor, head of the Department of Bacteriology, was appointed as executive assistant to Dean Moorman, who had acquired the additional title of superintendent of University Hospitals as a result of political manipulations. As of January 1, 1933, Bert Keltz was named director of the outpatient department of the hospitals, succeeding Dr. Langston; John Archer Hatchett was given the title of professor emeritus of obstetrics and was succeeded by Walter W. Wells as head of the Department of Obstetrics; Hugh G. Jeter returned to the medical school campus as director of hospital laboratories and supervisor of interns; and Kitty Shanklin was appointed as an assistant professor of medical social work and the director of social services at the University Hospitals.

In their June 27 meeting at the state capitol, the regents voted that members of the faculty should be assigned half-time duties and given half salaries upon reaching the retirement age of seventy years.

There were 147 members on the faculty of the Medical School in 1933–34 and ten members on the nursing faculty. Newly appointed faculty members were:

Mary Elizabeth Borella, G.N.
  instructor in principles and
  practice of nursing
Ralph Bowen, M.D.
  instructor in medicine
Leo F. Cailey, M.D.
  instructor in ophthalmology
Coyne Herbert Campbell, M.D.
  instructor in anatomy and
  pathology
Ralph Edward Chase, M.A.
  instructor in anatomy
Francis Edward Dill, M.D.
  instructor in gynecology

Onis George Hazel, M.D.
  instructor in epidemiology and
  public health
Minard Friedberg Jacobs, M.D.
  instructor in medicine
Wilbur Floyd Keller, M.D.
  instructor in medicine
Patrick Henry Lawson, M.D.
  instructor in genitourinary
  diseases and syphilology
Mary Jane Martin, R.N.
  instructor in operating room
  technique
Stanley Francis Wildman, M.D.
  instructor in genitourinary
  diseases and syphilology

The faculty authorized its admissions committee, on June 22, to limit the number of students accepted for the first-year class. Apropos of closer accord between premedical students and the faculty of the School of Medicine, Dean Moorman pointed out that a plan had been initiated the previous year whereby each premedical school in the state of Oklahoma had a premedical advisory committee.

In regard to the curriculum in the School of Medicine in 1933, the courses of applied biochemistry and clinical physiology, which had been instituted in 1929, were transferred from the basic science years to the second semester of the third year, with the applied biochemistry course lengthened to thirty-two hours. An applied pharmacology course was also added to the curriculum, and a weekly medical and surgical clinic for medical students was commenced in the

Central State Hospital at Norman. Concurrently, the Home of Redeeming Love and St. Anthony Hospital remained affiliated with the School of Medicine.

When the university regents met on September 29, the recurring question of unpaid county accounts due University Hospitals was discussed yet another time, because the total in accounts due was still in excess of $300,000. Finally, Regent Eugene Kerr made the motion that the governor be requested to instruct the attorney general to file suit on behalf of the University Hospitals in order to test the legality of the regents' attempts to have unpaid accounts collected for the hospitals; the motion carried.

The contract between the School of Medicine and Oklahoma City and Oklahoma County, to care for their indigent sick at the University Hospitals, was terminated in 1933. University Hospital continued to operate its dairy on a one-thousand-acre farm in Oklahoma County until 1939.

Appropriations to the medical center for 1933–34 were $66,000 for the School of Medicine, $125,000 for Crippled Children's Hospital, and $198,000 for the University Hospital, but the regents cut these allocations as follows: $9,405.39 from the School of Medicine budget, $28,352 from the University Hospital budget, and $7,718.75 from the Crippled Children's Hospital budget.

During this fiscal year, 3,608 patients were admitted to the University Hospital and 2,448 to Crippled Children's Hospital. The obstetrical department at the main hospital reported 466 births, aside from 674 home deliveries in which medical students assisted; and the outpatient department treated a total of 11,231 cases.

There were 243 medical students and 79 nursing students enrolled at the medical center for the year 1933–34; and in June, 1933, 56 graudates of the School of Medicine received the M.D. degree, and 39 graduates of the School of Nursing received certificates of Graduate Nurse. It should be noted also that the first approved list of medical technologists at the University Hospitals was prepared by the American Society of Clinical Pathology Board of Registry in 1933.

The whipping boy of the year was the postgraduate medical program, organized in 1924 by Luther Kibler of the University of Oklahoma Extension Division in cooperation with the Oklahoma State Medical Association, and with the dean of the School of Medicine acting as chairman of an advisory committee.[9] Since little or no appropriation by the state of Oklahoma was made for medical teaching under the extension plan in 1933, more than two thirds of the expense connected with postgraduate medical education in the state was defrayed by the physicians themselves.

A report made by the Committee on Postgraduate Extension Teaching of the State Medical Association shows that the association invested $770 in the program and that were 698 doctors in attendance at the clinics in 1933. The cancer teaching clinics were especially popular, with a total of 1,137 people in attendance. There were about 57 physicians at a meeting held for the southeast-

[9] Everett, *Medical Education in Oklahoma*, I, 196, 199, 234, 235.

ern part of the state in Hugo, and some 80 physicians attended a clinic held in the panhandle, for Texas, Cimarron, and Beaver counties.[10]

Continuation of the program depended upon the amount of cash available, as did other programs clamoring for state appropriations, so three members of the Committee on Public Policy and Legislation of the Oklahoma State Medical Association went before the governor in an effort to prevent elimination of $3,000 to pay the salary of the director of postgraduate medical study, Mr. Kibler. The first part of the visit with Governor Murray was "a little stormy" according to the report, but on the whole it was "profitable," although he made no promises other than to say that he would "give the matter due consideration and do whatever he thought was right."[11]

The fact that there is no mention of postgraduate courses in medical education in the 1934 catalog of the University of Oklahoma speaks for itself, as far as any use of state money was concerned for a program which physicians thought was right, not only for themselves but for the people at large in Oklahoma.

This was not only the third consecutive year of executive interference in medical education from the governor's office, it was also the third consecutive year of declining morale at the medical center, marked as it was by reduced budgets for the various departments of the School of Medicine and even lower than usual salaries for members of the faculty.

Pressure applied to the university regents to divide the administration of the University Hospitals by appointing a separate business manager who was totally unacquainted with hospital operations and then not making him responsible either to the superintendent of the hospitals or to the dean of the School of Medicine but directly to the regents of the university was an unwise change boding trouble.

Curtailment of the developing postgraduate program of the university and the Oklahoma State Medical Association by withdrawal of partial state funding for the 1933 joint project was another very shortsighted action, because it terminated the effectiveness of a worthwhile program which actually made few demands on the state treasury. Such ill-advised actions made it more and more certain that within a few years, under existing circumstances, the Council on Medical Education and Hospitals would, of necessity, place the University of Oklahoma School of Medicine on probation.

During 1934, the fourth and last year of Governor Murray's administration, he continued systematically to plague the University of Oklahoma medical center with his unsavory political influence, as the record testifies. For example, the question of a full-time dean of the School of Medicine to replace Dr. Moorman popped up for the first time at a meeting of the university regents on March 30, 1934. After lengthy pros and cons, President Bizzell was handed yet

---

[10.] *Journal of the Oklahoma State Medical Association*, Vol. XXVI (1933), 209.
[11.] *Ibid.*, 220.

another time bomb and charged with the task of investigating the possibilities of making such an administrative change.

The regents also decided that a separate bookkeeping system and method of accounting should be established for the School of Medicine, apart from that of the hospitals, because they felt it was unsatisfactory to keep the school's accounts in the University Hospital, which was controlled by the business manager. Here again, President Bizzell was requested to investigate the prospects of making this change and to report back to the regents at a later date. Surprisingly enough, at their regular meeting on June 2 the regents set aside any decision about changes in the accounting system of the medical center. Furthermore, after President Bizzell reported on his findings regarding the possibilities of engaging a full-time dean, it is recorded that the consensus of the university regents was unfavorable to the idea and that the then current arrangement of having a part-time dean should be continued until such time as additional appropriations became available.

This decision, however motivated, in no way lightened Dean Moorman's burdens, for, of all years, 1934 proved to be the most trying for him in regard to the incompatible behavior of Mr. Bostic, the business manager. Appointed by the university regents, under pressure from the governor, Mr. Bostic attempted to manage the financial affairs of the hospitals without any supervision by the dean and superintendent. It is an understatement to say that his policies in almost no time at all, resulted in downright confusion, lack of coordination, and diminished morale of everyone connected with the hospitals. Consequently, the unpalatable predicament which evolved required so much of Dean Moorman's time that his only alternative to working untold hours was to rely for assistance on a small advisory committee which he pressed into service.

There is a brief on the plight of the administration of the medical center at the time in the files of the office of the dean, written by Lewis J. Moorman. A sampling of excerpts from this rather long document will suffice for the history of medical education in Oklahoma. From early conferences with Mr. Bostic and from observation of his hostile attitude and devious methods of procedure, it soon became apparent to Dr. Moorman that no satisfactory cooperation with the business manager could be expected. Basically, Mr. Bostic failed to appreciate the professional problems inherent in the management of a large teaching hospital, a failure which could justifiably be attributed to his lack of knowledge of hospital administration in general and to a real need for special training and experience with the highly specialized and technical phases of teaching hospitals. Ludicrous as it may seem now, the minor incident of how to distribute the incoming mail exemplifies how frustrating even a simple action proved to be to the superintendent, Dean Moorman.

For some strange reason, Mr. Bostic ordered that all mail coming into the hospital should be placed on *his* desk. When this unaccountable decision was made known to the hospital board in a regular meeting, at which President Bizzell was present, the board summarily directed Dr. Moorman to seek a conference with the business manager and explain to him that priority required that the mail should go first to the superintendent's office and thence be distributed to the various departments. But when Dr. Moorman requested a conference on the subject with Mr. Bostic, even though he was in his office only a very short distance away, he declined to grant the interview on the ground that he was signing papers. His failure to cooperate on even so elementary an issue as this was reported to his immediate superior, the president of the university, but the mail continued to first cross the desk of the unrelenting business manager.

Thomas R. Ponton, representing the American College of Surgeons, inspected the University and Crippled Children's Hospitals on April 9, 1934. When he had completed his work, he came to the superintendent's office and said he would have to place one serious criticism of the hospitals in his record—"a divided administration." Then, in response to an inquiry as to how he had discovered that secret, he said he had known about it before he came to Oklahoma City.

In his brief of these problems, Dean Moorman enclosed a copy of a letter from Malcolm T. MacEachern, director of hospital activities for the American College of Surgeons, containing several comments about Dr. Ponton's inspection. "The only criticism of this hospital is in the administrative organization," he wrote, adding that the duties of the dean of the School of Medicine were confined to the professional activities of the hospital, whereas the business management was in the hands of a business manager directly responsible to the board of regents. "This dual management will sooner or later lead to friction," he said, "which will react against the best interests of the hospital. . . . There can be no doubt that the dean should be the one in authority, with the business manager subordinate and responsible to him, in conformity with the enabling act."

Several respected members of the medical faculty "joined the choir invisible" in 1934. Abraham Blesh, professor of surgery at the School of Medicine and head of the plastic surgery service, died in February, and in due time John Burton was appointed to fill that vacant chair. W. J. Wallace, professor of urology, and Lloyd M. Sackett, associate professor of gynecology, died in the fall of the year.

There were 135 members of the faculty, not including teachers in the School of Nursing and in dietetics, during the academic year 1934–35. New appointments included:

Ernest Lachman, M.D.
  assistant professor of anatomy
George Thomas Allen, M.D.
  instructor in obstetrics
Dan Roy Sewell, M.D.
  instructor in anatomy

Beatrice Edwards, M.A.
  research associate in biochemistry
Mathille Elizabeth Bjerregaard, M.S.
  assistant in bacteriology

This small reinforcement of the faculty was obviously a reflection of the rather austere financial restrictions with which the medical center had been encumbered for several years. The maintenance funds for the department of biochemistry and pharmacology, for example, had been cut from $4,000 to $1,700 per year.

Further evidence of inadequate funding of the school is evident in a letter addressed to President Bizzell from Dean Moorman in November, 1934, in which the dean said that the number of medical student admissions had been reduced from a maximum of 78 to 60 "as the years passed," in keeping with the recommendations of the Council on Medical Education. In the selection of students for enrollment in the School of Medicine, careful consideration was given to the results of the aptitude test required of all applicants for admission. Questions asked on this test were furnished by the Association of American Medical Colleges, and applicants were advised as to when and where the test was given.

At the graduation exercises in June, 1934, 61 medical students received the M.D. degree and 33 nursing students received the certificate of Graduate Nurse. During the academic year 1934–35, 237 medical students and 105 nursing students were enrolled at the medical center.

The total amount appropriated by the fourteenth legislature for the University of Oklahoma at Norman for the fiscal year 1934–35 was $1,140,049 as compared to a total appropriation of $389,000 for the medical center in Oklahoma City: School of Medicine, $66,000; University Hospital, $198,000; and Crippled Children's Hospital, $125,000. These figures were identical to the 1933–34 appropriations that were cut considerably by the regents. The dean's office promptly filed a complaint with the State Budget Committee stating that the medical center had been running on a greatly reduced budget for the past four years.

In answer to a request made by the university regents in September, 1933, for an opinion of the attorney general concerning the requirement for county funds for the University Hospitals, the attorney general cited the recent decision of the Supreme Court in the case of *Chicago, Rock Island and Pacific Railroad* vs. *Excise Board of Stephens County*. He ruled that, in his opinion, that part of the Crippled Children's Act which attempted to impose a portion of the burden of maintenance of crippled children at the University Hospital on the county from which a patient was committed to the hospital was unconstitutional and inoperative. It necessarily followed that neither the University Hospital nor the Crippled Children's Hospital should make further attempts to collect any funds from the various counties in the state, although the University Hospital and Crippled Children's Hospital were holding approximately $50,000 worth of warrants on trust from the several counties, when the decision was handed down. Some of these counties were liquidating their warrants, some were holding them while awaiting legal advice, and some were requesting the return of their warrants for cancellation.

Quite fully apprised by now of the very real financial dilemma, the regents of the university at their October meeting voted that the next budget for the School of Medicine should include requests for increases in a ratio commensurate with increases for the University of Oklahoma at Norman, namely 20 per cent. Furthermore, the regents voted that a request be made for a 20 per cent increase in funds for each of the hospitals, taking into consideration the amount of any supplemental appropriation for the hospitals for the purpose of completing the year.

There were 6,160 admissions to the University Hospitals representing 163,320 hospital days in 1934–35. There were 523 obstetrical patients in the hospital and 790 home deliveries. The total number of outpatient cases for the same period was 8,494.

Fortunately, termination of the Murray administration was heralded in the fall of 1934 by the election of a less prejudiced governor, and the era of confusion and lowered morale at the medical center, which had been engendered by political interference for the past four years, appeared at long last to be ending.

The decision of the attorney general that the University Hospitals should no longer attempt to collect costs for hospitalization of charity patients from the counties was a serious blow financially in 1934, and the termination of state assistance to the postgraduate program for physicians was one more example of the short-sightedness of the university regents during the Murray years.

While it is true that Governor Murray had not commanded a majority vote on the board, it was obvious that the university regents supported his schemes pretty consistently, evidently reluctant to thwart him regardless of the outcome.[12] Such temporizing could only guarantee a probationary status for the School of Medicine by the Council on Medical Education and Hospitals.

On the credit side of the ledger, an agreement was made during the year between the School of Social Work of the University of Oklahoma and the University Hospitals to institute supervised formal medical field work at the hospitals, even though the business manager was of the opinion that this was not a professional service.

It is with a feeling of relief that we now leave behind this era of governmental fatuity.

[12.] Contrariwise, a governor did not necessarily ssupport the political schemes of any regent, as evidenced by an incident which occurred rather early during Dr. Everett's deanship, when a regent attempted to force a prospective medical student's admission to the School of Medicine. (About eighty legislators had earlier engaged in the same tactic in one year.) Word was out one morning that the university regents, meeting at the medical school, would be discussing "admission," and Dean Everett was alerted to be available if needed. Imagine his surprise when his secretary announced that Captain ———— from the governor's office was in the outer room! A moment later, a tall, uniformed military man handed to the dean a sealed envelope and a letter from Governor Johnston Murray instructing the dean to hold the sealed "executive order" intact until he might be informed of any attempted interference with the admission policy of the School of Medicine. Whereupon, the dean was to open the envelope and hand the secret weapon to the erring regent—his official dismissal notice. Otherwise, the sealed letter was to be destroyed. Fortunately, the regents kept their own counsel and the episode ended happily, with the admission board of the faculty continuing to make all decisions relative to entrance to the University of Oklahoma School of Medicine.

Chapter II.
Stormy Weather Breeds
Full-time Dean:
1935–36

In 1932, Ernest W. Marland was elected as the first democratic congressman from the Eighth District of Oklahoma since statehood. After serving one term in the House of Representatives—with the support of President Franklin D. Roosevelt and his advisers—Marland entered the democratic primary in the race for governor of Oklahoma. He made his campaign slogan, ''Bring the New Deal to Oklahoma.'' and easily won the gubernatorial election in the fall of 1934.

A native of Pittsburgh, Pennsylvania, Marland had studied law at the University of Michigan before entering the oil business and migrating to Oklahoma in 1908. Over the years, he built an oil empire from Oklahoma black gold and made a fortune, valued at one time at $85,000,000. Though he lived in a manor house, he was a generous man who made contributions of considerable magnitude to various charitable enterprises. In time his ''nose for oil and the luck of the devil'' failed him, and ''Marland retired from his baronial mansion on the outskirts of Ponca City to live in the gate lodge of the estate.''[1]

The fifteenth legislature assembled in January, 1935, and on February 13 the senate appointed a special committee (Resolution No. 7) to investigate the administration of the University Hospitals. As originally constituted, the committee was composed of legislators Joe M. Whitaker, chairman, with Bower Broaddus, H. W. Wright, and H. M. Curnutt, members—all friends of P. B. Bostic, the troublesome business manager of the University Hospitals. When Louis A. Ritzhaupt found this to be the case, he requested that he, too, be placed on the committee; his request was granted.

Presently, an absurd controversy was precipitated because Mr. Bostic, who had been placed in charge of nonmedical personnel in 1933 by a resolution of the board of regents, never had made any effort whatsoever to cooperate with Dr. Moorman, dean of the School of Medicine and superintendent of University Hospitals. Therefore, during the one and one-half years in which Dr. Moorman

---

[1] *Oklahoma, A Guide to the Sooner State*, American Guide Series (Norman, University of Oklahoma Press, 1941), 189.

had attempted to carry out his duties in a dual capacity, he had been thwarted at every turn by Mr. Bostic, who assumed the role of top man on the totem pole. Most of the clinical faculty gradually became incensed by the impasse, so that opposition eventuated, and lines formed for the Bostic versus Moorman dilemma, as the political air of Oklahoma became heavy with charges and countercharges.

Concurrently, agitation for a full-time dean developed, which, from all appearances, was initiated by Dr. Ritzhaupt and a member of the university regents, Eugene M. Kerr, in an attempt to dislodge Dr. Moorman. L. S. Willour of McAlester, secretary of the Oklahoma State Medical Association, wrote President Bizzell that the only doctor he had ever heard express dissatisfaction with Dean Moorman was Dr. Ritzhaupt, and that, so far as he knew, the doctors throughout the state were satisfied with Dr. Moorman's conduct of affairs at the University School of Medicine. "Those who are working from a selfish interest," Dr. Ritzhaupt retorted, "to protect a friend or to keep someone in a position, will probably constantly watch for some place to attack me."

Caught in the middle, President Bizzell explained that he had only one concern, "to clean up this mess which has become a statewide scandal. . . . The fact that this situation resulted in appointment of a senate committee to make an investigation is unfortunate, not only for the School of Medicine, but also for the entire University."

Judge George L. Bowman was president of the university regents at this time, succeeded by Claude C. Hatchett in June. Other members of the board were Eugene M. Kerr, Eugene P. Ledbetter, Joe C. Looney, Lloyd Noble, and Malcolm E. Rosser, Jr. At their meeting in January the regents discussed problems of the School of Medicine, and Regent Kerr presented a resolution for securing closer supervision of the medical services in the University Hospitals through the creation of a medical director, subject only to supervision by the dean-superintendent, with full authority in all medical matters, including assignments and discipline of interns. President Bizzell concurred, suggesting that the recommendation of a person for the appointment of medical director be requested of the dean of the School of Medicine.

Then, in response to a complaint from the Crippled Children's Society that there were nearly 800 crippled children on the waiting list who were unable to secure admission to Crippled Children's Hospital, Mr. Kerr made a second resolution: "Be it resolved by the Board of Regents that at least ninety percent of the beds at the Crippled Children's Hospital be allocated for exclusive use of cases coming under the general designation of orthopedic, plastic or corrective surgery." The resolution was unanimously adopted.

The regents met again on February 12 in the Skirvin Hotel, Oklahoma City, and Judge Bowman divulged that Governor Marland had contacted him before the meeting about complaints of friction and lack of cooperation between the dean of the School of Medicine and P. B. Bostic, business manager of the hospitals. The governor was disturbed by rumors that the conflict resulting from divided authority had affected the morale and efficiency of the entire medical center organization, though he made no suggestions as to how to cure the situation, merely requesting that the board follow the recommendations of Dean Moorman and the president of the university.

President Bizzell introduced several resolutions which he had received from the full-time faculty, teaching clinicians, and house staff, pertaining to the divided administration of the University of Oklahoma School of Medicine and asked that they be read into the record. The theme of the resolutions was that the very existence of the School of Medicine was dependent upon the centralization of authority of all departments under the control of the legally designated head, the dean of the School of Medicine, subject to the approval of the president of the university.[2]

One resolution stipulated that "in this type of institution, established for the dual purposes of treatment and care of indigent patients," there could be no division of administrative authority "without a resulting disharmony detrimental to the teaching of scientific medicine and efficient handling of the sick committed to the institution." Another resolution requested that "the administration of this institution be made to conform to the principles and rules set forth in the enabling act,[3] in order that the former harmony and efficiency can be restored and that we may not be further subjected to the risk of sacrificing our established A rating, and also the loyalty which has played such an enormous part in the work of the School of Medicine and University Hospitals."

The full-time faculty presented an official petition to President Bizzell similar to the resolutions of the teaching clinicians and house staff; and the president of the fourth-year class sent an SOS letter to physicians throughout the state.

In light of these declarations, Judge Bowman finally called for some kind of action from the regents in regard to the School of Medicine controversy, since the governor was awaiting a decision and was insistent that something be done. Regent Hatchett immediately became riled because he felt he "was being stampeded"; he thought "very highly of Dr. Moorman and of Mr. Bostic" too. However, he honestly felt that someone other than Mr. Bostic should be appointed business manager, though he had no idea whom to suggest.

Eugene Ledbetter made known that he had been brash enough to think that he could get the differences between Mr. Bostic and the superintendent of the hospitals settled somehow and had talked at some length with Dr. Goodwin, supervisor of clinical clerkships, only to learn that "the esprit de corps had been destroyed over there," and that the impasse was by no means all Dr. Moorman's fault. "We are going to have about three investigations," Regent Ledbetter predicted, "and we have to have some friends along the line. We may make our peace with the Governor or try to control the legislature, but Senator Jim A. Rhinehart is hot as a firecracker to get in here on the medical school."

President Bizzell quelled the discussion by saying that the governor had told

[2] Mark R. Everett, *Medical Education in Oklahoma*, (Norman, University of Oklahoma Press, 1972), I, 161.
[3] *Ibid.*, 131, 132. House Bill No. 366 of the Sessions Laws of 1917.

him that he wanted the regents to run the university; whereupon, Eugene Kerr suggested they ought to wait about making any decision, since the senate would pass a resolution in regard to the whole issue anyway. And no decision was made.

The medical profession in general and organized medicine were open in their support of Dr. Moorman, as evidenced by available records.[4] Acting as influential referees of the imbroglio were Fred Zapffe, secretary of the Association of American Medical Colleges, and the press.

Dr. Zapffe kept in touch with Dr. Moorman during this stressful period, supporting the thesis that complete control and responsibility for all professional services in a teaching hospital should rest with a single individual—the administrative officer of the medical school. Whether a medical school's teaching hospitals were owned or merely controlled by the medical school, the responsibility from an educational viewpoint was the same, since the hospital was part of the teaching equipment of the medical school. "I am hopeful," Dr. Zapffe wrote in February, "that the information that has come to me with regard to University Hospital is wholly wrong. Deans occupying similar positions in other state university educational systems have full powers and responsibility, and thus far their administrations have met with universal satisfaction to all concerned."

Writing again in March, Dr. Zapffe commented that the position of superintendent of university-owned hospitals was often connected with politics, and that the fight for management of such hospitals by the medical schools had been a long one; and that even though deans were slowly being appointed superintendents of teaching hospitals, as in Oklahoma, a dean was not always competent to superintend a hospital. "Why then, if he cannot look after the details of hospital management (which do not directly concern education)," Dr. Zapffe asked, "can he not secure services of someone to help him? . . . Custom, politics, and experience determine the appointment of a superintendent."

Eugene M. Kerr, vice-president of the university regents and supporter of Governor Marland on institutional matters, testified before the Senate Investigating Committee in April that the university regents had been responsible for the appointment of Mr. Bostic, business manager of the University Hospitals, who had been given specific instructions to economize. Regent Kerr stated that Mr. Bostic was unanimously appointed by the regents after careful consideration, yet Regent Ledbetter testified he had never voted for Mr. Bostic.

In a further negative approach to the School of Medicine and University Hospitals, Vice-President Kerr criticized the admission to Crippled Children's Hospital of medical cases as opposed to surgical cases, reflecting a prejudice of

---

[4.] In the March issue of the *Journal of the Oklahoma State Medical Association*, Vol. XXVIII (1935), 105, the editor asked, "Why is it that a so-well-conducted institution of higher learning cannot be managed by its Dean, the President of the University and its Board of Regents? . . . If the medical department is booted about by investigating committees composed of men not acquainted with medical education, it will become a political institution."

the regents as evidenced by the resolution in January that the children's hospital should be used primarily for crippled children, and that the number of other cases should be kept down to 10 per cent. Moreover, Regent Kerr felt that the affairs of the medical school were dominated by the older doctors and that it would be a good thing if some "new blood were injected into the personnel of the faculty." When asked by a member of the Senate Investigating Committee for positive suggestions, the vice-president had said he was in favor of a full-time dean "from outside the state, with wide experience and knowledge concerning medical education," but that it would not be advisable to seek one right away because, "wittingly or unwittingly, considerable information would leak out of the state of Oklahoma that the medical school was under the dominance of politicians and any full-time dean would feel subject to the whims and wishes of the politicians, without any guarantee of permanency in his position." Truer words were never spoken, as the ensuing full-time dean was to learn to his dismay and despair.

Most of President Bizzell's testimony to the investigating committee was aimed at policies inaugurated under the Murray regime, which caused the president to believe the School of Medicine was in danger of losing its A rating as a result of the lowered morale of the faculty and personnel in the medical center. He advocated reestablishment of the dean of the School of Medicine as the administrative head. "For 22 years," Bizzell said, "the Medical School has been operated without serious internal friction of any kind under the policy of unified administration, and," he continued, "if the Regents are given a free hand . . . without interference from political sources, the situation that has brought this long and tedious investigation will not occur again."

The report submitted by the Senate Investigating Committee[5] concluded that there had been considerable unrest among the students at the School of Medicine—"fostered by some members of the Faculty"—and that there was a large amount of dissension among doctors throughout the state regarding the possibility that the School of Medicine might again lose its class A rating, which had been established by the Council on Medical Education of the American Medical Association in 1907.

The committee was of the opinion that a written complaint made by the dean of the School of Medicine to the university regents involved matters that were petty and trivial and should never have disturbed the morale or the operation of either the medical school or the University Hospitals. The members of the committee thought that the business manager had, at all times, endeavored to carry out the orders of the regents, who, through him, "accomplished material and magnificent savings to the state of Oklahoma in the operation of the two hospitals."

The committee made the following recommendations: that the medical school faculty and hospital staff members be selected and promoted on the basis of merit, ability, training, and research endeavor, rather than on the basis of seniority; that faculty members be retired at the age of 65 with the honorary

[5] See page 28.

position and title of professor emeritus; that members of the faculty, at the age of 60 years, start to relieve themselves of their more arduous duties and give the advantage of their knowledge (in an advisory capacity) to the younger staff members; and that all things pertaining to the medical and surgical care of those who required admittance to the hospitals be under the direct control of one man, and that he should have an M.D. degree. If the dean of the medical school were to assume the detailed work of the superintendency of the hospitals also, then he should be required to devote full time to the medical school and hospitals. In case the Board of Regents of the University of Oklahoma did not favor the employment of a full-time dean, the committee recommended employment of a medical superintendent to work in conjunction with the dean of the medical school, and that, under any arrangement, separate books and accounts should be maintained at all times for the hospitals and for the medical school.

Recommendations were also made by the senate committee that necessary steps be taken before the next legislative session to ascertain the appropriations needed for surgical and medical research and new buildings on the campus of the medical school. They also advised that the orders and instructions of the university regents be followed by all persons connected with the School of Medicine and University Hospitals and that any person refusing to comply therewith should be summarily discharged.

The splendid work and untiring efforts of the staff physicians, who had given of their time to carry on the duties of the medical school and hospitals, was acknowledged, as were the "constructive testimony and recommendations given by the physicians and surgeons and medical personnel of the hospitals" who came before the special committee.

The university regents held a recess session on June 17, 1935, with C. Hatchett presiding. This was a rather momentous meeting at which President Bizzell spoke out for the administration, and the regents took some positive actions.

Finally, the regents did something about an executive order from the Murray administration (reactivated earlier by Governor Marland), which provided for the transfer of the Union Soldiers Home to the university, as an annex to Crippled Children's Hospital. "It is the sense of the Board," the minutes state, "that we either continue the present arrangement in connection with the Union Soldiers Home—with the Union soldiers under separate care elsewhere—or take into the University Hospital all the present inmates who need hospitalization in return for the exclusive use of the property, as an annex to Crippled Children's Hospital. In the event that neither of these propositions is acceptable, the President of the University is authorized to return the property to the State Board of Affairs"—an ultimatum of determination by the regents.

President Bizzell then called attention to some recommendations made by the Senate Investigating Committee concerning faculty and hospital staff promotions and pointed out that selection and promotion of faculty and staff "on the basis of merit, ability, training, and research endeavor, rather than on the basis of seniority," had, in his opinion, been a policy followed consistently and conscientiously throughout the history of the School of Medicine. He differed with the committee recommendation that members of the medical school faculty and staff retire at age 65 with honorary position and title, saying that it was his opinion that the present policy of retiring at age 70 was sound, and that there was no reason to change that age limit. The committee's recommendation that admissions to the hospitals be under the direct control of one man having an M.D. degree was superfluous, since that policy was already being followed.

President Bizzell's preference for a full-time dean of the School of Medicine was embodied in a specific recommendation "that the Dean of the School of Medicine be given full authority to administer the School of Medicine and the Hospitals, subject to the approval of the President of the University."

The regents approved this recommendation and the simmering fat was in the fire; Regent Kerr immediately moved that the position of dean of the School of Medicine be declared vacant, whereupon Regent Bowman triggered the other barrel by amending the motion to read that the positions of medical director and business manager also be declared vacant. So it came to pass on June 17, 1935, that the positions of dean and business manager were declared vacant effective July 1, 1935, and that the president was authorized to recommend an acting dean and acting business manager to serve until a full-time dean was recommended, a position which the regents directed be filled. They further ordered that the dean elected have full authority to select the faculty and other employees of the School of Medicine and University Hospitals, subject to the approval of the president.

President Bizzell responded rather insensately by saying, "You have just dismissed Dr. Moorman, and I think you have done the best thing under the circumstances." He felt that they could look forward to having a full-time dean by September. He then recommended that Dr. Turley be made acting dean of the School of Medicine for the months of July and August, and that Hugh Jeter be made director of medical service and business manager for the same period. The motion carried and President Bizzell thanked Judge Bowman, retiring chairman, for the gratifying encouragement he had given during the very difficult past four years. Regent Kerr next moved that R. Q. Goodwin, supervisor of clinical clerkships in University Hospitals, be stricken from the salary list on July 1,[6] and that motion carried.

[6.] When Dean Moorman heard of this motion, he addressed himself to President Bizzell in a letter dated June 20, 1935, in which he said, "this seems an unwarranted action on the part of the Board. . . . Dr. Goodwin was in no way to blame for the conference with medical students during the Senate Committee investigation. . . . Dr. Goodwin has achieved a national reputation. . . . The Board's action is not only an injustice to Dr. Goodwin but a serious blow to the school."

This commentary is important in light of a statement made two years earlier, by Fred Zapffe, secretary of the Association of American Medical Colleges, that Dr. Goodwin was doing good work and that it would afford him pleasure to speak of it in circles where the opinions regarding the School of Medicine of the University of Oklahoma had been greatly at variance with the facts as he had found them when he visited the school.

The resignation of Dr. Moorman from his position as dean of the University of Oklahoma School of Medicine became effective on August 3, at which time the regents appointed Louis Alvin Turley, professor of pathology, as acting dean for the months of July and August. Immediately following this action, the regents, in "rapid fire," unanimously elected General Robert Urie Patterson as dean of the School of Medicine and superintendent of the University Hospitals at a salary of $7,500 per year, commencing September 1, 1935; but very little is recorded concerning the search for this first full-time dean of the School of Medicine. A reasonable assumption can be made. Senator Ritzhaupt and Regent Kerr had agitated continually for such an appointment and both the senate committee and president Bizzell finally concurred. On June 17 the position was officially made available by the university regents, and they directed President Bizzell to find a candidate, which he did with unprecedented dispatch. This would seem to have required the assistance of one of General Patterson's many friends.

Dean Patterson received his M.D. degree from McGill University, Montreal, Canada, in 1898, and an honorary LL.D. degree from McGill University in 1932. He was a fellow in both the American College of Surgeons and the American College of Physicians and had spent approximately 35 years with the United States Army. During those years of service, he had received many citations of a military nature, and when he came to Oklahoma City in 1935, General Patterson was surgeon general of the United States Army, retired.

On this same August 3, the regents accepted the resignations of Edward P. Allen, associate professor of obstetrics, and Horace Reed, professor of clinical surgery. On September 28 they designated Millington Smith professor emeritus of gynecology and appointed Bert F. Keltz, an instructor in the Department of Medicine, supervisor of the clinical clerkships. The death of M. M. Roland, associate professor of dermatology and radiography, occurred late in the year.

A request by Dean Patterson that all the financial records for the School of Medicine and University Hospitals should be kept at the University Hospital, for reasons of convenience, was also approved.

On November 24 the regents appointed Louis A. Turley assistant dean, as of October 1, 1935, a title he was holding for a second time, and Hugh Jeter was returned, as of December 1, to his former position as director of laboratories and supervisor of internships at the University Hospitals.

At the same time, Egil T. Olsen was appointed medical director and assistant superintendent of the University Hospitals. Before this appointment Dr. Olsen had been director of the Teaching Hospitals of the Detroit College of Medicine and Surgery, and before that he had been in private practice in Chicago, where he became chief of the Bureau of Hospitals of the Chicago Health Department, following a tour of duty as a member of the United States Public Health Service combating yellow fever in Cuba. Dr. Olsen was a physician especially adept at helping younger members on the staff, which resulted in professional benefits that were passed on directly to the patients.

Dean Patterson presided at a faculty meeting on October 10, at which he announced that Leo J. Starry was being appointed secretary of the faculty to succeed Edmund S. Ferguson. Dean Patterson told the faculty that he would depend largely upon their interest and support to assist him in maintaining the school in its present grade A position, and he also stated that it would be advisable to have an executive committee of the faculty to pass on emergency situations, the action of this committee to be reported to the faculty for confirmation at its succeeding meeting.

Having found that there were very few regulations on record that covered the conduct of the School of Medicine, Dean Patterson felt that such regulations should be formulated and also he would make it his practice to appoint committees annually. He told the faculty that he had requested that each of the School of Medicine's classes should meet and appoint a president and a secretary. He also announced that members of the clinical faculty should record their time spent in giving instruction in the School of Medicine in a ledger provided for that purpose. The same procedure should apply at the University Hospitals.

In regard to student advisers, Dean Patterson suggested that it was wiser to permit a student to select a member of the faculty of his own choosing than to have a faculty adviser assigned to him. In the dean's opinion, rules and regulations governing the use of library books, pamphlets, and journals were definitely needed, and plans were already in process for drawing up standards.

During the academic year 1935–36 there were 155 members of the faculty of the School of Medicine including the faculty members of the School of Nursing. There were 15 new faculty members appointed during the year:

Wayne McKinley Hull, M.D.
  director, outpatient department
Egil Thorbjorn Olsen, M.D.
  lecturer in hygiene and public health
  and assistant
  superintendent of University
  Hospitals
Frank Pitkin Bertram, D.D.S.
  instructor in dental surgery
Charles Arthur Brake, M.D.
  instructor in psychiatry
Donald Wilton Branham, M.D.
  instructor in genitourinary diseases
  and syphilology
Helen Carr, B.A.
  instructor in medical social work
Stearley P. Harrison, A.B.
  graduate assistant in physiology

Goldia Hermanstoffer, G.N.
  instructor in principles and practice
  of nursing
John F. Kuhn, Jr., M.D.
  instructor in anatomy and
  gynecology
Ruth Lacy, R.N.
  instructor in operating room
  techniques
William Gerald Rogers, M.D.
  instructor in gynecology
LeRoy Huskins Sadler, M.D.
  instructor in gynecology
Joseph J. Seifter, M.D.
  instructor in pharmacology
Wendell Logan Smith, M.D.
  instructor in medicine
Carl T. Steen, M.D.
  instructor in psychiatry

The Department of Biochemistry and Pharmacology was separated into two departments in 1935, with Mark R. Everett as professor and head of biochemistry, and Harold A. Shoemaker as professor and head of pharmacology. In this same year, Rex Bolend became head of the Department of Urology, and Willis

K. West became the acting head of the Department of Orthopedic Surgery, assuming the duties of Samuel R. Cunningham who was granted a leave of absence for reasons involving his health.

Several curricular changes were instituted during the year, notably in clinical subjects. A course in medical jurisprudence was organized, and arrangements were made for students in clinical medicine to attend psychiatry sessions on Saturday afternoons for 16 successive weeks at Central State Hospital in Norman. In addition, two applied courses in biochemistry and physiology, already given in the third year, were increased to 32 hours of study each; a course in applied pharmacology was added; and 160 clock hours of electives became a requirement for all medical students in 1935.

The fifteenth Oklahoma legislature took some important steps relevant to the School of Medicine and the University Hospitals in this period. Senate Bill No. 15, sponsored by Senator Ritzhaupt,[7] was made into a statute which modified the Crippled Children's Law enacted in 1927 and clarified the function of the law as it pertained to the Crippled Children's Hospital; it also enlarged the scope of private hospitals to participate in accepting such patients. In order to do this, the new act provided for a committee of standardization composed of five physicians appointed by the governor, whose duty it was to approve and classify hospitals eligible under the law for the care of child patients.

The decision of the attorney general in 1934 in respect to the constitutional right of a state institution, such as the Crippled Children's Hospital, to charge a county for charity hospital services, embedded the administration of the law in a tangle of confusion. One saving grace was that the supreme court had upheld the tenth mill county levy as applicable to other hsopitals, although not to state hospitals. In the December issue of the *Newsletter* for the Society for Crippled Children is to be found a statement that nearly all the bus lines in Oklahoma had agreed to extend half-fare rates to all children committed to an approved hospital under provisions of the law—the same rate to apply, in addition, to one escort for each child. This was a privilege, however, available only to patients in those counties collecting the pertinent mill levy.

The Commission for Crippled Children was created to supervise the entire hospital program, the commission members to be the state superintendent of health, chairman, the dean of the University of Oklahoma School of Medicine,

---

[7.] Louis H. Ritzhaupt, state senator from Guthrie, had become notorious in medical circles through his promotion of the Crippled Children's Act, his participation in the Moorman-Bostic affair (in which he continued to play a curious role, vacillating between support and attack, but always politically motivated), and his acquittal on charges of "unprofessional conduct toward the cults" by the Oklahoma State Medical Association during his bitter struggle for the presidency of that association. Dr. Ritzhaupt was even credited by some with having instigated the senate investigation of the University Hospitals for personal reasons, which resulted in the resignation of Dean Lewis J. Moorman and the appointment of General Robert U. Patterson as the first full-time dean of the School of Medicine. One of the authors recalls that more than a dozen years later the senator said he had been responsible for this appointment.

and the state superintendent of public instruction. The executive secretary of this commission was to be appointed by the president of the University of Oklahoma. The commission was designated as the official agency to cooperate with federal authorities in regard to provisions that might be enacted by Congress for the care of children. This new arrangement resulted in a 30 per cent increase in the number of patients committed to approved hospitals during the year 1935–36.[8]

Joe N. Hamilton was appointed executive secretary of the Crippled Children's Commission, a position similar to that which he had held in the Oklahoma Society for Crippled Children since 1926. Lew H. Wentz, Ponca City oil man and philanthropist, personally paid Mr. Hamilton's salary from 1926 to 1936.[9] The new Crippled Children's Act provided that the salary of the executive secretary should be included in the regular appropriation for support of the University Hospital or the Hospital for Crippled Children. However, no salary claim was ever made against the university by Mr. Hamilton, who gave valuable and efficient service to Oklahoma; and when federal funds became available, even though he filed monthly claims against the commission funds for his salary, without exception the respective warrants were endorsed by Mr. Hamilton to the Society for Crippled Children. During his long tenure as executive secretary of the Crippled Children's Commission, he never received one penny in salary in excess of the amount he had received as executive secretary of the Crippled Children's Society, which had been donated by his benefactor, Mr. Lew Wentz.

The purpose of the new Anatomical Law which was enacted by the fifteenth legislature was to provide bodies for dissection in the state universities. Since the School of Medicine of the University of Oklahoma was the main benefactor of this law because of its courses in anatomy, the Board of the Anatomical Commission was composed of Dean Patterson of the School of Medicine, Charles DeGaris, professor of anatomy, and Robert M. Howard, professor of surgery in the School of Medicine.

In 1935, for the first time in history, the legislature made an appropriation for medical research of $10,000 per year for the biennium to be used by the School of Medicine. Dean Patterson immediately appointed a committee to oversee this project, of which Dr. Turley was chairman and Dr. Everett a member. Two fellowships were established at an annual stipend of $1,200 each and one of $1,500, applications to be made to the dean of the School of Medicine.

A breakdown of appropriations for the University of Oklahoma is to be found in the 1935–36 university catalog of April 4, 1936. The main branch of the University at Norman was allocated $1,548,372; the Oklahoma City campus, $103,000 for the School of Medicine, $330,000 for the University Hospital, and $240,000 for the Crippled Children's Hospital, all monies from state funds.

At this time the main University Hospital was credited with 210 beds and the

---

[8] *First Annual Report* of the Oklahoma Commission for Crippled Children, July 20, 1936.
[9] Everett, *Medical Education in Oklahoma*, I, 205.

Crippled Children's Hospital with 243 beds. There were 2,387 admissions to Children's Hospital and 3,692 to the University Hospital in 1935; 14,483 patients were admitted to the outpatient department, and there were 522 births at the University Hospital and 728 home deliveries, according to the report to the president. Coupled with this report was a letter containing this statement: "It has not been the custom heretofore to make an annual report for the University Hospitals to the Regents of the University."

Fifty-five graduates received the M.D. degree in June, including Glenn J. Collins, who later became deputy surgeon general of the United States Army. Twenty-eight nurses received the Graduate Nurse certificate. During the academic year 1935–36 there were 241 medical students and 100 nursing students at the medical center.

In the records of the registrar, Helen Kendall, are to be found the numbers of students admitted to the School of Medicine during the preceding decade: 46 students in 1925; 62 in 1926; 53 in 1927; 66 in 1928; 65 in 1929; 74 in 1930; 57 in 1931; 75 in 1932; 65 in 1933; 63 in 1934; and 66 in 1935. These figures indicate that of the 63 students admitted in 1934 only 55 graduated.

An inspection of the University of Oklahoma School of Medicine by the Council on Medical Education and Hospitals and the Association of American Medical Colleges, the official accrediting agencies for medical schools and their hospitals, took place during the fall of 1935. Among other recommendations by the committee were three significant ones: that the school remain entirely free of political domination; that the student body be reduced until such time as more clinical facilities were made available; and that adequate financial support should be made available for the development of the School of Medicine.

A description of the curriculum for the School of Nursing is given in that school's 1935 bulletin. In addition to the customary lectures and classes by members of the School of Medicine faculty, courses were given in the theory and practice of nursing by specially prepared instructors. There were also courses in dietetics in cooperation with the department of dietetics of the hospitals.

The prerequisite for admission to the School of Nursing required ranking in the upper third of the graduating class in an accredited high school. The hospitals provided full maintenance for students at the Nurses Residence, but an investment of about $70 was required from each student for uniforms.

The academic personnel of the School of Medicine of the University of Oklahoma welcomed the new year with its change of administration at the state capitol. While it is true that the fifteenth legislature passed two laws favorable to the School of Medicine—a new state Anatomical Act and a new version of the Oklahoma Crippled Children's Act—and appropriated $20,000 in research funds for the next bienium, the special committee appointed by the senate to investigate the administration of the University Hospitals engendered such a plethora of biased attacks and counterattacks as to dwarf the importance of all other considerations.

The prejudiced report of the senate committee presented in May favored Mr. Bostic. The assertion that he "had accomplished magnificent savings" was a manipulated prevarication, and recognition of "the splendid work of the staff physicians" was a tongue-in-cheek commendation. When all the dust settled, the fact remained that Dean Long, Dean Moorman, Dr. Langston, Dr. Goodwin, and Mr. Smith had all been shoved out within a period of four years as the result of meddlesome political finagling and delay in positive University action.

It is from Dr. Moorman's summary of these years (in the files of the office of the dean), that we glean the kernel of his position relative to the aggravating situation in which he found himself enmeshed—frustrated and/or acquiescent. Without the dean's approval, the business manager moved the interns into University Hospital quarters, taking over 12 or 14 rooms formerly used for the isolation of infectious disease cases, and Dr. Moorman, weary of all the haggling, assented tacitly rather than jeopardize, as he saw it, the hard-earned accreditation of the School of Medicine. "Through the fine spirit of cooperation and untiring efforts of the faculty members in both the preclinical and clinical departments, the school has made some progress," he declared, as all worked, waited, and hoped for a harmonious relationship of the School of Medicine and its hospitals through restoration of administrative authority to the dean.

"If the citizens of Oklahoma need and want a medical school," Dr. Moorman continued, "they should decide to finance it adequately, place it on a sound educational basis, and free it from the dangers of political interference." This was exactly the same prescription given by the Council on Medical Education after a preliminary inspection in the fall of 1935. "Finally," Dr. Moorman said in closing his remarks, "may I call your attention to the fact that a businessman without training in hospital management, occupying a position of authority and basking under the William H. Murray administration, can embarrass and handicap approximately 150 physicians and other professional workers in their efforts to offer medical students adequate, credible medical school advantages."

Lewis J. Moorman, an accomplished physician and scholar with marked literary talent, began his practice of medicine in Oklahoma in 1901 in the little village of Jet in Alfalfa County. He became one of the first members of the clinical faculty of the School of Medicine in 1910, when he was appointed professor of physical diagnosis. He established his first tuberculosis sanitarium on the outskirts of Oklahoma City in 1914 and, four years later, built a larger sanitarium at N.W. Forty-Third Street and Western Avenue, moving farther north in 1925 where he continued to specialize in diseases of the chest. In 1942 the University of Chicago Press published his well-known book, *Tuberculosis and Genius*.

Chapter III.
Confidential Probation:
1936–37

 On January 1, 1936, Dean Patterson reported to the regents that the use of the former Union Soldiers Home as an annex to the Children's Hospital (by executive order of former Governor Murray) was quite unsatisfactory from the standpoint of inadequate facilities and inaccessibility. Unexpectedly on March 17, the state fire marshal terminated any contrary illusions by condemning the building for hospital use. Whereupon, the university regents adopted a resolution that the property be vacated as soon as possible, and by June 20, Dean Patterson had withdrawn all patients from the home. The regents then returned the property, which ultimately became the headquarters for the State Board of Health, to the State Board of Affairs on June 30, thus ending three years of monkeyshines.

The University of Oklahoma School of Medicine was placed on confidential probation when the survey committee of the Council on Medical Education and Hospitals made its report following the January, 1936, investigation, justifying the personal fears of former Dean Moorman.

The committee, composed of Herman Weiskotten and Charles W. M. Poynter, indicated that suspicion was prevalent that Dr. Ritzhaupt had offered to assist osteopaths and chiropractors in achieving admission of their patients to University Hospitals, as well as appointment of themselves to the faculty of the School of Medicine in return for political support. This charge had certainly heightened the running feud between Dr. Ritzhaupt and the Oklahoma State Medical Association.[1]

The survey team further indicated that it was quite obvious that Senator Ritzhaupt was antagonistic to Dean Moorman and biased in favor of the business manager of University Hospitals. They thought that it was also evident that Dean Patterson had no experience in medical education—in all deference to his war record—though President Bizzell was convinced that he would "have no difficulty in making very definite progress."

[1.] One wonders whether such gerrymandering may have been the basis for Governor Murray's executive order on July 27, 1931, regarding nonmedical practitioners. See Mark R. Everett, *Medical Education in Oklahoma*, (Norman, University of Oklahoma Press, 1972), I, 286.

There were specified requirements to be fulfilled in order that the School of Medicine might regain a grade A rating: (1) complete freedom from political interference; (2) adequately and competently staffed preclinical departments; (3) organization of the faculty in such a way as to afford opportunity for carrying on a satisfactory educational program; (4) adjustment of the curriculum to provide circumstances favorable for meeting the requirement for adequately supervised clinical training; (5) reduction in the size of the student body until sufficient clinical facilities could be made available; and (6) assurance of accessible financial support for further development of the school.

On December 7 the university regents authorized Mr. Ledbetter to draw up two bills for building needs at the School of Medicine campus, inasmuch as Governor Marland had earlier approved a six-year building program for certain institutions, including additions and new buildings for the medical school and its two hospitals. The second bill provided that oil bonuses, derived from oil drilling operations on the medical center campus, be set up in a special fund for buildings and equipment at the School of Medicine.

In a letter to Governor Marland, December 12, 1936, Dean Patterson said that he understood, or had been advised, that monies accruing as lease monies to the state as a result of these oil operations would almost certainly be reappropriated by the legislature for the specific benefit of the School of Medicine and its hospitals.

In that same letter, Dean Patterson recapped some of the remarks and recommendations which had come out of the January inspection of the medical center. He emphasized the restoration of salaries to levels reached before 1934, when Governor Murray had caused them to be reduced markedly, the need for increased funds to meet requirements for salaries for at least five new assistant professors, the necessity to have done with political interference, which had been so lethal during the previous administration, and for an increase in the capacity of the teaching hospitals, which would entail a building program.

The full scale of Dean Patterson's envisioned building plan was as follows: a new addition to the School of Medic building and the necessary funds to remodel the present building; a student union building for medical students (the only students at the university without available housing); and a residence for the dean of the School of Medicine on the campus. In addition to these proposals, there were others for the University Hospitals, which included a new residence to house staff nurses and student nurses; funds to remodel the old Nurses Residence, thereby converting it into both an outpatient department building for the hospitals and quarters for interns and residents; a new power plant; a new laundry; utility shops to be housed in one building; an additional wing for Crippled Children's Hospital; a convalescent building to increase the capacity of Crippled Children's Hospital; an isolation building to care for contagious diseases in the two hospitals; a residence for the medical director of the hospitals on the grounds; and an addition to the University Hospital to provide increased capacity and better segregation of cases, a truly remarkable prospectus by a man ahead of his time.

When the faculty of the School of Medicine met in January, 1936, Dean Patterson advised those assembled that hereafter the faculty would meet only twice a year, and that intermittently there would be an executive committee to take action on recommendations for faculty confirmation at the ensuing regular meeting. By September 4 the committee was known as the faculty board. At the meeting of this group, Dean Patterson discussed a new course in medical jurisprudence and confirmed that some clinical instruction would be given to third- and fourth-year classes, both at Wesley Hospital and at St. Anthony Hospital. He also outlined plans for future improvement of the library through a faculty library committee, of which Dr. Turley was named chairman.

A meeting of the entire faculty followed on September 25, when Dean Patterson announced that the next faculty meeting would be held shortly before commencement in the spring. A gracious innovation was then proposed by the dean—a faculty fund for the purpose of making appropriate floral tributes in honor of deceased faculty members. Joseph M. Thuringer was subsequently appointed custodian of this fund, with a small committee to draw up proper resolutions respecting the death of members of the faculty.

Members of the faculty who died in 1936 were Doctors Millington Smith, emeritus professor of clinical gynecology, who had begun his teaching career in the School of Medicine in 1910; H. Coulter Todd, professor of otology, rhinology, and laryngology, who also commenced his faculty service in 1910; Arthur Brown Chase, professor of clinical medicine, who joined that department in 1917; and Samuel R. Cunningham, professor of orthopedic surgery, who had begun his career in 1910 as professor of gynecology.

Resignations from the faculty during the year included those of Fannie Lou Brittain Leney, instructor in pediatrics, and Austin Lee Guthrie, assistant professor of otorhinolaryngology.

Everett Lain was named professor of dermatology and syphilology and head of the department; Willis K. West, acting head and professor of orthopedic surgery, was designated head of that department;[2] John Evans Heatley was named professor and head of radiology; and Rex Bolend became professor of urology and head of the Department of Urology. George Garrison and Wendal D. Smith were appointed to assist in the supervision of the clinical clerkships, and Lee K. Emenhiser, acting chairman of the Department of Anatomy, was given a leave of absence for one year.

Certain changes in names of departments in the School of Medicine were

[2.] In a March 2, 1936, memorandum Dean Patterson stated that in November, 1935, Samuel R. Cunningham sustained a leg fracture which kept him immobilized until February, 1936, during which period the department was under the charge of Willis K. West. Dean Petterson added, "I have observed that the department . . . is largely divided against itself. . . . I understand that the head of the department had been advised, before the new dean arrived, to achieve harmony, but it was not done. I found a tendency on the part of several to feel that some were not doing their work, particularly Dr. McBride. The latter has assured the dean that he would see that his service was carried on effectively."

approved by the regents, effective February 1, 1936: epidemiology and preventive medicine became hygiene and public health; dermatology, radiology, and roentgenology became dermatology and syphilology, with radiology being made a new department; urology and syphilology became urology.

Dean Patterson, at a regents meeting on June 1, presented a list of new titles for clinical faculty members, including a new title of associate for a number of positions.[3] He also requested that an additional assistant professor be appointed in each of the following departments: anatomy, biochemistry, histology, pathology, and pharmacology; and that a full-time professor be appointed in the Department of Orthopedic Surgery. The regents approved these appointments but withheld their sanction of a full professorship in hygiene and public health. Regent Looney was delegated to draw up a separate bill to provide an annual appropriation of $7,500 for the position of professor of orthopedic surgery.

At the same June meeting of the regents, a resolution was passed setting the retirement age for teachers on the clinical staff of the School of Medicine at 65, effective at the beginning of the academic year in 1937. The regents also voted that no member of the permanent staff of the School of Medicine should remain on the active list after attaining the age of 65, although a teacher might be reappointed from year to year for exceptional reasons. This ruling was applicable to preclinical as well as clinical faculty members.

During the year 1936–37 there were 161 faculty members for the School of Medicine, eight faculty members for the School of Nursing, and four faculty members for the Department of Dietetics. Thirty-six new appointments to the School of Medicine faculty are given in the following tabulation:

William Hotchkiss Bailey, M.D.
    professor of medical
    jurisprudence
Charles Francis DeGaris, M.D.
    professor of anatomy
Arthur Alfred Hellbaum, Ph.D.
    assistant professor of physiology
Darrell Gordon Duncan, M.D.
    associate in therapeutic radiology
Tullos Oswell Coston, M.D.
    instructor in ophthalmology
George R. Felts, M.D.
    instructor in medicine
Ferdinand Rudolph Hassler, M.D.,
    M.P.H.
    instructor in hygiene and public
    health

Jesse Lester Henderson, M.D.
    instructor in neurology
Virgil R. Jobe, M.D.
    instructor in hygiene and public
    health
John Henderson Lamb, M.D.
    instructor in dermatology and
    syphilology
George Seanor Mechling, M.D.
    instructor in anesthesiology
Bert Ernest Mulvey, M.D.
    instructor in medicine
Milam Felix McKinney, M.D.
    instructor in medicine
Robert Leonard Noell, M.D.
    instructor in orthopedic surgery

[3] It should be stated that at this time, and earlier, it was customary that all original appointments of physicians to the volunteer clinical staff of the University Hospitals were made in the outpatient department for a probationary period of from one-half to one year before inclusion of the name of the appointee on the rolls of the faculty.

Hudson Swain Shelby, M.D.
  instructor in anesthesiology
Howard Bruce Shorbe, M.D.
  instructor in orthopedic surgery
Ella Smith, B.S.
  instructor in physical education
O. Alton Watson, M.D.
  instructor in otorhinolaryngology
Joe Henry Coley, M.D.
  clinical assistant in obstetrics
Clifford Cannon Fulton, M.D.
  assistant in surgery
Jess Duval Herrmann, M.D.
  assistant in surgery
Waldo Philip Hitchcock, B.A.
  assistant in physiology
William Knowlton Ishmael, M.D.
  assistant in medicine
George Henry Kimball, M.D.
  assistant in surgery
Joseph Fife Messenbaugh, M.D.
  assistant in surgery
Vern Herschel Musick, M.D.
  assistant in medicine

Emil Patrick Reed, M.D.
  assistant in surgery
Charles Andrew Smith, M.D.
  clinical assistant in psychiatry
Ralph Argyle Smith, M.D.
  assistant in medicine
Gregory Everett Stanbro, M.D.
  assistant in surgery
John Powers Wolff, M.D.
  assistant in surgery
Henry Joseph Darcey, B.S.
  lecturer in hygiene and public
  health
Harold Martin Hefley, Ph.D.
  fellow in bacteriology
George M. Kalmanson, B.S.
  fellow in bacteriology
Charles Merrett Pearce, M.D.
  lecturer in hygiene and public
  health
Norvell Edwin Wisdom, B.S.
  research associate in
  pharmacology

A new School of Medical Technology at the medical center was approved in 1936 by the Council on Medical Education and Hospitals, with Hugh Jeter as director. The first course of this type leading to a B.S. degree was started at the University of Minnesota in 1923.

The council, which had commenced approval of individual internships in hospitals in 1915 and of residencies in 1927, approved the following residencies at the University of Oklahoma Hospitals prior to 1936: one in anesthesia, two in medicine, four in obstetrics, one each in ophthalmology, otolaryngology, and in orthopedics, and three in surgery. During the year 1936, residencies in pathology and in radiology were also approved.

Wann Langston was chairman of the curriculum committee at this time. There were 16 hours of electives for second-year students, 32 for third-year students (limited to preclinical subjects), and 48 hours of electives, in addition to 32 hours of applied biochemistry and 16 hours of advanced physiology, in the fourth year.

There were 210 beds in operation at University Hospital and 243 at Crippled Children's Hospital during the year; 4,070 patients were admitted to the main hospital with an average stay of 22 days, and 2,385 patients were admitted to Children's Hospital. There were 569 obstetrics admissions to the medical center in 1936 and 521 births. Home deliveries numbered 673. New outpatient cases totaled 9,979.

The chief political criticisms of the University Hospitals were being directed at the care given patients on the veterans' ward and to a belief that the hospital accepted too many patients from Oklahoma City. The latter complaint was one that was to be kept aflame habitually by certain legislators.

A number of teaching clinics were conducted at St. Anthony Hospital with 300 beds, at Wesley Hospital with 150 beds, and at Central State Hospital in Norman with 2,675 beds. The diagnostic clinics of the Commission for Crippled Children beginning February 1, 1936, were under the joint auspices of the commission and the Oklahoma Society for Crippled Children, who were also jointly responsible for the expenses.

The appropriated funds for the School of Medicine and University Hospitals for fiscal year 1936–37 were as follows: School of Medicine, $103,000; University Hospital, $320,000; and Crippled Children's Hospital, $240,000, making a total of $663,000. Funds for the University of Oklahoma on the Norman campus amounted to $1,193,200.

During the 1936 commencement exercises in June, twenty graduates of the School of Nursing were awarded Graduate Nurse certificates, and 58 graduates of the School of Medicine received M.D. degrees, one of whom, Dr. Charles Harold Gingles, became a brigadier general in command of Letterman General Hospital in San Francisco in 1965. There were 242 students enrolled in the School of Medicine and 115 in the School of Nursing during the academic year 1936–37.

The action of the Council on Medical Education and Hospitals placing the School of Medicine on probation was an inevitable result of the political tinkering occurring during the preceding five years. The council thus posed a definite challenge to state and university officials to improve their attitudes toward and to exhibit an active interest in their School of Medicine.

An important factor at the outset was that President Bizzell no longer hesitated to assume a more peremptory posture, once there was an end to political threats, and to display some optimism about future conditions.

On their part, the regents of the university welcomed Dean Patterson to their meetings to exchange information, and they increased the budgetary provisions, thus making it possible to add a number of additional faculty members to the teaching staff. Furthermore, they delegated one of their members to draw up two bills relative to the governor's six-year building program for state institutions, which included additions to the University Hospital.

A third factor in effecting change was Dean Patterson's own initiative and integrity and his patient devotion to some immediate needs of the institution—capable administrators of the hospitals, improved reorganization of some of the clinical departments, and his progressive ideas concerning the relations of the basic science teaching staff to the clinical departments, such as mutual participation in discussions of clinical cases at staff meetings.

Among the attributes of General Robert U. Patterson may be listed honesty; in fact, he was a fiercely honest man. To illustrate the nature of his extraordinary forthrightness, some excerpts from a copy of a letter which he wrote to President Bizzell in May, 1936, concerning a former employee of the University Hospital are quoted here verbatim:

I have never heard this man's name mentioned before I received your letter. . . . How he became recommended for employment I do not know. Rumor seems to indicate that it was through the influence of a relative who was a friend of one of the members of the Board of Regents. If that is true, it was of course, not in the interest of good administration, and in conflict with the present policy of the Board of Regents as indicated in August, 1935. . . . I find on file a letter written by you to Dr. Jeter, in which you stated that you were instructed by the Board not to dismiss this man, and that you were asking that he be retained in his present position or transferred to some other department. . . . The Board, without hearing Dr. Jeter, decided to have this man retained and he was granted a leave of absence. . . . for a year.

The situation at present is that there is no vacant position at the University Hospital that this man can fill unless he desires a laborer's position, which can be created for him, though at unnecessary expense. If the Regents feel they are obligated to reemploy this young man in some capacity, I recommend that he be given a vacancy in a department of the University other than the medical school and its hospitals. . . . Let it be distinctly understood that the undersigned is not interested in politics in any way whatsoever. . . . Respectfully submitted, Robert U. Patterson.[4]

To the faculty of the School of Medicine, all of this was like an encouraging breath of fresh air, as General Patterson made his frequent "tours of inspection" throughout the medical center. It is true that his aura of militarism did not appeal to some sensitive souls, but most faculty members and employees came to appreciate the executive ability of "the General."

[4] A more gratifying reference to a former employee may be found in a news item in the *Oklahoma City Times*, October 19, 1936, to the effect that Paul H. Fesler, a former administrator of the University Hospitals and later superintendent of the University of Minnesota Hospitals, was to become administrator of one of the most modern hospitals in the world—Wesley Memorial Hospital, near the campus of Northwestern University in Illinois.

Chapter IV.
No Room in the Inn:
1937–38

Early in January a house committee appointed to review conditions at the University Hospital and the Hospital for Crippled Children for the sixteenth legislature expressed confidence in Dean Patterson as an efficient director of the School of Medicine who should be commended for his untiring efforts to uphold the high standards set for the school. The committee also expressed appreciation to H. R. Dickey, chief clerk of the institution, for the accomplished clerical work that was being carried on in a very crowded and cramped area in the basement of University Hospital.

The committee found that the hospitals' facilities were woefully inadequate to care for the 5,000 patients coming from all over the state each month for treatment and observation and further reported that apparently there were only 30 beds for black patients in the whole hospital—10 each for males, females, and children.

"Our visit to Crippled Children's Hospital," the report continued, "was indeed heartsickening and a sad aspect to behold. Crippled bodies, twisted limbs, anxious expressions and, behind it all, untold suffering—a picture that would soften a heart of iron and cause your eyes to moisten for your need to help them share their suffering. We were told that there were over 300 children waiting for admission but . . . 'There is no room in the inn.' . . . We believe that investment in human lives is far better than placing it on prisoners in reform schools . . . and we sincerely believe the Hospital for Crippled Children should be doubled in capacity at once."

The committee also recommended that University Hospital should be expanded either by building wings or enlarging the present building in order to accommodate the growing demands from the 77 counties of the state, and that a more suitable nurses' residence should be constructed. Legislative action, which would earmark for building purposes some of the funds that were being obtained from oil on the University Hospital grounds, was also proposed.

And such a construction bill was introduced in the sixteenth session of the legislature. It provided that proceeds and income derived from oil operations on the Medical Center campus should be paid to the state treasurer and deposited to the credit of "a special fund to be known as the University Hospital Fund, set apart and designated for the use and benefit of the University Hospital, the

Crippled Children's Hospital and the School of Medicine.'' The bill stated that this income could be used for building additions to any of the hospitals or for purchasing such equipment and instruments as might be deemed necessary.

In spite of the fact that this bill had been written as a result both of action taken by the board of regents in December, 1936, regarding ''oil bonuses'' and the report of the house committee, the legislature never made any pretense of passing it, thereby depriving the medical center of a substantial ancillary source of income. According to the state budget officer, the proceeds from these oil wells, as reported to the board of regents in November, amounted to $124,989.

An editorial appearing in the April 25, 1937, edition of the *Oklahoma News* made the observation that ''most of the legislators just don't like the University and the Medical School. . . . The mere fact that the Board of Regents opposed the Clinton purchase (of a bankrupt hospital) is enough for some legislators to vote for it.''

On May 17, Dean Patterson wrote a letter to Dr. MacEachern, director of hospital activities of the American College of Surgeons, saying that the legislature had just closed after a very long and stormy session on salaries and maintenance, and that the medical profession had managed to secure the passage of a basic science law which, though not perfect, was a definite step forward. However, Dean Patterson was greatly disappointed that the legislature fell down absolutely on his construction program, which it had endorsed or approved in principle, failing to provide for even so much as one building. It was ''largely due,'' he agonized, ''to the fact that the legislature will probably go down in history as one of the worst in recent years in this State. Several hospitals that were not being run successfully were unloaded on the State. Money went for such purposes when they failed to support the state institutions they already had.''

Despite the very niggardly response to the dean's building requests, he was able to build a one-story addition at the south end of the old outpatient department, which had been largely remodeled, in order to provide a social service room, a waiting room, a new fluoroscopic room, and a clinical laboratory for the outpatient department. This new addition extended almost to the nurses' current residence, providing nineteen small examining rooms for patients, with new examining tables and other equipment.

Dean Patterson had reconstituted the faculty board by 1937 to include heads of all teaching departments, seven senior members, the dean, and the assistant dean, and he appointed in addition eleven other working committees during the year.

Consequent to the legislature's failure to make necessary appropriations, the question of modifying admissions to the School of Medicine was thrashed out in regents meetings, faculty board meetings, and faculty meetings on numerous occasions during the year.

A recommendation that not more than ten students from outside the state should be accepted in the first-year class of the School of Medicine, and that the nonresident fees for out-of-state students should be fixed at $250 per year was endorsed by the regents in April. In May, they reconsidered action taken the previous December, limiting the admission of first-year students from any one county to 11 per cent of the total enrollment, and fixed the new limit at 20 per cent.

In June and again in September the faculty discussed the possible requirement of a baccalaureate degree with not less than a B average for admission to the School of Medicine. In spite of the fact that no university school of medicine in any state appeared to be making this requirement, a resolution that such a requirement be instituted was approved.

The reaction of President Bizzell to the requirement of a B.A. or B.S. degree for entrance to medical school was that raising the standards would prove to be too sudden and too drastic, affecting the number of applicants to study medicine. Dean Patterson felt that it was a waste of state and private funds, as well as of the time of the student concerned, to encourage a poorly educated student to study medicine, ''only delaying his start in life in some vocation or business for which he is better suited.''

The end result of many discussions and resolutions was that the faculty finally approved a 1.5 grade average as a necessary requirement for entrance to medical school in 1937; not less than 90 semester hours of college credit (excluding physical education and military science) starting with the class entering in 1939; and not less than a baccalaureate degree with the necessary scholastic standing in the fall of 1940. But, no matter how the cloth was cut, there was no choice but to reduce the number of students entering the School of Medicine for the year 1937–38 from 72 to 65.

With reference to applications of students from a B grade medical school for admission to advanced standing in our medical school, Dean Patterson was advised by the secretary of the Council on Medical Education and Hospitals that, ''while a strong institution might feel free to exercise this prerogative once in a great while, it would be a very risky thing indeed for the University of Oklahoma, with its current status, to take chances of this sort.'' This opinion left few illusions regarding the ''confidential probation'' imposed on the school in 1936.

In order to meet the criticism of the council, outlined in its official report (apropos of its inspection in January, 1936), certain positive steps were taken in 1937: arrangements were made for two classrooms in the University Hospital in addition to the old amphitheater classroom on the second floor and for greater use of available clinical facilities in St. Anthony Hospital and in Wesley Hospital, where six to eight students could be accommodated in the laboratories. Additional facilities were also readied for use by the University Hospital clinical pathology laboratories, and the clinical faculty commenced conducting weekly ward walks and teaching sessions for third-year students at Wesley Hospital and for fourth-year students at St. Anthony Hospital. Furthermore, Dean Patterson stressed the importance of clinical clerkships by outlining a plan for future use which would include making physical examinations, following cases step by step throughout a patient's stay in the hospital, even to performing all ordinary laboratory tests.

At the close of the faculty board meeting on November 19 a resolution was passed authorizing the dean to communicate with the Council on Medical Education, apprising the secretary of the positive steps which had been taken in an effort to comply with some of the requirements necessary to avoid jeopardizing publicly the status of the medical school. The dean was also authorized to say that the faculty would welcome another inspection of the University of Oklahoma School of Medicine at the convenience of the council.

There were several changes in faculty appointments in 1937: Floyd Bolend was made associate professor emeritus of medicine and emeritus head of the Department of Anesthesia, while John Moffett, instructor in anesthesia, was promoted to the rank of associate professor and head of the Department of Anesthesiology as of February 1. George Barry became director of the outpatient department, replacing Wayne Hull, who was made assistant director of the hospital laboratories; David Paulus and William W. Rucks, Sr., were appointed as associates in medicine for the purpose of giving clinical supervision to students at Wesley Hospital. William Fowler, who had resigned as professor of obstetrics in 1929, succeeded former dean, C. S. Bobo, as director of the University of Oklahoma Student Health Service. Onis Hazel resigned as lecturer and temporary head of the Department of Hygiene and Public Health but continued to serve as an associate professor of dermatology and syphilology.

Hiram D. Moor succeeded L. A. Turley as chairman of the library committee; Jane Marie Melgaard was appointed director of the dietary department of the University Hospitals, following the resignation of Margery Sewell as chief dietitian. Edythe Triplett, a graduate of the School of Nursing, instructor in nursing education, and assistant superintendent of nurses, was appointed superintendent of nurses March 16, following the resignation of Candice M. Lee, the director of the School of Nursing and superintendent of nurses, a position which she held from 1919 to 1924 and again from 1929 to 1937. Mrs. Lee, who received a Graduate Nurse certificate from the University of Oklahoma in 1921, had served her alma mater long and well.

There were 172 faculty members in the School of Medicine during the year 1937–38, including seven teachers in the School of Nursing and one dietitian. Because of a misconception in certain parts of the state that all of these people were on the state payroll, Dean Patterson found it necessary to inform the public that, with only three exceptions, no members of the attending or visiting staff of either the University of Crippled Children's Hospital received any remuneration for care and treatment of patients in these institutions. On the contrary, their professional services to patients were free to the state and their remuneration for teaching purposes practically negligible, an average of approximately $90 per year, a mere token payment.

The names of 32 new members who joined the faculty in 1937 are:

Paul Crenshaw Colonna, M.D.
professor of orthopedic surgery
Berry Campbell, Ph.D.
assistant professor of anatomy

Irvin S. Danielson, Ph.D.
assistant professor of
biochemistry

Francis Cornelius Lawler, D.Sc.
assistant professor of bacteriology
Arnold John Lehman, Ph.D., M.D.
assistant professor of
pharmacology
Albert John Sheldon, D.Sc.
assistant professor of bacteriology
Onie Owen Williams, M.D.
assistant professor of pathology
David Dare Paulus, M.D.
associate in medicine
William Ward Rucks, Sr., M.D.
associate in medicine
Alfred Joseph Ackermann
instructor in radiology
George Newton Barry, M.D.
instructor in medicine
Ernst John Dornfeld, Ph.D.
instructor in histology and
embryology
Brunel DeBost Faris, M.D.
instructor in obstetrics
Hervey Adolph Foerster, M.D.
instructor in dermatology and
syphilology
Ora Fuchs, G.N.
instructor in nursing education
Opal Willard Gray
instructor in massage and
physiotherapy
Grace Ellen Clause Hassler, M.D.
instructor in anesthesiology

Frances Victoria Henry, R.N., B.A.
instructor in nursing education
Sybil Hubbard, R.N.
instructor in practical nursing
education
Wayne McKinley Hull, M.D.
instructor in clinical pathology
Freda Schroeder Johnson, B.S.
instructor in diet therapy
Jane Marie Melgaard, M.S.
instructor in dietetics
Andrew Parks McLean, M.S.
instructor in pharmacology
Milton John Serwer, M.D.
instructor in obstetrics
Effie Katherine Smith, G.N.
instructor in pediatric nursing
Mary Wilkinson, B.A.
instructor in foods and nutrition
Henry Washington Harris, M.D.
assistant in obstetrics
Austin Holloway Bell, M.D.
lecturer in surgery
Carl Albert Bunde, Ph.D.
research fellow in physiology
Thomas Francis Dougherty, Jr.,
M.A.
research fellow in pathology
J. P. Hart, M.S.
research fellow in biochemistry
Patrick Armour Nuhfer, B.A.
research associate in
pharmacology

A notable appointment was that of Paul Colonna as the first full-time clinical professor in the School of Medicine, at a salary of $7,500. This professorship, approved by the university regents, June 1, 1936, was made possible through a special appropriation by the sixteenth legislature in Senate Bill No. 91. In addition, the legislature again appropriated $20,000 for the biennium for medical research, to be used solely for purposes under the direction of the dean of the school. This fund had assisted 23 research projects at the Medical Center since its inception in 1935.

According to the 1938 university catalog, revenue available for the academic year 1937–38 for the university at Norman was $1,663,020. For the School of Medicine and its hospitals in Oklahoma City, the state appropriations were reported as $124,928 for the medical school, $360,225 for the University Hospital and $283,470 for Children's Hospital. Faculty salaries which had been cut 15 to 30 per cent in 1930 by order of Governor Murray were happily restored and the university regents raised the salary of Dean Patterson to $8,000 effective September 1, 1937.

Fifty-nine M.D. degrees were awarded at the commencement exercises in 1937, and 23 certificates of Graduate Nurse were conferred. For the academic year 1937–38, 223 students were enrolled in the School of Medicine and 125 in the School of Nursing.

A total of 6,923 admissions to the hospitals, was reported, including 477 black patients, of whom 198 were children. The average hospital stay was 17.2 days for adults and 30.6 days for children. There were 471 deliveries on the obstetrical service (where 540 patients were accommodated during the year) and 697 home deliveries. The total number of patient visits in the outpatient department was 49,992. The professional staff included 20 interns and 14 residents in 1937–38.

A new, comprehensive plan recommended by Dean Patterson for the admission of patients to University Hospital had been approved by the university regents on April 5. It embodied the following pertinent points: patients whose condition might be improved by hospital care and treatment were eligible for admission but not those suffering from tuberculosis, contagious communicable diseases, venereal diseases, mental conditions, or alcoholism; members of the faculty of the School of Medicine and the attending staff in the hospitals and their immediate families (as well as interns, student nurses, and those nurses employed for one or more years) were to be admitted without charge; and all other employees of the School of Medicine and hospitals were to be furnished care and treatment by members of the attending staff at a clinical rate of $15 per week. Medical students, whose health care was actually under the supervision of two clinicians appointed by the dean, were entitled to examination and treatment, including hospitalization for a period not to exceed five days each semester. Admission of a private patient (subject to a request by a member of the attending staff) was at regular hospital rates.

In the third annual report of the Commission for Crippled Children, for the year 1937–38, Joe Hamilton, secretary to the commission, mentioned the outbreak of poliomyelitis during the summer of 1937 and some of the problems that it posed. In the preceding year or two, 44 special clinics had been held in the state for the examination of 459 children suffering from the aftereffects of poliomyelitis, under the supervision of the Oklahoma Crippled Children's Commission.

During the eleven years since the passage of Senate Bill No. 75 in 1927,[1] according to the report, 29,086 children had been afforded hospitalization in University Hospitals, far exceeding the expectations of the most sanguine legislator or enthusiastic worker who had had anything to do with the passage of the bill. Payment for the care of some 1,250 of these children had been made from funds of the Public Welfare Commission.

[1] Mark R. Everett, *Medical Education in Oklahoma*, (Norman, University of Oklahoma Press, 1972), I, 203; Sessions Laws, 1927, Chapters 19 and 20.

Postgraduate work, which had been brought to a halt in 1933 as far as support by the legislature was concerned, was resuscitated in 1937 by recommendation of the Postgraduate Committee of the State Medical Association that the School of Medicine conduct a two-year program in obstetrics. The Commonwealth Fund made a generous contribution for this purpose, and the State Health Department also gave funds derived from the federal Children's Bureau. The total budget for the program amounted to $19,500 per year. A manual was printed and distributed, and certificates were given upon completion of the course. L. W. Kibler continued to be the field director of this extension work and Edward N. Smith, as instructor, gave his untiring effort to the success of the program, traveling more than 78,000 miles over the state. All counties were represented, with 805 physicians enrolled in the course. There were 1,293 private consultations with physicians, and 57,000 persons attended 220 lay lectures. Of the 805 physicians who initially enrolled in the program, 637 received certificates upon completion of the course.

However genuine the concern of the House Investigating Committee appointed by the sixteenth legislature to review conditions at the University Hospital and the Crippled Children's Hospital (''a picture that would soften a heart of iron and cause eyes to moisten''), it was converted to crocodile tears and a hypocritical show by callous legislative inaction. When the votes were counted, neither enough hearts of iron had been softened nor a sufficient number of eyes made wet with tears to make the necessary appropriations for expansion of the space and services of University Hospitals, and so ''there was no room in the inn.'' Even the number of students entering the School of Medicine for the fall term had to be reduced.

Despite this heartless response by the legislature, Dean Patterson managed to make some improvements in the outpatient department and to negotiate other positive steps to diminish the impact of the criticism of the Council on Medical Education, which had resulted in a probationary status for the University of Oklahoma School of Medicine. He felt that the printed report, together with a comparison of the medical school's activities with those of other schools seemed unjustifiably critical of some of the clinical departments, especially of the Department of Orthopedic Surgery, ''one of the strongest departments to be found at any medical school in the country.''

There was a great absence of any organized alumni activity immediately following the Murray fiasco. Recognizing this deficiency, Dean Patterson urged the faculty to cooperate with the medical profession of the state and with the alumni in an effort to obtain their good will and support in establishing the fact that the School of Medicine was not run by a clique of physicians in Oklahoma City, and that the hospitals tried to admit patients on the basis of need and worth rather than on the basis of political sponsorship.

Chapter V.
Inexorable Indifference
to Medical Education:
1938–42

 The spring of 1938 was rather calm for the Board of Regents of the University of Oklahoma, but clouds commenced gathering in May as the case against the librarian of the School of Medicine, Ruth Thompson Hughes, began building up to a crescendo. Mrs. Hughes had been appointed in September, 1931, under false qualifications, for example, "Assistant, St. Louis Public Library."

As early as October 5, 1931, President Bizzell notified Dean Moorman that officials of the St. Louis Public Library had advised him that there was no record there that Ruth Thompson (Mrs. Ruth Campbell Hughes) had ever been on their staff; and on March 29, 1937, the registrar of Washington University in St. Louis advised Dean Patterson apropos of Ruth Thompson, upon whom Washington University was supposed to have conferred the degree of Bachelor of Arts in Library Science, that Washington University had never offered a course leading to a degree in Library Science. Furthermore, the registrar's office at St. Louis University had no record either of any individual under the above names who had ever been enrolled there. In fact, St. Louis University had no School of Library Science at all and offered no courses in library training.

Confronted with this testimony and mounting complaints about Mrs. Hughes' performance, her lack of training as a librarian, and her repeated absences from duty in the library, General Patterson issued an executive order concerning the duties of the librarian, warning Mrs. Hughes that such unremitting conduct would only lead to her release. So it was no surprise that President Bizzell, on June 6, reported to the regents that Ruth Thompson Hughes had been notified of her dismissal effective June 1. That she had asked for a hearing before the regents and "was waiting" came as no surprise to anyone either.

It was the consensus of the regents that Mrs. Hughes should be granted a hearing, and General Patterson immediately asked that he be excused; at 5 o'clock Regent Hatchett asked that he be excused; and, following Mrs. Hughes' statements, she was excused. Whereupon, Dean Patterson recommended that "the services of Ruth Thompson Hughes be discontinued May 31, 1938," and that she should receive her regular salary for the months of June and July; said recommendation being officially approved by the regents.

But Mrs. Hughes made a second request for a hearing before the regents on September 24 and, though no new information or facts bearing on her case came to light, she requested yet another hearing. This time, the regents voted that she be requested to submit any new material in writing, together with documentary evidence, to the secretary of the regents before the next meeting. When no further material was submitted on November 5, a motion was made, seconded, and carried unanimously that the case of Mrs. Hughes be ordered closed.

The plaintiff's case was not quite closed though, for Mrs. Hughes sent a copy of a brief, which she said she had sent to Governor Phillips, to Regent Hatchett in August, 1939, that brought this sharp riposte:

> "To begin, let me get you straight on one matter: No employee of the State University has any tenure of position. Under the law the regents have a right to dismiss with or without cause at any time. The matter of a hearing before the Board . . . is not a matter of right . . . but a matter of grace. . . . You refer to various charges. As far as I know no charges were preferred nor any bill of indictment setting forth such was presented nor was it at all necessary that such be done. . . . The Board acted as it thought for the best interest of the University in dismissing you. The matter of your case is a closed book so far as I am concerned, and I am sure the Board feels the same way."

However, the book was not finally closed until April, 1940, when Mrs. Hughes' petition to the district court for damages and a judgment against William Bennett Bizzell and Robert Urie Patterson, "each of them for $50,000 and costs," was duly denied and dismissed by the court, after considerable personal expense to the defendants.[1]

All along, the need for the funding of building projects on the medical school campus was constantly on Dean Patterson's mind, culminating in the presentation of an itemized request for a construction and remodeling program totaling $1,654,400 to the university regents on September 24, 1938. A bit galled by the magnitude of the request, the regents belatedly informed General Patterson on December 7 that it was "the sense of the Board that the request for buildings at the medical school and hospitals should not exceed approximately $300,000." Whereupon, Dean Patterson wrote to the President of the regents, Eugene Kerr, that there were certain things to be done if we were to continue on the list of merely *confidentially unapproved* medical schools; and he mentioned the fact

---

[1.] This case has been described in some detail because it illustrates hazards involved in administration of official duties at that time and emphasizes the need for insurance against any such attempts to collect damages. Coverage of this nature was later provided and helped materially in the case of another false claim during the administration of Dean Mark R. Everett.

that the University of Arkansas School of Medicine had recently been put on probational status publicly. Furthermore, the University Hospital School of Nursing had been found ineligible for national accreditation by a survey committee from the National League of Nursing Education—an added minus point.

Another concern of the dean was the great service rendered by the volunteer hospital and outpatient staff, which would have amounted to $1,000,000 a year if the state had been charged for the services—more than double the entire amount appropriated by the legislature. Incredible as it may seem today, with only three exceptions, the teaching in the third and fourth years of the School of Medicine was done entirely by physicians who volunteered their services. "I do not know of any medical school in the United States," the dean said, "which does not have a few full-time teachers occupying the key positions in the clinical departments, with a nucleus of part-time instructors sufficient in number to insure that the teaching in the hospitals and the actual care of patients is carried out efficiently at all times; augmented by the assistance of a volunteer clinical teaching staff."[2]

The regents of the University of Oklahoma awarded honorary titles of professor emeritus to volunteer professors retiring in 1938 as follows: Doctors John Mosby Alford, who had served on the faculty since 1911, Edmund Sheppard Ferguson, John Frederick Kuhn, and William Merritt Taylor, heads of the Departments of Ophthalmology, Gynecology, and Pediatrics, respectively; and appointed Doctors Leslie M. Westfall, Grider Penick, and Clark Hall to succeed Dr. Ferguson, Dr. Kuhn and Dr. Taylor. J. A. Moffett, who resigned the post of head of the Department of Anesthesiology on June 30, was succeeded by Hubert Eugene Doudna at a salary of $3,500 as of August 11. Grace Robeson Sigerfoos was appointed librarian of the School of Medicine for a twelve-month period to replace Ruth Thompson Hughes, and Lila B. Heck became assistant librarian for a like period, succeeding Ida Lee Warner, who resigned on July 14.

Francis J. Reichmann, assistant professor of oral surgery and stomatology became president of the Oklahoma State Dental Association in 1938. Since 1928 he had worked tirelessly toward the establishment of a dental college on the School of Medicine campus.

There was a total of 196 faculty members in the School of Medicine during the academic year 1938–39, exclusive of the School of Nursing and teachers of dietetics. The 22 new appointments made to the faculty during this time are:

Donald Bard McMullen, D.Sc.
 assistant professor of bacteriology
 and associate professor of hygiene
Lois Lyon Wells, M.D.
 associate in anesthesiology

Rudolph Fink Nunnemacher, Ph.D.
 instructor in histology and
 embryology
Evelyn Stephens, R.N., B.A.
 instructor in practical nursing

[2.] Volunteer physicians had performed 4,288 major and minor operations in the two hospitals during the fiscal year ending June 30, 1937, including 1,700 fractures and applications of plaster casts.

Jack Paul Birge, M.D.
  assistant in surgery
Augustus Malone Brewer, M.D.
  assistant in urology
John Ashby Cunningham, M.D.
  assistant in surgery
Louis Najib Daril, M.D.
  assistant in medicine
Harry Linnell Deupree, M.D.
  assistant in medicine
Harry Cummings Ford, M.D.
  assistant in otorhinolarngology
Allen Gilbert Gibbs, M.D.
  assistant in medicine
Melvin Philip Hoot, M.D.
  assistant in otorhinolaryngology
Robert Bruce Howard, M.D.
  assistant in surgery
Virgil R. Jobe, M.D.
  assistant in surgery
James Polk Luton, M.D.
  assistant in ophthalmology
William Carl Lindstrom, M.D.
  assistant in obstetrics
Everett Baker Neff, M.D.
  assistant in surgery

Cannon Armstrong Owen, M.D.
  assistant in surgery
Raymond Delbert Watson, M.D.
  assistant in surgery
Tom Lyon Wainwright, M.D.
  assistant in surgery
Neil Whitney Woodward, M.D.
  assistant in surgery
Hubert Eugene Doudna, M.D.
  lecturer in anesthesia
Carrie S. Gillaspy, B.A.
  graduate assistant in anatomy
James K. Gray, M.D.
  fellow in pathology
Lilah Bell Heck, M.S.
  assistant librarian
Dan Roy Sewell, M.D.
  lecturer in surgery
Grace Robertson Sigerfoos, B.A.
  librarian
Arthur Stephenson Spangler, B.S.
  research fellow in pharmacology
Frederick H. Von Saal, M.D.
  fellow in orthopedic surgery

The salary scale for faculty members during the fiscal year 1938 to 1939 was as follows: professors, $3,800 to $4,500; associate professors, $3,000; assistant professors, $2,500 to $3,000.

Dean Patterson conceded in 1938 that, in spite of all the handicaps, teaching methods were gradually improving in the School of Medicine and that a balance of didactic and clinical work was being maintained. It was his opinion that the greatest improvement in the teaching of any preclinical course in recent years had been made in the Department of Anatomy under the direction of Ernest Lachman. In recognition of Dr. Lachman's special talent and dedication, the faculty approved the introduction of a new course in his department on June 3, 1938, to be known as Normal Anatomy Demonstrated by X-ray, a course which proved to be very successful in the ensuing years.

The Department of Histology and Embryology was separate from the Deaprtment of Anatomy at this time. Joseph Thuringer, the chairman, was an accomplished artist in photographic work. During his tenure he made a valuable contribution to his department in the form of 25,000 classified, microscopic slides of tissues and a complete card index of many bibliographic titles referring to histology and embryology.

Dean Patterson was genuinely interested as well in the Department of Biochemistry, one of the youngest departments (organized by Mark R. Everett in 1924),[3] whose members were actively affiliated with eight national scientific scoeities and institutes. By 1938 they had published over 40 articles in scientific journals and several books, in addition to directing graduate work which resulted in 12 theses.

The Department of Biochemistry worked closely with the clinical staff, actively assisting in investigations undertaken in such fields as allergy, dermatology, medicine, orthopedics, surgery, and urology, as well as in clinical conferences for fourth-year students (conducted jointly by members of the clinical staff and the students themselves) in quarter sections of the class. By means of such informal discussions the fundamental principles and metabolic aspects of disease were reviewed. The University of Oklahoma was one of the pioneers in this method which, at the time, was being adopted by a number of medical schools.

Active research at the University of Oklahoma School of Medicine had proceeded at a rather slow rate in earlier years, but, with the first appropriation of $20,000 for research by the legislature in 1935, the spirit of scientific investigation spread until by 1938 there were no fewer than 44 research projects being undertaken with some aid from this particular fund. This was at a time when federal funds for medical research were unavailable.

One important step toward future aid in the way of grants and gifts for the university and its various schools was the establishment in the spring of 1938 of the University of Oklahoma Foundation for receiving gifts and bequests and for administering these donations.

The University Hospitals had three senior residencies—one each in medicine, orthopedics, and surgery—with thirteen other residencies and two research fellowships; and the university regents approved a recommendation by Dean Patterson for the creation of a fellowship in orthopedic surgery effective July 1, 1938, as well as the title fellow in pathology, a position to be occupied by one of the residents in pathology.

According to the University of Oklahoma catalog for 1938–39, University Hospital had 210 beds, and Children's Hospital had 243 beds at that time. Fortunately, the medical school was able to use beds in affiliated hospitals for purposes of instruction because of the shortage of beds in general medicine. The Holme's Home of Redeeming Love was also available for obstetrical cases.

A contract with the Oklahoma State Soldier's Relief Commission, allotting Ward 3 of the University Hospital for veterans' care, was continued in 1938, and a contract with the United States Veterans Bureau for care of veterans at the University Hospital was also renewed.

Admissions to University Hospitals during the year amounted to a total of 6,527, of which number 2,624 were admissions to Children's Hospital.

[3.] Dr. Everett was a member of the research committee of which Dr. Langston was chairman, a member of the electives committee together with J. T. Martin and R. M. Howard, and chairman of the curriculum committee in 1938.

George Barry, director of the outpatient department, reported that 11,488 new patients, including 3,183 children, were examined during the same period, with the total number of visits in the outpatient department amounting to 50,740. This provided for clinical instruction a wealth of cases distributed throughout the following departments: general medicine, various medical specialties (such as gastrointestinal, cardiorespiratory, neurology, endocrinology, arthritis, and diabetes), radiology, dermatology, general surgery, gynecology, urology, neurosurgery, orthopedic surgery, ophthalmology, otorhinolaryngology, plastic surgery, rectal surgery, pediatrics, obstetrics, and dental surgery.

Included in the fourth report of the Oklahoma Commission for Crippled Children for the year 1938–39 was a special report by Paul C. Colonna, director of the Department of Orthopedic Surgery in the University of Oklahoma School of Medicine. In it Dr. Colonna stated that the Department of Orthopedic Surgery consisted of a 150-bed service at the Hospital for Crippled Children and a 15-bed service for adults and colored children in University Hospital.

A letter transmitted by Joe Hamilton, secretary of the Oklahoma Commission for Crippled Children, in the above cited report, contained some rather disparaging remarks about the governor's inattention to the distressing lack of hospital beds available to black children with crippling conditions, of which he had been apprised previously. The Commission urged that this "unfair situation be alleviated" by some legislative provision for a reasonable increase in facilities for colored patients in the Crippled Children's Hospital.

The Rotary Club, cognizant of the "lack of beds available to Negro children in crippling conditions," passed a resolution petitioning the next legislature and the hospital authorities to face up to this need by making more beds available to colored children.

In 1938–39 the staff of the Department of Orthopedic Surgery consisted of one full-time director, six attending staff surgeons, and a house staff of seven members. Two doctors well trained in orthopedic surgery, who had finished their residencies in orthopedics at this or some other institution, were assigned to the department for a year or more; and three physicians, John F. Burton, Don H. O'Donoghue and C. R. Rountree, who had been accepted for three-year residencies in orthopedics after completing a two-year general internship, were salaried through the Crippled Children's Commission.

The Social Service Department in the University Hospital was established in 1921 under the direction of Virginia Tolbert, a registered nurse, as a stepchild of the social service department of the University of Oklahoma in Norman.[4] By 1934 the school was well organized and ready to seek accreditation. In 1938, Helen Carr, supervisor of the field work for University Hospitals, became director of the ancillary department in Oklahoma City. And beginning in 1938 a course in the social aspects of nursing was offered by the School of Nursing.

According to the 1938–39 university catalog, the income for the year ending

    [4.] Mark R. Everett, *Medical Education in Oklahoma*, (Norman, University of Oklahoma Press, 1972), I, 158, 179, 237–38.

June 30, 1939, was $1,584,088 for the Norman campus. Separate legislative appropriations provided $142,000 for the medical school in Oklahoma City, $338,375 for the University Hospital, and $253,100 for the Crippled Children's Hospital.

There were 52 graduates of the School of Medicine who received the M.D. degree in 1938; 28 students in the School of Nursing received the certificate of Graduate Nurse. During the academic year 1938–39, 114 nursing students and 230 medical students were enrolled at the medical center.

Medical students selected for the first-year class in 1939 were required to have completed three years or 90 hours of college credit from an accredited college or university for admission to the School of Medicine; a resident fee of $100 per year was voted by the regents, and the nonresident fee was raised from $250 per year to $350. Emphasis on the scholastic average of the applicant was the main factor in selecting candidates rather than on the aptitude test used nationally for some years as a compulsory test for any candidate seeking admission to a medical school. This test was of value only as a guide.

Though the standards for admission to the University of Oklahoma School of Medicine had been raised gradually over a period of eight to nine years in conformity with similar actions at other schools of medicine, the records proved that there had been a definite reduction in the number of students in the first-year class who had had to be dropped later for scholastic failure. This may have been due, in part, to the fact that the head of each department of the School of Medicine was acting in an advisory capacity to any student who elected to take his course, and to the fact that there was a special committee on electives available to students, for guidance in the selection of courses.

A new code of professional conduct for students, adopted by the faculty in 1938, was also a clear-cut innovation whereby each instructor in the School of Medicine was asked to keep a record on individual students, under the heading of general and professional attitude. Observation of any irregularity or undesirable quality of character was first brought to the attention of the student concerned; secondly, to the attention of the faculty at the end of each semester, provided the attitude of the student remained unchanged, and finally, to the attention of the dean of the School of Medicine. Whereupon, the dean was expectcd to officially notify the student of his or her possible dismissal from medical school.

According to the 1938–39 university catalog, 60 per cent of the semester grade of a third- or fourth-year student depended upon professional attitude, which included approach to patients, attitude toward fellow students and associates, and personal appearance—standards acceptable to the faculty.

All lectures for third- and fourth-year students on Friday afternoons were open to any practicing physician in the state of Oklahoma, and all county medical society members were invited by the faculty to attend these lectures.

One sympathizes with General Patterson in his persistent efforts to secure appropriations for buildings on the medical center campus and for a appointments of full-time and part-time teachers in the clinical departments. Merely to read his correspondence, memoranda, and various reports for the year 1938 is to realize how earnestly he faced up to the problems of patient care and the relationship of these problems to standard quality medical education.

One can sense a note of despair but not of defeat in his report to the president and regents of the university in December, wherein he stated that "many cases have to be refused accommodations to the embarrassment and regret of the hospital administration . . . but without control of these two teaching hospitals by the School of Medicine, to furnish necessary clinical teaching material, this medical school would immediately be down graded . . ."—especially since the sixteenth and seventeenth legislatures had not provided any monies for buildings.

This, in spite of the fact that the dean had specifically pointed out that just the isolation of affected children and all contacts for the entire period of incubation took considerable time, making much-needed beds unavailable in the Children's Hospital because of the need to use part of one whole floor for isolation cases.

Undaunted by these reverses, Dean Patterson never ceased to plead the cause of the University of Oklahoma School of Medicine, facing the future with perseverance and hope. At the same time, he found time to look back, and he merits our gratitude for making an earnest effort to collect historical data concerning the school. One such gem is a letter written to Dean Patterson under date of January 18, 1938, by Roy P. Stoops, director of the medical department in Oklahoma in 1904:

> Several days ago I finally sent the photograph of myself which you requested of me some months ago, for placing upon the wall of the faculty room. . . . I have had a number of pictures taken in the last two or three years for similar purposes, the usual fault being that the photographer expended so much effort in obliterating the wrinkles that my features were hardly recognizable. . . .
>
> President Boyd was always opposed to delegating executive authority or to having any deans presiding over autonomous colleges. But it was necessary to use the title when we entered the Association [of American Medical Colleges][5] so the term "Acting Dean" was invented for the occasion. . . .
>
> Now Dr. Patterson this is the first time I have expressed my opinion on anything connected with the medical school since thirty years ago. The time is long past when personalities and factional quarrels have any importance, if they ever had any. Oklahoma may be turbulent but there are forty-seven other states just as turbulent.

The voters of Oklahoma elected Leon C. Phillips governor of the state of Oklahoma in the fall of 1938, a choice which promised a grim outlook for medical education; for the governor's attitude of opposition to the School of

_____
[5] *Journal of the American Medical Association*, Vol. XLVII (1906), 633.

Medicine had been stated lucidly in newspaper accounts, and the governor himself had openly criticized the methods and procedures used by the school in determining admission of candidates.

Consequently, all members of the faculty board of the School of Medicine were urged by Dean Patterson on January 27 to get in touch with their friends and legislators at their earliest convenience and to inform them of the serious situation confronting the School of Medicine and hospitals, both in regard to construction of new buildings and sufficient funds to meet salaries and maintenance costs.

Furthermore, it was the unanimous opinion of the faculty board on February 25 that a reinspection of the School of Medicine by the Council on Medical Education and Hospitals, as requested in November 1937, should be postponed until fall. While this opportunity for reinspection would have been most welcome under ordinary circumstances, it seemed wise then to ask the secretary of the council for postponement. The appearance of representatives of the council on the School of Medicine campus might give the governor the false impression that they were there for the sole purpose of counteracting him.

In an effort to bolster the shrinking budget, the regents of the University of Oklahoma convened in the capitol building with Governor Phillips on March 27, and they formulated a bill for introduction into the legislature which would provide some funds by requiring a tuition fee for entrance to the School of Medicine. The fee for residents of Oklahoma was set at $50 per semester and for nonresidents at $175 per semester, or $350 per year—a raise of $100 over the present year—effective in September, 1939.

The next order of business was a discussion about the need for construction of an isolation ward at Crippled Children's Hospital, and when the regents left the meeting, it was with the understanding that an appropriation of $67,000 for that purpose would have the governor's approval.

Four days later, in an evening meeting with Governor Phillips, Dean Patterson expressed some misgivings in a letter to Regent Eugene M. Kerr, about a suggestion made by J. M. Holliman, state representative from Washington County. "It seems to me," Dean Patterson wrote, "that both the Governor and Mr. Holliman . . . should be advised that they cannot push the medical students onto any independent hospital such as St. Anthony . . . with only 20 per cent of its beds allotted to the public . . . entirely insufficient for our needs." And the dean continued by saying that the very fact that we controlled our teaching hospitals placed the University of Oklahoma School of Medicine among the main medical schools, thereby meeting in this respect the higher standards set for teaching hospitals. "I cannot think that the suggestion of Mr. Holliman was made seriously," he said. For the very idea that the top echelons of state government would so much as contemplate abandoning an excellent plant such as the University Hospital, thereby reducing the capacity of the state to care for its indigent patients in the superior way that it has been doing over the last 20 years, was beyond the comprehension of General Patterson. "I think," he said, "the Irish dividends that would result by that practice would be sufficient to defeat the political ambitions of anyone who advocates it in this state."

At the next meeting of the regents on April 10 a motion (biennially resurrected) was made and carried that the legislature appropriate a pool out of oil royalties and bonuses from medical campus properties to be used by the regents for the purpose of erecting an isolation building at Crippled Children's Hospital and a nurses' residence at University Hospital.

This time the seventeenth legislature actually did pass such a bill, earmarking $68,000 in oil royalties for use of the regents, but the old snare and delusion about an oil royalties fund still held. Governor Phillips chose to veto the bill! And, as if that were not harassment enough, the governor curtailed the budget for the University of Oklahoma and its School of Medicine in deference to other state functions, "due to the poor financial situation of the state treasury."

The fact of the matter was that the seventeenth legislature had slashed appropriations for education across the board by 20 per cent at a time when there was still hope that self-interest and frontier type politics would no longer prevail. But under the impact of the 20 per cent reduction, and a still further reduction for the first quarter of the fiscal year, nothing could possibly be done about construction of any buildings, the appointment of a full-time faculty member in the Department of Medicine, or of six faculty members for the outpatient department.

"We have had many disappointments during the past four years," the dean told his faculty on September 23, "and the outlook for the future is not very bright." Yet, for the third time in as many months (if not days) he mentioned the governor's promise that funds for a new nurses' residence would be appropriated during the next legislative session. For some reason, perhaps his own rigid honesty, Dr. Patterson still kept his faith in the governor's word.[6]

Because of another bleak picture, the university regents discontinued operation of the University Hospital dairy, on termination of its lease to the University Hospital on June 30, 1939, during a special session with Governor Phillips in the Blue Room in the state capitol building on April 17. A financial review by Howard Dickey, business manager of University Hospitals, showed that, whereas the dairy had operated at a profit from 1931 to 1935, from then on it had begun to show losses because of the drought and the resulting necessity of having to purchase cattle feed. And the losses had increased considerably during 1937–38, when 65 cattle expired because of an epidemic of Bang's disease, a plague which had also affected other dairies.

[6.] An interesting footnote to the financial crises of 1939 may be found at the end of a letter dated October 3, 1939, from former Governor Robert L. Williams to General Patterson. "I hate to see the meager appropriations for the University Hospital reduced," Governor Williams wrote. "Of all appropriations, the ones for the University Hospital and the asylums and the feeble minded institutions are the last that should be reduced. Better to close the colleges, and let these institutions run on full appropriations. The fact is that half of the students that go to these colleges ought never to be in college. . . . Of all the achievements of my administration as Governor, I am most proud of the fact that I backed the proposition to build the University Hospital and sometime, when I have the opportunity, I want to tell you with what difficulty that appropriation was obtained."

On recommendation of Dean Patterson, the regents replaced L. A. Turley, assistant dean of the School of Medicine, with the appointment of Harold A. Shoemaker, professor of pharmacology, effective July 1, 1939.

The faculty of the University of Oklahoma School of Medicine was shocked and deeply grieved by the accidental death on February 16 of Andrew Parks McLean, instructor in pharmacology, in the medical school building,[7] the only fatal laboratory accident of record during the existence of the University of Oklahoma medical center.

Floyd Jackson Bolend, who had joined the faculty as an instructor in children's diseases in 1912, died on June 22, 1939, when he was associate professor emeritus of medicine and head of the Department of Anesthesiology.

There were 218 members of the faculty during the academic year 1939–40, seven of whom were teaching in the School of Nursing and three in dietetics. Fifteen persons were newly appointed to the faculty by the university regents, as follows:

Kenneth Murrell Richter, Ph.D.
  assistant professor of histology
Irwin Clinton Winter, Ph.D.
  assistant professor of pharmacology
Benedict Ernest Abreu, Ph.Dl
  instructor in pharmacology
Marie Garrett, R.N., B.S.
  instructor in nursing education
Edna McElvogue, G.N.
  instructor in pediatric nursing
Charles Marion O'Leary, M.D.
  instructor in surgery
Moorman Paul Prosser, M.D.
  instructor in psychiatry
Joseph Anton Rieger, M.D.
  instructor in mental diseases

Ruby Allen Wortham, M.A.
  instructor in histology
James Richard Huggins, M.D.
  assistant instructor in medicine
John William Records, M.D.
  assistant in obstetrics
Robert Irvine Trent, M.D.
  assistant in ophthalmology
Evan Leonard Copeland, M.S.
  research fellow in physiology
Lowell Thomas Crews, M.S.
  research fellow in biochemistry
Grady Fred Mathews, M.D.
  lecturer in hygiene and public health

The University of Oklahoma awarded 52 M.D. degrees to graduates of the School of Medicine at commencement in 1939, with both Fratis Lee Duff and Robert W. Kahn being granted degrees with cum laude distinction for successfully completing honors assignments.[8] Twenty-nine certificates of Graduate Nurse were issued in the School of Nursing.

In concurrence with a resolution passed by the faculty in 1938, the regents

[7] Mark R. Everett was a personal witness to the events following Mr. McLean's fatal accident in his research laboratory when a large flask containing alcohol, which he was heating, exploded. Upon hearing the foreboding boom, Dr. Everett grasped a fire extinguisher and dashed down the hall, only to see his fellow scientist rushing headlong for the stairway, with all his clothes aflame. He was stopped by friends on the stair landing, who tried desperately to smother the flames with a blanket, but to no avail.

[8] Dr. Duff later became a brigadier general in the United States Air Force. Another graduate in the class of 1939, George Munroe Davis, Jr., achieved the distinction of

voted on February 6 that a degree of bachelor of science in medicine should be discontinued after the 1940 commencement exercises in Norman, in view of the new requirement of three years, or 90 hours, of college credit for admission to medical school. This step was in conformity with the established trend among medical schools requiring a longer period of premedical matriculation.

During the academic year 1939–40, there were 237 medical students and 131 nursing students on the campus of the medical center in Oklahoma City.

A number of new residents were accepted at the University Hospital in September in addition to eight residents who were continuing their training. These new appointments were in the Departments of Obstetrics, Medicine, Surgery, Pathology, Dentistry, Radiology, Orthopedic Surgery, and Anesthesiology.

A grant of $3,000 was made to the Department of Orthopedic Surgery from the National Foundation for Infantile Paralysis to be used for research and study in cases of paralytic scoliosis (infantile paralysis leaving curvature of the spine). Under a plan formulated by the department, case studies of the course of development of this disease were to be made and then a conclusion drawn as to the best method of treating such cases.

According to the 1939–40 catalog of the University of Oklahoma, the revenue for the university at Norman was $1,555,770, and the funds for the support of the School of Medicine were as follows: School of Medicine, $132,722; University Hospital, $331,948, and Crippled Children's Hospital, $253,243. Hospital statistics for the same period included 5,909 patients admitted to both hospitals, 3,873 to University and 2,036 to Crippled Children's Hospital. The total number of deliveries was reported as 489 and the total number of outpatients treated at both hospitals as 21,424, of which 10,508 were new patients.

It is to the credit of the university regents that they authorized their president on September 9 to request the governor to at least make a deficiency grant of $5,000 to meet the need for braces and shoes for children at the Crippled Children's Hospital.[9]

During the year, Dean Patterson compiled a brief history of the University of Oklahoma School of Medicine and its teaching hospitals. Among other assertions, he claimed that 964 students had graduated from the School of Medicine

---

becoming a vice admiral in the United States Navy.

Admiral Davis received a commendation ribbon for his part in the landing on Iwo Jima. He was named commanding officer of the Bethesda Naval Hospital in Maryland in 1965 and surgeon general of the Navy in 1968.

There were two other generals of the United States Army who graduated from the University of Oklahoma School of Medicine in 1925, namely, Brigadier General Emery Ernest Alling and Major General Alvin Levi Gorby. Both retired from the army in 1955.

[9.] E. C. Hopper, Jr., of Eufaula attended the meeting of the regents on September 9, replacing Eugene M. Kerr. Claude S. Chambers of Seminole, who was also appointed by Governor Phillips, attended for the first time on March 27, replacing Malcolm E. Rosser, Jr.

since 1910, and that 58.2 per cent of those graduates had been practicing medicine in 90 cities and towns and in 54 counties in Oklahoma in the last ten years. These figures were slightly in error for he had inadvertently included seven 1910 graduates of Epworth University College of Medicine in his enumeration. As determined from the lists of graduates at commencement each year, the figure should have read 949 graduates rather than 964. The dean figured that 42.3 per cent of the faculty members of the School of Medicine were its own graduates, "teaching oncoming generations of physicians," and that 55 per cent of the staff of the two teaching hospitals was made up of graduates of the University of Oklahoma School of Medicine.

Dean Patterson tried once more in 1939 to secure the appropriations from the legislature which he felt were necessary for the development of a Class A medical center but, alas, without success. He even consulted with Senator Mike Monroney in Washington, D.C., about the possibility of WPA projects, including such things as a new wing for the University Hospital, the Isolation Hospital, the nurses' residence, a Crippled Children's Hospital addition, utility buildings, and a School of Medicine building addition, but with negative results.

Despite this wholesale set of disappointments, we find Dr. Patterson writing to a prospective candidate for the position of medical director and assistant superintendent of the University Hospitals on December 21, 1939, saying that "the climate of Oklahoma is fine and the people are kindly and hospitable"; then going on without any intimation of discouragement to outline the separation of duties between a medical director of the hospitals and the dean and superintendent of the medical center. He promised his prospective assistant administrator a free hand, except in cases of important policy making affecting either the administration or the teaching, in such a way as to result in criticism of the hospitals or bad relations for the medical center. "Because of local conditions," the dean added, "it is desirable that the physician undertaking the work be one who possesses tact and the ability to get along with his colleagues. Such qualifications are needed anywhere in the country."

But no matter what the qualifications of an administrator should be—and General Patterson's were ample—the key to the impasse at the medical center was money, and there appeared to be no surplus of that commodity in Oklahoma in 1939. At least none was being diverted to education and health, as evidenced by an editorial in the *Woodward Republican* on November 9, 1939, entitled "To the Glory of the State," "In dictator countries, the life of the individual does not count. It is all secondary 'to the glory of the State.' If it is too expensive to repair a handicapped child, don't bother—it's cheaper to raise another." We claim superiority for democracy, but listen to this. "For the first time in several years," says Joe Hamilton, director of the Oklahoma Commission for Crippled Children. "It appears that there is a strong probability that physically handicapped children and others suffering from acute surgical conditions are to be denied medical and surgical care in time of need. The administration of the Oklahoma Hospital for Crippled Children has been forced to make a radical reduction in the number of available beds; 47 have been removed from active service—a situation which is not due to failure of the hospital authorities to do what they can, but to lack of funds.'' And a similar article appeared in the November 11 issue of the *Oklahoma City Times*:

> It has been charged that we have been spending too much on hospitals. So it seems children who are now crippled are to remain cripples all their lives. . . . No one is more conservative than Mr. Joe Hamilton. . . . It's just that they do not have the money . . . in spite of cuts for hospitals, for schools, for every service possible. . . . So Oklahoma must retreat . . . some 15 to 20 years into the past, if the budget is to be balanced.
>
> One of the peculiar features of the situation is that state's righters, like Governor Phillips, who are pledged to aid the sick and the crippled and the children in the weak school districts, and who find the state utterly unable at the present time to do the work, are bitter opponents of bills pending in Congress for federal aid to education and health, in those states and sections which of themselves cannot provide funds from their own resources.

Small wonder that Dean Patterson could bring himself to say, though without rancor, only three complimentary things about our state: ''the climate of Oklahoma is fine and the people are kindly and hospitable . . . $4,500 per year is considered a very large salary in the southwest.''

According to the 1940 federal census of Oklahoma, the ''grapes of wrath'' exodus in the 1930's resulted in a marked decrease in the population of the state by about 60,000 to 2,336,434. However, the severe drought which caused the farmers to leave Oklahoma was not the only culprit. Another contributing factor was the use of mechanized farm equipment which enabled a farmer to cultivate many more acres singly than had ever been possible previously. Furthermore, many who had not already left the state moved to the urban areas. The population of Oklahoma City increased to 204,424, that of Tulsa to 142,157, and that of Norman to 11,429. But no matter how the statistics tallied, the situation was one that only added to the woes of the state treasury.

Possibly certain circumstances could not have been avoided by the governor in his efforts to live within the state budget, but the fact that the seventeenth legislature had reduced available appropriations for the operation of state institutions could not be overlooked either. In addition to the difficulties already existing because of inadequate salaries for all classes of professional and technical hospital personnel, the medical school was faced with the double dilemma of being unable to compete successfully with like institutions in other states, not only in attracting suitable staff but in retaining what they had, all of which interfered with maintaining continuity of policies and teaching methods.

A delay was requested in the inspection of the School of Medicine, which had been scheduled for April 1 and 2 by the Council on Medical Education and Hospitals of the American Medical Association. Dean Patterson became especially apprehensive about the school and its hospitals being ''derated'' by the council, which set up and maintained standards for the United States and Canada, and by the State Board of Medical Examiners.

While it is true that some improvements in the curriculum had been made—lectures in medicine in the third year, a formal course of 144 hours in hospital clinical clerkships (in medicine, surgery, and pediatrics) as well as outpatient clinical clerkships, bedside teaching in the fourth year, and training of medical technologists as part of the basic science degree program—there was still much to be desired. The attorney general had ruled that the appropriation of $68,750 (Senate Bill No. 201) by the seventeenth legislature was dependent on matching federal funds, and no portion of it could be used for the purpose for which it was appropriated unless the federal funds were procured. This was a prelude to darkness, for the university regents, after much discussion on March 20, voted to hold the matter of building an isolation ward at Crippled Children's Hospital in abeyance "for the time being," although it had been set up as a WPA project.

Dean Patterson's fears were not unfounded, for Dr. Cutter, secretary of the Council on Medical Education, notified him on July 8 that the University of Oklahoma School of Medicine was indeed being continued on probation as ruled in 1936.

Meanwhile, President Bizzell notified the university regents on May 13 of his desire to retire from the presidency of the University of Oklahoma as of July 1, 1941, and the regents accepted his resignation, making William Bennett Bizzell president emeritus of the university and head of the Department of Sociology at a salary of $6,000 per year.

All of this was very discouraging to Dean Patterson who had done everything in his power to improve standards of medical education in Oklahoma. And on July 19 we find him writing to Claude S. Chambers, regent of the University of Oklahoma, in a despairing tone about two most urgent construction projects. He enclosed a pamphlet which he had prepared and sent out "to a good many people" in an effort to show some persons with means and philanthropic desires how they might help the School of Medicine and its hospitals by contributing directly to the proposed building program. "I have had letters of courteous acknowledgement," wrote the dean, "but nothing else so far."

The regents had appointed Lewis L. Reese medical director and assistant superintendent for the University Hospitals effective April 1, 1940, replacing E. T. Olsen who retired on March 31. Dr. Reese had received his M.D. degree from Boston University School of Medicine, served internships in the Massachusetts Memorial Hospital, the Haynes Memorial Hospital in Boston, and the Boston City Hospital, where he later served as night superintendent and executive assistant. Dr. Reese was a diplomate of the National Board of Medical Examiners.

By this time, Dean Patterson was very sensitive about the medical center's public relations image, and he advised Dr. Reese that any emergency memoranda and/or orders, which he thought should be issued, should first be approved by the dean since in the end he was responsible for anything that happened as a result of emergency measures.

Fortunately, "that little spark of celestial fire—conscience," was kept alive,[10] and the training of doctors continued valiantly within the walls of the too few buildings, under the direction of the executive board, which consisted of Dean Patterson, Dr. Reese, Dr. Clymer, Dr. Langston, Dr. Wails, and Dr. Hall, with Dr. O'Donoghue as an alternate. There was necessarily some cutting of corners to lighten the work load, for example, reports on general and professional attitutdes of students were discontinued except in cases where attitudes were unsatisfactory; but many indispensable burdens were, for the most part, accepted more cheerfully than might have been expected.

There were two deaths among the faculty in 1940—that of Darrell G. Duncan, associate in therapeutic radiology, on March 1, and of John Archer Hatchett, professor emeritus of obstetrics, on August 16.[11] Appropriate resolutions in memory of these men were made by the faculty, as well as in memory of W. J. Jolly, deceased, a former dean of the School of Medicine.

The regents awarded honorary titles to two professors during the calendar year: Leander A. Riely became professor emeritus of clinical medicine, and David Wilson Griffin became professor emeritus of mental diseases.

Owen Royce was appointed director of the outpatient department at both hospitals in February, thus filling the vacancy caused by the resignation of George N. Barry, who was reappointed assistant director of the department effective July 1.

Edward N. Smith was appointed a full-time associate professor of obstetrics at the School of Medicine effective February 1, with the understanding that his salary would continue to be paid by the State Department of Public Health and Federal Children's Bureau funds, through an arrangement with Grady Matthews, commissioner of health for the state of Oklahoma. Dr. Smith's services were initially available as a full-time instructor in 1937 for the inauguration of a School of Medicine postgraduate course in obstetrics available to physicians in Oklahoma. His new appointment was of great help to the obstetrics department which had never been able to take full advantage of clinical teaching opportunities because of the lack of a full-time member of the department.

There were also several other changes in appointments: Charles R. Rayburn was made professor and head of the Department of Mental Diseases in January, following the resignation of James Jackson Gable; Russell L. Moseley was appointed assistant professor of anatomy during the leave of absence of Berry Campbell; and Wayne Hull's title was changed to instructor in medicine as of November 15.

Dean Patterson was unsuccessful in trying to secure a full-time director of the clinical laboratories of the University Hospitals, but he did report to the faculty on September 27 that there were then five full-time faculty members in the Departments of Medicine and Surgery. For the academic year 1940–41 there

---

[10.] Rule from the copybook of George Washington when a schoolboy. See John Bartlett, *Familiar Quotations*, Boston, (1943), 268.

[11.] Dr. Hatchett had been inducted into the Oklahoma Hall of Fame in 1933. An article of appreciation concerning him was published in the Sunday edition of the *Daily Oklahoman* (September 24, 1939).

was a total of 225 faculty members, including nine in the School of Nursing and three in the Department of Dietetics. The 22 newly appointed faculty members were:

Francis Cornelius Lawler, D.Sc.
  assistant professor of bacteriology
Russell LeRoy Moseley, Ph.D.
  assistant professor of anatomy
Edward Needham Smith, M.D., D.Sc.
  associate professor of obstetrics
Ruby Duff, R.N.
  instructor in operating room
  technique, School of Nursing.
Curtis Howard Epps, M.D.
  instructor in clinical pathology
Elizabeth Fair, B.A., G.N.
  instructor in nursing education
Hugh Malcolm Galbraith, M.D.
  instructor in neurology
Owen Royce, Jr., M.D.
  instructor in medicine and director
  of outpatient department
Frank Thomas Siebert, Jr., M.D.
  instructor in clinical pathology
Meredith Marcus Appleton, M.D.
  assistant in urology
Marion A. Flesher, D.D.S.
  clinical assistant in dental surgery

Meyer Kurzner, M.D.
  assistant in pediatrics
Richard C. Mills, M.D.
  assistant in obstetrics
Aileen Petway, M.D.
  assistant in anesthesiology
Harvey Randel, M.D.
  assistant in ophthalmology
Delbert Gilmore Smith, M.D.
  assistant in obstetrics
Charles Burton Broeg, M.S.
  research fellow in biochemistry
Sue Elizabeth Browder, B.A.
  graduate assistant in anatomy
Richard Michael Burke, M.D.
  visiting lecturer in medicine
Eugene A. Gillis, M.D., M.P.H.
  lecturer, contagious diseases,
  School of Nursing
Dorothy Omundson, B.A.
  research fellow in bacteriology
Lewis Laban Reese, M.D.
  lecturer in medicine, assistant
  superintendent and medical director
  of University Hospitals

The whys and wherefores of the position of the Council on Medical Education regarding the status of the University of Oklahoma School of Medicine were outlined in great details by its secretary, William D. Cutter, in a letter to Dean Patterson on September 12, 1940. Dr. Cutter said that the council appreciated the fact that both the clinical and preclinical faculty had been strengthened since Dr. Weiskotten's visit in 1936, and that the hospital plant had been enlarged and imrpoved. However, in view of an approaching session of the Oklahoma Legislature, Dr. Cutter took the liberty of pointing out "what appear to be the most urgent needs of the institution at the present time."

The five major suggestions offered by Dr. Cutter were: (1) the operation of the School of Medicine and its hospitals must be free from political interference of any kind—that the dean and faculty were responsible solely to the board of regents and to no one else; (2) the legislature should realize that larger appropriations were needed for the School of Medicine, maintained on a fairly permanent basis, so that a recurrence of recent fluctuations would be impossible; (3) one reason that appropriations had to be increased was because salaries had to be increased in order to secure and retain competent teachers; (4) the facilities of the teaching hospitals also needed to be increased "both for the purpose of providing sufficient variety in the clinical material available for teaching and in order to render adequate service to the people of the state of Oklahoma. Neither the University Hospital nor the Children's Hospital is anywhere near adequate to meet this demand''; and (5) it was necessary to realize the importance of the principal features of a building program.

"Without question," Dr. Cutter emphasized, "the State should operate on a balanced budget and when its income declines, some of its activities must be cut. But the operation of the medical school is one of the activities that must be maintained on a satisfactory level or it must cease. The budget of the school must be stabilized on a long-term basis, otherwise the school cannot maintain satisfactory standards and would be obligated to close.''

When Dean Patterson discussed this communication at the October meeting of the university regents, they voted that a copy of the letter from Dr. Cutter should be presented to the chairman of the Committee on Appropriations in the house and to the chairman of the committee in the senate, as well as to the budget officer at the convening of the legislature in 1941. Subsequently, a committee consisting of Regents Claude S. Chambers, E. C. Hopper, and John Rogers, appointed on May 13 to study the problems of the Medical Center, met with Dean Patterson to go over the budget and to formulate recommendations to be presented at the meeting of the regents on December 2. The committee then recommended that the regents should approve the medical center budget for submission to the budget officer of the legislature for its next session.

The first annual Phi Beta Pi lecture, sponsored by the local chapter in honor of the late Dean Long, who served the School of Medicine faithfully for 16 years, was given in March by Chauncey E. Leake, professor of pharmacology at the University of California.

Fifty-two graduates received the M.D. degree in 1940, one of whom, Lloyd Nance Gilliland, Jr., was graduated cum laude for completing work as an honors student in the Department of Biochemistry. Thirty-one graduates were with the army at the time, fourteen with the navy, and two with the United States Public Health Service.

Thirty-seven nurses received the Graduate Nurse certificate at commencement; and, according to a School of Nursing bulletin published in January 1940, the school was supplying nursing service to the University Hospital, Crippled Children's Hospital, and the outpatient department. Classes were admitted twice yearly, in September and in January, to a three-year course in nursing. Scholastic requirements for admission included graduation in the upper third of the class from an accredited high school. Costs cited for uniforms, books, and incidentals over the three-year period amounted to $143.

During the academic year 1940–41 there were 238 medical students and 123 nursing students enrolled on the Oklahoma City campus. Fees for the four-year course in the School of Medicine amounted to $279.50.

The revenue for the University of Oklahoma in Norman for the year ending June 30, 1941, was $1,555,770. Separate appropriations for the Institutions on the Oklahoma City campus for the same period were $132,722 for the School of Medicine, $326,948 for the University Hospital, and $248,243 for the Crippled

Children's Hospital.[12] The total budget for the library of the School of Medicine was $8,015. As a matter of record, the librarian, Miss Sigerfoos, in a letter to the library committee, stated that no complete accession records were available prior to the ninth month of 1938 when she took charge.

Patient statistics for the University Hospitals in 1940–41 were as follows: 6,775 patients were admitted to both hospitals, 4,094 to University Hospital and 2,681 to Crippled Children's Hospital. There was a total of 546 obstetrical deliveries, and the average stay in the hospital for a patient was twenty days. Outpatient care was extended to 18,500 individuals, 10,799 of whom were new patients. Studied in the light of former years, these figures indicate that seven hospital records were broken during this fiscal year, with more patients than in any previous year. It should be mentioned that grants from the National Foundation for Infantile Paralysis were given to the University Hospitals during this period, chiefly at Children's, and that during the year plans were under way at the instigation of Joe Hamilton to change the orphanage at Bethany, on the outskirts of Oklahoma City, to a children's convalescent home.

The resident staff at University Hospital consisted of 36 physicians, and the nursing staff numbered 160. Many of the physicians who were faculty members of the School of Medicine were also members of the staff of Wesley Hospital, with a capacity of 150 beds. This hospital granted teaching privileges as an affiliate, and it held clinics at stated times.

Henry J. Turner, chairman of a committee of the Oklahoma State Medical Association on postgraduate education in medicine, made a review of the program in 1940,[13] in which he mentioned that when political interference by the governor of the state had terminated the university's participation in the postgraduate program, the Oklahoma State Medical Association became the sole sponsor of the program to which Oklahoma physicians had already contributed $91,325 in fees. The committee then decided in 1937 that a two-year educational project in obstetrics should be undertaken, and the State Medical Association granted $4,000 for this purpose.

A full-time instructor was essential to the intensive program that was contemplated, and Edward N. Smith was particularly qualified for the position because of his valuable experience in private practice in a rural community, his years of extensive postgraduate study, and his experience as a lecturer in obstetrics for the Oklahoma State Medical Association over a period of two years. Following this experience, when he was in charge of the graduate program in obstetrics at the School of Medicine, he established the first intramural postgraduate course ever offered at the school, May 1, 1940. He also conducted a mother's class in an obstetrical annex at 1210 N. Phillips Street in Oklahoma City, which was most successful, with over 900 mothers attending.

[12.] Statistics concerning the 1940–41 academic year for the School of Medicine may be found in the university catalog covering that period.
[13.] A summary of Dr. Turner's remarks may be found in the *Journal of the Indiana State Medical Association*, Vol. XXXIII (1940), 126.

During the two-year postgraduate program in obstetrics, the practicality of Dr. Smith's lectures, the number of free consultations, and the large attendance at the lay lectures attest to his untiring efforts to insure the success of the program.

By 1940 final arrangements were completed for a postgraduate program in pediatrics similar to the one just completed in obstetrics. It included lectures in 46 centers throughout the state, starting on February 1, 1940, with James C. Hughes as instructor and L. W. Kibler as field director.

Possibly the most significant single action taken by the staff of the University Hospitals in 1940 was the resolution passed on May 3, to wit: "Resolved that the University Hospital agrees to comply with the request of the Surgeon General of the United States Army to organize Evacuation Hospital No. 21, United States Army, for service in any national emergency, as outlined by the Surgeon General of the Army in his letter of March 25, 1940, and in accordance with tables of organization promulgated by the War Department from time to time."

On May 4, Dean Patterson apprised President Bizzell of events leading to the hospital staff's resolution and of the surgeon general's request for our cooperation, together with that of a number of similar institutions throughout the country. He drew the president's attention to the fact that the 56th General Hospital for service in time of national emergency had been organized at the University Hospital in 1922; and, on behalf of the staff of the University Hospitals, requested that approval be given by the regents for such an evacuation hospital unit, even though 38 of the 158 members of the hospital staff would be required to staff it in the event of a national emergency.

When President Bizzell presented the resolution to the regents on May 13, their approval was immediately granted. A committee appointed by Dean Patterson then selected Cyril E. Clymer as the original director of the unit (No. 21). He was later replaced by H. D. Collins, when Dr. Clymer was physically disqualified for military service. Members of Evacuation Hospital No. 21 were as follows:

Lt. Col. Herbert Dale Collins
Major Austin Holloway Bell
Major Jess Duval Herrmann
Major George Henry Kimball
Major Robert Leonard Noell
Major Paul Brann Lingenfelter
Major Bert Ernest Mulvey
Major Ward Loren Shaffer, D.C.
Major John Powers Wolff
Captain Allen Gilbert Gibbs
Captain Samuel Ewing Franklin
Captain Robert Bruce Howard
Captain John Frederick Kuhn, Jr.

Captain Cecil Willard Lemmon
Captain Ray Harvey Lindsey
Captain Everett Baker Neff
Captain Floyd Smith Newman
Captain Rudolph Joseph Reichert
Captain John Millard Robertson
Captain William Ward Rucks, Jr.
Captain Chester Randall Seba
Captain Evans Edward Talley
Captain Jim Mabury Taylor
Lieutenant Felix M. Adams
Lieutenant John DeWitt Ashley
Lieutenant D. R. Bedford

Lieutenant Marion Allen Flesher   Lieutenant Harvey M. Richey
Lieutenant John Andrew Graham   Lieutenant Owen Royce, Jr.
Lieutenant Daniel Bester Pearson

This unit was not called to active duty until July 5, 1942, so its activities will be discussed later in this volume.

Dean Robert U. Patterson began the new year by marshaling his forces for an appeal to the eighteenth legislature of the state of Oklahoma to accept its responsibility to meet stipulated standards for medical education by providing some kind of material assistance for the University of Oklahoma's School of Medicine.

Early in January, 1941, by direction of the university regents, he sent a copy of the September 12, 1940, letter from the secretary of the Council on Medical Education and Hospitals to the governor, the president pro tem of the senate, the speaker of the house, the state budget officer and the members (about 80 in all) of the appropriations committees of both the house and the senate. But obviously this letter, setting forth unmistakably "in kindly but clear language" the importance of adequate support for both the medical school and its hospitals, was not appreciated. Incredible as it may seem, during the eighteenth session of the legislature, not more than two representatives, senators, or officials of the state administration visited or inspected the buildings forming this important humanitarian educational group, located less than one mile from the capitol of the state, thereby demonstrating an unusual indifference and lack of appreciation of the needs of a large group of wards of the state by those in responsible positions.

Altogether, the eighteenth legislature appropriated $1,900,182 for buildings at other state institutions, to be expended during the next biennium, but not one cent for the erection of any single project in the building program of the School of Medicine. "Apparently," the dean said, "these matters are not considered important compared with certain other state activities. . . . Every representative and senator consulted about the matter has excused himself on the ground that it was the duty of the senators and representatives of Oklahoma County to look out for the interest of the medical school and its hospitals."[14]

Yet Dean Patterson had had an interview early during the legislative session with Creekmore Wallace, representative from the district in which the medical school and hospitals were situated. He had given Mr. Wallace tentative drafts of two bills—one providing for the appropriation of $56,250 for an isolation building promised by Governor Phillips, in addition to the previous $68,750 appropriated by the seventeenth legislature, and the other for monies for a new nurses' residence—which Mr. Wallace agreed to put into the proper phraseology and introduce in the house. But "for want of a horse the rider was lost" somewhere along the usual runaround. Instead, approximately $450,000,

---

[14.] Report to the president of the university, July 14, 1941.

which had accumulated from oil royalties and leases on the campus of the School of Medicine was placed in the general fund of the state; and it was that money, together with other funds, that was appropriated *for the use of other institutions*, when every moral consideration entitled the School of Medicine and its hospitals to money accrued from the activities of the oil industry on its own campus.

It was this action that provoked Dean Patterson into expressing the opinion that the great majority of the members of the legislature (and many other citizens of the state) had no conception or realization of the value and importance of the dutues that were being carried on for Oklahoma by the hospitals' provision of care for indigent citizens. So once more Dr. Patterson pointed out that professional care and treatment was given to approximately 7,000 patients in the wards of University Hospitals every year, in addition to the examination and the treatment of around 20,000 persons in the outpatient department of the hospitals. He added that, on June 25, 1941, there were 2,051 persons on the waiting list for admission to the University Hospital.

Dean Patterson declared,

> I am making these statements as a matter of record so that it may not be said that the present Dean and Superintendent failed to bring the situation to the attention of higher authority. He has done so in his annual reports as well as in written communications to and personal interviews with committees and members of the Sixteenth, Seventeeth and Eighteenth Legislatures. I wish also to be on record as holding the opinion that unless hereafter there is developed a sincere interest in the welfare of the medical school and hospitals, not only by part of the University, but by the whole University, together with concentrated action by the senators and representatives from every county . . . they will be responsible for the probable disapproval or loss of accredited rating of this medical school, to the real disgrace of the State of Oklahoma.[15]

The fact that no building has been provided at the University's medical center since 1928 was a glaring commentary on the forgetfulness of the legislators toward medical care and medical education. The only bill passed by them in 1941, relating in any way to medical education, was Senate Bill No. 13 which made clarifying amendments and better definitions for the duties of the Crippled Children's Commission, provision for payment for exceptional medications, and provision for the appointment of a dentist to the Committee of Standardization.

In a less than noble gesture they recognized the dean of the School of Medicine only as a member designate on the appeal board of the State Board of Medical Examiners created by the eighteenth legislature. Moreover, a real indignity was perpetrated when all hope of securing federal matching funds for

[15.] *Ibid.*

construction of the long-promised isolation building for children with communicable diseases—in the days before antibiotics—went up in thin air, because appropriations made on a contingent basis by the seventeenth legislature lapsed on November 11.

Meanwhile, Dean Patterson found time to write a considerate letter to Leo Blondin, long-time clown and jester for the Oklahoma City zoo, saying that it had been his privilege, on several occasions, to observe Mr. Blondin's kindly activities in connection with entertainment of children in the Children's Hospital. "I am sure that 'Uncle Leo,' " Dr. Patterson wrote, "is as much a source of pleasure to every child in the Crippled Children's Hospital as their anticipation and actual contemplation of Santa Clause when he arrives. You may be sure that the administration is deeply appreciative of your kindness and your deep interest in the welfare of the children committed to its care."

On March 11 a constitutional amendment was adopted by the people of the state establishing the Board of Oklahoma State Regents for Higher Education, consisting of nine members with authority to coordinate all institutions of higher learning supported wholly or in part by state appropriations. Three members of the newly appointed board were alumni of the University of Oklahoma, namely, Frank Buttram, James E. Perry, and John Rogers.

Dean Patterson felt that the creation of the Board of Regents for Higher Education offered a ray of hope for the future in that this group of men, in dealing with the legislature, might be able to secure more adequate support for medical education in Oklahoma—another way of saying one must live with hope to survive.

At a meeting of the university regents on May 30, John M. Craig of Idabel was appointed a member of that board to replace John Rogers who had resigned to become a member of the new State Regents for Higher Education, and Mr. Craig in turn was appointed a member of the Medical School committee of the regents in place of John Rogers.

In accordance with the approval of the university regents, a memorial tablet honoring LeRoy Long, former dean of the School of Medicine, was placed in the entrance hall of the medical sciences building on May 19, 1941; and in compliance with the desires of the donors, the regents accepted the tablet in the name of the University of Oklahoma during the dedication ceremonies. The second annual LeRoy Long Memorial Lecture, sponsored by the local chapter of Phi Beta Pi, was given about this same time by Earnest Sachs, professor of clinical neurological surgery at Washington University School of Medicine.

Joseph August Brandt, a graduate of the University of Oklahoma in 1921, became its seventh president in August, 1941. President Brandt had served as director of the University of Oklahoma Press from 1928 to 1938, when he left to become director of the Princeton University Press. According to Roy Gittinger, President Brandt worked to bring about several changes in university administration during his presidency.[16] For one thing, he thought that the general

[16.] Roy Gittinger, *The University of Oklahoma: 1892–1942* (Norman, University of Oklahoma Press, 1942), 167–68.

faculty should be organized to assume a larger share in the determination of university policy, and secondly, that the younger members of the staff should be trained for a greater participation in the direction of university affairs. Many who consider Oklahoma a radical state thought the educational institutions of the state of Oklahoma were ''as unstable as the shifting sands of factional politics,'' and that the university authorities were conservative and unwilling to experiment with new and untried schemes. For reasons such as this, President Brandt felt that reorganization of all departments was rather essential and that there should no longer be heads of departments but rotating chairman serving for short terms instead.

Dean Patterson immediately took issue with the new president on this stand in a letter on September 13, in which he wrote as follows:

> I am apprehensive that your policy with respect to chairmen of departments will not work efficiently at the medical school. For example, the head of our department of biochemistry who is well qualified has been with the school 17 years. If it means that next year he would not be the chairman of his department but that one of his younger assistants, perhaps a man who had come here only within the last year or two, would be in charge, [then] I do believe that would not work successfully, especially among members of a professional group. In fact it would be contrary to all administrative procedure in medical schools all over the country.

Changes within the administration of the School of Medicine and its hospitals also occurred during the year, including the resignation on November 20 of Dr. Reese as medical director of the University Hospitals, after only about eighteen months of service, and that of Owen Royce, director of the outpatient department, after about fifteen months of service. In the continuing game of musical chairs, George Barry was appointed acting medical director of University Hospitals—his second appointment to the identical position; and Dr. Hall assumed the duties of chief of staff of the Convalescent Home for Crippled Children in Bethany. Following the resignation of Helen Carr, Ketourah Foulks became director of the social services department of the University Hospitals at a time when the department had not yet achieved academic status.

L. A. Turley was made chairman of a committee to study and present an acceptable course leading to the degree of bachelor of science in medical technology (acceptable to the regents) in time for the beginning of the scholastic year in 1942; Mark R. Everett was appointed chairman of the research committee (an appointment which he held until 1946); and Arthur Hellbaum succeeded Hiram Moor as chairman of the library committee.

There were 230 faculty members of the School of Medicine in the year 1941–42, including nine faculty members of the School of Nursing and one dietitian. The twenty-nine newly appointed faculty members during the year are given in the following tabulation:

Homer Floyd Marsh, Ph.D.
 assistant professor of bacteriology
Paul Winston Smith, Ph.D.
 assistant professor of pharmacology
Clare Marie Jackson Wangen, M.A.
 director of the School of Nursing
 and superintendent of nurses
Olga Broks Dittig, M.A.
 assistant director of the School of
 Nursing
Margaret Bolton
 instructor in nursing education
Elaine L. DeBorra, R.N., B.S.
 instructor in nursing education
Charles W. Freeman, M.D.
 instructor in pediatrics
Elizabeth Rose Hall, M.S.
 instructor in bacteriology
Alice Olson Swenson, B.S.
 instructor in nursing education
James Mabury Taylor, M.D.
 instructor in urology
James Asa Willie, M.D.
 instructor in neurology
Henry Garland Bennett, M.D.
 assistant in gynecology
Lorenzo Matthew Farnam, M.D.
 assistant in surgery
Charles Edward Leonard, M.D.
 assistant in medicine

Lawrence Stanley Sell, M.D.
 assistant in orthopedic surgery
William Turner Bynum, M.D.
 visiting lecturer in medicine
Earl Rankin Denny, M.D.
 visiting lecturer in medicine
Louis Edward Diamond, M.S.
 research associate in biochemistry
Frederic Griffin Dorwart, M.D.
 visiting lecturer in medicine
William Patton Fite, M.D.
 visiting lecturer in surgery
Douglas Meharg Gordon, M.D.
 visiting lecturer in medicine
Walter Alonzo Howard, M.D.
 visiting lecturer in medicine
Clark Hawkins Ice, M.S.
 research fellow in pharmacology
Ray Harvey Lindsey, M.D.
 visiting lecturer in surgery
Tracey Holland McCarley, M.D.
 visiting lecturer in medicine
Russell Clarke Pigford, M.D.
 visiting lecturer in medicine
Carl Puckett, M.D.
 visiting lecture in medicine
Arthur Strohm Risser, M.D.
 visiting lecturer in surgery
Henry Clarence Weber, M.D.
 visiting lecturer in surgery

Edmund Sheppard Ferguson, who joined the faculty of the School of Medicine of the University of Oklahoma in 1910, died in Oklahoma City on June 28, 1941. Before 1910, Dr. Ferguson had been professor of otology, rhinology, and laryngology in the old Epworth University Medical School in Oklahoma City and was secretary of the School of Medicine faculty for many years.

Edward N. Smith prepared and published in 1941 a history of the Department of Obstetrics of the University of Oklahoma School of Medicine in which he pointed out that the service at the Holmes Home of Redeeming Love had been in charge of W. R. Bevan in 1912, and that the Department of Obstetrics in the School of Medicine at that time consisted of two faculty members now deceased, John A. Hatchett and R. E. Looney, and also W. A. Fowler, who was actively engaged in promoting the out-patient aspects of the department and was in charge of deliveries at the Holmes Home of Redeeming Love—a task fraught with numerous risks. In order to arrive at the home, it was customary for the ''deliverer'' to ride to the nearest station on the interurban train for El Reno, where he hoped to be met by a horse and rig. However, it was not uncommon for the physician to miss this connection, in which case the last mile of the journey had to be negotiated on foot. Understandably, both doctors and patients were dubious about this sort of obstetrical service, so it grew slowly at first. But in a relatively short time the university was able to promise each senior student the opportunity to deliver six "outpatient" obstetrical cases in homes.

As the obstetrical services of the University Hospitals saw a steady growth away from those early days, the difficulty was reversed, and the admission of patients to the hospital had to be limited to a number which could be cared for properly. By 1941, Dr. Smith pointed out, the Department of Obstetrics staff had increased from three initially to fifteen members in 1941.

In spite of the fact that the clinical staff was greatly reduced, because fourteen visiting staff physicians and seven interns and residents were called into active military service early in 1941, 6,602 patients were admitted to the University Hospitals with an average stay of nineteen days during the teaching year 1941–42, and the outpatient department of the hospitals counted 8,888 new patients.

In the seventh annual report of the Oklahoma Commission for Crippled Children for the fiscal year 1941–42, Joe Hamilton reported to the governor that there had been a marked decrease in the number of children committed to hospitals for remedial treatment, and that the great backlog of long-neglected cases had been largely removed, with more and more efforts being confined to the newer cases. He mentioned, however, that there were a few black patients above the age of twelve with orthopedic and plastic conditions who were in need of attention and who had to be hospitalized in crowded wards in University Hospital where beds were quite limited.[17]

Statistics issued May 4, 1942, show that the following funds were available to the Oklahoma City campus for the year 1941–42: $135,453 for the School of Medicine, $326,400 for the University Hospital, and $247,725 for the Crippled Children's Hospital.

Three cum laude honors students were announced on June 6, 1941—Edward Merige Farris, who was engaged in research work in the Department of Biochemistry, and James Ottley Asher and William Robert Flood, who prepared a joint thesis in the Department of Pharmacology. Fifty-four M.D. degrees were granted to graduates of the School of Medicine, and thirty-three Graduate Nurse certificates were awarded to graduates of the School of Nursing in June.

The Board of Regents of the University of Oklahoma complied with a request that all medical schools increase their enrollment for the year 1941–42 by agreeing to increase the admission of the next first-year class from sixty-five to seventy students. All members of the incoming class were required to attend matriculation ceremonies held at the university in September.

There were 240 medical students enrolled in the School of Medicine, 133

[17.] Mr. Hamilton's report contained a comprehensive table showing the yearly commitment of crippled children to the hospitals from 1927 to 1942.

students in the School of Nursing, and 8 dietitians serving internships during the 1941–42 academic year.

Clare Wangen, a graduate of the Johns Hopkins School of Nursing and superintendent of nurses at the University of Virginia Hospital, became director of the School of Nursing and Nursing Services in the University Hospitals on July 14, 1941.

Dean Patterson set his sights high for a long-range building program for the medical center, only to be thwarted in his efforts to obtain support by certain citizens: the president of the university, most members of the regents, three legislatures, and two governors; because money for expansion was the real issue—money, which in its effects can be "as beautiful as roses"; and because of a prevailing attitude that the School of Medicine and the University Hospitals belonged to Oklahoma City.

"We must educate the people of Oklahoma," he told his faculty in 1941, "that the medical school and its hospitals do not belong to Oklahoma City but to the entire state." And he told them that he envisioned an active alumni association as a powerful political force to get this message to every county and every legislator in the state; that with the alumni and the faculty working together, "we can put on a campaign that will produce better results when the Nineteenth Legislature meets in January, 1943."

Possibly General Patterson's frustrations with being unable to realize his hopes and expectations are best summed up in his own words, in his letter of September 13 to President Brandt:

> I feel that the time has come for very plain speaking as far as the medical school is concerned and I wish to be on record that I feel that there must be aggressive action on the part of the University as a whole, as well as by all alumni, to have any kind of effect on the legislature in the future that will result in this School receiving the attention and financial backing that it requires. I am sure that you will be able to do much to remove the general feeling that exists here, within the faculty of the School of Medicine and the staff of the hospitals, that this medical school is simply a step-child instead of an integral, important and necessary part of the university.

Chapter VI.
Old Soldiers Never
Die: 1942–43

 While on several occasions there have been comments upon Governor Phillips' lack of interest in the School of Medicine and the University Hospitals, there were some extenuating circumstances which should not go unmentioned. First, in all honesty it must be conceded that the effects of the financial depression of the late thirties were rather devastating; and secondly, that the involvement of the United States in World War II, just before the close of Governor Phillips' administration, diverted attention from state political battles to the larger task of winning a world battle.

In January, Dean Patterson reported to the faculty that everything possible had been done to induce the local draft boards to defer medical students, and that the matter had been settled by the director of selective service. Third- and fourth-year students would be deferred in order to complete their education but would be expected to take a commission either as a second lieutenant in the medical administrative corps of the army or as an ensign in the navy after being graduated from the School of Medicine.

In May, 1942, Dean Patterson advised the faculty and staff of the hospitals that 69 members of the faculty and 76 members of the hospital staff had been certified to the armed forces. Those uncertified were considered essential to the operation of the medical institutions, and anyone who wished to be removed from the essential list had an obligation to provide a substitute to fill his place.

In order to partially replenish the depleted staff, the dean recommended to the university regents that all emeritus and retired teachers of the School of Medicine who were still able to perform further duties for the hospitals be requested to do so "for the duration"; and that the regents confirm such appointments as soon as possible, since the institution was losing many residents and interns who normally carried on the bulk of the professional care of patients under the supervision of the visiting staff.

Medical authorities throughout the country had repeatedly stated that under no circumstances should standards for admission to medical schools, or the character or quality of the instruction in medical schools be lowered by reason of the military situation. However, the regents of the university approved, as an emergency measure, a recommendation (confirmed by the Council on Medical

Education and Hospitals) that the requirements for entrance to the School of Medicine be reduced to a minimum of sixty academic hours or two years of premedical college work, including the prescribed subjects.[1]

On May 29, Dr. Patterson informed the faculty that the Association of American Medical Colleges had recommended in December, 1941, that medical colleges put their schools on an accelerated basis as soon as possible. Whereupon the faculty unanimously passed a resolution, which was subsequently approved by the president and regents of the university, in favor of an accelerated program in the School of Medicine with three semesters a year for the duration of the war, making it possible to graduate a student after approximately three rather than four scholastic years.[2]

The dean then reminded the faculty that the legislature would have to provide additional funds to enable the school to operate on an accelerated basis, saying that this school was not one that would wish to be slow in trying to do its part in any effort essential to the national defense. And he suggested that the alumni of the school should use their influence to bring about the election of a legislature friendly to the School of Medicine. "As long as I live," the General said in conclusion, "I shall always be interested in the welfare of this School of Medicine and its teaching hospitals."

The last words were apparently an intimation from Dean Patterson that he was about to resign, for within a month (on June 24, 1942) his letter of resignation as dean of the School of Medicine and superintendent of University Hospitals effective September 1 was read before the regents of the university. In the course of the letter Dean Patterson said, "At our next commencement, seven classes of physicians will have been graduated from the School of Medicine under my direction."

In the many documents concerning the administration of the medical center during this period, a July 22 letter was found which uncovered one of the more compelling reasons as to why Dr. Patterson resigned a year before he was 65 years of age. "I would like to avoid," he explained, "going up against the legislature which meets in January. That has been one of the most objectionable features of the duties connected with the school and hospitals. I have begun to develop some hypertension and it seems wise, at my age, to drop activities which involve so much detail and so many annoyances."[3]

---

[1] This recommendation had previously been adopted by the faculty of the School of Medicine with a proviso to return to a 90-hour minimum entrance requirement after the war.

[2] The accelerated teaching program was designed to supply additional doctors and nurses for the armed services of the United States.

[3] On September 18, Dean Patterson spoke to the faculty of his resignation from the deanship as having been tendered to the university regents in March, but that he had agreed to stay on while a committee appointed by the regents canvassed the field for his replacement. "I will probably never again meet with this fine body of men as a group," he said, "so I want to wish you all good luck. Remember I will always have these institutions close to my heart."

Dean Patterson made a lengthy report to President Brandt on July 31, in which he mentioned certain observations in the interest of the future welfare of the School of Medicine, especially in regard to the very poor financial support given to the medical school and its teaching hospitals during the seven years that he had been dean and superintendent. With general recognition of the need for more adequate salaries for members of the teaching profession in grade and high schools, it was disturbing to Dean Patterson that there was so little awareness of a like need for teachers in the professional schools and colleges. "In the medical school of a nearby state," he said, "the salary of full professors is $6,000 per annum and for heads of departments, $8,000," adding that in a number of other medical schools no larger than this one there were often three or four full-time teachers in each major clinical department—a very real need—as well as at least one part-time clinical teacher in each of the medical specialties, in order to stabilize a dependable nucleus around which the volunteer visiting staff could work.

And he voiced the opinion that senators and representatives were often annoyed that there were no beds available for a constitutent in whom they were interested, when the remedy lay in their own hands and not in those of the superintendent or medical director. The very idea that only the senators and representatives from Oklahoma County were the ones who should interest themselves in the medical center was unwarranted and a source of considerable irritation to General Patterson. "Apparently, it has been a delusion upon which the legislature has been acting for many years," he said.

President Brandt was quoted as saying that General Patterson had done "a magnificent job as dean and supervisor of the hospitals," and that he had "worked miracles in the face of serious difficulties caused by an unreasonably low budget."[4]

Robert U. Patterson's resignation effective November 15, 1942, was accepted during the October 6 meeting of the university regents. The regents asserted that Dean Patterson had been loyal and faithful in the performance of his duty, and that "he could leave his position with the knowledge that he had helped the advancement of the Medical School of the University of Oklahoma and its hospitals toward the high goals held by the medical profession of America."

Meanwhile, President Brandt had traveled to Chicago for conferences with Fred Zapffe and H. G. Weiskotten, secretaries of the Association of American Medical Colleges and of the Council on Medical Education and Hospitals, respectively, regarding the appointment of a part-time or full-time dean. These doctors were rather firm in their belief that it would be unwise to appoint a dean on a part-time basis.[5] However, in a discussion of the matter with Dean Bachmeyer, University of Chicago Medical School, and with President Robert

[4.] *Sooner Magazine*, August 26, 1942.

[5.] A liaison committee on medical education was established under joint supervision of the American Medical Association and the Association of American Medical Colleges in 1942, so that surveys of medical schools would be conducted jointly in the future

Hutchins, it appeared there would be difficulty in finding a full-time dean, unless the University of Oklahoma could offer a considerable increase in salary to a prospective candidate for the position. President Hutchins said that many professors in the University of Chicago were enjoying incomes of as much as $18,000 a year.[6]

The net result was that, at the meeting of the university regents on October 6, President Brandt proposed that Thomas Claude Lowry be named dean of the School of Medicine, November 15, 1942, to July 1, 1943, which was approved; and the president of the university was instructed to continue his search for a permanent full-time dean.

Dr. Lowry was born in Rockwall, Texas, August 19, 1891. He received his B.S. degree from the University of Oklahoma in 1914 and his M.D. in 1916. He was awarded the first Letzeiser medal given to a university student for scholarship, and he was a member of the Pe-et honorary scholastic society for men on the Norman campus. Dr. Lowry served as a captain in World War I with the 24th Evacuation Hospital in France. His first official affiliation with the School of Medicine began in March, 1920, as an instructor in medicine; and, when appointed to succeed General Robert U. Patterson as dean of the School of Medicine, he was a professor of clinical medicine.

"Tom Lowry," as he was affectionately called by his many friends among the medical profession and the faculty of the school, was in rather poor health, but a man of great integrity and courage, with an abiding loyalty to his alma mater. In deference to his chronic illness, the regents authorized Harold A. Shoemaker, professor pharmacology and assistant dean since 1939, to act as dean of the School of Medicine and superintendent of University Hospitals, commencing concurrently on November 15. The salary for Dr. Shoemaker was increased $100 per month.

With both Dr. Lowry and Dean Patterson present at this meeting, President Brandt voiced the opinion that the regents hoped something could be done during the next legislative session to relieve the financial crisis at the School of Medicine. Whereupon Dean Patterson remarked that he was leaving the position of dean of the School of Medicine with a great deal of personal regret, because he was deeply interested in Oklahoma and would always have an interest in the university.[7]

Dr. Shoemaker was born in New Ringgold, Pennsylvania, in 1896. He received his undergraduate degree in pharmacy from Valparaiso University in Indiana and his masters degree in pharmacy from the University of Washington

---

in an effort to achieve concerted action and to guard against "guild control" by the profession or "ivory-tower control" of medical education by the professorial scientists in the colleges of medicine.

[6.] Minutes of the board of regents, September 15, 1942.

[7.] General Patterson had the single satisfaction of believing that a $125,000 venereal hospital would be constructed on the grounds of the Crippled Children's Hospital through a grant from the Federal Works Agency, but even that turned out to be a Pyrrhic victory because it never materialized (University regents minutes, June 1, 1942).

in Seattle. He was awarded a Ph.D. degree in pharmacology and toxicology from Yale University in 1931. Dr. Shoemaker was assistant professor of pharmacy at the University of Oklahoma from 1923 to 1925. He became assistant professor of biochemistry and pharmacology in the School of Medicine in 1925, and in 1935, when pharmacology became a separate department, he was made professor of pharmacology and chairman of the department.

There were major changes in the profile of the faculty during the year, too, either by demise, by resignation, or by appointment. John Frederick Kuhn, Sr., professor emeritus of gynecology, who had joined the faculty in 1912 and was professor and head of the department from 1924 to 1938, died on February 14; and Herbert Dale Collins, associate in the Department of Surgery, met an untimely death at the age of 41 years on October 12. Dr. Collins' death came as a great shock to the School of Medicine community for he was head of the newly organized evacuation hospital unit which had been called to active duty only three months previously on July 5.

Everett S. Lain, who had served for more years than any other member of the faculty, became professor emeritus of dermatology and syphilology in 1942, with special commendation from the dean; and Charles P. Bondurant was promoted to the position vacated by Dr. Lain.

Paul Colonna, professor of orthopedic surgery and head of the department, resigned as of August 1 to accept a similar appointment at the University of Pennsylvania School of Medicine, which apparently came as no surprise to the dean. "Naturally, I do not want to see him leave here," he confided to a friend, "but I have recognized the extreme difficulty any man in orthopedics who comes from outside the state has to face, with the tremendous jealousies that exist. . . . It will be some years before the orthopedic surgeons here will be willing to recognize that a man who comes to this University from another state is not a 'foreigner'. . . . I may say that situation hardly exists among the general profession or among other specialties." W. K. West, associate professor of orthopedic surgery, was promoted to the rank of professor and acting head of the department as of August 1.

Clark H. Hall became director of the rheumatic fever program at Children's Hospital, and George Barry, who had been acting director of the hospitals as well as director of the outpatient department in 1941, again played musical chairs as he accepted the position of medical director of University Hospitals. H. Thompson Avey moved into one of the chairs vacated by Dr. Barry to become the new director of the outpatient and admitting departments.

An important appointment, at an annual salary of $6,000, was that of Béla Halpert as professor of clinical pathology and director of the clinical laboratories and of the School of Medical Technology, following the resignation of Dr. Jeter. Dr. Jeter had arranged for the training of graduates with a B.A. or B.S. degree in our laboratories as medical and x-ray technologists; and both the laboratories of the University and Crippled Children's Hospitals were approved for this training course in 1942. One year of practical and theoretical instruction was required to qualify for a certificate as a laboratory technician from the American Society of Clinical Pathology. The laboratories of the University Hospitals performed approximately 25,500 examinations during the year 1942–43: 12,000 urine analyses, 6,300 blood chemistry tests, 3,880 bacteriology examinations, 8,812 serologic tests, 2,141 blood typings, 1,460 cross-matchings, 445 electrocardiographic examinations, and 519 basal metabolic rate determinations.

There were 232 members of the faculty of the School of Medicine during the academic year 1942–43, including ten teachers in the School of Nursing and one in dietetics. The eighteen newly elected faculty members were:

Béla Halpert, M.D.
  professor of clinical pathology,
  director of laboratories of the
  University Hospitals
Harry Thompson Avey, M.D.
  assistant professor of medicine
Samuel Abraham Corson, Ph.D.
  assistant professor of physiology
Alton Clair Kurtz, Ph.D.
  assistant professor of
  biochemistry
Harold Jacob Binder, M.D.
  associate in pediatrics
Ella Marie Henke, B.S.
  assistant superintendent of nurses
Hulda Gunther, B.S.
  instructor in nursing arts
Ollie Boyd Houchin, Ph.D.
  instructor in pharmacology

Mary Lucille Asling, B.A.
  assistant in clinical pathology
Lasla Kendey Chont, M.D.
  assistant in therapeutic radiology
Harry Anthony Daniels, M.D.
  assistant in medicine
Walter Henry Dersch, M.D.
  clinical assistant in medicine
Albert R. Drescher, D.D.S.
  clinical assistant in dental surgery
John Martin Parrish, M.D.
  assistant in obstetrics
Alvin L. Swenson, M.D.
  assistant in orthopedic surgery
James William Finch, M.D.
  visiting lecturer in medicine
John Theodore Jacobs, M.D.
  research fellow in orthopedic
  surgery

The honors courses in the basic science departments in the School of Medicine were included in the lists of elective courses from 1931–43, and much of the elective course system was due to the efforts of Edward Mason, professor of physiology. An elective course in tropical medicine was added to the curriculum for the first time during this year.

According to a report released in March from the main library of the university in Norman, the total accessions in the library of the School of Medicine on the Oklahoma City campus amounted to 258 current journals and 16,595 books and bound volumes, with a working staff of one librarian, two assistant librarians, and two assistants. Lilah B. Heck was promoted to the position of librarian on August 1, 1942, following the resignation of Miss Sigerfoos. Donald McMullen succeeded Dr. Hellbaum as chairman of the library committee.

The University of Oklahoma awarded 54 M.D. degrees to graduates of the School of Medicine in 1942 and 24 Graduate Nurse certificates in the School of Nursing. For the academic year 1942–43 there were 232 medical students and 145 nursing students enrolled on the medical center campus. By 1941–42 there were 1,125 alumni of the School of Medicine with 54 per cent of them practicing medicine in 67 counties and 139 cities and towns in Oklahoma.[8]

The income for the university during the fiscal year 1942–43 was $1,660,035 for the Norman campus and $129,403 for the School of Medicine—$320,450 for the University Hospital and $245,575 for the Crippled Children's Hospital. In addition, the W. K. Kellogg Foundation made a grant of $10,000 to the School of Medicine—$2,500 for scholarships and $7,500 for student loans—plus a grant of $4,000 to the School of Nursing for fourteen loans and three scholarships to student nurses.

An inventory taken in 1942 on the Oklahoma City campus showed that the value of equipment belonging to the School of Medicine and the University Hospitals amounted to $647,655, and that of buildings and grounds, $1,197,424, making a total investment of $1,845,079.

There were 200 patient beds in operation in University Hospital and 242 beds in Crippled Children's Hospital during the year, a total of 16,464 x-ray treatments, 5,744 physiotherapy treatments, and 4,034 surgical operations in the hospitals.

The surgical situation at Crippled Children's Hospital had improved somewhat because of the employment of a surgical nurse who devoted full time to the patients in the plastic surgery department. Consequently, the plastic surgeons were able to care for a larger number of patients than formerly. This resulted in a marked decline in the waiting list over the previous year.

Four hundred and ninety-five childbirths occurred in University Hospital and there were 125 deliveries in the Holmes Home of Redeeming Love, with 370 deliveries in district homes. In the outpatient department a total of 15,265 patients received 53,335 treatments.

The training of interns and residents had been curtailed considerably by this time. Moreover, the rotating internship had been limited and reduced from two years to nine months. The new plan, as formulated, called for a nine-month internship and a nine-month residency—in line with the acceleration program. During 1942–43 there were only ten interns and fourteen residents on duty in the University Hospitals. The internship for dietitians turned out eight full-fledged dietitians each year for responsible positions in hospitals throughout the country.[9]

Five nursing schools in Oklahoma were affiliated with the University School of Nursing during this particular year for instruction in pediatrics, outpatient techniques, and diet kitchen training. And the School of Nursing participated in the Cadet Nurse Corps program conducted under the supervision of the United States Public Health Service. This program precipitated an increase in enrollment from 114 to 150 students who, upon graduation, received the certificate of Graduate Nurse.

[8.] A. C. Scott, "The University of Oklahoma School of Medicine," paper for Oklahoma City Chamber of Commerce, February 22, 1943.

[9.] Mark R. Everett, *Medical Education in Oklahoma*, (Norman, University of Oklahoma Press, 1972), I, 226.

A civilian defense and medical service was organized in Oklahoma City early in the year, with Chester McHenry as the director and Dr. Colonna as commander. The Emergency Medical Unit No. 1, as it was designated, was comprised of personnel from the University Hospitals and School of Medicine.

On July 23, 1942, Evacuation Hospital No. 21 of the United States Army, formed from the staffs of University and Crippled Children's Hospitals, left Oklahoma City for desert maneuvers in the vicinity of Needles, California. Major Bert Ernest Mulvey assumed command of the unit because of the illness of Lieutenant Colonel Herbert Dale Collins who had completed the organization of the unit.[10]

On August 5 the personnel of Evacuation Hospital No. 53 left Camp San Luis Obispo in California for the same desert maneuvers and arrived in Needles, where an evacuation hospital with a 750-bed capacity had already been installed. Twelve days later, the two evacuation hospital units were combined as Evacuation Hospital No. 21.

On September 7, Erneze F. Pope was appointed chief nurse of Evacuation Hospital No. 21 and sworn in as first lieutenant in charge of securing nurses to be attached to the hospital in Needles. Lieutenant Pope, who had received her nursing training in Oklahoma City, succeeded in recruiting 42 nurses for assignment to the unit. Military authorities were generous in their praise of the faculty of the medical school and the staffs of the University Hospitals for having organized a unit such as No. 21 from rather limited personnel.

The coming of Major General Robert U. Patterson to the University of Oklahoma School of Medicine in 1935 added considerable local prestige to the office of dean because of General Patterson's background. Although he became a civic leader in Oklahoma City, he devoted most of his energy toward effecting an expansion of the School of Medicine and its hospitals through the appointment of full-time faculty members, the implementation of his envisioned building program, and the eradication of the school's probationary status.

It is an understatement to say that he was disappointed over his failure to enlist governors and legislators in his "deeply cherished ambition." But he never displayed any bitterness publicly, because his concept of "a dependable nucleus of full-time teachers around which the volunteer staff could work" had not eventuated. On the contrary, it is to his everlasting credit that he started the cogs moving in that direction.

As General Patterson faded away to the east, to become dean of the University of Maryland School of Medicine, Robert S. Kerr was elected as the first native-born governor of the state of Oklahoma. The steadfastness of Dean Patterson against any and all political interference for seven years with that sector of higher education entrusted to his stewardship and the election of Governor Kerr marked an end to a turbulent and violent type of politics that had plagued the state of Oklahoma at intervals for all too many years.

[10.] The 31 physicians and dentists comprising the unit are listed on pages 62 and 63 of this volume.

Chapter VII.
Medical Men in
Uniform: 1943–44

 The inauguration in 1943 of Robert S. Kerr as the twelfth governor of Oklahoma terminated more than a generation of turmoil in the administration of state government, years wrought with the seize-and-overpower tactics of a frontier era. The postwar period of Scott Fitzgerald in the 1920's and the depression of the 1930's had doubtless brought disillusionment to many who had witnessed these phenomena, and one suspects that the majority of Oklahomans had achieved a measure of political maturity by 1943.

Robert S. Kerr was born in Pontotoc County (Indian Territory) where he attended public schools on land that his family had leased from a Chickasaw Indian. He later studied at Central State Teacher's College, Oklahoma Baptist University, and the University of Oklahoma; and he had served ten months in France during World War I. About 1926 he became interested in the oil drilling business and soon acquired extensive oil interests of his own. Kerr was a large tall man with an impressive personality. It is said that "special beds were installed in the governor's mansion in Oklahoma City to accommodate his family." As governor, he traveled a great deal outside the state, selling the industrial potentialities of Oklahoma to likely investors, thus bringing favorable publicity to the striving young state.

The new governor recognized the importance of medicine in his message to the nineteenth legislature and appeared to be intensely interested in the welfare of the School of Medicine. At least, the legislature passed several pieces of legislation favorable to the University of Oklahoma School of Medicine: an appropriation of $50,000 was made for "an annex to the colored ward" (the south ward of the University Hospital); another appropriation of $40,000 was made for the purchase of an annex immediately west of the School of Medicine for a dormitory, in order to alleviate some of the pressure for space on the Oklahoma City campus; House Bill No. 297 was enacted vitalizing the constitutional amendment establishing teacher retirement; and two other constitutional amendments, which made the Board of Regents of the University of Oklahoma and that of the Agricultural College constitutional rather than statutory bodies, were approved and later endorsed by the voters.

President Brandt was authorized by the university regents on April 14 to conclude the necessary negotiations for securing a $40,000 annex to the School of Medicine, and when the regents met on June 9, the president reported that Lot 22 of Block 8 (Howe's Capitol Addition apartment building) was purchased by the State Board of Affairs as temporary quarters for a nurses' home across the street and west of the School of Medicine building. By August 15 the new dormitory had at long last been equipped to accommodate 70 nurses at a total cost of $67,826.

The nineteenth legislature might have been a trifle more generous had the newly created State Regents for Higher Education, in their recommendations to the legislature, not made marked reductions in the requests submitted to them for funds for the University of Oklahoma School of Medicine and University Hospitals.

In a letter addressed to the State Regents for Higher Education on January 25, 1943, Harrington Wimberly, president of the university regents, reminded them of their dereliction.

> If we are going to require additional teaching from the members of the faculty, and if we are going to continue with an increased class, we must provide additional instructors as well as increased salaries. The salary scale for members of the Faculty of the School of Medicine is entirely too low for us to compete with other schools of medicine in securing and retaining competent teachers . . . the salaries paid nurses and technicians are below those which they can obtain in the various government services, defense industries, and private industries, and there are vacancies which we have not been able to fill.

Joseph A. Brandt had been president of the university for five months when he addressed the faculty of the School of Medicine on January 15. He apologized for his tardiness, saying that that was one of the penalties of having two campuses although he was "thoroughly aware that the School of Medicine was part of the University of Oklahoma" (shades of tutoring by General Patterson).

With Dr. Lowry in the audience, President Brandt then said he regretted that the burden of ill health had made it necessary for Dr. Lowry to request a leave of absence from his deanship on November 15, 1942, the day of his appointment, and that Harold A. Shoemaker would be acting dean "until otherwise ordered."

In traveling about the country during the intervening months, the president said he had learned that our medical school actually had a very high standing and he felt that the medical schools of the United States were the "most important adjuncts of higher education at the time." He congratulated the faculty as far as its excellent teaching was concerned but hoped that the medical school would take a much more active leadership in research than in the past. "Research goes hand in hand," he said, "with scholarship and outstanding medical administration."

Aware of the tragedy that the school and the hospitals had never been adequately financed, he was particularly distressed by the lack of development "at this critical period of the war." But he was quick to say that he appreciated the fact that those who had been placed on the essential list had consented to remain (at a sacrifice) and that he hoped they would continue to do so. For the University of Oklahoma had been designated as one of 27 schools in the country with the distinction of having both army and navy trainees.

Dr. Shoemaker reported at this same meeting that 63 members of the faculty and staff of the hospitals had entered the armed forces, placing a very heavy burden on the remaining essential teachers and hospital staff.

While Tom Lowry's appointment as dean had been on a part-time basis— November 15, 1942, to July 1, 1943—President Brandt recommended to the regents on June 9 that Dr. Lowry remain as dean of the medical school in an advisory capacity without salary until such time as a permanent dean might be obtained. But on October 13 the president informed the regents that he had written to Dean Lowry asking him to take over the deanship on a full-time basis as a solution to one of the problems.

Meanwhile, the whole area of administration had evidently become a nightmare to President Brandt for he tendered his resignation as president of the University of Oklahoma effective January 1, 1944, at a special meeting of the board of regents on October 2.

President Brandt revealed that he had accepted a position as director of the University of Chicago Press. "When this Institution was compelled to take a 15 per cent reduction in appropriations last spring," he said, "and to my knowledge, Oklahoma was the only state which reduced appropriations for higher education, I knew there was little hope for the future. . . . I would be doing myself and my family a grace injustice if I were to reject this offer for the will-o-the-wisp future which the financing of Oklahoma's higher education holds. If Oklahomans would only gain a vision of the real service their university could render, they would feel no pride in the $7,000,000 balance in the State Treasury, a balance largely achieved at the expense of education."

Eleven days later the regents unanimously adopted a resolution that, upon the termination of Mr. Brandt's tenure as president of the university, the affable Joe W. McBride, then president of the university regents, was to become acting president of the university, to serve until a permanent president had been chosen and until such time as a new president assumed the responsibility of the office. However, Joe McBride was relieved from serving as acting president of the university on November 29, "for personal reasons, stated by the president and the Board of Regents"; and George Lynn Cross, acting dean of the Graduate School of the University of Oklahoma, was elected to serve as acting president effective January 1, 1944, at a salary of $7,500 per annum, until a permanent president for the university could be chosen.

This sudden departure of President Brandt was less than inspiring to the university faculty members, but there were certain official actions in regard to them too in 1943, as recorded in the university regents' minutes. One important item in regard to the basic science faculty was that their appointments were changed that year from a ten-month to a twelve-month schedule, with corresponding salary increases; a chairman of a department received $6,000 per annum with the new timetable. Arthur A. Hellbaum was promoted to professor of pharmacology and acting chairman of the department, effective January 1, 1944.

Robert M. Howard, who was named professor of clinical surgery when the School of Medicine was organized in 1910, became professor emeritus of surgery upon reaching retirement age; and Cyril Clymer succeeded Dr. Howard as head of the Department of Surgery. C. B. Taylor was promoted to professor of urology and acting head of the department, effective July 1; and John F. Hackler was appointed professor of hygiene and public health at a salary of $6,000 per annum effective December 1. Bert Keltz was appointed supervisor of clerkships, with George H. Garrison and M. F. Jacobs as assistant supervisors. Appointments were approved for eleven physicians who had been working for some time in the outpatient department without titles: two instructors and six assistants in medicine, one assistant in obstetrics, and two instructors in surgery. Charles M. Bielstein became a resident in pediatrics.

There were 247 faculty members of the School of Medicine in the year 1943–44, including six members of the faculty of the School of Nursing and one dietitian. The twenty-eight newly appointed faculty members during the year were:

John Fielden Hackler, M.D.
   professor of preventive medicine
   and public health
John William Cavanaugh, M.D.
   assistant professor of surgery
Allan John Stanley, Ph.D.
   assistant professor of
   physiology
Jack Louis Valin, M.D.
   assistant professor of
   anesthesiology
Kathlyn Allison Krammes, M.N.
   director of the School of Nursing
   and superintendent of nurses
Ralph Otis Clark, M.D.
   instructor in surgery
Juanita Granger
   instructor in nursing arts
Bertha Marion Levy, M.D.
   instructor in pediatrics
Ruth Alden McKinney, Ph.D.
   instructor in clinical pathology
Michael Victor Moth, M.D.
   instructor in medicine
John Augustus Roddy, M.D.
   instructor in medicine
Bessie Souders, R.N.
   instructor in surgical nursing

Noble Franklin Wynn, M.D.
   instructor in pharmacology
Alton Brooke Abshier, M.D.
   assistant in dermatology and
   syphilology
Ethel Maxine Bastion, G.N.
   assistant in nursing
Lucille Spire Blachly, M.D.
   clinical assistant in medicine
Margaret Cleverdon, B.S.
   assistant in clinical pathology
Marvin Brown Glismann, M.D.
   assistant in medicine
Newman Sanford Mathews, M.D.
   assistant in medicine
William Charles McClure, M.D.
   assistant in medicine
Thomas Craig Points, M.D.
   assistant in obstetrics
Rudolph Joe Reichert, M.D.
   assistant in medicine
Peter Ernest Russo, M.D.
   assistant in roentgenology
Mary Kate Schmelzenbach, B.A.
   assistant in nursing arts
Donovan Tool, M.D.
   assistant in medicine

John Walter Barnard, Ph.D.
　research fellow in anatomy
Frank Hladky, Jr., B.S.
　research fellow in biochemistry

Ivo Amazon Nelson, M.D.
　visiting lecturer in clinical
　pathology

During a faculty meeting in August a report was presented by Mark R. Everett, chairman of the curriculum revision committee, of which Doctors H.D. Moor, Arthur Hellbaum, Bert Keltz, and G.E. Stanbro were also members. Dean Lowry complimented the committee for performing an excellent task in revising the curriculum for the first-year class adding, ''You all realize that the compressed teaching program, combined with the terrific heat, has worked an increased hardship on every member of the faculty.''

Howard R. Dickey became assistant superintendent and business director of the University Hospitals on June 19, a valuable addition to the administration. The University Hospital was recipient of $3,975.93 from the estate of Kristina Preston, deceased; and Children's Hospital was bequeathed approximately one-half the estate of William Noble of Oklahoma City—an estimated amount of $44,136.24—for the benefit of crippled children.

Training for medical technologists in the University Hospital was in the name of the pathologist until 1943, when prospective technologists were required to take training in approved laboratories of medical schools. Consequently, Béla Halpert, director of the laboratories, became director of the School of Medical Technology of the University of Oklahoma.[1]

Poliomyelitis reached epidemic proportions again in 1943, and as early as July 29 the regents of the university had reviewed its effects on admissions to the Crippled Children's Hospital, coming up with the decision that the emergency was under control. One month later five wards in Children's Hospital were being utilized to accommodate the many poliomyelitis patients. With health care becoming one of the largest industries in our society, Dean Lowry found it imperative to appoint a committee to draw up bylaws and articles of organization for the University Hospitals in November.

According to the June 15, 1944, University of Oklahoma catalog, the total income of the university for 1943–44 was $2,106,083. Appropriations for the campus in Oklahoma City amounted to $189,700 for the School of Medicine, $370,986 for the University Hospital, and $270,000 for the Crippled Children's Hospital, making a total of $830,686.

The University Hospital functioned with a 200-bed capacity and the Crippled Children's Hospital with a 242-bed capacity during the year 1943–44. There were 6,115 admissions to University Hospitals. The average stay was 19.6 days—27 days for children, 15 days for adults. There were 43,518 outpatient visits; technicians performed 81,417 laboratory tests; obstetrical deliveries totaled 541 in University Hospital and 315 in the outpatient service; 6,648

[1.] In 1937 the College of Arts and Sciences of the University of Oklahoma had organized a School of Applied Biology, and a curriculum for a B.Sc. program in medical technology, was made available the following year.

physiotherapy treatments were given; 16,739 x-ray examinations made; and 2,948 surgeries performed.

There were fourteen residents, ten interns, and five dietetic interns at the University Hospitals during this period. A serious wartime depletion of the nursing staff of the hospitals is evidenced by the fact that there were only 46 registered nurses on the payroll on July 1, 1943, compared to 73 on the same date in 1942.

One hundred and ten graduates of the School of Medicine received the M.D. degree, and 32 nurses were given Graduate Nurse certificates in 1943. There were 334 students in the School of Medicine and 186 in the School of Nursing for the ensuing term.

Before a midwinter commencement on December 23—because of the accelerated program—a special faculty meeting was held on December 22. At the close of the meeting Dean Lowry commented that it had been customary in the past for the oath *Sponsio Academica* (a modification of the Hippocratic oath) to be administered to members of the graduating class by the dean in a private ceremony, but that the decision had been made to present the formality before the faculty on this particular occasion. So the meeting was closed with the graduating class standing and repeating the *Sponsio Academica* in unison with Dean Lowry—a very impressive ceremony.[2] Commissions as first lieutenants were given to the medical graduates the following day.

There was a separate annual University of Oklahoma bulletin for the School of Nursing beginning in 1943, listing the director, the faculty, outline of curriculum, et cetera. A schedule of estimated fees approved for the school on July 14 was $200 for the first year, $90 for the second year, and $35 plus a

[2.] *Sponsio Academica* or physicians' oath, "I, _____, having received the required instruction in medical science, and now qualified to receive a degree, do promise in the presence of a Holy God, Searcher of Hearts, that I will to the last breath of life continue in the duties of one grateful to the University, and that furthermore I will employ my skill in medicine cautiously, conscientiously and honorably and, that so far as in me lies, I will faithfully look after all those things that are helpful in bringing about the health of bodies that are sick, and finally that I will not without urgent reason, divulge those things either seen or heard during medical practice which should be kept secret, so may the Divine Being be present to witness my oath."

Acting Dean H. A. Shoemaker prepared a brief history of the *Sponsio Academica*. The administration of this oath, considered more modern than the Hippocratic oath, was commenced in the School of Medicine of the University of Oklahoma in 1937. It is practically the same as the *Sponsio Academica* given at the University of Edinburgh, where it was introduced in 1705 when the university began to confer degrees in medicine, and before the formation of the medical faculty. In its original form it was practically a literal translation of the Latin Hippocratic oath. But in 1731 that long, cumbersome arrangement was shortened to where it became very much like its present structure, a change made because of certain objections by religious groups; and in 1803 the *Sponsio Academica* was reduced to its present form in Latin. The oath administrered to our graduates is a literal translation of the *Sponsio Academica* used at McGill University in Canada, which was prepared by Professor J. W. Sturgis, professor of Latin at the University of Oklahoma.

graduation fee of $8.00 for the third year, a total of $333. Classes were admitted three times yearly (in June, September, and February) for the duration of the war. A candidate for admission was given a date to come to the University Hospital for prenursing tests and a personal interview with the superintendent of nurses, after having received favorable preliminary consideration.

There were 80 cadets in the local United States Cadet Nursing Corps in 1943,[3] and both a navy contract and a United States Nurse Cadet Corps Training contract were entered into by the School of Nursing on July 1, 1944. President Brandt reported to the regents that $93,408 had been allocated to the School of Nursing under the Bolton Act for the current fiscal year ending June 30, 1944, to pay for incidental maintenance expanses.

Evidently most dietitians did not 'go to war' but they were responsible for the control of general, therapeutic, and metabolic diets in the University Hospitals. There was one chief dietitian, one teaching dietitian, one therapeutic dietitian, and one assistant dietitian at the University Hospital and two assistant dietitians at Crippled Children's Hospital.

There had never been any serious complaint about any of the hospitals approved to accept orthopedic patients under the Crippled Children's Act of 1927 before the nineteenth legislative session, when a Tulsa house member attempted to amend a proposed bill to establish new hospital rates, with the intimation that there was something wrong in his home town, specifically at Hillcrest Hospital.[4] So the accounts and reports of Hillcrest Hospital were scrutinized, and when the air cleared there was no proof that any surgeon had been paid for the 20 orthopedic patients treated at that hospital during the previous year. But the report states that "possibly no other institution in Oklahoma had been more careless in its accounts . . . nor more prone to keep patients over extended periods of time''; thus hinting that the hospital had been collecting even though "no orthopedic surgeon was paid.''

As a matter of record, it should be noted that when the Crippled Children's Commission was first founded, the advisory committee of the federal children's bureau recommended that the minimal qualifications for an orthopedic surgeon were that he had either passed the national orthopedic board examinations or was eligible to pass them. Later, the commission's Committee on Standardization of Hospitals and Physicians ruled that no additional surgeons would be approved for orthopedic work in Oklahoma who had not passed the board examinations. However, the committee failed to make the ruling retroactive, so some surgeons continued to practice who were not diplomates of the American Orthopedic Board.

Regardless of this oversight, only those physicians who were diplomates had ever been approved to receive pay for their surgical services by the Oklahoma

[3.] This corps was established by Congress in 1943. Those volunteering were required to be available for military or other federal service during the war.

[4.] Hillcrest Hospital in Tulsa was approved in 1927 under the name of Flower Hospital and later designated Morningside Hospital. St. John's Hospital was approved about the same time.

Crippled Children's Commission. And the aftereffect of the investigation of Hillcrest Hospital was that most of the orthopedic surgeons in Oklahoma began taking their board examinations.

The total number of admissions to Crippled Children's Hospital on the School of Medicine campus was 2,205. There were 6,710 orthopedic outpatient visits and 403 plastic visits. The total amount of money available for the County Crippled Children's Fund was $119,208, and the total expeditures certified amounted to $50,818. The total available in the State Assistance Crippled Children's Fund was $110,838, and total expenditures for the Oklahoma Hospital for Crippled Children were $321,065.[5]

Colonel Rex Bolend, professor of urology at the School of Medicine on leave of absence since October, 1940, was in command of the 21st Evacuation Unit Hospital in January, 1943. The personnel of the unit consisted of 46 officers, 326 enlisted men, and 42 nurses. However, on March 27, in a reorganization of Evacuation Unit No. 21, male technicians were authorized in place of the previously authorized nurses, who were transferred to Corvallis, Oregon, with Evacuation Unit No. 71.

Doctor Shoemaker quieted some fears that "the army was taking over the medical school," at a faculty meeting on May 5, by saying that we were merely in the process of negotiating a contract for the training of a certain number of medical students for a service unit to be known as #3865 under the Army Specialized Training Program (ASTP).

This medical school unit was activated on May 12, with Captain Lyman F. Barry as its commander, and on the same day President Brandt reported to the regents that we were said to be "the first school in which the medical students were enlisted and put in uniform." He added that "86 per cent of all students being trained for the degree of Doctor of Medicine would eventually be in either the army or the navy, and that only 14 per cent would remain civilians."

By August 25 there were 161 men on active duty with the army and 59 with the navy, with both programs in motion and operating smoothly, as well as being the source of additional funds for the School of Medicine. A check of alumni about this time indicated that more than 30 per cent of our living graduates of the School of Medicine were also in the armed forces.

Governor Kerr was a graduate of the University of Oklahoma, class of 1916, and by 1943 was well aware of the status of institutions of higher education in the state. He was sympathetic to their problems, but he had set as a goal for his administration what he called "puritan economy"; and the net result of that economy was the same old tune. Budgets of educational institutions of higher learning were, with only one or two exceptions, cut 15 per cent across the board, causing Joe Brandt to resign as president of the University of Oklahoma.

While the governor was adamant regarding the financial crisis on the Norman campus, he was sincere about the needs of the School of Medicine, and

[5] *Ninth Annual Report*, 1943–44, of the Oklahoma Commission for Crippled Children.

provision for some emergencies was made: $40,000 for purchase of real estate for a dormitory for nurses, a $50,000 appropriation toward the construction of a Negro ward annex to the University Hospital, and revitalization of the constitutional amendment establishing teacher retirement.

On the public relations side, the Oklahoma City Chamber of Commerce sponsored the preparation and printing of a brief article by Dr. A. C. Scott entitled *The University of Oklahoma School of Medicine*, to which several references are made in this work. In acknowledging receipt of a copy of Dr. Scott's history on April 19, 1943, Dr. Shoemaker, acting dean, wrote: "I have read this story with a great deal of interest. This will make a valuable addition to our archives. . . . I hope some day we will have someone with sufficient time and energy to write a complete history of this school."

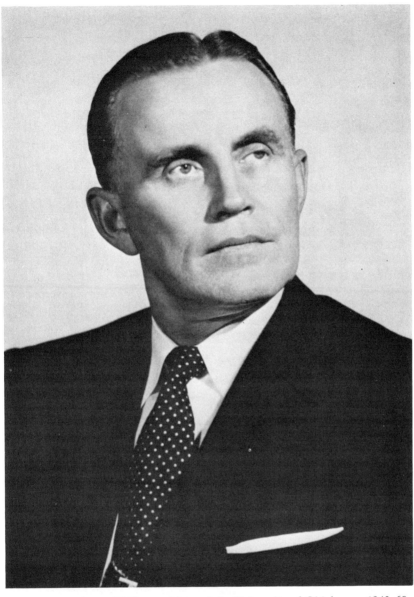

George Lynn Cross, Ph.D., president of the University of Oklahoma, 1943–68.

Courtesy University of Oklahoma Medical Center

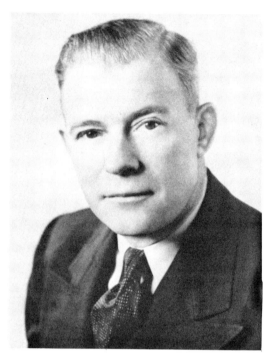

Roy J.Turner, governor of
Oklahoma, 1947–51.

*Courtesy University of
Oklahoma Medical Center*

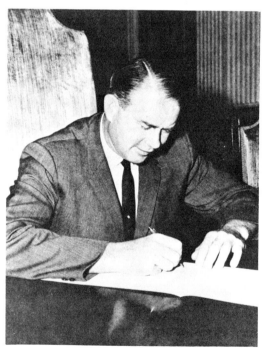

Governor Henry S.
Bellmon, 1963–67.

*Courtesy University of
Oklahoma Medical Center*

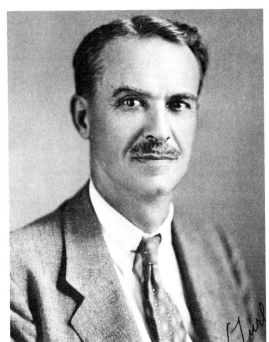

Louis Alvin Turley, Ph.D., acting dean of the School of Medicine, July 1, 1935, to September 1, 1935, and chairman of the Department of Pathology, 1909–44.

Courtesy Sooner Medic

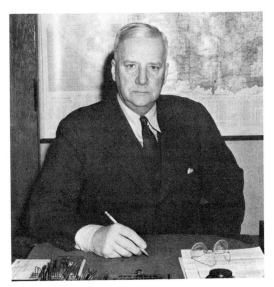

General Robert Urie Patterson, M.D., C.M., LL.D., dean of the School of Medicine, 1935–42.

Courtesy University of Oklahoma Medical Center

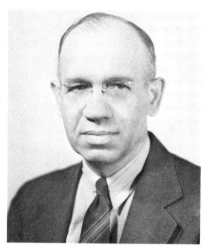

Harold Adam Shoemaker, Ph.C.,
Ph.D., acting dean of the School of
Medicine, 1942–43, and chairman of
the Department of Pharmacology,
1935–44.

Courtesy University of Oklahoma
Medical Center

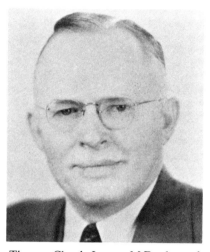

Thomas Claude Lowry, M.D., dean of
the School of Medicine, 1942–45.

Courtesy Sooner Medic

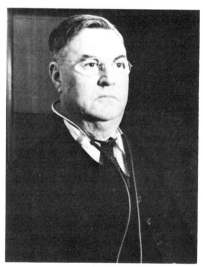

Wann Langston, M.D., dean of the
School of Medicine, 1945–46, and
chairman of the Department of Medicine, 1944–47.

Courtesy Sooner Medic

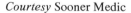

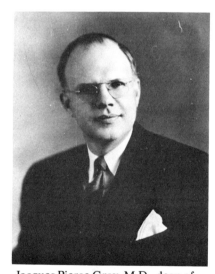

Jacques Pierce Gray, M.D., dean of
the School of Medicine, 1946–47.

Courtesy Sooner Medic

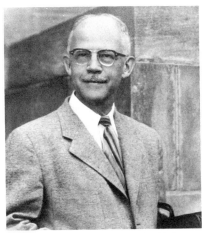

Mark Reuben Everett, Ph.D., D.Sc.,
dean of the School of Medicine,
1947–64; director of the Medical
Center, 1956–64; chairman of the
Department of Biochemistry,
1924–(64).

*Courtesy University of Oklahoma
Medical Center*

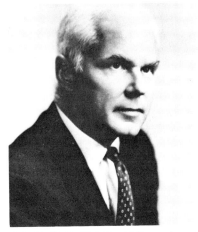

Merlin K. DuVal, Jr., M.D., assistant
director of the Medical Center,
1962–63.

*Courtesy University of Oklahoma
Medical Center*

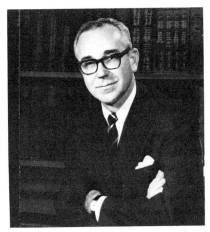

Joseph M. White, M.D., acting dean of
the School of Medicine and acting
director of the Medical Center, July 1,
1964, to August 1, 1964, and chairman
of the Department of Anesthesiology,
1956–(64).

*Courtesy University of Oklahoma
Medical Center*

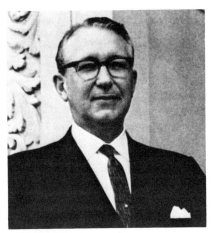

James Lowden Dennis, M.D., dean of
the School of Medicine and director
of the Medical Center, (1964).

Courtesy Sooner Medic

91

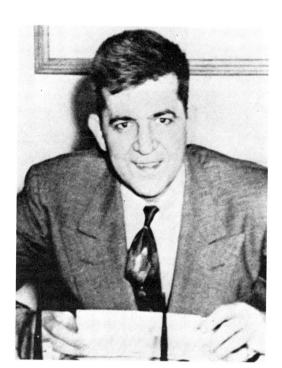

Homer F. Marsh, Ph.D.,
associate dean of students,
1947–52, and head of the
Department of Bacteriol-
ogy, 1951–52.

Courtesy Sooner Medic

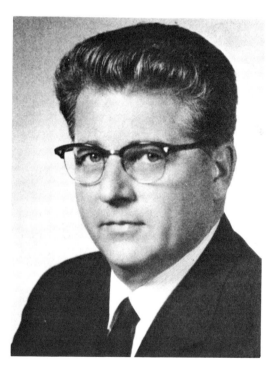

Ardell Nichols Taylor,
Ph.D., associate dean of
student affairs, 1952–60,
and chairman of the
Department of Physiology,
1947–60.

Courtesy Sooner Medic

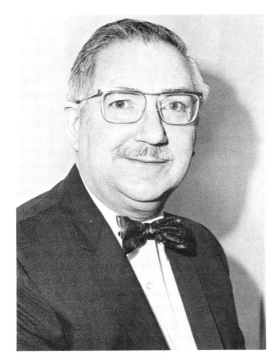

Philip E. Smith, D.Sc.,
associate dean of student
affairs, 1960–(64).

*Courtesy University of
Oklahoma Medical Center*

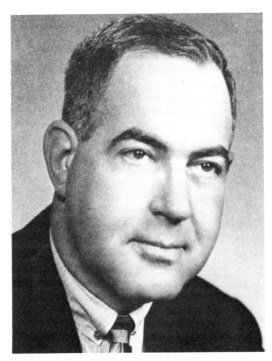

Samuel Newton Stone,
M.D., associate dean of
clinical instruction,
1951–(64).

Courtesy Sooner Medic

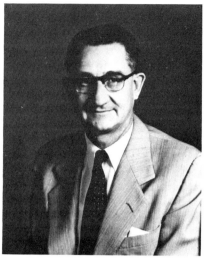

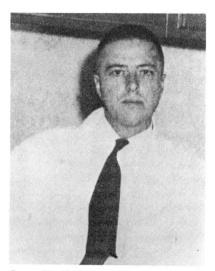

Arthur A. Hellbaum, Ph.D., M.D., associate dean of graduate studies and research, 1947–57, and chairman of the Department of Pharmacology, 1944–57.

Courtesy University of Oklahoma Medical Center

James W. H. Smith, M.D., associate dean of graduate studies and research, 1954–56.

Courtesy University of Oklahoma Medical Center

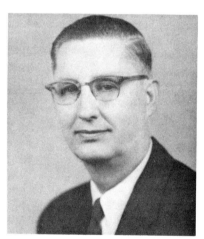

Kirk T. Mosley, M.D., D.P.H., associate dean of special training and research programs, 1959–60, and chairman of the Department of Preventive Medicine and Public Health, 1952–60.

Courtesy Madelon B. Katigan

Chapter VIII.
A New University
President: 1944-45

 George Lynn Cross, professor of plant sciences and acting dean of the Graduate School, became acting president of the University of Oklahoma on January 1, 1944. The immediate problem which President Cross inherited in 1944 was a university budget that had been reduced by over 15 per cent from the previous 1942-43 budget; and, with the approval of the regents, he proceeded to appoint a university planning commission. Tom Lowry, dean of the School of Medicine, was made a member of two sections of the commission, the building plans and campus development section and the personnel statewide tuition plan section.

When the university regents met on March 31, with Dr. Claude Chambers of Seminole presiding, President Cross again broached the subject of the budget and the resulting financial crisis on the Norman campus as the initial issue; whereas the School of Medicine on the Oklahoma City campus had received some encouraging support from the nineteenth legislature. Furthermore, a $73,000 grant from the Federal Works Agency in June guaranteed completion of the "annex to the colored ward" at a total cost of $114,963, toward which the legislature had appropriated $50,000.

The enthusiasm derived from this accomplishment was somewhat diminished, however, when President Cross advised members of the university regents in November that the State Regents for Higher education had tentatively reduced the requests of the School of Medicine and its hospitals, suggesting that the revenues for the hospital should be separated from the revenues for the School of Medicine. In support of their recommendation, the state regents reasoned that only in this way could the estimated 20 per cent of the operating costs of the hospitals be truly calculated on a per capita educational cost basis as the cost of instruction of medical students.

At this same meeting a change in the rate of pay for members of the volunteer clinical staff of the School of Medicine was authorized—an increase from three to five dollars per lecture hour for professors and associate professors.

Meanwhile, Dean Lowry had replaced the executive committee set up by Dean Patterson at the medical school in 1935 with an advisory council composed of representatives from the basic science and clinical departments of the School of Medicine. During the first meeting on April 27 the main topic of discussion was directed to the question of retirement of members of the faculty. First, the retirement of Louis A. Turley, age 65, head of the Department of Pathology, was discussed, for Fred Zapffe, secretary of the Council on Medical Education and Hospitals, had earlier recommended to Dean Lowry that a clinician should be installed as chairman of the Department of Pathology in order to properly encompass all areas of the subject in the School of Medicine and its hospitals.

There had been for some time a rather prevalent impression that the Department of Pathology should be reorganized under one man, so Dean Lowry initiated the discussion by saying that there was a great deal of difficulty "between the two sides of the street"—basic science and clinical. Whereupon, Dr. Langston, chief of the medical service, immediately stated that he felt very definitely that there should be a clinical pathologist in charge of the hospital laboratories who was "interested in living pathology rather than dead pathology;" and that there was no actual supervision of the clinical pathological laboratories. "Our clinical laboratories are, in may opinion," Dr. Langston added, "as low as they have ever been in the history of the school. . . . In most of the teaching hospitals, the clinical pathologist heads the laboratory set-up, with the exception of tissue."

Dr. Keller then asserted that Dr. Turley had been one of his best friends, but that he felt that the Department of Pathology was one of the weakest in the School of Medicine, adding that he had had this brought home to him rather forcefully when he attempted to take some postgraduate work and found out how little he actually knew. "I had to start from the ground up," he said. "I think the professor of pathology should be in charge of both sides of the street."

Now, no member of the council cared to disassociate Dr. Turley, who had been connected with the School of Medicine for thirty-six years (during which time he rendered a great deal of service), even though he was subject to retirement according to the regents' ruling. Therefore, the recommendation to the regents by Dean Lowry was that Dr. Turley be retained on a part-time basis.

The next consideration was in regard to members of the volunteer faculty who had reached retirement age and wished to resign in order to be relieved of administrative responsibilities. "They have all rendered a good service," Dean Lowry said. "If we do accept their resignations, we feel that we should give them something to indicate that we appreciate it."

Subsequently, the following retiring faculty members received professor emeritus certificates at a faculty meeting on September 13, 1944: Doctors John Mosby Alford, medicine; David Wilson Griffin, mental diseases; Robert Mayburn Howard, surgery; Everett Samuel Lain, dermatology and syphilology; George Althouse LaMotte, medicine; Leander Armistead Riely, clinical medicine; William Merritt Taylor, pediatrics; Louis Alvin Turley, pathology; and Arthur Weaver White, clinical medicine—"all grand men" who had joined the faculty in the early days of organization of the School of Medicine.

Following the awarding of these certificates, Dean Lowry called on President Cross to address a few remarks to the faculty, saying that Dr. Cross had spent at least one day out of every month at the School of Medicine assisting in the task of solving some of the current problems.

Dr. Cross assured the faculty that he was greatly interested in the history of the School of Medicine and that the progress of the school since 1928 had been remarkable. He said that whenever he felt pessimistic, he thought of the progress that had been made in the school in the last 20 years, and that he was 100 per cent behind the faculty and its program. "I am very much impressed with what you are doing here," the president declared, "and I congratulate you, You can depend upon my support in every possible way."

Howard C. Hopps, assistant professor of pathology at the University of Chicago was appointed professor of pathology and chairman of the department at the University of Oklahoma School of Medicine by the regents on July 12 at a salary of $7,000 per annum effective September 1, 1944; and Dr. Turley, for part-time service, was granted a title of professor emeritus of pathology at a salary of $3,600 per annum. On September 1, Dr. Langston became professor of medicine and chairman of the department, and Robert H. Bayley was appointed professor of clinical medicine and vice-chairman of the department at a salary of $7,500 per annum.

A two-month leave of absence was approved by the university regents on March 15 for John F. Hackler, professor of preventive medicine and public health, to visit the DeLamar Institute of Public Health at Columbia University for a period of eight weeks, with all expenses paid by the Commonwealth Fund. Before 1944 the Department of Preventive Medicine and Public Health was the Department of Hygiene and Public Health.

There were 253 members of the faculty in the School of Medicine in the year 1944–45, including seven members of the faculty of the School of Nursing and two dietitians. The eleven newly appointed faculty members during the year were:

Robert Hebard Bayley, M.D.
　professor of clinical medicine
Howard Carl Hopps, M.D.
　professor of pathology
Anderson Nettleship, M.D.
　associate professor of pathology
Florene Cora Kelly, Ph.D.
　assistant professor of bacteriology
Charles Allen Winter, Ph.D.
　assistant professor of physiology
Clara Wolfe Jones, R.N.
　acting director of the School of
　Nursing, acting superintendent of
　nurses

Mary Leidigh
　assistant administrative dietitian
William Bradford Carroll, M.D.
　instructor in neuropsychiatry
Howard George Glass, Ph.D.
　instructor in pharmacology
Bonnie Hewett, G.N.
　instructor in nursing arts
Frances Williamson
　assistant in histology and
　embryology
Lieonnir Janeal Villet, B.S.
　graduate assistant in biochemistry

At the faculty meeting on September 13, Mark R. Everett, chairman of the curriculum committee, presented a final report and recommendations in connection with revision of the medical school curriculum, after having visited ten other medical schools in pursuit of a basic guide for this proposed revision. The chairman expressed appreciation to the committee for its splendid cooperation and careful deliberation for over one year and for the assistance given to solving the many problems encountered in revising the curriculum. As a result of the comparative study, a total of 4,700 curriculum hours was reduced to 4,200 hours; the rotating clerkship hours were extended to full time on a broader basis; and more free time was made available in the preclinical years. Dr. Clymer moved that the report be accepted as read, and the motion, seconded by Dr. Burton, was passed.

President Cross reported at this same faculty meeting that Coyne H. Campbell had independently made the first significant gift to medical research in Oklahoma to be known as the John Hatchett Memorial Research Fund. He specified that the chairman of the Department of Biochemistry of the School of Medicine be authorized—with the approval of the dean—to order expenditures under this fund, and Dr. Cross stated that the regents had voted to accept the gift with the attending stipulation.

As early as April 25, 1944, preliminary plans were under way by a committee appointed by the Alumni Association of the School of Medicine, of which Wayman J. Thompson of Oklahoma City was chairman, to create an endowment fund for research in medicine. The details of how this dream eventualized may be found in *Pioneering for Research—Origin of the Oklahoma Medical Research Foundation*, by Mark R. Everett of the University of Oklahoma Medical Center. Mark Everett wrote:

> They began modestly in 1944, at which time Dr. James William Finch of Hobart was the fifth president of the Alumni Association of the School of Medicine and Dr. Ennis M. Gullatt of Ada, the vice-president. Dr. John H. Lamb had become secretary-treasurer of the association in 1943, a most provident occurrence, since his vigorous crusade was to provide the key to the founding of the research institute. . . .
>
> The first result of action taken by the Alumni Association was to stimulate the appointment of a cooperating Endowment Committee in the School of Medicine. In October 1944, Dean Tom Lowry [the first alumnus to become dean of his school] designated such a committee, with Dr. John Lamb as chairman, and Dr. Ray Balyeat, Dr. John Burton, Dr. Tullos Coston and Dr. Mark R. Everett as members. . . .
>
> The School of Medicine Endowment Committee met with Dean Lowry in October to discuss its task and decided that the research needs of the School of Medicine should be proposed by the heads of departments. . . . By November the committee had ascertained from the university authorities that legislative financial support should not be sought for such projects and that the endowment program could best be developed through the Alumni Association of the School of Medicine . . . and in December of the same year, upon request by the Alumni Association, the University of Oklahoma Foundation prepared a trust

declaration for a Fund for the Advancement of Medical Science in Oklahoma to provide for the acceptance of gifts.

According to the University of Oklahoma bulletin, catalog issue 1944–45, there were three fellowships available in the School of Medicine to properly qualified applicants for prosecution of research in medical sciences—two fellowships with an annual stipend of $1,200 and one fellowship with a stipend of $1,500.

In line with all the activity on behalf of medical research, the regents of the University of Oklahoma authorized President Cross on August 9, 1944, to proceed with the establishment of a Graduate School of Public Health in accordance with a recommendation which the president had made previously. A. G. Fletcher was an instructor in surgical diagnosis, 1944–45, and L. W. Kibler was again employed as field director of the medical school's post-graduate program.[1]

George N. Barry was named medical director of University Hospitals in 1944. During the year there were 6,595 admissions to the hospitals with an average stay of 18.9 days and 14,230 patients coming to the outpatient service for a total of 44,366 visits. The number of new outpatients equaled 7,836 according to the 1944–45 catalog of the University.

The appropriations for the university's Oklahoma City campus for 1944–45, as listed in the catalog, were as follows: for the School of Medicine, $178,950; for the University Hospital, $370,986; and for the Crippled Children's Hospital, $270,000; making a total allocation of $819,936.[2]

In addition to University Hospital with 180 beds and the Oklahoma Hospital for Crippled Children with 220 beds, the following hospitals were listed as having granted to the School of Medicine teaching privileges: Wesley Hospital, a general hospital with a capacity of 150 beds; Central State Hospital with a capacity of 2,675 beds; and the Deaconess Hospital with favorable circumstances for practical training in obstetrics.

Dean Lowry advised Sister Mechtildis, St. Anthony Hospital, on October 3, 1944, that, because of a change in the curriculum of the third and fourth years of the University of Oklahoma School of Medicine, there was no longer any necessity "to impose on you for the use of operative clinics." At the same time Dr. Lowry expressed deep appreciation to Sister Mechtildis for St. Anthony's "hearty cooperation and help in our teaching program."

The Chamber of Commerce was active during 1944 in endeavoring to bring a Veterans Administration Hospital to Oklahoma City, and several members of the faculty who had endorsed the proposition were on a medical center committee working with the chamber on this important project. A brochure was

[1.] *Abstracts of lectures*, Oklahoma State Medical Association, published by the Commission on Postgraduate Medical Teaching (1938–1951).
[2.] The will of William Noble, probated on March 15, 1944, set up funds to acquire and equip a clinical investigation laboratory in the Crippled Children's Hospital in 1948.

prepared for the purpose of obtaining facilities for such a hospital in Oklahoma City.

On the student side of the ledger, there were 56 graduates of the School of Medicine who received the M.D. degree, and 27 nurses received Graduate Nurse certificates in 1944. There were 353 students enrolled in the School of Medicine and 210 students in the School of Nursing for the year 1944–45.

A detailed program on a collegiate basis was proposed for the School of Nursing in 1944 on a separate budget from that of the School of Medicine. A leave of absence was granted to Kathlyn Krammes, director of the School of Nursing and superintendent of nurses, for one year without pay beginning August 1, 1944, in order that she might work toward a Master of Science degree at the University of Washington in Seattle.[3]

President Cross reported to the university regents on February 9, 1944, that plans for the admission of a higher percentage of women to the School of Medicine were under way, and on July 14 the regents approved two resolutions pursuant to recommendations made by the executive council of the Association of American Medical Colleges, which were endorsed by the faculty: (1) that the School of Medicine continue to admit students to the first-year class at nine-months intervals during a period of acceleration, but that the size of the class should be reduced from 75 students to 60 students; (2) that the prewar requirement of 90 semester hours for admission, as voted by members of the faculty, be reinstated effective January 1, 1946. Students who were nonresidents of the state of Oklahoma were required to pay a tuition fee of $50 for each semester in all schools and colleges except the School of Medicine in which the nonresident tuition fee was $175 a semester. A promising development on the Oklahoma City campus in 1944 was the formation of a student council composed of two representatives from each class and an advisory member from the faculty, approved by the dean, to act as a liaison with the faculty, staff, and alumni.

Seventy-seven students (44 army, 23 navy) were enrolled in the first-year medical school class of January to September 15, 1944. From September 15 to March 31, 1945, 77 students were again enrolled, with 31 in the army and 21 in the navy.

President Cross was present at the faculty meeting on September 13 when the dean of the School of Medicine, as chairman of the committee on promotions, composed of Doctors John F. Burton, R. Q. Goodwin, Mark R. Everett, and Homer F. Marsh, presented the committee report regarding graduates. Following the meeting, the members of the fourth-year class and the faculty gathered in the auditorium of the medical school for the administration of the *Sponsio Academica*, or doctor's oath, by Dean Lowry. Subsequently commencement exercises were held for the graduating class on September 15 in the auditorium at Oklahoma City University.

Information pertinent to the operation of the Oklahoma Commission for Crippled Children may be found in the tenth annual report, fiscal year 1944–45.

[3] Clara Wolfe Jones was appointed acting director of the School of Nursing during Miss Krammes' absence.

While "the relationship of the Commission to the counties, the Committee on Standardization, the Oklahoma Hospital for Crippled Children, and other hospitals, is defined by law," the report reads, "the Commission has worked closely with other public and private agencies on a purely cooperative basis. . . . as the fiscal year ends, Oklahoma is experiencing once more an unusual number of acute infantile paralysis cases."

The total number of new patients admitted to the Oklahoma Hospital for Crippled Children in 1944–45 was 1,812, with 694 return cases, making an overall total of 2,506 entrances to the hospital. There was a total of 6,011 orthopedic visits to the outpatient department and 474 plastic surgery visits. Services for children under the age of 21 with orthopedic, plastic, and rheumatic fever conditions for the calendar year 1944 were as follows: outpatient department, Oklahoma Hospital for Crippled Children, 2,327 individuals, 7,200 visits; physical therapy, 189 individuals, 5,723 visits. Total expenditures at the Oklahoma Hospital for Crippled Children for the year 1944–45 amounted to $364,181.

The 21st Evacuation Hospital Unit[4] arrived at Guadalcanal in the South Pacific on October 3, 1943, and the hospital was opened on December 6 for only a brief period, closing on January 15, 1944. During that 42-day period 2,175 patients were admitted to the hospital. A change of command was effected on January 10 when Colonel Bolend was recalled to the United States and Lieutenant Colonel Robert E. Allen assumed command of the unit.

During the latter part of January preparations were made for moving the hospital unit, and on February 2 the last of the personnel departed from Guadalcanal arriving at Empress Augusta Bay, Bougainville, on February 4, where a dense jungle had to be cleared and drained before a hospital site could be established. Notwithstanding, the hospital began receiving patients on February 15 and in the nick of time, as an impending Japanese offensive against the perimeter materialized on March 8. Thirty-five battle casualties were received in a five-hour period the next day, when "the hospital was operating under strict black-out conditions and under a heavy and constant artillery barrage." Captain James M. Taylor, in his June 22, 1945, letter to Dean Tom Lowry, said, "We had two underground wards for the most critical cases and a larger underground surgery. Casualties were pouring in steadily. . . . the shock tent was a madhouse of organized confusion. Every morning the place looked like a saloon after a big night. Plasma bottles piled high in the corner, piles of clothes off the wounded and a general litter of odds and ends."

On November 3, 1944, the Bougainville hospital station was closed, and on December 22 the unit departed for a destination "somewhere in the Philippines."

From January 5, 1944, to September 15, 1944, army and navy medical student trainees at the University of Oklahoma School of Medicine were

---

[4.] The following information was obtained largely from a report by Lieutenant Colonel Allen G. Gibbs, M.D., *A Brief History of the 21st Evacuation Hospital* (1945); and from a letter by Captain Jim M. Taylor, M.D., to Dean Tom Lowry, June 22, 1945.

enumerated as follows: first-semester army 171, navy 72; second-semester army 169, navy 71.

Students in the School of Nursing who joined the United States Nurse Cadet Corps, with which the University of Oklahoma school was affiliated, had all their expenses paid by the United States Public Health Service and in addition received a monthly stipend and outdoor uniforms as in the year 1943–44.

Receipts under federal trainee contracts from December 7, 1941, to December 31, 1944, at the School of Medicine and University Hospitals amounted to a total of $286,803 as follows: army contract (School of Medicine), $180,153; navy contract (School of Medicine), $66,452; U.S. Nurse cadet Corps training contract (School of Nursing), $40,197.

A resolution by the executive council of the Association of American Medical Colleges on postwar medical education reads as follows: "RESOLVED, that the Executive Council of the Association of American Medical Colleges recommends that each member of the Association endeavor to formulate a program for postwar graduate and postgraduate medical education, in affiliation with the hospitals in its area, which can provide satisfactory advanced clinical training."

The appointment of George L. Cross as president of the University of Oklahoma and the acceptance by Tom Lowry of the full-time duties of the dean's office brought a certain amount of equilibrium to administrative spheres in 1944, which resulted in improvement of the spirit on both campuses. President Cross attended all faculty meetings at the School of Medicine during the year and was optimistic even when he felt pessimistic. Dean Lowry, himself an alumnus, backed the quickening interest among the alumni of the School of Medicine in the establishment of an endowment fund for research.

The heavy-handedness from governors and legislators regarding selection of students for admission to the School of Medicine, to which former Dean Patterson had been subjected during his administration, appears to have diminished with the advent of Robert S. Kerr as governor of Oklahoma. Certainly, "Dr. Tom" symbolized the epitome of honesty and integrity as an administrator, and he left us a philosophical legacy following the recitation of the *Sponsio Academica* with the fourth-year class at the faculty meeting on September 13.

"Truly, the teacher lives forever and has a sort of immortality which comes through service," Dean Lowry affirmed; and quoting from Oliver Wendell Holmes, Jr., Dr. Lowry continued.

"Riders in a race do not stop short when they reach a goal. There is a little finishing canter before coming to a standstill. There is time to hear the kind voice of friends and to say to one's self: 'The work is done.' " And so with a line from a Latin poet, who uttered the message more than 1,500 years ago, "Death plucks my ears and says live I am coming," and I think that is a creed we can apply to all medical men.

Chapter IX.
The Dean Called
Dr. Tom: 1945–46

In his message to the twentieth session of the Oklahoma legislature, Governor Robert S. Kerr recommended increasing the capacity of the University of Oklahoma and expanding the training of doctors, nurses, and technicians at the School of Medicine. Furthermore, he was a pioneer in his efforts to secure more adequate facilities for black patients at the University Hospitals—one of his campaign promises.

The Oklahoma Statutes were amended in 1945 (House Bill No. 463), definitively designating the School of Medicine as "The School of Medicine of the University of Oklahoma," formerly referred to in the statutes as "medical department," "medical school," and "medical college," without a clear definition of title. This bill also amended the statutes to designate the University Hospital by that title. It also specified the site and location of the School of Medicine of the University of Oklahoma . . . "a tract comprising fifteen and sixty-four one hundredths (15.64) acres, more or less . . . belonging to the state and being a part of what is known as the capitol lands" (Section 1251).

Section 1256 of Bill No. 463, pertaining to the admission of patients to the University Hospital, included a statement that "the Dean of the School of Medicine of the University of Oklahoma is authorized to make such further rules and regulations as may be approved by the Board of Regents of the University or their successors, for the management of the hospital, provided that such rules and regulations . . . shall not prohibit the use of the hospital to any physician or surgeon licensed to practice in this State by the Board of Medical Examiners." The bill, passed without a dissenting vote, apparently eliminates cults from attempting to practice in the University Hospital.

Of significant importance to alumni, and to the state as a whole, was the passage of Section 1 of Appropriations Bill No. 101 (by Creekmore Wallace of the House, and J. C. Nance and Robert Burns of the Senate), which appropriated from the general revenue funds of the state to the Oklahoma state regents the sum of $247,500 "for buildings, improvements and purchase of equipment for and at the University of Oklahoma School of Medicine and its hospitals." The appropriation included the sum of $1,432,503 to the Oklahoma state regents from the public building fund of the state of Oklahoma, for the fiscal year ending June 30, 1946, ''for construction of buildings, improvements, and purchase of equipment for and at the University of Oklahoma School of Medicine and its hospitals.'' It included the newly affiliated Southern Oklahoma Hospital at Ardmore (formerly the Oklahoma Confederate Home), which the twentieth legislature established as an auxiliary to the University Hospital, transferring its property to the Board of Regents of the University of Oklahoma on July 1, 1945.

A concurrent resolution was passed which stipulated that, of the above appropriations of $1,680,000, it was the intent of the legislature that the State Regents for Higher Education allocate $250,000 to the Southern Oklahoma Hospital to be used in matching contributions from municipal and county governments, private citizens, and civic or other organizations for the construction of said hospital.

Dean Lowry told the faculty on June 14 that citizens of Ardmore were raising $250,000 for this project, and that the sum might in turn be matched by $500,000 of federal funds, to provide $1,000,000 for the care of chronic tuberculosis and general patients. This complicated maneuver had certain political undertones in the light of Dean Lowry's revelation that the hospital was comprised of three buildings, with only about 40 patients.[1]

House Concurrent Resolution No. 8 by the House Appropriations Committee transmitted to the Oklahoma State Regents for Higher Education the operational budget needs of the various institutions comprising the Oklahoma state system of higher education, which were considered as the basis for appropriations to the state regents by the twentieth legislature. ''The list of items and amounts of needs of each of the institutions, as transmitted, truly reflects the items and amounts considered by the twentieth legislature in making the consolidated appropriations, as set forth in House Bill No. 101, for the fiscal year ending June 30, 1946: University of Oklahoma, Norman, state appropriations $1,899,885 (out of a total income of $2,224,885); for the School of Medicine, $236,640 from state funds (out of a total income of $281,885); and for University Hospitals $765,580 from state funds (out of a total income of $825,580).''

At the beginning of the legislative session on January 10 the regents of the University of Oklahoma had discussed the building program of the School of Medicine and its hospitals. But they were also justifiably concerned with the question of revenues for the Norman campus and entered the following opinion in their minutes: ''While we concur in the building program at the School of Medicine in Oklahoma City, there are other needs of the University that are just

---

[1] Responsibility for the administration of the Southern Oklahoma Hospital was placed under the supervision of the School of Medicine of the University of Oklahoma on October 29, by an opinion of the attorney general. And with the approval of the State Regents for Higher Education, the university regents passed a resolution in November, ''declaring the Southern Oklahoma Hospital to be part of the functions of the University Hospitals'' and directed the president of the university ''to take charge of the Southern Oklahoma Hospital.''

as vital as the needs of the medical school.'' The regents then agreed that this statement should be signed by the president of the board and that it should be sent to the State Regents for Higher Education and also to the governor; for, at long last, political winds appeared to be favoring the university's Oklahoma City campus.

In November the university regents belatedly authorized President Cross to file a request with the State Regents for Higher Education for an allocation of capital funds totaling $1,090,503 for the School of Medicine and the University Hospitals, as suggested by Dean Lowry.

Under provision six of House Bill No. 463, the Board of Regents of the University of Oklahoma was given authority to prescribe rules and regulations for the School of Medicine and its hospitals, and on September 12 the regents requested President Cross to recommend appropriate rules and regulations for operation of the newly created Negro Division of the University Hospital—politically important to Governor Kerr. One month later the following resolution was unanimously adopted by the board: The recently completed addition to University Hospital, constructed with funds appropriated by the nineteenth legislature and an allotment by the Federal Works Administration, is known as the Negro or South Ward Division of the University Hospital. Its administration will be under the dean of the School of Medicine and the administrative officials of the University Hospitals. ''Insofar as possible the nurses, aides, and janitors serving their respective departments in the Negro wing, should be Negroes. The training of Negro nurses is to be instituted as soon as feasible in the Negro Division, under the direction of the School of Nursing of the University. Certificates or diplomas for the Negro nurses are to be issued by Langston University.''

W. L. Haywood, was named chief of staff of this division of the University Hospital at a salary of $100 per month effective October 1. An adjunct staff of Negro physicians for the south ward, consisting of accredited physicians who were members of the Oklahoma State Negro Medical Association, was also set up by the regents but with no teaching duties. In a report to the superintendent of the hospitals, Dr. Haywood stated that the program actually commenced on September 17, and that he had received ''good treatment from white doctors and officials.''

Dr. Lowry, presiding at a faculty meeting on June 14, asserted that the Alumni Association of the School of Medicine had been vitally interested in the endowment program of the school during the past year and a half, and that their committee had appointed key doctors in each district of the state to further the project; and that a declaration of trust had been prepared for the University of Oklahoma to accept endowment gifts earmarked for special purposes. Since John Lamb, chairman of the School of Medicine endowment committee was out of town, John Burton made a brief report, naming the members of the committee—Dr. Balyeat, Dr. Burton, Dr. Coston, and Dr. Everett—and stating the purposes of the endowment committee of the alumni association as follows: to establish a medical endowment fund; to supervise private donations for research; to organize various research projects and supervise the spending of such funds; to oversee the selection of fellows to carry on the work; to provide funds for guest lectureships throughout the year; to help raise money for a needed building, such as a library or research building, through possible memorial contributions; and to finance special chairs in experimental medicine.

This endowment fund for the School of Medicine, set up as a part of the Oklahoma University Foundation, in no way took the place of appropriations, nor was it tied in any way with the state's financial policies for the school. At that time the School of Medicine had only $20.847 in endowment funds, which included $4,000 in the Hatchett Fund originated by Coyne Campbell for the Department of Biochemistry, $2,995 in the Rosalee Powell Estate Fund, $3,438 in the Kristina Preston Estate Fund for the purchase of equipment for the polio ward in Children's Hospital, and $19,164 from the William Noble estate held in trust for the benefit of Crippled Children's Hospital.

The balance in the W. K. Kellogg Foundation Loan Fund for medical students at the University of Oklahoma School of Medicine was $3,079, and the balance in the scholarship fund was $1,600 on September 30, 1945. Previous grants totaled $15,000. The balance in the loan fund at the School of Nursing on the same date was $1,840 and in the scholarship fund $600 from the original grants of $3,000 and $1,000.

Turning our attention to the teaching staff of the School of Medicine and its hospitals, we find that the regents made numerous academic changes during the year 1945. Possibly one of the more far-reaching in its effects was the appointment of Paul Fesler[2] as the administrator of the University Hospitals at a salary of $7,000 as of May 15, since George N. Barry, who had applied for a commission in the navy, had resigned as medical director. Following Mr. Fesler's appointment, the regents named a committee on the medical school and hospitals composed of Lloyd Noble, chairman, Regents Don Emery and Harrington Wimberly, members.

On recommendation of Dean Lowry and President Cross, the following changes in titles were approved by the regents: Basil Hayes was promoted to professor of urology effective January 1 and acting chairman of the department during the absence of Rex Bolend; Ernest Lachman was promoted from the rank of associate professor to professor of anatomy effective February 11 and also chairman of the department at a salary of $6,000 to succeed Charles DeGaris; Albert Douglas Foster, Jr., was appointed professor of anesthesiology effective February 1 at a salary of $5,000, replacing Hubert E. Doudna, who had been granted leave for military service; Charles Rayburn, professor of mental diseases, who had been on leave of absence with the army, returned to active status

[2.] Paul Fesler was a charter fellow of the American College of Hospital Administrators, a past president of the American Hospital Association, and chairman of the Teaching Section of the American Hospital Association for a number of years. After returning to Oklahoma in 1944, he served as executive secretary of the Oklahoma State Medical Association. See also Mark R. Everett, *Medical Education in Oklahoma*, (Norman, University of Oklahoma Press, 1972), I, 207; II, 106.

with the School of Medicine, also effective February 1; James Patton McGee was promoted to professor of ophthalmology and chairman of the department, when Leslie M. Westfall reached retirement age on May 1; Edward Pennington Allen, professor of clinical obstetrics, became chairman of the department on June 1, when Walter W. Wells reached retirement age; W. L. Haywood was appointed chief of staff of the South Ward Negro Division at a salary of $100 per month on October 1; Bert Ernest Mulvey, assistant professor of clinical medicine, was appointed to serve as assistant supervisor of clinical clerkships, November 1; and Robert Bayley became acting chairman of the Department of Medicine on December 13.

The following faculty members achieved professor emeritus status in 1945: Charles B. Taylor, urology; Leslie M. Westfall, ophthalmology; and Walter W. Wells, obstetrics. At a faculty meeting on June 14, Dean Lowry paid special tribute to these men for their 28–35 years of service to the University of Oklahoma School of Medicine and also to Robert M. Howard, professor emeritus of surgery.

Professor emeritus of clinical medicine Arthur Weaver White, a graduate of Rush Medical College in 1902, who joined the faculty of the School of Medicine in 1910 as an instructor in gastrointestinal diseases, died June 11, 1945.

There were 245 members of the faculty of the School of Medicine in the year 1945–46, including four members of the School of Nursing. The 12 newly appointed faculty members during the year are shown as follows:

Albert Douglas Foster, M. D.
    professor of anesthesiology
John Walter Keys, Ph.D.
    professor of speech and director
    of speech and hearing clinic
William Arlin Loy, M.D.
    associate professor of preventive
    medicine and public health
Henry Wade Hooper, M.S.
    instructor in histology and
    embryology
Harvey Mac Richey, M.D.
    instructor in surgery
Florence H. Muelhauser, R.N.,
    B.S.
    educational director

Doris J. Stranathan, R.N.
    instructor in orthopedic nursing
Lewis Carroll Taylor, M.D.
    instructor in anesthesiology
Paul Merton Vickers, M.D.
    instructor in surgery
Johnny A. Blue, M.D.
    clinical assistant in medicine
Alberta Webb Dudley, M.D.
    assistant in medicine
Wiley Thomas McCollum, M.D.
    fellow in pathology

A ruling on the question of nepotism was made by the regents for the University of Oklahoma on September 12 to the effect that in the future ''no two members of any family related within the third degree, either by blood or by marriage, should be employed by the University or any branch of the University.''

Wesley Hospital, with a bed capacity of 150, extended teaching privileges to the School of Medicine again in 1945–46, making a total of 640 available teaching beds, including 270 beds at University Hospital and 220 at Crippled Children's Hospital.

There were 4,506 patients admitted to University Hospital in 1945–46 (720 to the Negro Division) making a total of 67,354 hospital days and an average stay of 14.9 days; the number of patients admitted to Children's Hospital equaled 2,438[3] with 62,172 hospital days and an average stay of 27 days, the total number of polio patients being 149; 14,136 individuals visited the outpatient department for a total of 46,403 treatments. Nursing services for the two hospitals totaled 302,982 hours—56,243 hours by staff nurses, 38,783 hours by ward aides, and 207,956 hours by nursing students. In all, 7,384 physical therapy treatments were administered. The hospital laboratories provided 81,044 examinations, including 1,777 surgical specimens in pathology, 11,999 x-ray examinations, and 10,102 treatments in radiology. There were 3,585 operations in surgery and 736 deliveries on obstetrical services.

There were 279 students enrolled in the School of Medicine and 179 in the School of Nursing for the year 1945–46. A significant ruling by the board of regents, apropos of admissions to the University of Oklahoma, was made on November 7, 1945, to wit: "that the Board of Regents instruct the President of the University to refuse to admit anyone of Negro blood as a student of the University for the reason that the laws of the State of Oklahoma prohibit enrollment of such a student in the University."

At a faculty meeting on June 14, Dean Lowry announced that special commencement exercises would be held in the municipal auditorium on June 15, with the Chamber of Commerce assisting in making the arrangements. Dr. Lowry congratulated the fourth-year class, which was asked to attend the faculty meeting, and the student body at large on publication of the yearbook and the *Apex Beat*, a monthly publication by the students of the University of Oklahoma School of Medicine. Then Dr. Lanston addressed the fourth-year class with a few pertinent remarks about the changes confronting them in a world with a social revolution in progress.

> Medical practices have changed from the empiricism of the Dark Ages to a highly technical and scientific profession within sixty-five years, and we cannot hold to the identical practices of even 20 years ago. You are going to be confronted with perplexing problems, not only in diagnosis and treatment, but ethical problems as well. . . . In the practice of medicine, the welfare of the patient is the first consideration and must stand out above every other obligation. If you keep this thought in mind you will make no errors. Not everyone can be a renowned teacher, researcher, surgeon, or internist, but it is within the power of each of you to become a good doctor and attain high standing in your community as an able practitioner of medicine and the most

[3.] The *Eleventh Annual Report*, Oklahoma Commission for Crippled Children, fiscal year 1945–46.

respected citizen in the community, a high standing that carries with it great responsibilities.

Following Dr. Langston's remarks, 69 men and three women—members of the class of 1945—stood, and with right hands upraised, repeated the *Sponsio Academica* in unison with the dean, as Jaundice, the students' mascot, stood by with a proper "solemn" demeanor.

The commencement exercises and the commissioning formalities were held as scheduled on the following evening in an impressive ceremony, with Major General George F. Lull, assistant surgeon general, U.S. Army, as guest speaker.[4] Major General Lull, wearer of the Purple Heart for wounds in action, spoke on the wartime progress of medicine and surgery and "the problems arising from this nation's first mass contact with the dread scourges that afflict the Orient." Army and navy reserve commissions were awarded to 65 graduates before they left for their internships, and 36 nurses received cadet corps certificates.

Major General Raymond S. McLain, in Oklahoma City on a short leave before returning to his commend in Germany, expressed the congratulations of the army to the graduates receiving commissions and appreciation to the community for the excellent training program that was being carried out by the state's School of Medicine—encouraging words to Oklahoma Cityans looking forward to an expansion and enlargement of the School of Medicine located here.

The military program on the Oklahoma City campus of the University of Oklahoma was still active in January when Major Carl E. Anderson inspect Army Student Training Unit No. 3865 and reported that it was one of the best in the nation. There were 168 medical students enrolled in the army program on February 3, and 74 in the navy program. In Dean Lowry's report to the president of the university, May 7, 1945, he stated that there were 66 faculty members, 535 graduates of the School of Medicine, and 13 graduate nurses serving in the armed forces.

The navy program at the School of Medicine ended on October 27, 1945, and all students enrolled under the program were discharged at that time. The United States Nurse Cadet Training Corps was also terminated in October.

As early as June, Dean Lowry announced the appointment of a postwar educational committee for the purpose of making a preliminary study and of outlining a tentative schedule for a one-month postgraduate refresher course to be offered to doctors returning from government services. The School of Medicine commenced this postwar training program on December 3, 1945. The first course was in general medicine, consisting of a total of 134 hours over a period of four weeks, and the second course of similar length began January 7, 1946. This was a course in general surgery and its specialties.

[4.] A colorful musical program preceded the principal address with "a chorus of 350 voices under the direction of James Neilson of Oklahoma City University and the Navy band from Norman."

Tom Lowry, dean of the University of Oklahoma School of Medicine, superintendent of the University Hospitals, and professor of clinical medicine, died at his home on December 11, 1945, at the age of 54. His last appearance at a medical meeting was with his faculty on the previous evening. Therefore, it seems fitting to record here the memorial tributes from the faculty and clinical staff of the hospitals, the students of the School of Medicine, and the regents of the University of Oklahoma.

A resolution drawn up on behalf of the staff of the hospitals and the faculty of the School of Medicine embodied in part, as formulated, these thoughts:[5] that Tom Lowry, our dean and friend, succumbed to a coronary occlusion on December 11, 1945, in the same dramatic way as did his twin brother, Richard Clyde, four years ago; that Dr. Lowry was loved and respected because of his ability in his chosen profession, his sterling qualities as a man, his irreproachable character, his friendly manner, and his religious background; that Dr. Lowry had carried on very much aware of what fate had in store for him, often speaking of his impending doom; and that his fortitude and equanimity were ennobling.

"While these thoughts cannot adequately portray the deep and sincere affection which the faculty had for Dr. Tom," the resolution concluded, "the members of the Faculty of the School of Medicine of the University of Oklahoma treasure the memory of Dr. Tom Lowry who worked with and for us so graciously and unselfishly."

The *Apex Beat* carried an "In Memoriam" feature article on Tom Lowry on the front page of its December 21 issue (Vol. 2, No. 6), with a photograph and this statement: "We, the medical students, will remember this man of courage, ability and humbleness. We will never forget the dean who asked us to call him 'Dr. Tom.' "

And a commemorative acknowledgment of esteem may be found preserved in the minutes of the regents of the University of Oklahoma for January 6, 1946, which reads as follows:

Dr. Thomas Claude Lowry, beloved father, alumnus of the University of Oklahoma, dean of the University Medical School, leader in his profession, patron of civic affairs, and honored citizen of the State of Oklahoma, departed this life in Oklahoma City December 11, 1945, and whereas his life in every respect has been one of earnest devotion to his fellow man and whereas his efforts to advance the cause of medical education have been a constant source of inspiration, now therefore be it resolved that we, the Regents of the University, record permanently our profound respect and admiration for the life and influence of Dr. Lowry, that we manifest our appreciation of the great service he has rendered,

---

[5.] At a meeting of the University Hospital clinical staff on December 21, a motion was made and passed that a resolution in reference to the death of Dean Lowry be drawn up by a committee consisting of Lea Riely, Gregory Stanbro, and Mark Everett.

that we express our deep sense of personal loss on the occasion of his death.

Because the play must go on, the university regents, in session the day following the death of the dean of the School of Medicine, authorized President Cross to approach Wann Langston on the possibility that he would be willing to step into the breach caused by Dr. Lowry's death. And within a week (on December 21), when the regents met in special session in the University Hospital to consider the appointment of a temporary dean of the School of Medicine, President Cross reported that Dr. Langston had agreed to accept the duties of the office at a salary of $500 per month, but that he did not wish to continue in that capacity for any length of time.

Wann Langston, professor of medicine, was appointed dean of the School of Medicine of the University of Oklahoma on December 17, 1945. He was graduated from the University of Oklahoma School of Medicine in 1916, and in 1944 he became professor of medicine and chairman of the Department of Medicine at the University of Oklahoma.[6]

Having appointed a new dean of the School of Medicine, the university regents turned their attention to a new order of business, reinforcing the chain of command in administration of the university by unanimous support of the following resolution:

Resolved that the president of the university be authorized and directed to take such steps as are necessary to require that the conduct of all the affairs of the schools, colleges, and departments of the university requiring approval of this board be submitted to the regents through the president of the university, and further that any public contacts contemplated by any college, school, or department of the university, or their representatives, such as a statement to the press, be made only after submission to and approval of the president of the university.

Progressive legislation in 1945, including appropriation of $1,432,503 for the School of Medicine, was enthusiastically supported by the Oklahoma State Medical Association and the alumni of the School of Medicine. Representative Creekmore Wallace of Oklahoma County and the whole twentieth legislature worked in harmony with Governor Kerr to win favorable action on many of Dean Lowry's recommendations. And Tom Lowry was the first to say that the whole program was due to the foresighted ambitions of Governor Kerr, who wanted the people of Oklahoma to have a health set-up equal to that of any state in the Union.

With the phasing out and actual termination of the military programs on our

---

[6.] In 1918–19, Dr. Langston served with the army—nine months of his service being overseas. After the armistice he remained in the service as a member of the faculty and as an organizer of the Department of Bacteriology at the A.E.F. University, Beaune, France.

campus by the end of October, let us speak briefly of the 21st Evacuation Hospital Unit's overseas service—lest we forget.

It will be recalled that the 21st Evacuation Hospital had been in operation in Bougainville (Solomon Islands) for about ten months before departing for service in the Philippines. The initial landing was at Lingayen Gulf, Luzon Province, on January 11, 1945. Following a short-term bivouac in that area, the hospital unit moved to San Carlos, Pangasinan Province, and "set up shop" in an ancient cathedral that dated back to 1581. "Here, for the first time overseas, we met civilized women; Filipino nurses joined us, and shortly afterward we drew a consignment of American nurses who had been in another hospital in New Guinea."[7]

The hospital had been in operation for about one month in San Carlos— running considerably over its quota of patients—when orders were received to move to Manila which was then under fire. The new hospital site was New Bilibid Prison, about 20 miles southeast of Manila proper. Operation of a hospital commenced immediately with such facilities as were available, and very soon the unit's quota of patients was exceeded three times. "Furthermore, over a period of approximately three months, in addition to operating a hospital with a bed capacity of 2,000 at times, the medical unit also assumed the responsibility of furnishing mess facilities and medical care for about 2,000 civilian internees, rescued from a near-by camp."[8]

The unit closed its station at the New Bilibid Prison on June 2 and moved to the Wack Wack Country Club in the vicinity of Manila, going into bivouac pending the completion of a hospital being constructed by the army engineers. On June 18, Lieutenant Colonel Lawrence B. Hanson assumed command of the unit, replacing Lieutenant Colonel George H. Kimball who had occupied the position only temporarily; and on August 6, 1945, before construction of all of the hospital building was completed, the doors of an installation promising to be "one of the finest of its type in this area" were opened for the reception of patients.

---

[7] Capt. Jim Taylor, M.D., in a letter to Dean Tom Lowry on June 22, 1945.

[8] Lieutenant Colonel Allen G. Gibbs, M.D., "A Brief History of the 21st Evacuation Hospital" (1945).

Chapter X.
Discouraging Problems:
1946–47

Wann Langston was no novice when he became dean of the School of Medicine at a salary of $500 per month. With the exception of two years of military service, he had performed administrative duties of one kind or another at the medical center since 1916. But when he sat in the dean's chair he was like the old woman who lived in a shoe; he had so many problems he knew not what to do. There was a critical shortage of nurses because of inability to pay salaries comparable to those in other institutions; there was criticism of hospital records in a recent audit; there was neither a director for the outpatient department nor a medical director of the hospitals, "much needed as a lieutenant to the dean," and no director of the clinical laboratories, a seemingly unsolvable operational budget problem; and there was a lagging building program.

Meeting with the faculty of the School of Medicine on January 11, President Cross disclosed that the sum of $1,059,000 in capital funds had been belatedly allocated to the School of Medicine and its hospitals by the State Regents for Higher Education for the fiscal year ending June 30, 1946—far short of the approximately $1,679,500 intended by the legislature. President Cross explained that the allocation was in two parts—$247,500 earmarked by the legislature and the remaining $811,500 from the building fund for the entire state system.[1]

Cross assured the medical faculty that he had had no knowledge that the Norman campus had profited at the expense of the School of Medicine, and that he was very much disturbed "that the medical school was coming out on the short end of the appropriations," saying that he was just as interested in one part of the university as in another. Obviously the State Regents for Higher Education agreed with the university regents that there were "other needs of the university that are just as vital as the needs of the medical school."

On February 13, President Cross advised the university regents that the current rate of expenditures at the medical center would result in a deficit at the end of the year and that this situation was, for the most part, due to the fact that

---

[1.] The $811,500 in capital funds was allocated as follows: power plant, laundry, and equipment, $159,575; School of Nursing addition and equipment, $478,720; and additions to University Hospitals, $173,205.

no appropriations had been provided for operation of the South Ward Negro Division of University Hospital, for the operation of the Southern Oklahoma Hospital, or for the purchase of penicillin, the new effective antibiotic for curing infectious disease. Whereupon, President Cross was instructed by the regents to advise Dr. Langston and his administrative staff that immediate steps would have to be taken to restrict expenditures to the available funds because of the constitutional prohibition against incurring deficits, even if restriction of expenditures resulted in limitation of services in the hospitals.

Frustrated by the rejoinder from the president and the regents that the only solution to the problem of the budget was to limit services (reduce the bed capacity for a period of three months at least) Dean Langston wrote to Governor Robert S. Kerr on March 27 informing him that there was an emergency situation caused by an inadequate operational budget, and that closing the hospitals would amount to a catastrophe.

Two days later there was a special called meeting of the university regents in the Skirvin Tower Hotel, at which time the financial difficulties of the University Hospitals were discussed at length and with some concern. The regents finally resolved that the Oklahoma State Regents for Higher Education should be requested "to make a supplementary allocation of $85,000 for salary and maintenance, including University Hospital, Crippled Children's Hospital, and the Southern Oklahoma Hospital, for the remainder of the fiscal year, and that in the event the State Regents have no funds out of which to make a supplemental allocation, that they should request the governor for an allocation of funds from his contingency fund for the aforesaid purposes." And by April 10, $85,000 from the governor's emergency fund had been allocated to the University Hospitals by the State Regents for Higher Education, making it possible to carry on for the remainder of the year 1945–46.

While regulations and bylaws for the University Hospitals had existed before 1946, Dr. Langston said that these rules were for type-three hospitals of the American College of Surgeons, and early in 1946 he had expressed the need for formally adopted bylaws for the staff of the hospitals. He appointed a committee to propose a revision of the former rules and regulations. On February 29 new "Bylaws, Rules and Regulations for the Organization and Conduct of the Staff of the University Hospitals and the School of Medicine of the University of Oklahoma" were signed by Wann Langston, dean, and Paul H. Fesler, administrator, and adopted by the staff of the University Hospitals on March 8, 1946. A supplement, "Negro Division Rules and Regulations," was approved and adopted by the hospital board and the staff of the University Hospitals on February 20 and March 8, respectively.

The holdover advisory committee to the dean from Dr. Lowry's administration took action on January 2 to terminate the accelerated teaching program of the School of Medicine (in operation since September, 1942) on March 22, the day set for commencement exercises in Oklahoma City. The faculty followed this action on January 11 by voting a return to the normal university calendar year beginning the next scholastic term on September 16, 1946.

Meeting for the first time on March 21, a reorganized advisory committee recommended that certain beds be allocated for private patients at the University Hospitals; that annual reports be sent to the dean from each department of the School of Medicine; and that an honor system for examinations, on petition of the student council, be instituted in September when the new class entered the School of Medicine.

A faculty meeting was held the same evening, as customary preceding the day for commencement exercises, and on this particular occasion Dr. Langston very graciously conceded that much of the legwork for the administration was being done by the assistant dean, Dr. Shoemaker, "including preparation of a brief history of the oath, *Sponsio Academica.*"

With the fiscal year winding down, be it ever so precariously, the search for a permanent dean continued, and on May 25 we find Dr. Langston writing to President Cross:

> I am aware of, and greatly appreciate, the attitude expressed by the committee of Heads of Clinical Departments toward my continuing in the deanship. I told them that I had accepted the deanship on a temporary basis and that, around the first of March, I had asked you to be prepared to relieve me on the first of July. . . . I do not want you to consider me a candidate for the position.
>
> There are a great number of problems, some of them extremely delicate, awaiting solution. The solution of these problems must bring distressing repercussions. Since I am not continuing in the position of Dean, I will not tackle some of these problems because I must live among these people.[2]

Dean Langston hung on a while longer, and on his recommendation President Cross appointed a planning committee for the School of Medicine. But the outlook was bleak in the face of another deficient budget for the fiscal year 1946–47, as allocated by the State Regents for Higher Education. The University of Oklahoma was assigned $1,695,517 out of a total income of $5,865,427; the School of Medicine, $211,714 (total income $302,083), and the University Hospitals, $993,938 (total income $1,231,746, not including $306,641 in capital funds).

On July 10 of the new fiscal year President Cross reported to the regents that financial problems continued to plague the University Hospitals as outlined in a letter from Dean Langston and Paul Fesler, in which the dean stated that the budget for the year 1946–47 had been made on the assumption that additional funds would be made available from the governor's contingency fund. With that understanding, the dean revealed, he had requested the State Regents for Higher Education for an allocation in the amount of $138,444 to cover the

[2] For example, it fell to Dr. Langston's lot to write all full-time members of the clinical faculty in June that they were to have no consultation privileges on private patients in the University Hospitals.

period from July 1 to December 31, 1946, for operation and maintenance of the University Hospitals. The university regents realizing that the appropriations which were made previously were totally inadequate in the face of increasing costs of hospital supplies, employment of personnel, and general operational expenses, passed a resolution approving the request for the additional funds from the State Regents for Higher Education.

In accordance with recommendations submitted in the agenda, Dr. Cross next presented the name of Jacques Pierce Gray for the position of dean of the School of Medicine. Following discussion, Oscar White (who had been appointed to the university regents in April) made the motion, seconded by Mr. Emery, that Dr. Gray be appointed dean of the School of Medicine at an annual salary of $10,000 effective on the date of his arrival in Oklahoma City. This motion passed unanimously.

Important staff changes also occurred during the year. For one thing, several doctors on military leave of absence returned from the service, namely, Lee K. Emenhiser, Hervey Foerster, Onis Hazel, Robert Noell, John W. Records, and Howard Shorbe. H. Thompson Avey, director of the outpatient department, resigned on July 31, 1946, creating a pressing need, although he did reamin as assistant professor of medicine; in February Robert C. Lowe, acting director of the outpatient clinics, became a full-time assistant professor of medicine at a salary of $5,000 per year; Albert Foster, professor of anesthesiology and chairman of the department, resigned his post effective November 1, 1946; Basil A. Hayes was appointed chairman of the Department of Urology for the year ending June 30, 1947, during the absence of Rex Bolend. New appointments for 1946–47 in the following tabulation, included the assignment of academic rank to Dean Gray:[3]

Jacques Pierce Gray, M.D.
  professor of public health medicine, dean and superintendent
Robert Chester Lowe, M.D.
  associate professor of medicine, director of the outpatient department
David Von Brown, M.D.
  assistant professor of pathology
Alice M. Brues, Ph.D.
  assistant professor of anatomy
Zola Katherine Cooper, Ph.D.
  assistant professor of histology and embryology
Jack Milowsky, M.D.
  assistant professor of anesthesiology

John William Shackleford, M.D.
  assistant professor of preventive medicine and public health
Robert Douglas Anspaugh, M.D.
  associate in obstetrics and gynecology
Porteous Elmore Johnson, M.D.
  associate in orthopedic surgery
Margaret Dewar, R.N.
  teaching superintendent, operating room technique
Barbara Amdell Battles, R.N., B.S.
  instructor in communicable disease nursing

[3.] President Cross was authorized by the regents of the university in May to relax, temporarily, their previous ruling prohibiting employment of relatives and to revise it to read that ''no one related within the third degree be appointed to any position in which tenure is contemplated.''

Ruby Blakely, R.N.
  instructor in operating room
  technique
Ardell Benton Colyar, M.D.
  instructor in preventive medicine
  and public health
Margaret S. Hamburger, R.N., B.S.
  instructor in pediatrics
Effie Hughes, R.N.
  instructor in medical nursing
Willard Van Voorhis Thompson,
  M.D.
  instructor in medical jurisprudence
Bonnie L. Trinque, R.N.
  instructor in communicable diseases
Maxine Turner, M.S.
  instructor in preventive medicine
  and public health
William Howard Atkins, M.D.
  clinical assistant in medicine
Nasry Fayad Vander Barkett, M.D.
  assistant in surgery
Ben Bell, M.D.
  clinical assistant in psychiatry and
  neurology
Charles Max Bielstein, M.D.
  clinical assistant in pediatrics
Adolph Ebner Blatt, M.D.
  clinical assistant in medicine
George Sam Bozalis, M.D.
  clinical assistant in medicine
Harold W. Buchner, M.D.
  clinical assistant in pediatrics
John Richard Danstrom, M.D.
  clinical assistant in radiology
Louis Raynor Devanney, M.D.
  clinical assistant in surgery
Reba Huff Edwards, M.D.
  clinical assistant in medicine
Leon Ferber, M.D.
  clinical assistant in psychiatry and
  neurology
Phyllis Emmaline Jones, M.D.
  clinical assistant in dermatology and
  syphilology
Jordon Albert Kelling, M.D.
  clinical assistant in psychiatry and
  neurology

Robert Farris Loughmiller, M.D.
  clinical assistant in
  otorhinolaryngology
Elias Margo, M.D.
  clinical assistant in orthopedic
  surgery
Maude Merle Masterson, M.D.
  clinical assistant in medicine
Coye Willard McClure, M.D.
  clinical assistant in ophthalmology
James R. Miller, D.D.S.
  clinical assistant in dental surgery
Henry Clinton Morrison, M.D.
  clinical assistant in obstetrics
Roy Lawrence Neel, M.D.
  clinical assistant in
  otorhinolaryngology
Joe Marion Parker, M.D.
  clinical assistant in surgery
James Ira Payte, M.D.
  clinical assistant in medicine
James Ralph Ricks, Jr., M.D.
  clinical assistant in medicine
Elmer Ridgeway, Jr., M.D.
  clinical assistant in medicine
Charles Abraham Royer, M.D.
  clinical assistant in ophthalmology
Welborn Ward Sanger, M.D.
  clinical assistant in ophthalmology
Samuel Newton Stone, M.D.
  clinical assistant in surgery
Robert Theodore Sturm, M.D.
  clinical assistant in surgery
Lawrence McCoy Williamson, M.D.
  clinical assistant in
  otorhinolaryngology
Charles Hugh Wilson, M.D.
  clinical assistant in surgery
Andrew Merriman Young, III, M.D.
  clinical assistant in urology
Paul Martin Darden, M.D.
  graduate fellow in pharmacology
Ellen Corine Keaty, Ph.D.
  research fellow in pharmacology
John Barnhart Morey, M.D.
  visiting lecturer in medicine
Harold G. Muchmore, M.D.
  graduate fellow in pharmacology

James Leonidis Nicholson, M.D.
  visiting lecturer in preventive
  medicine and public health
Richard Weston Payne, M.D.
  graduate fellow in pharmacology

William Milton Prier, M.D.
  fellow in pathology
Marvin Ray Shetlar, Ph.D.
  research associate in biochemistry
A. Martyne Woods, R.N.
  acting instructor in nursing arts

Robert H. Bayley, vice-chairman of the Department of Medicine and an investigator of considerable stature, received a grant of $28,000 from the United States Public Health Service to carry on electrocardiographic research during 1946–47; and Dean Langston granted Dr. Bayley permission to collect fees for his electrocardiographic work in conjunction with private patients in the University Hospitals.

The real push for research at the medical center, however, continued to be sponsored by the alumni who were very interested in developing a foundation which would supply the medical center with a much-needed research facility. Action directed at achieving such an objective crystallized in August, 1946, with the establishment of the Oklahoma Medical Research Foundation incorporated under the laws of the state of Oklahoma.

The question of allocating part of the School of Medicine campus for a research institute and cancer hospital building was brought before the university regents by President Cross on August 14. Dr. Cross stated that the park board of Oklahoma City had been advised that block 11, Sixth State Capitol Addition, formerly belonging to Oklahoma City, now belonged to the state of Oklahoma, and that the request from the alumni was for acquisition of that particular portion of land immediately adjacent to the School of Medicine building at 801 N.E. 13th Street. The consensus of the regents was that the proximity of a research facility to the heart of the medical center would enhance the efficiency of the teaching staff engaged in research activities, and they passed a resolution recommending to the State Board of Affairs that the above described tract of land be allocated to the Oklahoma Medical Research Institute. In the resolution, the board commented on its enthusiastic support of the objective and purposes expressed in the articles of incorporation of the research institute and hospital, and later Regent Noble asked that each member of the board be furnished with a copy of the bylaws of the articles of incorporation. It is of note that the American Cancer Society granted a total of $189,879 for research at the University of Oklahoma medical center over a period of five years, 1946 to 1951 inclusive.

On October 14 also, Howard Dickey, chief clerk in the University Hospital, requested approval by the regents of an application for the hospital to become a member in the Blue Cross Hospital Service, and approval of the application was granted. About this time, one senses a bit of uneasiness on the part of the dean regarding Paul Fesler, administrator of University Hospitals. For one thing, Mr. Dickey was put in complete control of the budget in April, and there are other references in the dean's files to the diminishing responsibilities of Mr. Fesler.[4]

Meanwhile, in an exchange of letters between Dean Langston and Jacques P. Gray, dean designate, we sense a note of despair rather than encouragement in Dr. Langston's responses. "I think the most pressing problem connected with the Institution," he wrote on August 23, "is the selection of a medical director for the hospital and the outpatient department at the earliest possible moment. I think the situation is critical. It seems to me that the work in these institutions is becoming more and more disorganized." And on August 30, Dr. Langston wrote,

> During the early months of my administration, I found a $100,000 deficit for the year, and the nursing situation became so short, because of our inability to pay adequate salaries, that it was necessary to close certain wards at both the University and Children's Hospitals. I was able to go to the Governor and secure $85,000 to complete the fiscal year with the understanding that we will reopen the wards that have been closed. Now that has not been done. . . . Everywhere I have turned, I have been met by the stone wall of a shortage of nurses (mentioned as early as December, 1941 by Dean Patterson).

When the faculty of the School of Medicine convened on September 5, with Jacques P. Gray and Harold A. Shoemaker present, President Cross opened the meeting by saying that the death of Dean Lowry had created a real crisis for the School of Medicine which seemed insurmountable until Dr. Langston agreed to help. "When I first asked him if he would help," Dr. Cross said, "he made some laughing remark about finances but he has been magnificient. . . . I feel the Faculty of the School of Medicine appreciates all his very fine efforts."

Dr. Cross then introduced Jacques P. Gray as "your new dean" and Dr. Gray replied that, though he had been in Oklahoma City but a short while, he found himself "already so deep in things that I now have to reach up to touch bottom."

One of the new dean's first disillusionments was to learn that the School of Medicine of the University of Oklahoma was on unpublished probation. Dean Gray stated that he had learned more or less by accident several weeks after assuming the post of dean that the Council on Medical Education and Hospitals had placed the school on tacit probation early in 1936 after a 1935 inspection; that in response to certain admonitions in the report, the next entering class of students had been reduced from 77 to 65; and that adequate financial provision was still a big must. Dean Gray said he was not aware of a letter from Dr. Weiskotten under date of February 22, 1943, mentioning the probationary status of the school, nor could he find any official reply in the file. Neither could

[4.] Howard Dickey later resigned as chief clerk of the School of Medicine and University Hospitals effective January 1, 1947.

he find the 1936 survey report (although there is now in the file a complete copy of the survey committee's report). However, upon inquiry, Dean Gray did receive a letter from Victor Johnson, secretary of the Council on Medical Education and Hospitals, verifying the authenticity of such a survey report and the fact that the School of Medicine "had been placed on confidential probation in 1936."

When Dean Gray first met the faculty on September 5, Dr. Shoemaker attempted to explain that a delay in the building program was occasioned by the necessity of trying to obtain federal aid, and that the ensuing months of deferment had resulted in increased building costs. However, the building program must have been under way by December 14, when Dean Gray advised President Cross that an oil well, which had not been producing for some time, directly east of the University Hospital, "was in the way of new construction" and that the Sun-Ray Oil Company had been requested to "plug the well, remove the derrick and all other structures."

At the same time (on September 5) the faculty abolished the academic titles of assistant and associate for clinical staff members (created during the administration of General Patterson); and three volunteer members of the clinical staff, Doctors Keltz, Jacobs, and Garrison, who had carried the load of the clerkships in the hospitals during the war emergency, asked to be relieved of those responsibilities. This was understandable, for the whole clerkship program was due for expansion under the newly improved curriculum as an integral part of the respective clinical departments. Moreover, instruction in the outpatient department (with the exception of obstetrics, gynecology and surgery) was being shifted from the third to the fourth year.

Advanced biochemistry and physiology were no longer included in the clinical curriculum, and the Departments of Physiology and Pharmacology were combined under one chairman at the beginning of the 1946 fall semester, because the two departments dealt with closely related subjects. It was the opinion of President Cross and Dean Gray that such a combination was not only feasible but would be conducive to the efficiency of both departments and an advantage economically.

Qualification for a Bachelor of Science degree in medical technology, following three years in the College of Arts and Sciences at Norman and 12 months of special laboratory instruction in University Hospitals, was authorized by the university regents in April, 1946.[5] Béla Halpert was director of the course.

Residencies in plastic surgery, neurosurgery, and urology in University Hospitals were approved by the Council on Medical Education during the year.

According to Dean Gray's report to the regents, 1946–47, there were, during the year, 492 employees in the University Hospitals; 366 available beds; 4,801

[5.] For development of the program over a period of years, see pages 74–75 and 82. St. Anthony Hospital in Oklahoma City and St. John's Hospital in Tulsa were approved for the training of clinical laboratory technicians in 1946.

admissions to University Hospital with an average stay of sixteen and one-half days; 45,866 visits in the outpatient clinics; 96,876 tests performed in the laboratories; 204 available beds in Children's Hospital; and, according to the Oklahoma Crippled Children's Commission report, 2,143 admissions (in spite of the closing of 35 beds), with an average patient stay of 30 days. Polio cases totaled 221, with the National Foundation for Infantile Paralysis contributing $15,000 toward the care of these unfortunate children. A new service program for children was the establishment of a hearing service clinic on the north campus in Norman by John W. Keys of the University of Oklahoma Department of Speech.

Of the total expenses for the medical center, $447,075 were for nursing services and $29,802 for nursing education. There were 140 students enrolled in the School of Nursing and 291 in the School of Medicine in 1946–47, with 69 graduates receiving the M.D. degree and 56 students receiving the Graduate Nurse certificate in 1946.

A larger number of applications were received for entrance to the School of Medicine in Spetember, 1946, than in any of the nine preceding years. Inasmuch as this was the first class to return to the decelerated program, a responsibility to veterans and to the residents of Oklahoma was taken into consideration by the admissions committee. Consequently, every one of the 85 members of the first-year class was an Oklahoman and 69 were veterans. Out of a total enrollment of 291, including ten graduate students, 111 were veterans. Graduate courses were offered in the medical sciences—anatomy, bacteriology and parasitology, biochemistry, histology and embryology, pathology, and in pharmacology and physiology.

The School of Nursing offered both a three-month and a six-month course in pediatric nursing to students in affiliated nursing schools in 1946–47. Basic courses were taught by members of the faculty of the School of Medicine; lectures and classes in the various specialty fields of clinical medicine were conducted by members of the resident and visiting staff of the University Hospitals; and instruction in nutrition and diet therapy was given by the dietary staff under the direction of Vera Parman.

In the official file may be found a citation from the Armed Service Forces, Office of the Surgeon General, dated 20 February 1946, which reads as follows:

It is with a great deal of pleasure that we forward to you the enclosed Certificate of Appreciation as a token of our gratitude for your patriotic contribution to the successful prosecution of World War II. The excellent cooperation which we received from the University of Oklahoma and the outstanding service which was rendered by the 21st Evacuation Hospital contributed materially to the exceptional record of the Medical Department. It is with great pride that we record these compliments as a part of the history of the Army Medical Department.

/S/ Norman T. Kirk, Major General, The Surgeon General

A similar commendation was received from the Surgeon General, U.S. Navy, Rear Admiral C. A. Swanson (MC) on January 22, 1948.

At the request of the Veterans Administration early in 1946, a dean's committee was formed at the medical school to cooperate with the Veterans Administration in developing plans for staffing a veterans' general hospital at Will Rogers Field, although no official announcement had been made by the Veterans Administration. Members of the committee were: Wann Langston, dean, H. A. Shoemaker, assistant dean, R. H. Bayley, vice-chairman Department of Medicine, C. E. Clymer, chairman Department of Surgery, and W. K. West, chairman Department of Orthopedic Surgery.

A preliminary program for participation in medical education by the Veterans Administration had been initiated in 1944 under the guidance of General Omar N. Bradley and Dr. Paul R. Hawley, who endeavored to develop standards for affiliation of as many veterans' hospitals as possible with medical schools throughout the country. Almost at once, a committee of the Oklahoma City Chamber of Commerce and several members of the faculty of the School of Medicine—foreseeing a reciprocal benefit for the service programs of the Veterans Administration and the medical training programs of both a veterans' hospital and the medical school—requested the establishment of such a hospital in Oklahoma City.

However, under a change of administration in 1945, with General Carl R. Gray, Jr., administrator, and Paul B. Magnuson, medical director, the whole veterans' hospital program became a shambles. The projection for teaching beds had been unrealistic, and, though Dr. Magnuson made every effort to continue the program as originally outlined, he soon realized he had inherited a medical director's nightmare. Physicians and medical schools, with a growing sense of uneasiness and distrust, began rebelling against the program instead of courting it because of the low standards of medical care which were in no small measure attributable to outmoded, rigid, insular, and completely uninspired principles of medical administration.

New life was given to the cooperative plan on January 3, 1946, when the Eightieth Congress passed Public Law 239. Under the terms of this law medical care of the American veteran and programs of research and education were assured. The most important element in the enlistment of the cooperation of the medical schools was the initiation of dean's committee administrative bodies. This was a unique operation wherein the executive branch of the United States government and the institutions of learning worked together harmoniously, without any contracts being required on either side. The terms of reference in this interesting relationship were set forth in Policy Memorandum No. 2 of the above law, to wit: the dean's committee was to be composed of the dean of the participating medical school and chiefs of the major clinical departments, with such representation from the laboratories and basic sciences as might be desired. This committee was charged with the supervision of the educational and research programs; but it also had a very important relationship to the quality of the medical care and was responsible for the nomination of all members of the medical staff to the manager of the veterans' hospital. In most instances such staff members, acceptable to the chiefs of respective services and to management, were utilized for instruction not only within the Veterans Administration Hospital but also in the medical school itself.

Dean Langston outlined the plan of the newly formed dean's committee to the faculty on March 21 assuring those present that, in order to preserve the teaching structure of the School of Medicine, the Veterans Administration had agreed to a system whereby alternate teams of consulting physicians would be exchanged every six months in order to correspond with the semesters of the School of Medicine.

Will Rogers Memorial Hospital, Will Rogers Base, Oklahoma City, was used temporarily as a veterans' general hospital, and faculty members who were veterans became the attending staff, with Dr. Langston as chief of staff and Dr. Clarence Bates as administrator.

On September 11, President Cross revealed that construction of a 1,000-bed hospital in Oklahoma City was under consideration by the federal government, and that government officials had already made inquiries about land east of the School of Medicine building.

Dr. E. H. Cushing, assistant chief medical director of Veterans Hospitals for Research and Education, Washington, D.C., was unfalteringly helpful during the year, and early in December a listing of Veterans Administration hospitals with residency training programs included the "Will Rogers Station Hospital" in Oklahoma City, with Jacques P. Gray as chairman of the dean's committee.

When Robert S. Kerr became governor of the state of Oklahoma in 1943 there was a state indebtedness of $37,000,000, but, owing to his administrative skills, Oklahoma was free of debt when he left office. And the School of Medicine—though still gasping—was better situated in some respects than other state institutions.

The school year 1946–47 was, in fact, an uphill year in many ways for the School of Medicine, beset by administrative and financial uncertainties month after month after month that would have tried the patience of Job. But Wann Langston, administrator, teacher, and physician, met the exigencies with courage and concerned compassion, at a time when the school was dependent on the free services of his peers in private practice for its clinical teaching program.

There were two significant occurrences on the plus side during the year, the establishment by the alumni association of the Oklahoma Medical Research Foundation, and the cooperation of the medical profession in setting up a Veterans Administration Hospital in Oklahoma City. Proposals for building a city-county hospital were floating around, too, only to disseminate in thin air until some future resurrection.

A state mental health board was established under the guidance of Charles A. Smith, succeeded later by A. A. Hellams, who was in turn succeeded by Director Charles F. Obermann. Furthermore, Floyd Keller worked on legislation presaging passage of a state medical examiner law during the administration of incoming Governor Roy J. Turner.

Jacques P. Gray, who became dean on September 1, 1946, soon found himself "so deep in things" that he had "to reach up to touch bottom," and there is little question but that he had accepted the appointment as dean on the basis of some false impressions in regard to available appropriations and public and professional interest in medical care and medical education.

"The impression was given and accepted," Dean Gray wrote in his 1946–47 report to the president of the university, "that with high interest and enthusiasm for the School and Hospitals, with an awakened and developed interest on the part of the populace, of the profession, and of the legislature, and with surplus incomes from taxes in the State Treasury, now was the time to request funds for essential needs for the Schools and Hospitals. It was even stated that 'It is now or not again for a long time.' " So Dr. Gray took up the gauntlet only to learn that he was too disenchanted for combat.

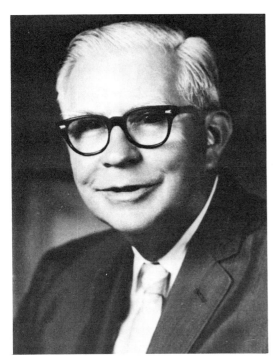

John F. Burton, M.D.,
professor of surgery.

*Courtesy University of
Oklahoma Medical Center*

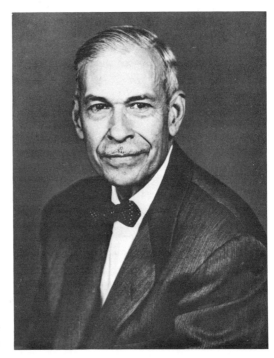

George H. Garrison, M.D.,
clinical professor of
pediatrics.

*Courtesy University of
Oklahoma Medical Center*

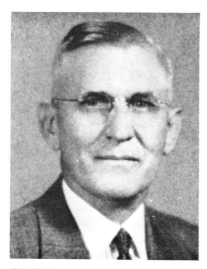

Emil R. Kraettli, secretary of the
University of Oklahoma.

*Courtesy University of Oklahoma
Medical Center*

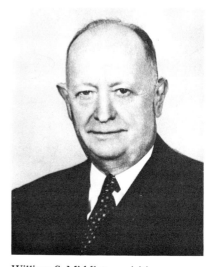

William S. Middleton, visiting
professor of medicine.

*Courtesy University of Oklahoma
Medical Center*

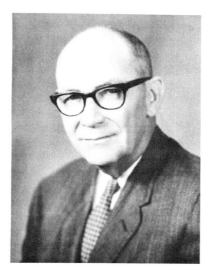

Ben H. Nicholson, M.D., clinical
professor of pediatrics.

Courtesy Commentary

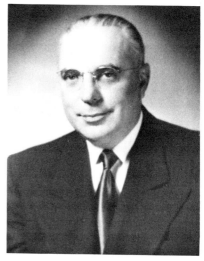

Hugh G. Payne, executive vice-
president of the Oklahoma Medical
Research Foundation.

*Courtesy University of Oklahoma
Medical Center*

126

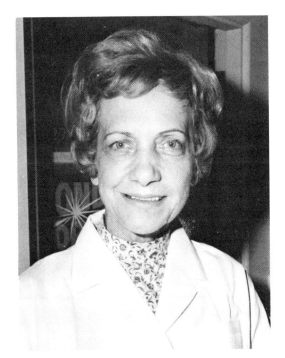

Thelma Pedersen, M.A., director of the School of
Physical Therapy.

Courtesy Sooner Medic

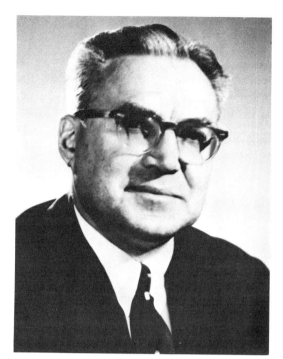

Lawrence W. Rember,
LL.B., secretary of the
Alumni Association of the
University of Oklahoma
School of Medicine.

*Courtesy University of
Oklahoma Medical Center*

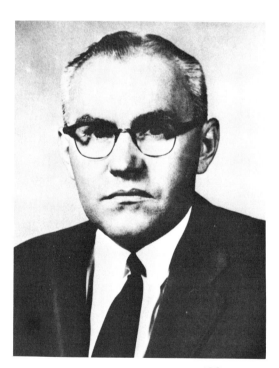

Oren T. Skouge, M.D.,
manager of the Veterans
Administration Hospital.

*Courtesy University of
Oklahoma Medical Center*

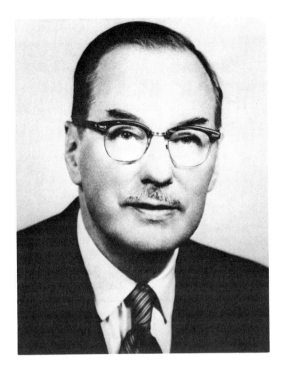

Harry Wilkins, M.D.,
professor of surgery.

*Courtesy University of
Oklahoma Medical Center*

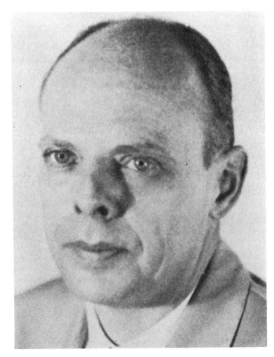

Bert F. Keltz, M.D.,
director of the Outpatient
Department, 1933–35.

*Courtesy Oklahoma City
Academy of Medicine*

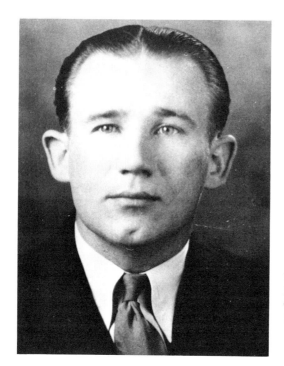

Wayne McKinley Hull,
M.D., director of the
Outpatient Department,
1935–37.

*Courtesy State Board of
Medical Examiners*

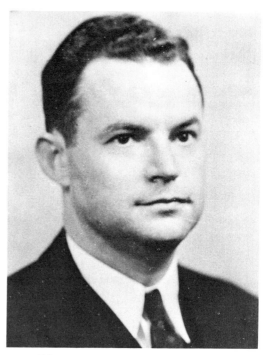

Owen Royce, Jr., M.D.,
director of the Outpatient
Department, 1940–41.

*Courtesy State Board of
Medical Examiners*

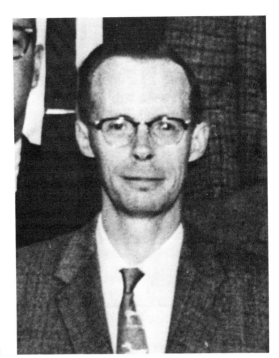

Harry Thompson Avey, Jr.,
M.D., director of the Outpatient Department,
1942–46.

Courtesy Sooner Medic

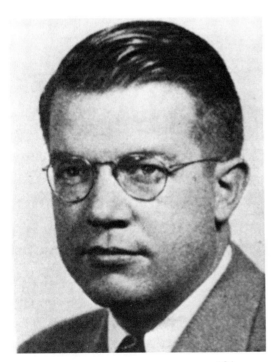

Harold G. Muchmore,
M.D., acting director of the
Outpatient Department,
1949–52.

Courtesy Sooner Medic

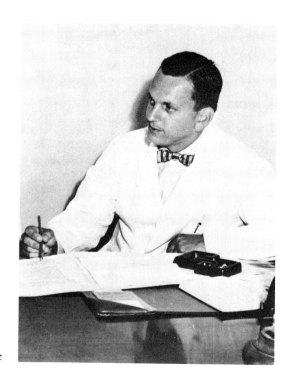

John P. Colmore, M.D.,
director of the Outpatient
Department, 1952–61.

Courtesy Sooner Medic

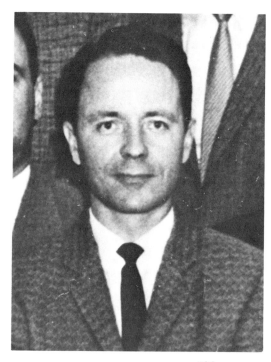

Carl W. Smith, M.D.,
director of the Outpatient
Department, 1961–(64).

Courtesy Sooner Medic

Chapter XI.
The Grey Year:
1947–48

 Roy J. Turner, veteran of World War I, was the second native son to be elected to the state's highest office. He was born on the claim his father staked in the "Run," learned accounting, worked at several different jobs, prospered in the oil business, and took up ranching as a lucrative sideline. And he encouraged young people in farm clubs to raise livestock by selling good stock to them at fifty dollars a head. According to some of his friends, Governor Turner was "slow in decision, not deciding a question until the last half of the ninth inning with two out and two strikes on the batter; but when he did, the decision stuck."[1]

The twenty-first legislature (with James C. Nance president pro tempore of the senate and C. R. Board speaker of the house) formed an organization very early in the session that was friendly to Governor Turner and his institutional building program. A referendum for a $36,000,000 bond issue for colleges and universities across the board, endorsed by the legislature, was later approved by the voters. The people also voted approval of a recommendation by former Governor Kerr that the University of Oklahoma and Oklahoma State University regents be removed from politics by extending their terms to seven years with "dismissal for cause only."

In a gesture toward an expanding medical center, the legislature authorized the conveyance of a portion of land available at the site of the School of Medicine (a parcel 250 feet wide on N. E. Thirteenth Street and 300 feet deep immediately adjacent to and east of the school) to the Oklahoma Medical Research Foundation, in order that the foundation might have complete control over its facility and get off to a successful beginning.

Similarly, legislation was passed authorizing the conveyance of nine acres (the major portion of the plot of ground east of the school and north of N.E. Thirteenth Street) to the Veterans Administration of the United States government as the site of a proposed 1,000-bed VA Hospital to replace the Will Rogers Memorial Veterans Administration Hospital located at Will Rogers Field. This

---

[1.] Angie Debo, *Oklahoma: Foot-Loose and Fancy-Free* (Norman, University of Oklahoma Press, 1949), 51, 87.

$15,000,000 to $18,000,000 structure was scheduled for erection during the 1947–49 biennium.

However, with the second half of the fiscal year 1946–47 scarcely begun, the University Hospital was still operating in the red. So the university regents adopted a resolution on January 8 requesting a deficiency appropriation of $138,444 from the governor's contingency fund—via the State Regents for Higher Education—to cover the last six months of 1946–47.

The state regents, meanwhile, had made their customary reduction in the budget requests for the medical center in its recommendation to the legislature, which resulted in $320,822 for the year 1947–48 and $290,613 for the year 1948–49—very drastic reductions from the amounts submitted by the university regents as necessary for operational expenses. So on February 13 the university regents unanimously adopted a resolution requesting the state regents to revise and reinstate the items and amounts deducted for the next biennium, advising them that the School of Medicine had been on a probational status for some time because of inadequate facilities and that the American Medical Association had stated publicly that a survey of American Schools of Medicine would be made in 1947 and that the School of Medicine of the University of Oklahoma could not continue to function either on a probational basis or unapproved status.

With his request for improved facilities in the amount of $4,650,000 cut to the bone, Dean Gray declared to members of the faculty on January 30, "If the state regents' recommendations for appropriations are to be the basis for improvement, then plans should be made for the discontinuation of the School of Medicine, the School of Nursing, and the University Hospitals. . . . Unless there is adequate financial support, Oklahoma had better not attempt to stay in the field of medical education." And he further stated that he felt the time had come very definitely when there must be a showdown on the budget; that he had told Mell Nash, chancellor of the State Board of Higher Regents, he doubted that we could meet the standards of the Council on Medical Education.

Wann Langston; dean emeritus of the School of Medicine, then rose to the occasion,

> I should like to go on record here and now as to what I think our attitude should be. I have given much time and study to this situation. For a third of a century the faculty has begged for money to run this school. And, at the same time, we the clinical faculty have donated each year, in free service, an amount equal to the appropriated amount for this school. We ought not to have to make this fight for money to run our school. We should let them know we are not prepared to make any compromises and I suggest that the faculty go on record as not being prepared to accept any reduction in our request for financial support for the School of Medicine; that we believe the budgetary requests as made and approved by the University Regents are conservative and reasonable requests to the State Regents, and that they merit respect as the basis of

appropriations and allocations. . . . We cannot continue the school even at its present size with inadequate support.[2]

Several faculty members expressed the opinion that an effort might be made to create an interest in the School of Medicine among legislators, especially those on the appropriations committee, inasmuch as the alumni, the Oklahoma Medical Research Foundation, the Oklahoma State Medical Association and the Oklahoma City Chamber of Commerce were all interested in seeing adequate funds made available for the medical school. But at this point Dean Gray counseled, "Gentlemen, I must remind you that we are in a faculty meeting and we cannot take action, or enter into any political arrangement and I must rule you out of order."

Dean Gray was thwarted on another issue by the state regents when he championed a degree program leading to the Bachelor of Science degree for the School of Nursing "under the College of Medicine," which had been unanimously approved by the university regents. But the state regents refused to designate the School of Medicine as the "College of Medicine," with the School of Nursing "organized under it," even though financial support for the School of Nursing had been taken out of the hospitals' budget and set up as an autonomous item. This fact was brought out in a presentation to the State Regents for Higher Education, but, unbelievable as it may seem, there was no provision at all for the School of Nursing in the recommendations for higher education by the state regents. Small wonder that their board was a thorn in Dean Gray's side that nettled him continously.

"There is serious doubt as to whether the real needs in medical care, medical research, and medical education in Oklahoma are realized, or appreciated, or understood," he wrote to President Cross on May 6. "Until these are understood . . . the attempt probably will be made to continue in status quo, a policy which can lead only to correction at a later date or discontinuation of the school. . . . already, the exodus of members of the faculties, both in medicine and in nursing, has begun."

In May also, Dean Gray sent a memorandum to the members of the alumni association emphasizing the fact that he had not known about the unpublished probationary status of the School of Medicine when he assumed the deanship, and that the recurring deficiency appropriations were discouraging to say the least. "The establishment of the Research Institute, in itself, will not save the School," he said, "but it will play an important role in enhancing the status of the school locally and nationally, as a regional source for medical investigation."

Dean Gray gradually developed a sort of phobia about not having been informed of the unpublished probationary status of the School of Medicine in

---

[2] This statement was unanimously approved as an expression from the faculty to be sent to the president, the Board of Regents of the University, the Oklahoma State Regents for Higher Education, and the legislature.

1936 and again in 1943. He introduced the subject again and again, always saying, ''I did not know of the probationary status of the school when I came to Oklahoma.'' On one occasion he said to the faculty, ''I learned of it in October, 1946. . . . Dr. Langston assumed that the President would inform me and discuss this situation with me, and Dr. Cross assumed that Dr. Langston had told me.''

Inevitably, little by little, rather severe criticism was leveled at the dean for his suggestion that ''if medical education is not adequately supported, it would be better to close the school.'' An alternative to closing the school, which developed in hearings before the appropriations committee but was extremely unpopular with the State Regents for Higher Education and with members of the legislature, called for a reduction in the size of the entering classes in order to achieve a more favorable student-faculty ratio, with the incumbent dean recommending that the entering class be limited to 52. The Regents of the university finally limited the size of the class entering the School of Medicine in Setpember of 1947 to not less than 64 students, with the state regents favoring many more. In the end 66 applicants were admitted—all of them residents of Oklahoma.

Obviously, Dean Gray was fed up, disgusted, and frustrated by a succession of unsurmountable obstacles when he wrote in June, ''It is, indeed, a discouraging future that presents itself for the School of Medicine of the University of Oklahoma and University Hospitals under conditions which have obtained, which obtain at present, and which will obtain for the biennium of 1947–49, possibly for a longer period.''

Notwithstanding the grim appraisal by Dean Gray, the establishment of a speech and hearing clinic on the medical center campus showed signs of becoming a reality in May, when the regents authorized an expenditure of $2,500 from the revolving fund of the School of Medicine to remodel a portion of the ground floor in the east wing of the Oklahoma Hospital for Crippled Children as quarters for the clinic. In addition, an unearmarked contribution of like amount was granted by the regents; and District No. 124 of Rotary International made $3,000 available for purchase of equipment for a speech and hearing clinic. Furthermore, the Oklahoma Commission for Crippled Children agreed to support the new program on an annual basis. John W. Keys was designated director of the hearing clinic, and Carl Ritzman was director of speech correction.

Early in June a contract was let for a diagonal wing at University Hospital to accommodate surgeries, 26 medical beds, and radiology; and construction commenced on the School of Nursing building, which would cost $478,968 and house 88 students. By October a $20,000 allocation was announced for the purpose of constructing animal quarters on the roof of the School of Medicine building.

A report of the Oklahoma Division of the American Cancer Society, covering the period from September 1, 1947, to August 31, 1948, substantiates the fact that research continued to be carried on effectively in the School of

Medicine regardless of impediments. Research projects by Mark R. Everett, J. M. Thuringer and Zola Cooper, and by Howard C. Hopps were funded in amounts of $14,000, $3,675, and $2,984, respectively, by the American Cancer Society, and tumor clinics were established in University Hospital and at St. John's Hospital in Tulsa, by two grants of $10,000 per hospital from the Oklahoma Division of the American Cancer Society. Henry G. Bennett, Jr., was appointed director of the tumor clinic at the School of Medicine and University Hospitals on a half-time basis effective December 14, 1947, at a salary of $4,200 per annum—all payments from grants.

On May 14 the university regents accepted a deed of gift representing stocks valued at $5,000 from Mrs. Sadie H. Edwards in appreciation of the care given her late husband, R. J. Edwards, by Charles B. Taylor over a period of years. Mrs. Edwards stipulated that the profits made from these stocks be used to maintain a lectureship in the School of Medicine to be called the Charles B. Taylor Lectureship.

The appointment of Laurence H. Snyder as dean of the University of Oklahoma Graduate College, at a salary of $10,000 per annum, was made on June 11 with the School of Medicine budget absorbing $2,500 of Dean Snyder's salary as recompense for a collateral teaching assignment in medical genetics at the medical center.

Coyne Herbert Campbell was appointed associate professor of psychiatry and neurology effective November 12, 1947, and Ada Crocker, former director of the School of Nursing, returned to the Medical Center on a temporary basis as director of the School of Nursing, December 11, 1947, to March 31, 1948.

By special arrangement with the surgeon general of the army, Colonel Alfred H. Bungardt was assigned to the School of Medicine with the title of professor of military science and tactics, with an opportunity to take training in orthopedic surgery at the Crippled Children's Hospital.

A complete list of appointments to the School of Medicine faculty in 1947–48 follows:

Laurence Hasbrouck Snyder, D.Sc.
  professor of medical genetics.
Garmon Harlow Daron, Ph.D.
  associate professor of anatomy
Henry Bonheyo Strenge, M.D.
  assistant professor of pediatrics
Audray Delbert Ward, M.D.
  assistant professor of orthopedic
  surgery
Perry J. Cunningham, M.D.
  instructor in anesthesiology
Vernon Cushing, M.D.
  instructor in medicine
James Gartrelle Phillips, M.D.
  instructor in urology

Harlan Keith Sowell, M.D.
  instructor in anesthesiology
James Robert Walker, M.D.
  instructor in anesthesiology
Ellis Edwin Fair, M.D.
  clinical assistant in surgery
Harold Waton Hackler, M.D.
  clinical assistant in psychiatry and
  neurology
Robert C. Lawson, M.D.
  clinical assistant in medicine
Edwin Norris Robertson, Jr., M.D.
  clinical assistant in
  ophthalmology

George William Winkleman, M.D.
  clinical assistant in psychiatry and
  neurology
Harold Brian Witten, M.D.
  clinical assistant in psychiatry and
  neurology

John Woodrow Devore, M.D.
  graduate fellow in anatomy
Alfred Ian Rubenstein, M.D.
  graduate assistant in anatomy

As far as the hospitals were concerned, there was definite bias on the part of the state regents as evidenced in a communication from Dr. Gray to Paul Fessler in February, 1947, in which the dean stated that John Rogers, a member of the Oklahoma State Regents for Higher Education, had made the irresponsible remark that 50 per cent of all admissions to the University Hospitals were of patients of Oklahoma City residence. He also said that Oklahoma City and Oklahoma County were "really riding the general fund for service in the University Hospitals far in excess of a prorated amount to which the people of those two political subdivisions were entitled."

In view of the fact that the request for capital expenditures for the next biennium was emasculated by the Oklahoma State Regents for Higher Education and cut back to 14.3 per cent of the request, professional services and a paucity of beds for teaching purposes in the University Hospitals continued to present a very serious problem. So clinical members of the full-time faculty staff were granted permission to provide consultation services in cases where there was no other alternative (reversal of a former directive).

The university regents created the new position of purchasing agent for the School of Medicine and University Hospitals in March. They authorized the dean of the School of Medicine and University Hospitals to approve payrolls and claims for expenditures of funds for the school and the hospitals provided that, in the dean's absence, the assistant dean might sign claims.

There were 206 available beds, including 33 bassinets, at University Hospital during the year and 186 available beds at Children's Hospital, making a total of 392 beds in operation, with 75 beds closed. There were 5,306 patients admitted to University Hospital with an average stay of 12.1 days and 15,094 admissions to the outpatient department; 2,284 patients were admitted to Children's Hospital with an average stay of 24.5 days; clinical laboratory examinations totaled 117,010 in 1947–48, an increase of 39,041 from 1942–43.

The total income for the fiscal year 1947–48 for the School of Medicine was $381,279, of which $290,000 was appropriated by the legislature: and for the University Hospitals the income was $1,566,382, of which $1,051,687 was from the state. Capital funds totaled $786,658.

In 1947–48 there were 259 medical and eight graduate students enrolled in the School of Medicine, 171 of whom were veterans, and 132 students were enrolled in the School of Nursing. Seventy graduates in medicine received the M.D. degree, and 38 nurses received the Graduate Nurse certificate on June 2, 1947.

The annual report of the librarian, Lilah B. Heck, showed that the School of

Medicine had a depository of 572 periodicals and annuals, 23,180 accessioned volumes, that donations were received from the Oklahoma County Dental Society and $500 from the Oklahoma County Medical Society for books and journals. Miss Heck's staff consisted of an assistant librarian and two assistants. Allan J. Stanley was chairman of the library committee.

On September 18, Jacques P. Gray lowered the boom when he read a letter of resignation to the faculty on the eve of the scheduled release of the announcement of his resignation from the University of Oklahoma, to be effective not later than November 15, 1947. "My new affiliation," he said, "will be that of medical consultant in the Park-Davis Company organization, with headquarters in Detroit." Then, in the "may all that is good be yours" rhetoric so familiar to recipients of letters and memoranda (shorted to "mat-ig-by" by the facetious), Dean Gray wished the faculty "in all ways all that is good always." Dr. Gray's version of the major stumbling blocks to "all that is good" had to do for the most part with inadequate facilities and the attitudes of the state legislature and the State Regents for Higher Education—stumbling blocks for any dean of a school of medicine aspiring to break the spell of eleven years of probationary status hanging over the institution like an albatross.

Dean Gray presided at a faculty meeting for the last time on October 1, when President Cross addressed the faculty.

It has been suggested on several occasions that an advisory committee to work with the president in connection with the administration of the School of Medicine is desirable. You have read in the papers that I have planned for representation on such a committee from the alumni association, the Oklahoma State Medical Association, the Oklahoma Medical Research Foundation, the clinical faculty and the preclinical faculty. This committee will work with the president and not with the new dean. I shall ask for its advice in regard to appointment of a temporary or acting dean, but the final decision will be my own. The committee will also be asked to give advice and opinions in regard to selecting a permanent dean. I say permanent only in a relative sense, because we cannot seem to make our deans very permanent. There are a number of problems which should be settled. If the new dean is confronted with too many problems, he may become discouraged; if he undertakes to solve these problems vigorously, he may find a couple of strikes against him before he gets started.

President Cross met with the university regents on October 8 and reported that he had set up a committee as outlined above to act as an advisory body pending the appointment of a successor to Dean Gray, with Arthur A. Hellbaum as chairman. And under dateline "Norman, October 15," the *Daily Oklahoman* reported that

the University Administration plans to work out pressing internal problems [of the School of Medicine and University Hospitals] before appointing a new medical school dean. . . . Present plans do not call for appointment of a new dean until the beginning of the next term autumn [1948]. . . . It was learned Wednesday that the University Regents approved no faculty promotions for this school year because of a failure of the school to submit a definite policy of promotions.

And a follow-up article on October 28 stated that

this is one of the kinks which Dr. J. P. Gray, dean of the school who has resigned, explains he hasn't had time to straighten out. But Cross wants it straight before Gray's successor is appointed. . . . One of the more difficult situations, which nobody wants to talk about publicly, had to do with part-time teachers among Oklahoma City physicians. . . . The President's committee, being composed of doctors, can thrash out such touchy problems where a new dean would be on shaky ground. If this much of the weight can be lifted from the new dean's shoulders before he comes in, Cross believes the school will be able to move ahead with a steady step.

In the meantime, according to another article,

it would seem a fair diagnosis to say that the 'med school' needs a blood transfusion, a little plastic surgery. . . . After little more than a year Dr. J. P. Gray is resigning in deep disillusionment. . . . Three key figures in the school-hospital setup followed in the dean's lead; Kathlyn Krammes, Director of Nursing and two of her top associates walked out, protesting the lack of a five-year course to turn out nurses with college degrees.

And on another date we read in the local press,

While medical men themselves are raising funds for a great research center and while the federal government plans a large veterans hospital, the State Regents for Higher Education, acting with the intelligence of a bunch of kindergarten kids dealing in building blocks, are rapidly wrecking the University School of Medicine.

On November 10, 1947, President Cross announced through the press that Mark R. Everett had been appointed dean of the School of Medicine to succeed J. P. Gray who had recently resigned.[3]

___

[3.] Memoir by Mark R. Everett: I was surprised, while at work in my laboratory one November day, to have an important visitor—President George Lynn Cross, whom I had known and respected for years.

I was dumfounded when he began talking about the deanship of the School of Medicine, actually asking me to consider being a temporary dean, and I recall telling the

"Dr. Everett will serve until August 31, 1948," the president said, "and will have the full power and responsibilities of the dean during his term of office. He has accepted the position for a period of one year after which he hopes to devote all of his time to his present position as head of the Department of Biochemistry and to the establishment of a Research Institute."

Dr. Gray's resignation was accepted effective November 15, 1947, and Dr. Everett's appointment was officially authorized by the university regents in session on November 24; Dean Everett's salary was fixed at an annual rate of $10,000.[4]

---

president that I was not particularly interested in administrative work, although I thoroughly enjoyed my work among Oklahoma's friendly people. "Mark," George Cross said pointedly, "you have been here twenty-three years, a constant member of the faculty. During that time, you have attained a stature which permits you to identify yourself as willing to share administrative tasks of the University." It was agreed that I should take a week or so to consider his invitation before notifying him of my decision. My most disturbing thought was the possibility that, as dean, I would imperil many friendly relations with clinicians.

By chance, a former dean at Harvard University was visiting in our city at that time, and he permitted me to consult with him, but would answer neither yes or no to the question of my becoming dean. He showed me a book he carried entitled, *What I Learned as a University President*, by Lawrence Lowell. Among President Lowell's remarks were some very interesting ideas, including that of a president leading a faculty parade. "And suppose it was going down past the Boston Commons and that you suddenly became aware of an unexpected barricade across the street! What to do?" President Lowell said to turn either to the right or to the left—whichever opportunity presented itself—and to do so with spirit and speed as one curved back to the original road, never having lost sight of his true objective.

Another piece of advice was not to personally push ideals or plans upon a faculty, because the average faculty critic or governing board member might not be able to follow one's persuasion. Develop a commendable plan, yes, but then discuss it with a trustworthy friend or alumnus to obtain an objective evaluation. If his reaction proved favorable, get someone to present the proposition at the first suitable meeting without saddling it with an administrator's personal preference. Thus after appropriate approval by his peers, the dean should be in a position to push the idea, unlabelled with his name.

I finally decided to accept the position on the advice of an absent Lawrence Lowell and that of my family and friends; but I recall telling President Cross that I would not accept an appointment as temporary dean, acting dean, or interim dean. In my letter of acceptance, I assured the president and regents of the university that I would work only for the best interest of the School of Medicine, and that I would at all times adhere to the proper forms of official communication. Furthermore I stated that, if at any time the president and/or regents were of the opinion that it would be best if I resigned, they should inform me and I would do so; and vice versa, if I felt at any time that I was not receiving the necessary support from the president and/or regents I would submit my resignation my letter to take effect in 30 days.

[4.] Mark R. Everett was born November 2, 1899, in Slatington, Pennsylvania, and was graduated from Bucknell University in 1920 with a Bachelor of Science degree in chemical engineering. From 1920 to 1924 he was an Austin Teaching fellow in chemistry and biochemistry at Harvard Medical School, where he received a Ph.D.

On recommendation of the president, also, the administration of the School of Medicine was reorganized by the creation of three associate deanships to assist Dr. Everett: Homer F. March, associate professor of bacteriology, was designated associate dean of students, for a similar period as the dean's at a salary of $6,500; Henry Turner, associate professor of medicine, was designated associate dean of the faculty, effective November 10 to August 31, 1948, at a salary of $2,000; and Arthur Hellbaum, professor of pharmacology, was designated associate dean of the Graduate College and research at the School of Medicine for the same term, with his salary fixed at $8,000.[5]

Under the policy current at the time the dean of the School of Medicine was also superintendent of the University Hospitals (responsible in all matters pertaining to those institutions). President Cross recommended the creation of two additional positions to assist the dean-superintendent: (1) a medical director in charge of all professional services having to do with the care of patients, including interns, residents, and members of the full-time staff, (nurses, laboratories, dietitians, drugs, supplies, admitting office, record room, outpatient department, and members of the visiting staff); (2) a business administrator subject to the supervision of the dean-superintendent in full charge of all financial matters and such operational activities as were not the responsibility of the medical director.

A resolution was passed by the university regents discontinuing the title "Head of Department" in the School of Medicine in favor of the title "Chairman of the Department," with those then holding the title of "Head" officially appointed as "Chairman" for the remainder of the fiscal year ending June 30, 1948.

President Cross called a special meeting of the faculty on November 20, at which Mark R. Everett presided as the new dean. Dr. Cross discussed at some length the necessity for reorganization of the departments so that staff would

---

degree in medical sciences in June, 1924. In the fall of that year he moved with his bride to Oklahoma where he had accepted a position as professor and head of the newly formed Department of Physiological Chemistry and Pharmacology.

Dr. Everett soon became a vigorous scientific researcher, which resulted in the publication of many of his articles in scientific journals and his recognition as a medical educator. His *Medical Biochemistry*, published in 1942, merited national acclaim as a very adequate source of biochemical reference.

[5.] Dr. Marsh, recipient of a Ph.D. degree from Ohio State University in 1941, was engaged in bacteriological research in the Department of Bacteriology and was active in various student societies at the medical center campus. Dr. Turner was interested in endocrine research which he carried out so successfully that he became well known nationally as an endocrinologist. Dr. Hellbaum held a Ph.D. degree in zoology from the University of Wisconsin and was actively involved in research studies having to do with hormones of the pituitary gland and the adrenal cortex, in addition to his administrative and teaching duties in the Department of Pharmacology. While at the University of Oklahoma he completed his work toward a Doctor of Medicine degree which he received from the University of Chicago.

have a greater voice in departmental affairs, and Dean Everett suggested the need for an advisory committee elected in part and appointed in part to represent all departments. Dean Everett also said that he had reactivated the old hospital board with Dr. Turner replacing Dr. Shoemaker who had resigned as assistant dean; and that in the future Dr. Turner, associate dean of the faculty, would preside at faculty meetings.

In a letter addressed to Dean Everett on November 20, Fred C. Zapffe, secretary of the Association of American Medical Colleges, wrote:

I did wonder why you stuck your neck out and accepted the deanship. I hope when they get another dean they will not repeat the mistakes they made on two previous occasions. I know, people seek advice and ask for help, but too often they do not approach the right people. However, they are the ones who must pay the price for any mistakes they may make. My fear about you is that since administrative work demands so much time, you will find yourself forcibly detached from your chosen field of teaching. . . . If I can help you in any way, please consider me at your service.

In replay on December 18, Dr. Everett wrote:

The four of us retain our professorships and continue our teaching and research projects. For example, I meet three classes as before, and I am continuing to direct a research project, and to review biochemistry literature systematically. . . . In regard to the outlook, there is a greater state-wide interest in the institution than formerly. . . . Reports coming to me indicate that our alumni are cooperating actively in constructive efforts. . . . Personally, I am not fearful of pressure since it is known that I have no selfish interest to defend. It is in this spirit that I appreciate for the school as well as for myself the good will which you have always exhibited so generously.

On December 29, Dr. Zapffe answered,

You know, deans have a job to do nowadays that does not in any way concern teaching. They must promote and propagandize; this takes all their time so that if they have any interest in any one particiular field of science, that interest dies from inanition. Do not let that happen to you. . . . Of course, if you want to give up biochemistry and go into administrative work, here is your chance; personally, I think you would be making a very serious mistake. Do not let anyone rush you. Being a dean is not an honor; it is simply taking advantage of a trusting soul and ruining him for life. Do not forget that we have had 64 new deans over a period of four years. True, some of them have simply changed places, but more than 50 are actually new men. The life of a dean is a short and hard one—not a merry one. Wishing you a very Happy New Year, I am sincerely yours.

On December 30, Donald G. Anderson, M.D., secretary, American Medical Association Council on Medical Education and Hospitals, advised Dean Everett that the council had requested that a new inspection of the School of Medicine of the University of Oklahoma be made at an early date and that, in accordance with established policy, this inspection would be undertaken jointly with a representative of the Association of American Medical Colleges. The date for the inspection was tentatively set for the week of February 23, with Dr. Anderson conceding that ''an inspection coming so close upon your assuming the deanship may not be entirely convenient for you. On the other hand, it is possible that the findings of our survey may be of a real assistance to you as you undertake the development of the school.''

And Paul B. Champlin, president of the Oklahoma State Medical Association, writing in the December issue of its journal, complimented George Cross, president of the University of Oklahoma, on the aggressive attitude he had manifested in tackling the problems of the medical school.

The selection of Dr. Mark Everett, Ph.D., to serve as acting Dean brings to the position a man who knows the problems of the school from first hand knowledge and a popularity with both the pre-clinical and clinical staff that will bring about whole-hearted cooperation from both groups. . . . I am personally of the opinion that the Medical School has now entered a stage of development in which we will all be proud to have a part. May I suggest that everyone put his shoulder to the wheel, give the Medical School and its new administrative staff a pat on the back, and a pledge of full cooperation.

Chapter XII.
Reorganization and
Expansion: 1948–49

 On an inclement, snowy day in January, 1948, Dean Mark R. Everett met in Edmond with the State Regents for Higher Education in joint session with the legislative council's education committee.

The twelve-year probationary status of the School of Medicine was discussed, and Dean Everett revealed that this fact was "confidential" on the part of the Council on Medical Education in an effort to help the medical school and was never intended to have been made public or to have received the extensive publicity that appeared in the press in a struggle for additional appropriations from the twenty-first legislature.

The dean conceded, however, that the increased allocations were appreciated inasmuch as the cost of commodities was $204 compared with $100 in 1941, so that a dollar then was equal to 50 cents in 1948. "It now costs $5,100 a year including hospital allocations, to educate a medical student," the dean said, remarking that this calculation was made by dividing the combined state appropriations for both medical school and hospitals by the number of medical students; but that the cost would be approximately $1,000 per student per year, if one subtracted $4,000 per student for maintenance of University Hospitals. "One can either be sad at this figure or be happy that the thousands of patients being treated at the University Hospitals apparently incur no expense at all [for their care]," the dean added.

Regent Frank Buttram said that, in view of the efforts to make Oklahoma City a great medical center, the county indigent hospital problem ought to be solved, and that he thought it could be solved. This initiated a rather fruitless discussion about requiring counties to pay the cost of hospitalization of indigent patients sent to University Hospitals. But the state supreme court had previously ruled that county support was unconstitutional, and that care of the indigent was "strictly a state obligation." In any event, care of the indigent posed a dilemma for the State Regents for Higher Education and, in the words of one legislator "a heavy charity load."

Dean Everett added that Oklahoma was one of the few states in which the full costs of the university medical school and hospitals was paid with state appropriations, and he mentioned that it was then costing $5,000 per month for penicillin alone in University Hospital, and that the average pay for a staff nurse had risen from $1,040 to $2,280 annually in seven years.

With respect to patients from Oklahoma City, Dean Everett reported that 43 per cent of the beds and 28 per cent of the hospital days were assigned to them, but he also pointed out that 80 per cent of these patients were either obstetric cases necessary for teaching purposes or children requiring admittance into the hospital under the Crippled Children's Act. Otherwise, the city's figure was less than 9 per cent of the patients'. The dean then asserted that one of the reasons for locating the hospital in Oklahoma City in the first place was availability of patients for teaching purposes.

One of the more troublesome matters for the administration pertained to indigent patients who were admitted to the University Hospitals and then, because of inability or negligence on the part of relatives or of the counties in which they were legal residents, remained in the hospital for periods of time beyond which hospitalization was indicated. Since the requirement of the Council on Medical Education and Hospitals stipulated that each student should study a minimum of three new patients per week, Dean Everett emphasized that it was exceedingly important that a case requiring only nursing care (and presenting no valuable teaching aspects) should not be confined in the University Hospital when no further medical therapy was indicated. He should be discharged and placed in some other facility.

Dr. Everett pointed out that such trouble spots were of immediate concern in view of the fact that the accrediting agency of the American Medical Association would be inspecting the School of Medicine again on March 1 in an effort to restore full accreditation.[1]

By April the state regents evidenced a sincere interest and spirit of cooperation in trying to improve the School of Medicine, when they instructed Dean Everett to open approximately 100 beds in University Hospitals on or before September, 1948, and made funds available for the year 1948–49 in the amount suggested by Dr. Everett. They further agreed to assume the responsibility of endeavoring to obtain deficiency appropriations from the incoming legislature in January of 1949, if the medical school proceeded to open closed wards and to take in a class of not less than 64 students at the beginning of the next term.[2]

Meanwhile, rotation of department chairmen (a plan which had been used successfully on the Norman campus for several years) was evolving as part of the new program to obtain greater efficiency in the entire administration of the School of Medicine in Oklahoma City. Whereas formerly, the department head was appointed by the dean and his advisory council, under the new plan each clinical department nominated two or three men from whom the dean and his

---

[1] In separate letters dated January 27, John Rogers, member of the State Regents for Higher Education, and L. D. Melton, director of the Oklahoma State Legislative Council, expressed deep interest and appreciation to Dean Everett "for the excellent presentation yesterday of the status and needs of the medical school."

[2] John Rogers so informed Dr. Fred Woodson, president of the Alumni Association of the School of Medicine, in a letter dated May 18, 1948.

advisory council in turn elected a chairman. Rotation of chairmanships was perfected by repeating the process every two years, with chairmen and vice-chairmen eligible to succeed themselves. In any event, the rotation plan spread out the burden of administrative work and gave the clinical faculty more time for research and advanced study.

A ten-year projected building program for the medical school campus was approved by the university regents on May 25, and this projected plan received excellent coverage in the press, all of which was favorable. The units in the ten-year plan included an addition to the medical school (two wings); remodeling of the present hospital and an addition, $554,000; a new ten-story hospital addition, $2,300,000; an addition to Crippled Children's Hospital, $645,500, and an enlargement of its school facilities; shops and laundry; a tunnel to connect the main hospital and the medical school with the Oklahoma Medical Research Institute; a new nurses' home and remodeling of the present nurses' home.

Elmer Peterson, in a concurrent editorial in the *Daily Oklahoman*, commented that every factor was favorable to the establishment of an impressive medical center on East Thirteenth Street "except the finances needed to construct the units mentioned."

As a matter of fact, the local press and also the state press had spotlighted the medical school's financial predicament unstintingly for months, and articles appeared in the Oklahoma City papers almost daily, reporting complete data on many facets of medical education for scrutiny by the public eye.

Foremost among the by-line reporters was Mike Gorman who wrote a series of articles in the *Daily Oklahoman* on the obstacles to be overcome before the School of Medicine could enroll 87 first-year students, as recommended by the Oklahoma State Medical Association and the school's alumni association. Mike investigated every nook and cranny of the existing physical facilities in conjunction with expansion of the medical school's laboratories and surgical quarters, classrooms, office space, library, teaching beds, and nurses' home. In addition, he promoted a psychiatry ward and mental health clinic,[3] for which he later received a special Lasker Award from the National Committee for Mental Health Hygiene.

Early in Dean Everett's administration, President Cross endorsed plans for some kind of controlled public relations procedure, which finally culminated in the appointment of Harold Muchmore, Department of Pharmacology, as public relations assistant on a half-time basis. The policy, as determined by the president, was to release only items of a constructive nature, channeled through Dr. Muchmore, and President Cross admonished Dean Everett to inform Dr. Muchmore and his committee that the president was responsible for all news, and therefore, any news affecting general policies of the school which was subject to regents action should be cleared through him.

[3.] Grady Matthews, state commissioner of health, was very instrumental in assisting in the establishment of this mental health clinic, which was housed in the annex building of the School of Medicine, and Coyne Campbell became administrator of the program.

On May 17 the elected officers and counselors of the Alumni Association of the University of Oklahoma School of Medicine passed a resolution that Mark R. Everett be made permanent dean of the School of Medicine, to which President Cross replied on June 4. He agreed that the situation in the medical school had improved immeasurably during Dr. Everett's administration, but he said:

> The administrative changes made at the medical school and the hospitals, which to a significant degree are responsible for this improved condition, were not initiated by Dr. Everett. They were recommended to me by the Advisory Committee (composed of two clinical teachers, two preclinical teachers, two alumni, two members of the Oklahoma State Medical Association, two representatives from the Oklahoma Medical Research Foundation, and two persons at large). . . . By way of specific example, I should like to mention the proposed revision of departmental administration in the Medical School. Dr. Everett's doubts as to whether the new plan could be peacefully inaugurated at the school led to my appearance at a general faculty meeting where the problem was explained and the new plan discussed. It was my impression at the time that Dr. Everett's confidence in the proposal had been shaken as a result of pressure put upon him by certain members of the faculty who disapproved.
>
> On the other side of the ledger, I must commend Dr. Everett most highly for the smooth, tactful and efficient way in which the changes were put across after all doubt as to whether they should be adopted had been removed. He should be commended also for his unselfish and diligent effort in coping with many and diverse lesser problems of the institution. . . . I have not, however, seen him initiate an important idea concerning the school and independently bring the faculty to an acceptance of the idea.

President Cross went on to say that the thing most necessary to be done at the School of Medicine was to revise and modernize the curriculum of the clinical years, and that, if this could be achieved within the next few months, then we would be on our way toward a school of which all of us could be proud. "In my mind," Dr. Cross said, "this will test Dr. Everett's leadership and if he is successful in bringing about the revision of the curriculum, even though the matter came through the American Medical Association rather than himself, I shall feel that his initial efforts as Dean have been most successful."

On June 12 the university regents approved the recommendation of President Cross that Mark R. Everett be appointed dean of the School of Medicine for one more year, until June 30, 1949, at the same time continuing as professor of biochemistry. The budget of the School of Medicine and University Hospitals was approved as submitted.

In accepting the reappointment as dean of the School of Medicine for another year, Dr. Everett expressed his gratitude to President Cross and the university regents for the sympathetic aid and support he had received from them during the preceding months—"greatly appreciated factors in whatever improvements may have been accomplished"—especially the assured Class A accreditation.

When on July 10 official notice was released that the Council on Medical Education and Hospitals had indeed "voted to remove the University of Oklahoma School of Medicine from confidential probation," the stirring satisfaction which the doctor gains *when the patient lives* became an experience shared by the public and the many devoted believers in the School of Medicine. The survey committee remarked that Dr. Everett, with the full cooperation of Dr. Cross, had made marked improvement in faculty organization and opportunities for the faculty to participate in programs and policies, as well as having effected a "rather sweeping reorganization of the clinical departments." The committee noted further that the Oklahoma Medical Research Foundation had been established, and that political interference in the School of Medicine had ceased.

Understandably, suggestions were made for further improvements, such as expansion in all areas in the ten-year projected building program in order to accommodate classes of 80 to 100 students of medicine by 1951. The suggestion was also made to utilize the greatly expanded affiliated hospital teaching facilities which in the fall of 1948, justified an entering class of 64 students instead of only 52.

Under the affiliated plan approximately 260 beds in Wesley, Mercy, St. Anthony, and Veterans Administration hospitals—not financed by the state from educational funds—were made available for teaching purposes, in addition to 31 beds reopened at University Hospital in January and 34 in the new wing, plus 38 reopened at Children's Hospital in August. This was a considerable improvement over the 312 available beds when the year began.

Two hundred and fifty thousand dollars, requested from the State Regents for Higher Education for the period starting July 1, was apportioned into $200,000 to cover hospital maintenance expenses, salaries for nurses, interns, and maids, and for setting up diet kitchens. And $50,000 was allocated for the School of Medicine.

No sooner were more teaching beds available than the clamor for the training of a maximum number of physicians was under way—"up to 100 if possible, starting in 1949."[4] And busily breathing on the embers was the Alumni Association of the School of Medicine whose members rallied round Dr. Everett, because he had played such an active part in their organization of the

---

[4.] The 1947–48 directory of the Oklahoma State Medical Association listed only 297 physicians in 33 selected counties with an estimated population of 629,675 persons, or approximately one physician to each 2,500 persons. Oklahoma, as a whole, had an average of one active practicing physician to 1,226 persons, as compared with an average of one to 840 persons in the United States.

Oklahoma Medical Research Foundation.[5] This support included ladies, too, in the days before women's lib. Grace Clause Hassler wrote that "the girls felt quite fortunate in having someone who is sympathetic with women in medicine." And Dr. Ruth S. Stelle wrote from Albany, New York, "It is because of deans such as you that the young women who are undertaking the study of medicine can have faith in their choice. . . . It means a great deal to have [as dean] one who so well understands the situation."

The reorganization of the administration of the hospitals and the clinical faculty, begun during the preceding year, culminated in the appointment of Herbert C. O'Neil as superintendent of buildings and grounds in February, of Kenneth F. Wallace as business administrator of the School of Medicine and University Hospitals in March, and of Vernon D. Cushing as the University Hospital's medical director in June. Paul Fesler was named consultant to the dean and superintendent on a half-time basis at a recommended salary of $4,000 per year.

According to regulations adopted by the faculty in March, a full-time faculty member acting as a medical consultant was not allowed to have an office outside the University Hospitals or the School of Medicine and was permitted to receive fees only from patients who were under the care of another physician (to be collected directly by the consultant and to be regarded as a supplement to his salary). Moreover, the yearly income from all such consultant services was not to exceed the official yearly salary. But no restrictions were placed on other remunerative outside activities such as scientific or literary work.

Minimal standards for appointment to the part-time clinical faculty, adopted on September 5, were as follows: graduation from an approved Grade A medical schoolwith one year of internship and one year of residency (or five years of practice in the field to which the appointment was to be made) and five years of service at the grade of instructor, assistant professor, associate professor, or clinical professor before promotion. Furthermore, each clinical department was required to have a committee on promotions to advise its chairman, at least once a year, in regard to recommendations for promotions of members.

The organization of the preclinical departments was subject to instructions from the administration, and recommendations for promotion of members were made directly to the administration by the chairmen of the respective departments.

Robert H. Bayley was retired as head of the Department of Medicine (though retaining his professorial appointment on the teaching staff) in February, and R. Q. Goodwin was appointed to the chairmanship effective February 1, 1948, to June 30, 1950. Howard Allen Bennett was appointed professor of anesthesiology February 15 at a yearly salary of $7,500, and Lewis J. Moorman, professor emeritus, was appointed lecturer in the history of medicine and medical ethics in the Department of Medicine on March 1.

Joining the ranks of emeritus professors in 1948 were Edward P. Allen,

---

[5.] Mark R. Everett, *Pioneering for Research*, University of Oklahoma Medical Center, Oklahoma City (1966).

obstetrics, and C. J. Fishman and Joseph T. Martin, active members of the Department of Medicine since 1911, and Wann Langston.

New appointments to the faculty for 1948–49 were as follows:

Howard Allen Bennett, M.D.
professor of anesthesiology
Mary C. Zahasky, B.S.
associate professor of nutrition
Harrell Chandler Dodson, M.D.
assistant professor of surgery
Charles Frederick Obermann, M.D.
assistant professor of psychiatry and neurology
Mack Irvin Shanholtz, M.D.
assistant professor of preventive medicine and public health
Daniel Gilbert Costigan, M.D.
instructor in orthopedic and fracture surgery
Louis S. Frank, M.D.
instructor in pediatrics
Vera Iva Parman Peters, M.S.
instructor in dietetics
Fred August Quenzer, M.D.
instructor in surgery
Margaret F. Shackleford, M.S.
instructor in preventive medicine and public health
Barbara Wells, M.S.
instructor in bacteriology and preventive medicine and public health
Homer V. Archer, M.D.
clinical assistant in obstetrics
Cleve Beller, M.D.
research fellow in endocrinology
Vance Arthur Bradford, M.D.
clinical assistant in surgery
C. Alton Brown, M.D.
clinical assistant in medicine
Richard Allen Clay, M.D.
clinical assistant in ophthalmology
Jess Donald Cone, Jr., M.D.
graduate fellow in anatomy
Loyal Lee Conrad, M.D.
clinical assistant in medicine
Clarence Benton Dawson, M.D.
clinical assistant in urology
John J. Donnell, M.D.
clinical assistant in medicine

John Hartwell Dunn, M.D.
clinical assistant in urology
Edward Merhige Farris, M.D.
clinical assistant in surgery
Athol Lee Frew, Jr., D.D.S., M.D.
clinical assistant in dental surgery
James Jackson Gable, Jr., M.D.
clinical assistant in medicine
Tom Sid Gafford, Jr., M.D.
fellow in pathology
William Thomas Gill, M.D.
visiting lecturer in pathology
George Henry Guthrey, M.D.
clinical assistant in psychiatry and neurology
Richard Lowell Harris, M.D.
clinical assistant in obstetrics
Walter Kenneth Hartford, M.D.
clinical assistant in gynecology
Jack Van Doren Hough, M.D.
clinical assistant in otorhinolaryngology
Arthur W. Hoyt, M.D.
visiting lecturer in pediatrics
Dick Howard Huff, M.D.
clinical assistant in medicine
Leo Lowbeer, M.D.
visiting lecturer in pathology
Jess E. Miller, M.D.
fellow in pathology
William Arthur Miller, M.D.
graduate fellow in anatomy
Samuel Turner Moore, M.D.
clinical assistant in orthopedic and fracture surgery
Robert Jesse Morgan, M.D.
graduate fellow in dermatology and syphilology
John Edwin McDonald, M.D.
visiting lecturer in othrepedic and fracture surgery
James Newton Owens, Jr., M.D.
visiting lecturer in pathology
Emil E. Palik, M.D.
visiting lecturer in pathology

Robert Franklin Redmond, M.D.
  graduate fellow in pharmacology
William H. Reiff, M.D.
  clinical assistant in medicine
Robert Alvin Rix, Jr., M.D.
  clinical assistant in surgery
Harold G. Sleeper, M.D.
  clinical assistant in psychiatry,
  neurology, and behavioral sciences
Bryan Freemont Smith, M.D.
  clinical assistant in medicine
Hugh Albert Stout, M.S., M.D.
  clinical assistant in medicine and
  instructor in pathology

Ernest Martin Tapp, M.D.
  clinical assistant in medicine
Lal Duncan Threlkeld, M.D.
  clinical assistant in obstetrics
Reber Van Matre, M.D.
  clinical assistant in psychiatry and
  neurology
George A. Wiley, M.D.
  clinical assistant in ophthalmology
Leroy David Wright, D.M.D.
  clinical assistant in dental surgery
Edward W. Young, Jr., M.D.
  graduate fellow in pharmacology

In line with other medical schools, the designation of the Department of Art and Photography was changed to Department of Illustration as Applied to Medicine; and the department designated Orthopedic Surgery was changed to Department of Orthopedic and Fracture Surgery.

W. L. Haywood, director of the Negro Division of University Hospital, stated that his department "had no major problems they had not been able to solve amicably and satisfactorily because of the definite and positive cooperation of the Dean of this hospital and all of the subordinate departments."

On the research side of the ledger, the School of Medicine of the University of Oklahoma was one of 60 of the nation's 77 medical schools included by the Cancer Institute of the United States Public Health Service in a two-million-dollar program to improve cancer teaching nationally. Grady Matthews, commissioner of the Oklahoma Department of Health, who assisted during the year in establishing an outpatient tumor dlinic at the University Hospital, started the negotiations for these funds which resulted in a grant of $24,982.[6] In addition, an appropriation by the twenty-first legislature of $15,000 a year for research assured the beginning of clinical isotope studies at the University medical center.

By August the curriculum committee had entirely revised instruction in the clinical years in accordance with suggestions made by the Council on Medical Education, and the didactic hours were limited so that the students had a period when his major hospital clerkship was entirely uninterrupted. Members of the third-year class served for periods of several weeks on full-time inpatient clerkships, four in number in medicine, surgery, pediatrics, and obstetrics-gynecology.

Tom L. Wainwright was named coordinator of clerkships on September 9, and his associate coordinators were Doctor Cleve Beller, W. C. McClure, W. H. Reiff, S. N. Stone, and H. B. Strenge. The duty of the coordinators was to provide efficient management of the student inpatient clerkships and to refer any problem on a given clerkship to the chairman of the department concerned

[6] Dr. Matthews also assisted in equipping the new wing of the University Hospital by allocation of funds for that purpose.

or to his departmental representative. The chairman of the Department of Medicine was given a courtesy appointment to the staff of St. Anthony Hospital for the purpose of supervising the clerkship program there.

The fourth-year class, of 55 students, worked on outpatient services except for one-quarter of the class, which served successively on inpatient surgery and obstetrics-gynecology clerkships in order to make possible the shift in curriculum without entire loss of experience in these fields.

Changes were instituted in the outpatient department of both the University and Children's Hospitals whereby definite appointments were given to patients for visits to respective clinics, making it possible to operate certain clinics more efficiently on particular days. About 75 per cent of the appointments were kept.

According to the annual report of University Hospitals, July 1, 1948, to July 1, 1949, there was a total of 138,925 inpatient days of hospital care with an average of 381 patients per day, and a total of 55,045 visits to the outpatient department—7,719 new patients and 20,031 return patients. Total hospital admissions came to 6,135 at University Hospital and 2,264 at Children's Hospital, with 38 beds at Children's authorized for polio patients. The University of Oklahoma Hospitals house staff consisted of thirty-five residents and fifteen interns with an increase in veteran resident trainees.

There were 260 students enrolled in the School of Medicine and 101 in the School of Nursing in 1948–49. Sixty-two medical school graduates received the M.D. degree in June, 1948, and 44 nursing graduates received the Graduate Nurse certificate.

The total income for the fiscal year 1948–49 for the School of Medicine was $405,287, of which $300,000 was appropriated by the state, and for the University Hospitals, $1,657,758, of which $1,300,000 was appropriated. Capital funds for the University Hospitals totaled $178,119.

A resolution to merge the School of Medicine budget with that of the university was submitted to Dean Everett by President Cross on February 25 and, in turn, by Dr. Everett to the inspectors from the Council on Medical Education for their opinion during the first week in March. Subsequently it was also submitted to the advisory board, since the question involved basic policies of the School of Medicine. Consequently, on March 13, Dean Everett advised Dr. Cross that he was not in a position to sign the resolution because of uniformly unfavorable reception to it. So President Cross withdrew his recommendation, saying he would not present it to the regents because of the opposition expressed by the inspectors. Later, an agreement was reached to harmonize the business policies of the School of Medicine with those of the university through voluntary cooperation, insofar as it was beneficial to the medical school.

The period between July 1, 1947, and January 1, 1948, was a dark page in the history of the School of Nursing, due in part to the inability of the University Hospitals to retain nurses when the salary level of other hospitals and offices was pulling the graduates away. As a result, the severe nursing shortage became a stumbling block to progress in the hospitals until the press went to bat for the medical center once more. Then miraculously, because of the increased publicity, Mary Caron, director of the School of Nursing, was able to line up the largest class ever enrolled in nursing—67 recruits for the freshman class entering in September, out of a total of 85 applicants. In fact, the campaign for more nurses was so successful that Mrs. Caron began accepting applications for the classes entering the School of Nursing in March and September of 1949.

The newly opened $450,000 nurses' home was an attraction, to be sure, with an auditorium that seated 300 persons, dietetic and nursing laboratories, classrooms, office space, and a resident director and receptionist—quite an improvement on the residence still being maintained at "Old Main."

Mary Zahasky was promoted to the position of head of the dietary department, and Vera Parman was promoted from half-time to full-time status as a teacher.

The Speech and Hearing Clinic, now located at the Crippled Children's Hospital, became an associated clinic in the outpatient system of the School of Medicine in 1948; and John Keys, director of the hearing program, served also as director of the clinic, with the title of consulting audiologist in the Department of Otorhinolaryngology.

The three-fold purpose of the clinic—diagnostic and remedial services, teacher training, and research—was implemented on a state-wide basis, with 81 per cent of the clinic's activities supported by the Crippled Children's Commission. Twenty-one deaf children, ranging in age from three to six years, ten cleft palate cases and a dozen children with other types of speech defects were taught in the clinic every day. In the first year of operation 1,028 patients made a total of 5,952 visits to the clinic. Research, an integral part of the program, offered students opportunities for study toward a master's degree, and the staff trained prospective teachers of the deaf, as well as speech correction technicians.[7]

On September 8 representatives from the United States Children's Bureau in Dallas and the United States Public Health Service visited the medical center and commented favorably on the well-baby clinic, the rheumatic fever clinic, squint clinic, plastic clinic, and the outpatient departments in general.

A diagnostic and research laboratory for the treatment and study of physically handicapped children—known as the William Noble Memorial Clinical Investigation Laboratory—was opened at Children's Hospital in the fall of 1948. It was marked with a bronze plaque honoring the benefactor, William Noble, whose $20,000 trust fund made suitable equipment possible for differential diagnosis and study in connection with muscular dystrophy, as well as tracer isotope studies. The laboratory was staffed by adequate technicians from the School of Medicine and University Hospitals, with Henry B. Strenge director of the laboratory.

Looking at the other side of the coin, we find Crippled Children's Hospital faced with the problem every summer and fall of delayed admissions of other

---

[7] A committee, consisting of the chairman of the speech department at Norman, the director of the speech clinic, and the director of the hearing clinic in Oklahoma City, was responsible for coordination of the program.

sick and crippled children because of accessory need for beds for poliomyelitis patients in an emergency situation. The year 1948 was no exception. By September 8 the number of polio cases for the year had reached 230, with 14 deaths on record. On that same date there were 18 acute and 59 convalescent cases in Crippled Children's Hospital.

An editorial entitled "Shut-Eyed Waiting" in the October *News Letter* from the Oklahoma Society for Crippled Children stated:

> Once again, Oklahoma has been passing through the throes of a poliomyelitis epidemic. Once again, an almost complete arrest has been placed upon the general activities of the Oklahoma Hospital for Crippled Children because of the flood of actue patients entering the state's children's hospital. Patients with conditions other than acute poliomyelitis have been denied treatment. . . . Medical students for months have been quite limited by the decrease in patients for general pediatric training. . . . What is Oklahoma going to do about it? Is she going to follow the Boy Scout motto, or is she going to continue with her shut-eyed waiting?

In a year when the key words were reorganization and expansion, and the challenge was to pull a rabbit out of the hat, possibly excerpts from a letter to Governor Roy J. Turner are sufficient comment. Carl C. Thompson, state representative, Western Oklahoma, National Foundation Infantile Paralysis, wrote on October 28, 1948:

Dear Governor:

I know you have complaints of state agencies so often and compliments so seldom, that it behooves me to pay tribute to the Administration of University Hospitals for an amazingly good job of caring for victims of infantile paralysis during the epidemic now subsiding.

It was my duty and privilege to work with Dean Mark Everett, Dr. Vernon Cushing and Mr. Kenneth Wallace to see that every patient received the best possible treatment. I am happy to inform you that these gentlemen and their staff members devoted every effort toward that end. . . .

Not once since this epidemic started have I felt that the hospital staff was not making the most of limited facilities. . . . It is true that many improvements remain to be made, but definite progress is evident.

You and those other people responsible for the selection and employment of the present hospital administration can take pride in a job well done.

Sincerely yours,
Carl C. Thompson

Chapter XIII.
A Refreshing Governor:
1949–50

 Working quietly through the past twelve months on internal reforms and staff improvements, the administration of the School of Medicine succeeded in increasing enrollment from 52 to 64 students and succeeded also in having the probationary label removed; but the medical school still had a long way to go before achieving equal status with other topflight schools of medicine. So, very early in 1949, Dean Mark Everett appeared before both the House Committee on Appropriations and the Joint Legislative Appropriations Committee of the twenty-second legislature, urging that something be done immediately about emergency operating funds for the University Hospitals in order to complete the fiscal year ending June 30, and about facing up to the critical shortage of doctors in Oklahoma. He pointed out that, before he had become dean of the School of Medicine, hospital authorities, in an effort to keep up with rising costs, had closed beds one ward at a time until 100 beds were unoccupied. Since being installed, the new administration had opened those 100 beds and had acquired 260 additional teaching beds from outside sources, thus breaking the stalemate.

The House Committee on Appropriations straightway recommended that a bill be passed asking for emergency appropriations totaling $568,926 for the University of Oklahoma School of Medicine and other institutions of higher learning, with $200,000 allotted to the School of Medicine. By the end of January the emergency appropriation bill had passed both houses of the legislature—much to the credit of Paul Harkey of Idabel, chairman of the House Committee on Appropriations, who explained that these funds had previously been taken from original budgets of the institutions by the State Regents for Higher Education in order to meet emergency conditions at smaller institutions.

However, the State Regents for Higher Education actually boosted their appropriation requests for the School of Medicine in the spring of 1949; and John Rogers of Tulsa, a member of this board, lauded the administration at the medical school, when he appeared before the legislature. He said that the reorganization started more than a year ago had proved a success and that the medical school was in the best shape in its history. "If you gentlemen are generous with us," he added, "I think we can build one of the finest medical schools in the country in the next six to eight years."

The legislature came through with appropriation requests and, in turn, requested the State Regents for Higher Education to provide $1,150,000 for new buildings at the School of Medicine of the University of Oklahoma. Incredulous as it may seem, good fortune prevailed, and on July 13, President Cross reported that the State Regents for Higher Education had actually allocated $650,000 for an addition to the medical school building, $500,000 for an outpatient building and an addition to the nurses' building,[1] $15,000 for a water well, $15,000 for cancer research, and $425,700 for the operational budget.

Apart from the official budget requests, Dean Everett sought monies from various foundations to finance a broadened teaching program, and Mike Gorman wrote of these plans in the *Daily Oklahoman*, as well as of plans to strengthen the operation of the internship and residency programs of the affiliated hospitals of the university. He also mentioned plans to establish intramural postgraduate training of state physicians, with extramural short sessions and lectures in state cities and hospitals.[2]

The one person most entitled to wear a Santa Claus suit in 1949, as far as institutions of higher learning were concerned, was Roy J. Turner, governor of the state of Oklahoma. He fought an uphill fight against the usual legislative independence during a governor's second legislative session but, in spite of the opposition, persuaded the twenty-second legislature to vote to submit a $36,000,000 bond issue to the people of Oklahoma for a building program at state institutions. Then, with the odds heavily against him again, he took to the hustings in every county in the state with his story; and the people listened to him and believed him and gave their overwhelming approval to his bond issue in September—a great personal triumph for the governor.

Gradually, interest in the medical center became widespread, not only among the citizens of our state but throughout the United States and Canada, and medical foundations began visiting the medical campus on an exploratory basis. Such recognition, the dean believed, was the result of superb teamwork on the part of the president of the university, the university regents, the state regents, the legislature, the alumni, the profession, and the faculty, with the

---

[1] The request for an addition to the recently completed nurses' residence was necessitated by the record-breaking enrollment of 66 students the previous September. Mike Gorman, writing a feature article in the *Daily Oklahoman* on capital improvements at the medical center, avowed that Dean Everett was "determined to keep the School of Nursing on the upswing."

[2] Next to the Alumni Association of the School of Medicine, the medical school had no better supporter than Mike Gorman, who in company with many outside the organization worked to insure the successful passage of bills favorable to the School of Medicine—Paul Harkey, Guy James, Ted Warkentin, Hugh Payne, and Senators Gary, Jarman, Logan, Nance, and Ritzhaupt. In April, Senator Louis Ritzhaupt sponsored a bill in the legislature to assist in obtaining animals for research; and when the American Anti-Vivisection Society sent its legislative representatives to Oklahoma City to fight the bill, Dr. Ritzhaupt reacted by saying, "They are just a bunch of crackpots. . . . Other states such as California have to lie and steal about taking dogs for research because of their anti-vivisection laws. At least we are doing this in an open and above-board way."

news media cooperating in every phase of the institution's programs approved by the Council on Medical Education.

E. H. Cushing, assistant medical director for research and education in the Veterans Administration, after visiting the medical center, wrote that he would do all he could to expedite the development and building program of the Oklahoma City veterans' hospital, and that he would be most interested in knowing about the future of the Medical Research Institute. And Alan Gregg, director of medical sciences for the Rockefeller Foundation, said of the alumni-sponsored dream, "The Foundation will stand as a constant reminder to more than two million Oklahomans that a battle is being carried on to find the causes of many diseases that are taking such a tragic toll today. It is unique, by that I mean it is wonderful, and there is no other project of its kind that I know of."

The Oklahoma Medical Research Foundation was highlighted on Sunday, July 3, 1949, by participation of Sir Alexander Fleming in the dedication of the institute building.[3] Governor Turner, general chairman of the foundation's fund-raising drive, stressed the fact that the dedication ceremony was open to the public and not just to those who had received special invitations. "The Oklahoma Medical Research Foundation," he said, "is the greatest thing that has happened in Oklahoma since statehood. It is a cause in which I profoundly believe; it is a cause which I think will add credit and renown to our young state; it is a cause in which I shall have no hesitancy in asking my personal friends to take part."

A long article, which appeared in the *New York Times* on Tuesday, July 5, 1949, concerning the launching of the research institute and the preceptorship program at the University of Oklahoma School of Medicine prompted a few facetious remarks from Paul Hoeber of the medical book department of Harper & Brothers, in a letter to Dean Everett: "Congratulations on the launching the other day, and the lions you captured for the dedication ceremonies! As your clipping service has no doubt informed you, Oklahoma got a big play in the New York papers. . . . I marvel that you have been able to give any thought at all to [a new edition of] the textbook in the last few weeks."[4]

Dean Everett explained that the purpose of the preceptorship training program was actually a local effort to combat a problem of national scope, that is the growing tendency for the fourth-year medical student to think in terms of selecting a medical specialty in order to practice medicine in one of the larger cities as opposed to general practice in a small community. The attack on the problem was "three-pronged," the dean said, but the heart of it was the preceptorship plan, whereby the student was brought into intimate association with the general practice of medicine—in the home and in the office—as a supplement to the intensive clerkships in the larger hospitals in Oklahoma City.

---

[3] Mark R. Everett, *Pioneering for Research*, University of Oklahoma Medical Center, Oklahoma City (1966), 50.

[4] Mark R. Everett, *Medical Biochemistry*, (Paul B. Hoeber, Inc., New York and London, 1942).

The public and the prospective young doctors were very enthusiastic about the program, and in March 72 out of 75 members of the fourth-year class volunteered to participate in the experiment during their vacations; and 130 of the 1,000 practicing physicians in the state volunteered to serve as preceptors or guides.

Since the alumni had proposed the plan originally, there was no question about their cooperation and support, for 690 of the 1,241 graduates of the School of Medicine of the University of Oklahoma were practicing in Oklahoma, according to a survey made by the American Medical Association in 1949.

Under the Oklahoma preceptor program, each fourth-year student was required to spend 11 weeks (in addition to the regular 32-week session in the fourth year) in a selected community under the guidance of one of 19 preceptors named by the university regents. There were also approximately 50 associate preceptors, and the student had the privilege of participating in the practice of medicine to the extent deemed advisable by his tutors. In this way, the School of Medicine gave the student an opportunity to learn to apply the facts and principles learned in medical school to the practice of medicine under circumstances prevailing in outlying communities; to experience the problems of diagnosis and therapy without the support of all the facilities and personnel of the medical center; and, most important of all, to learn something about the physician's place in the community professionally, politically, socially, morally, and financially.

The essential requirements for a preceptor were that he be a member of the Oklahoma State Medical Association and a reputable physician in his community, with a definite interest in medical education and a willingness to assume responsibility for the appropriate organization and administration of a preceptorship.

Preceptors were selected by a committee composed of representatives from the alumni association, the State Medical Association, the Academy of General Practice, and the School of Medicine faculty, from applications submitted by physicians in the state. A system of periodic rotation of preceptors was practiced as a matter of policy. At the end of the general practice period, each preceptor submitted a written evaluation of the student professionally and personally to the administration of the School of Medicine. The student, in turn, was given the opportunity to express a preference as to his choice of a preceptor and the period in which he wished to serve his preceptorship.

The second prong of the program (to extend aid and interest to medical activities throughout the state) was the establishment of regional internships in general practice in small-town Oklahoma hospitals. This plan was greatly assisted by a grant of $130,000 from the W. K. Kellogg Foundation over a period of five years for "regional medical education," and only four other medical schools in the United States received a similar grant. The program, designed to develop general practitioners, included establishment of a two-year general practice residency at the university and its affiliated hospitals, the organization of new internships and residencies, and the establishment of postgraduate courses at the University Hospitals and elsewhere in the state.[5]

On November 15, 1949, eight candidates for the two-year general practice internship (to begin in 1950) were accepted—six of them from the University of Oklahoma School of Medicine—to spend one half year in Oklahoma City and the other half year in a hospital in one of the smaller communities in the state. Oklahoma, for the first time in its history, was fortunate to have a hospital outside Oklahoma City and Tulsa included in its residency training program schedule.

In addition to Cleve Beller, the staff for the Division of Postgraduate Education consisted of two associate directors, Hal A. Burnett, surgery, and George Winn, internal medicine. Moreover, the board of directors of the Oklahoma State Department of Public Health agreed to contribute $16,000 annually for the creation of two half-time professorships—one in obstetrics and gynecology and one in pediatrics, with George Garrison as adviser. The total budget for the division equaled $48,347 for the fiscal year 1949–50, $37,147 of which was for salaries.

The third step in an effort to encourage general practice by graduates of the School of Medicine was to train more doctors. Oklahoma's need for more medical services, based on authenticated data (2,266 living physicians in a population of 2,362,000 in June, 1948), was estimated to be 1,030 additional doctors in order for Oklahoma to provide its share of the total number of physicians in the United States. This was a deceptively low estimate, because Oklahoma had an unusually high ratio of aged physicians—the state's median age for physicians being 50.9 years as compared with 47.5 for the entire country. At the same time, there was an average attrition of 8 per cent in the student body of the School of Medicine. Oklahoma had an average, based on these data, of one physician to every 1,042 persons compared to 718 persons in the entire United States. Furthermore, only two other states had a higher median age than Oklahoma, and the beginning medical doctor had an active practice expectancy of no more than 35 years.

In the area of research, two laboratories for clinical investigation were developed in the University Hospitals during the year—the William Noble Memorial Laboratory in Crippled Children's Hospital and an investigative laboratory for the Department of Medicine located in the main hospital. The Noble laboratory, which was opened in October, was made possible by a gift from the estate of William Noble.[6]

---

[5] Amendments to the articles of affiliation of Oklahoma City hospitals with the university provided for affiliation of outlying hospitals for undergraduate as well as postgraduate educational purposes, and for the inclusion of the Central State Hospital at Norman.

[6] Mr. Noble had been a veteran of the Spanish-American War and had fought with Teddy Roosevelt's Roughriders. Later, President Roosevelt appointed him postmaster in McAlester, and then he moved to Oklahoma City to become industrial commission inspector, a position he held for fifteen years before retirement. He was a thirty-third degree Mason.

Applications for federal grant programs increased markedly during the year because of encouragement by C. J. Van Slyke of the National Institute of Health. In November the National Heart Institute granted $67,132 to the Oklahoma School of Medicine and a construction grant of $100,000 to the Oklahoma Medical Research Foundation. And the National Advisory Cancer Council recommended extension of a cancer training grant through June, 1950, in the amount of $25,000.

Don H. O'Donoghue was elected chairman of the faculty board on June 23, fulfilling the need for an adviser to the dean inasmuch as the position of associate dean of the faculty was officially terminated as of July 1. Although the position of chairman of the faculty board carried with it no administrative duties and no office hours, it was anticipated that the chairmen of departments, as well as individual faculty members, would feel free to speak to him in regard to policies of sufficient importance that they should be brought to the attention of the administration.[7]

Those members of the faculty who received the title of professor emeritus in 1949 were John Evans Heatley, radiology, and Louis Alvin Turley, pathology. Joseph Kelso replaced Grider Penick as chairman of the Department of Gynecology, A. N. Taylor became chairman of the Department of Physiology, J. B. Goldsmith acting chairman of the Department of Preventive Medicine and Public Health, and Cleve Beller director of postgraduate medical instruction for one year. Ellen Corine Keaty was named a consultant research associate in the Department of Dermatology, and Ella Mary George, after a year of post-graduate training in physical medicine at New York University's Bellevue Hospital, came to Oklahoma to chair the newly created Department of Physical Medicine. Other new appointees to the faculty were as follows:

Edgar Harold Hinman, M.D., Ph.D.
  professor of preventive medicine and public health
John Raymond Stacy, M.D.
  clinical professor of orthopedic and fracture surgery
Ella Mary George, M.D.
  assistant professor of physical medicine
Walter Joel, M.D.
  assistant professor of pathology
Joseph H. Perlmutt, Ph.D.
  assistant professor of physiology
Hal A. Burnett, M.D.
  instructor in surgery

Allan Alfred Katzberg, Ph.D.
  instructor in histology
James Charles Amspacher, M.D.
  clinical assistant in orthopedic and fracture surgery
Hubert M. Anderson, M.D.
  clinical assistant in surgery
Glen Lee Berkenbile, M.D.
  graduate fellow in anatomy
Kenneth Earl Bohan, M.D.
  clinical assistant in pediatrics
Maurice Philip Capehart, M.D.
  graduate fellow in neurosurgery
Richard Everett Carpenter, M.D.
  clinical assistant in medicine
Donald Gene Clements, M.D.
  fellow in oncology

[7.] The place of dentistry in the medical center was discussed about this time, although there was no immediate prospect of starting a dental program. However, the thought was there, to be encouraged to grow in future expansion plans for the medical center.

James Robert Colvert, M.D.
  clinical assistant in medicine
Daisy Van Hoesen Cotten, M.D.
  clinical assistant in obstetrics
Sterling Thomas Crawford, M.D.
  clinical assistant in gynecology
John Furman Daniel, M.D.
  clinical assistant in gynecology
Charles Shelly Graybill, M.D.
  fellow in orthopedic and fracture
  surgery
Charles Eugene Green, M.D.
  visiting lecturer in pediatrics
Walter Scott Hendren, M.D.
  clinical assistant in medicine
Robert Graham Hirschi, D.D.S.
  clinical assistant in dental surgery
Robert Perry Holt, M.D.
  clinical assistant in orthopedic
  and fracture surgery
Robert W. Kahn, M.D.
  clinical assistant in medicine
Achilles Courtney Lisle, M.D.
  clinical assistant in surgery
Robert Lowe Loy, Jr., M.D.
  clinical assistant in obstetrics

James Neill Lysaught, M.D.
  clinical assistant in pediatrics
William George McCreight, M.D.
  clinical assistant in dermatology
  and syphilology
Robert Doreck McKee, M.D.
  clinical assistant in obstetrics
Clarence Robison, Jr., M.D.
  graduate fellow in pathology
Paul Joseph Rosenbaum, M.S.
  research associate in radiology
Herbert Victor Louis Sapper, M.D.
  clinical assistant in pediatrics
Jerome Daniels Shaffer, M.D.
  clinical assistant in pediatrics
James Howard Snyder, M.D.
  clinical assistant in psychiatry and
  neurology
Herman Hull Stone, M.D.
  clinical assistant in medicine
William L. Waldrop, M.D.
  clinical assistent in orthopedic
  and fracture surgery
George Louis Winn, M.D.
  clinical assistant in medicine

On July 1, Harold Gordon Muchmore became assistant director of the outpatient department, at the same time retaining his part-time public relations appointment in the office of the dean. Robert Lowe assumed the duties of medical director of University Hospitals in October, filling the vacancy created by the resignation of Vernon D. Cushing.

Renown came to the Department of Surgery at the University Hospital when an entire issue of the *Southern Medical Journal*, published in Atlanta, Georgia, was devoted to a review of surgical practice at University Hospitals. The issue consisted of fourteen articles written by the faculty members of the Department of Surgery at the University of Oklahoma.[8]

The twenty-second legislature authorized the State Department of Health to use $35,000 in funds from that department to move five wooden buildings,[9]

[8.] Special mention should be made of Harry Wilkins and Jess Herrmann, professor and associate professor, respectively, in the Department of Surgery since 1946, and partners in the practice of neurosurgery. They personally supplemented the monthly salary and subsistence pay of residents in neurosurgery in the University Hospitals, up to a total of $200 per month. As of December 12, 1949, $4,505 had been paid by these two doctors to four fellows and residents in neurosurgery—concrete evidence of their abiding interest in medical education.

[9.] These buildings composed a unit of the Oklahoma medical center, a federally financed institution under the jurisdiction of the Oklahoma State Department of Health.

valued at $93,250, from the old Will Rogers Field site to the campus of the School of Medicine in 1949. The main motivation for this transfer was to provide certain services for venereal disease patients and to assist the School of Medicine in the care of large numbers of polio-myelitis patients—a recurring emergency to be expected every summer—and, at the same time, to provide more than 100 additional teaching beds. Two of the transferred buildings were used as wards for the treatment of communicable diseases and two for convalescent poliomyelitis patients.

Governor Turner and other state leaders appealed to the National Foundation for Infantile Paralysis for $75,000 in August for the care of Oklahoma's polio patients, when the hospital budget had been exceeded by $12,750 a month (including salaries for six physiotherapists, 26 recruited graduate staff nurses, and 23 ward workers).

President Cross said that we were actually straining the law a bit by spending money in excess of the budget allowances, but that there was nothing else to do in such an emergency. And, following a tour of the children's polio wards with Dean Everett, he remarked, "Troubles! *My* earthly troubles seem mighty small!"

On the brighter side, Warren Kingsbury, New York regional director for the National Foundation for Infantile Paralysis, assured President Cross and Dean Everett that ways would be worked out to provide needed funds, and interested citizens came through with flying colors. The Oklahoma sheriffs and peace officers contributed $1,000 for the purchase of an iron lung as did the Carpenter's Union; the State 4-H Clubs voluntarily raised approximately $11,000 during the year to equip the buildings for poliomyelitis patients; the Oklahoma City Trades and Labor Council contributed an annoxia photometer; the electricians bought a rocking bed to be used to simulate breathing; and the plumbers purchased a physiotherapy tank.

There were 1,299 cases of poliomyelitis reported in Oklahoma as of November 30, with a fatality rate of 7.5 per cent. Hillcrest Hospital in Tulsa and St. Mary's Hospital in Enid were the only hospitals in the state, other than Crippled Children's Hospital, admitting polio patients in 1949.

The actual cost of operating University Hospitals in 1949–50 was $1,699,712, including $1,125,241 for salaries and $504,715 for maintenance. The Soldiers Relief Commission was still functioning by virtue of its $50,000 per year appropriation for the care of veterans. The veterans' ward 3-W consisted of 32 beds for the exclusive use of veterans up until 1941, when four extra beds were designated for the use of Negro veterans on ward 1-E.

According to the comptroller's office, for 1949–50, $3,266,812 were appropriated for the University of Oklahoma in Norman out of a total income of $5,868,042; $452,700 for the School of Medicine out of a total income of $542,824, with capital funds of $996,218; and $782,471 for University Hospitals out of a total income of $1,584,888, with capital funds of $2,009,773.

During the fiscal year 1949–50 there were 6,584 patients admitted to University Hospital with an average stay of 12.8 days, and 2,513 children admitted to

Crippled Children's Hospital with an average stay of 23.7 days. This amounted to an average of 414 patients per day in the University Hospitals, while 15,697 individuals made 62,974 visits to the outpatient department, and the clinical laboratories conducted 180,848 examinations. The per diem cost for an inpatient was $12.24 and for an outpatient $1.74, which was 25 per cent less than for any other teaching hospital in the United States. The minimum value of professional services rendered gratuitously approximated $1,126,666.

There were 279 students enrolled in the School of Medicine for the academic year 1949–50 and 126 students in the School of Nursing. A total of fifty-four graduates including eleven women, received the M.D. degree in 1949, and twelve graduates received the certificate of nursing.

With the long premedical grind safely vaulted, 80 candidates, the largest number in history, were admitted to the School of Medicine of the University of Oklahoma in September, 1949. There were 253 applications from residents in Oklahoma, from which 60 veterans and 20 nonveterans were finally selected representing 33 counties.[10] The larger class was made possible by an increased appropriation and the prospects of a bond issue for a building program which would permit expansion of the School of Medicine and University Hospitals.

In choosing medical students, careful consideration was given to the results of the professional aptitude test as administered by the Educational Testing Service of Princeton, N.J. For the first time, all applicants were required to take this examination, which was offered once in the fall and again in the spring of the year.

Possibly the revamped mode of study in the last two years of the curriculum—a radical departure from the old lecture system—was the greatest innovation to date in the history of medical education in Oklahoma. There were only a few medical schools in the country placing as much emphasis on bedside work as the University of Oklahoma at a time when, ironically, the outpatient facilities were as deficient as any in the country. More than 60,000 patients a year were being handled in the outpatient departments of the two university hospitals, and they were even jammed into the hallways, leaving little room for clinical sessions, to say nothing of precious little office space.

The Speech and Hearing Clinic which was officially opened in October, 1947, had treated 1,145 patients from all over the state by January 25, 1950.[11] During that period, those patients made 14,893 visits to the clinic. Twenty-nine deaf youngsters, ranging from two and one-half to seven years of age, received daily instruction in the clinic, as did 15 children with cleft palates. The Commission for Crippled Children reimbursed the clinic for the care of eleven deaf children who lived in foster homes, but parents of many other children moved to Oklahoma City in order to take advantage of correct training in speech

[10] There were approximately 2,000 requests for admission to the School of Medicine from nonresidents, none of whom was considered for admission.

[11] Report by John W. Keys, director of the Speech and Hearing Clinic, January 25, 1950, to Arthur J. Lesser, M.D., Children's Bureau, Federal Security Agency, Washington, D.C.

and hearing for their children. Some 22 youngsters in all were receiving help in articulatory disorders in 1949. The staff of the clinic consisted of eight full-time persons—two speech correctionists, three auricular training teachers, a clinical audiologist, an acoustical engineer, and a director. In addition, a social worker and a secretary were employed on a full-time basis.

In order to meet the requirements of the National League of Nursing Education, that all students have psychiatry experience, affiliation was arranged with the Wichita General Hospital, Wichita, Kansas, making it possible for six senior nursing students to be sent to Wichita for three months on March 1, 1949, and six on June 1. Besides, through the combined efforts of the Oklahoma State League of Nursing Education and the State Mental Health Board, plans were also completed to have psychiatry affiliation at the Central State Hospital at Norman, Oklahoma, on September 1, 1949.

During the year, 79 students were admitted to the School of Nursing, almost doubling the student census of the preceding year. As the fall semester began, word was received that the school ranked with the top 25 per cent of the nation's basic programs in nursing, and that it had been placed in Group 1 of the 1949 interim classification of institutions offering such programs in nursing.

The $300,000 project for expansion of the nurses' home and teaching facilities at the medical center was approved in Washington on October 18, 1949, the federal contribution amounting to $100,000. This project virtually doubled the number of nurses who could be accommodated on the campus of the School of Medicine.

Governor Turner called a special session of the legislature in late November to vitalize the $36,000,000 bond issue which had passed in September, and the State Regents for Higher Education were immediately put on notice that a fight would be made in the legislature to build a $1,574,800 neuropsychiatric hospital addition here, out of the $36,000,000 building monies they wanted for colleges and universities. In fact, Representative Paul Harkey, chairman of the House Appropriations Committee, had previously proposed construction of such a neuropsychiatric hospital at the School of Medicine, and with him stood Representative J. D. McCarty of Oklahoma City, who said welfare of the mentally ill was "far more deserving than our cattle."

McCarty further stated that the State Regents for Higher Education had had two months to study the bond issue and that he was "surprised and shocked" at the cool reception being given the neuropsychiatric hospital bill by Chancellor M. A. Nash. "Most people who know the need for this hospital have assumed that the Higher Regents had included it as a must in their program, until Dr. Nash showed up hostile to it," he said.

Governor Turner had given his approval for the new hospital providing its financing could be worked out, and "J.D." (as Representative McCarty was usually designated) said that it was his belief that the amount necessary to build the hospital could be diverted from the $15,000,000 asked by the State Regents for Higher Education. But, at a hearing on the bill, Chancellor Nash was quite chary about the possibility that the legislature might decide to deduct money for this program from the amount suggested for higher education, and he said so.

Charles Obermann, state mental health director, spoke on the question before the appropriations committee, saying that Oklahoma had long needed such a hospital and that there would never be a strong Department of Psychiatry at the School of Medicine until the state built a facility such as this—all of which induced a heated discussion.

In an exchange between the Reverend J. Clyde Wheeler of Oklahoma City and Representative James Bullard of Duncan, Dr. Wheeler said, "We are going to have to have adequate facilities for training. We cannot educate people in a vacuum." "Do you think your reference to our mental hospitals as 'hell holes' is adequate?" Bullard asked. And the Reverend Wheeler replied, "Indeed I do."

A $36,000,000 program, with the governor's blessing, was made known at a press conference in December, which included the governor's recommendation that a $640,000 item for expansion of the Crippled Children's Hospital be cut to $320,000 and that $640,000 be provided for expansion of University Hospital.

While the element of personal victory for Governor Turner on the bond issue vote gave legislators no little respect for the program he handed them, there was the usual legislative independence which "caused some individual gagging." But in the end, the legislature accepted the program very much as it was presented. The final bill called for a lump sum appropriation of $10,749,010 to the State Regents for Higher Education with the senate committee writing a separate section into the bill, providing $500,000 for the neuropsychiatric ward and $320,000 for expansion of Crippled Children's Hospital.

"All we know is that all the money will be spent," declared Paul Ballenger of Holdenville, as Senator Ritzhaupt commented that in his opinion the State Regents for Higher Education had displayed "an imperialistic attitude." And someone else remarked facetiously that "the record would not chronicle the unusual spectacle of a governor exercising almost iron control over his third legislative session."

But newspaper pictures just before Christmas registered a sly grin on the face of Governor Turner as he signed the bill which provided an overall building program of over $38,000,000 for new construction, modernization, and repairs in state institutions—by far the largest building program ever undertaken in the state of Oklahoma at one time.

When the special legislative session closed after four tense weeks, the governor appeared in each house and sang his latest cowboy ballad. Then, giving a nod up the chimney he rose!

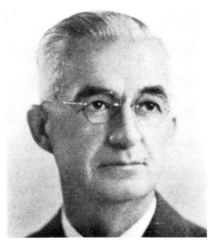

Edward P. Allen, M.D., chairman of
the Department of Obstetrics,
1945–46.

*Courtesy Oklahoma City Academy
of Medicine*

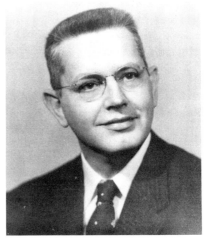

Robert H. Bayley, M.D., chairman of
the Department of Medicine, 1947–48.

*Courtesy University of Oklahoma
Medical Center*

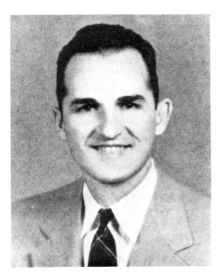

Howard A. Bennett, M.D., head of the
Department of Anesthesiology,
1948–55.

Courtesy Sooner Medic

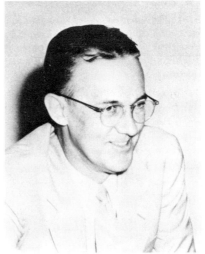

Frank P. Bertram, D.D.S., acting
director of the Department of Oral
Surgery, 1941–46.

*Courtesy Mrs. Margaret Bertram
Lemmond*

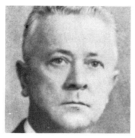

Rex George Bolend,
M.D., head of the
Department of Urology,
1936–43.

*Courtesy Oklahoma
City Academy of
Medicine*

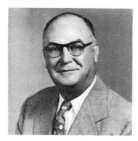

Charles P. Bondurant,
M.D., chairman of the
Department of Derma-
tology, 1942–56.

*Courtesy University of
Oklahoma Medical
Center*

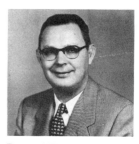

Donald W. Branham,
M.D., chairman of the
Department of Urology,
1954–61.

*Courtesy University
of Oklahoma Medical
Center*

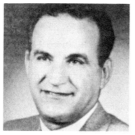

George M. Brother,
M.D., chairman of the
Department of Preven-
tive Medicine and Public
Health, 1951–52.

*Courtesy Madelon B.
Katigan*

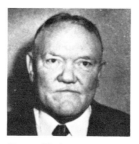

Coyne H. Campbell,
M.D., chairman of the
Department of Psychi-
atry, Neurology, and
Behavioral Sciences,
1948–54.

Courtesy Sooner Medic

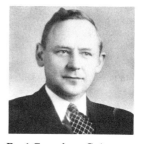

Paul Crenshaw Colonna,
M.D., chairman of the
Department of Ortho-
pedic and Fracture
Surgery, 1937–43.

*Courtesy University
of Oklahoma Medical
Center*

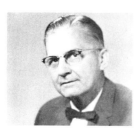

Tullos O. Coston, M.D.,
chairman of the Depart-
ment of Ophthalmology,
1962–(64).

*Courtesy University
of Oklahoma Medical
Center*

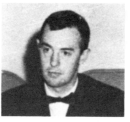

Marion deVeaux Cotten,
Ph.D., chairman of the
Department of Pharma-
cology, 1961–(64).

Courtesy Sooner Medic

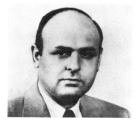

Martin M. Cummings,
M.D., chairman of the
Department of Bacteri-
ology, 1959–61.

*Courtesy University
of Oklahoma Medical
Center*

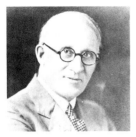

Samuel R. Cunningham,
M.D., chairman of the
Department of Ortho-
pedic and Fracture
Surgery, 1936.

Courtesy Dr. Joseph A.
Kopta

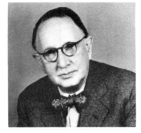

Charles F. DeGaris,
M.D., Ph.D., chairman
of the Department of
Anatomy, 1936–45.

Courtesy University
of Oklahoma Medical
Center

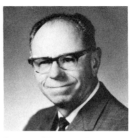

Hubert Eugene Doudna,
M.D., chairman of the
Department of Anesthe-
siology, 1938–48.

Courtesy University
of Oklahoma Medical
Center

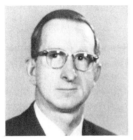

Albert R. Drescher,
D.D.S., chairman of the
Department of Oral
Surgery, 1955–61.

Courtesy Oklahoma
State Dental
Association

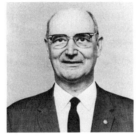

Lee K. Emmenhiser,
M.D., head of the
Department of Oto-
rhinolaryngology,
1959–62.

Courtesy University
of Oklahoma Medical
Center

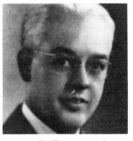

James B. Eskridge, Jr.,
M.D., chairman of the
Department of Obstet-
rics, 1946–54.

Courtesy Oklahoma
City Academy of
Medicine

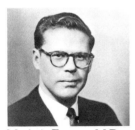

Mark A. Everett, M.D.,
chairman of the Depart-
ment of Dermatology,
(1964).

Courtesy University
of Oklahoma Medical
Center

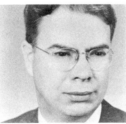

Shelby G. Gamble,
M.D., chairman of the
Department of Physical
Medicine, 1954–58.

Courtesy Oklahoma
State Board of
Medical Examiners

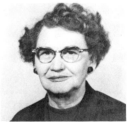

Ella Mary George,
M.D., chairman of the
Department of Physical
Medicine, 1952–54.

Courtesy University
of Oklahoma Medical
Center

169

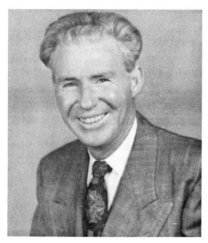

Joseph Benjamin Goldsmith, Ph.D., acting chairman of the Department of Preventive Medicine and Public Health, 1948–51.

Courtesy Madelon B. Katigan

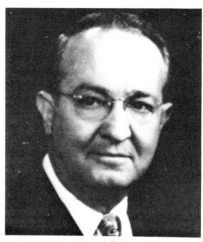

Rufus Q. Goodwin, M.D., chairman of the Department of Medicine, 1948–51.

Courtesy Oklahoma City Academy of Medicine

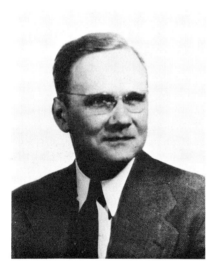

John F. Hackler, M.D., chairman of the Department of Preventive Medicine and Public Health, 1943–48.

Courtesy University of Oklahoma Medical Center

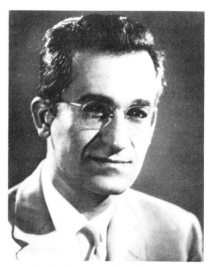

Francis J. Haddy, Ph.D., M.D., chairman of the Department of Physiology, 1961–(64).

Courtesy University of Oklahoma Medical Center

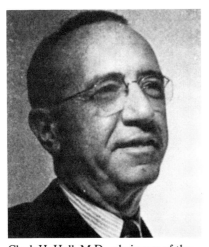

Clark H. Hall, M.D., chairman of the Department of Pediatrics, 1938–55.

Courtesy Sooner Medic

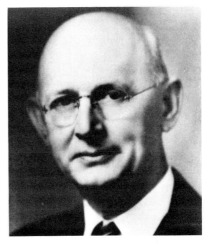

Basil A. Hayes, M.D., head of the Department of Urology, 1946–54.

Courtesy University of Oklahoma Medical Center

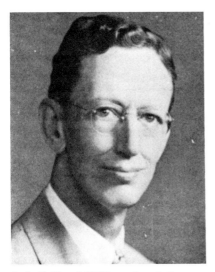

Onis G. Hazel, M.D., acting chairman of the Department of Preventive Medicine and Public Health, 1936–37.

Courtesy Oklahoma City Academy of Medicine

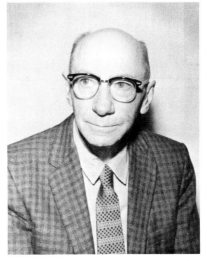

John E. Heatley, M.D., chairman of the Department of Radiology, 1936–48.

Courtesy University of Oklahoma Medical Center

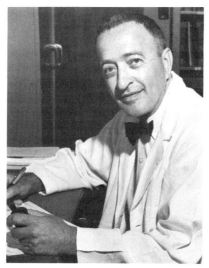

Ben I. Heller, M.D., head of the
Department of Laboratory Medicine,
(1964).

Courtesy Commentary

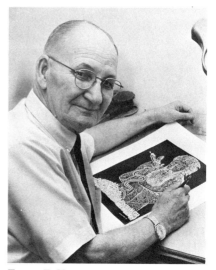

Ernest F. Hiser, B.A., head of the
Department of Medical Illustration,
1948–(64).

*Courtesy University of Oklahoma
Medical Center*

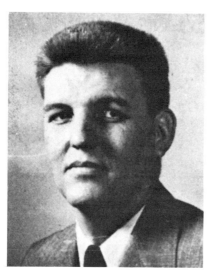

Howard C. Hopps, M.D., chairman of
the Department of Pathology, 1944–56.

Courtesy Sooner Medic

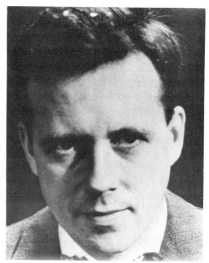

William E. Jaques, M.D., chairman of
the Department of Pathology,
1957–(64).

*Courtesy Oklahoma State Board of
Medical Examiners*

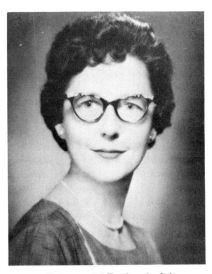

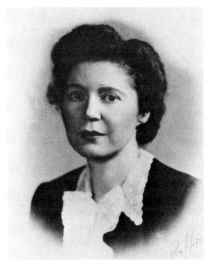

Phyllis E. Jones, M.D., head of the
Department of Dermatology, 1961–63.

*Courtesy University of Oklahoma
Department of Dermatology*

Florene C. Kelly, Ph.D., chairman of
the Department of Bacteriology,
1952–58.

*Courtesy University of Oklahoma
Medical Center*

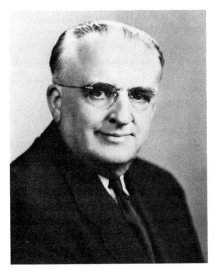

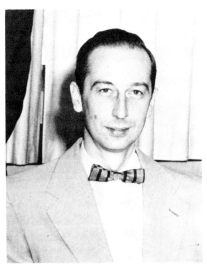

Joseph W. Kelso, M.D., chairman of
the Department of Gynecology,
1951–61.

*Courtesy University of Oklahoma
Medical Center*

M. Jack Keyl, Ph.D., chairman of the
Department of Physiology, 1960–61.

*Courtesy University of Oklahoma
Medical Center*

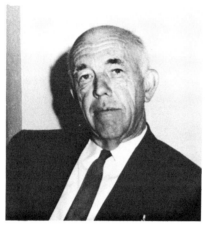

John W. Keys, Ph.D., head of the Department of Communication Disorders, 1960–(64).

Courtesy Sooner Medic

Gaylord S. Knox, M.D., acting chairman of the Department of Radiology, 1963.

Courtesy Dr. Sidney P. Traub

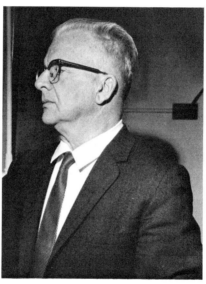

Ernest Lachman, M.D., head of the Department of Anatomy, 1945–(64).

Courtesy University of Oklahoma Medical Center

174

Chapter XIV.
Bona Fide Building
Blocks: 1950–51

 In 1950, January followed Christmas, as it had for hundreds of years, and members of the family of institutions for higher learning began wondering how the state regents were going to parcel out the gift certificates from the special session of the twenty-second legislature. The third ear of the State Regents for Higher Education was attuned to echoes of matching monies from the most bounteous Santa of them all—Uncle Sam.

After the lengthy study of the allocations to the School of Medicine, as of July 13, 1949, and the lump sum appropriation of $10,749,010 to the State Regents for Higher Education in December, the administration of the School of Medicine submitted a final revised request to the university regents for approval on March 8 for four major buildings on the medical school campus in Oklahoma City. This request included $500,000 for a neuropsychiatric addition to the University Hospital and $320,000 for expansion of the Crippled Children's Hospital (written into the state building bill by the senate in December, 1949), plus $250,000 for an addition to the medical school building and $214,000 for shop, laundry, and food services, making a total of $1,284,000.

Meeting on April 19, the university regents awarded the $1,284,000 from the $36,000,000 state building fund to the School of Medicine to commence its long-range expansion program. Moreover, they endorsed a tentative program for special modernization and repair of existing facilities ($300,000 for the University Hospital and $50,000 for the School of Medicine) and accepted the bid of the Charles M. Dunning Company in the amount of $767,870 for remodeling the School of Medicine building and construction of a new wing. By June 14 construction of classrooms and laboratories was underway, which would make it possible to admit an increased number of students to the School of Medicine in 1950–51, as requested by the twenty-first legislature.[1]

The administration was delighted that the regents had followed its requests "right down the line," and Dean Everett expressed gratitude (through the press) on April 20 to everyone who had helped to achieve this elusive goal. He

---

[1.] Two hundred fifty thousand dollars from the state building fund for the medical school addition, added to the $650,000 provided by the legislature, had made it possible to let the construction contract.

observed that the building program would afford adequate facilities for providing better medical service to the state of Oklahoma and for training medical students "By filling out some rough spots in our teaching program."

In the meantime, President Cross and Dean Everett were very concerned—not to say puzzled—over the 10.27 per cent reduction in the School of Medicine's budget, as indicated in a statement of approved budgets announced by the State Regents for Higher Education in April. For it appeared that the School of Medicine had been cut 14.0 per cent compared to 1949–50, while the average reduction for all institutions in the state system was only about 3.51 per cent.

Writing to President Cross on June 9, Dean Everett asserted that the state regents had stated repeatedly that they would assist in every way to prevent the curtailment of services in the University Hospitals and that their objective was to secure a fair proportion of the cost of operating the hospitals from agencies which should share some of the expense. On the contrary, they had simply reduced their allocations to the University Hospitals systematically since 1948–49, as follows: 1948–49, $1,300,000, 1949–50, $782,471, 1950–51 (proposed), $736,398.

According to the comptroller's office, the medical school finally received $408,722 and the University Hospitals, $920,170 in appropriations from the state for 1950–51, while the university at Norman received $3,500,574 compared with $2,662,385 in 1948–49, an increase of $838,189—obviously differential treatment.

Even though a shortage of operating funds was a dark cloud on the horizon, the building program continued to glitter. On June 13 the United States Public Health Service advised the administration of the School of Medicine that an addition to University Hospital of an outpatient department had been approved, as well as the expense of 75 beds for the neuropsychiatric ward at an estimated outlay of $1,407,000. The share of the federal government was to be $844,200, the remainder of the cost to be borne by the state of Oklahoma. And on September 16 the university regents accepted a bid of $1,264,431 to construct the outpatient building, with the neuropsychiatric addition incorporated therein.

It was now three years since the twenty-first legislature had given state land for an Oklahoma City veterans' hospital, and, in the meantime, more than $16,000,000 from several sources had been allocated for new construction on the medical school campus—putting the University of Oklahoma School of Medicine out front as one of the developing medical centers in the nation.

When on July 15, 1950, the contract for construction of a 500-bed veterans' hospital was awarded, at the low bid of $7,024,000, J. Wiley Richardson, president of the Oklahoma City Chamber of Commerce, exclaimed, "It is like a dream come true!" And the acting chief medical officer of the Veterans Administration regional office, Dr. Howard E. Martin, expressed the opinion that this veterans' hospital would "round off a truly great medical center."

Governor Turner was quick to say that Oklahoma was "on the threshold of the greatest period of advancement in the field of medical science" and, in dedicating the site for the veterans' hospital, given by the state of Oklahoma during his administration, he said in conclusion, "I hereby dedicate this oil of Oklahoma to perpetual service."

Governor Turner had proclaimed Thursday, February 16, as Oklahoma Medical Research Foundation Day, in support of a new campaign for a two and one-half-million-dollar expansion program. And Coyne H. Campbell and his wife, Margaret, transferred ownership of the $250,000 Coyne Campbell Psychiatric Sanitarium to the Oklahoma Medical Research Foundation, with all the net income from its operation of the 90-patient capacity sanitarium to go to the Oklahoma Medical Research Institute.[2]

Although the Oklahoma Medical Research Foundation was established and functioning as an organization independent of the School of Medicine, its full-time research personnel were given the opportunity to receive School of Medicine appointments as follows: (a) research professor in a department closely allied with his or her research, on recommendation by that department; (b) research associates, fellows, or assistants to conduct research work independently or in collaboration with members of a department, on recommendation by the department.

Meanwhile, autonomous research continued at the School of Medicine and the University Hospitals. The head of the $30,000 research program using radioactive isotopes as weapons in the fight against diesease (made possible by the twenty-second legislature) was war-trained Cleve Beller, who had traveled the army research route from Los Alamos to Oak Ridge. Radioactive phosphorus and radioactive iodine were supplied to the Medical Center laboratory by the Atomic Energy Commission, and the researchers were authorized to use P-32 for treatment in case of polycythemia vera and in blood dyscrasias.

The isotope committee of the Medical Center, consisting of Doctors Beller, Russo, Lowe, Conrad, and Rosenbaum, reserved the right to determine whether or not isotopes should be used in any particular case and, at a meeting on February 22, reached an agreement to establish an isotope clinic. Ambulatory cases received service in the isotope laboratory located on the third floor of "Main" at the University Hospital.

The second quarter was one of great significance for the laboratory, the institution, and the state. In addition to the completion of the acquisition of almost all of the basic radiation measurement and detection instruments during this time, medical history was made on March 14, when a radioactive isotope was administered to a patient for the first time in the state of Oklahoma. During the period from February 1 through April 30, twelve patients received radioac-

---

[2.] The *Daily Oklahoman*, February 23, 1950, said, "In explaining the gift, Dr. Campbell pointed to his lifelong interest in research, and recalled his establishment of the John Archer Hatchett Fund, at the University of Oklahoma School of Medicine. He remarked that that small fund of $3,000 had resulted in the publication of four excellent research papers in regard to cancer. 'I thought if $3,000 could bring me so much pleasure, a larger gift would result in proportionately more pleasure,' he said." See also Mark R. Everett, *Pioneering for Research*, University of Oklahoma Medical Center, Oklahoma City (1966), 50–51.

tive iodine and two, radioactive phosphorus for diagnosis and treatment of thyroid diseases, cancer, or certain blood diseases.

Numerous grants and grants-in-aid came to the medical center in 1950, at a time when research money was limited, and even small grants were meaningful and greatly appreciated—$24,996 for undergraduate training in cancer research and $26,500 from the National Institutes of Health for training in the fields of mental health and heart disease.

The chairman of the Department of Psychiatry stated that the grant in the field of mental health was very opportune, since it encouraged the development of the department at a time when the psychosomatic teaching program seriously needed it, and that it would be of considerable aid not only to students but also to staff members in their efforts to harmonize the psychiatric program with that of other clinical departments.

In his annual report, Arthur Hellbaum, associate dean in charge of graduate studies and research, reported that there were seven men holding postgraduate fellowships in various departments of the School of Medicine, in addition to two National Institutes of Health postdoctoral fellows; and that certificates had been issued to 35 residents, 23 interns, and 6 dietetic interns under the affiliated hospitals system. The research activities were summarized as follows: the research committee of the medical school granted funds for 21 research projects totaling $6,574. Nine United States public health grants were made to the School of Medicine totaling $63,378, four of them continued from previous years and five being new grants. Funds from other sources included three grants from the American Cancer Society totaling $19,534, and one from the Life Insurance Medical Research Fund for $3,874. Thus, a total of $93,360 was earmarked for research at the School of Medicine in 1949–50.

There were two deaths of members of the faculty in 1950: Walter W. Wells, who became professor emeritus of obstetrics upon his retirement in 1945, died on February 14, and Major General Robert Urie Patterson, the first full-time dean of the University of Oklahoma School of Medicine and a former surgeon general of the army, died at Walter Reed Hospital in Washington, D.C., on December 6. Upon leaving Oklahoma, General Patterson had become dean of the University of Maryland School of Medicine in Baltimore.

Dean Everett's salary was approved for the coming year by the university regents (April 13) at a total of $11,500—$8,500 as professor of biochemistry and $1,500 each for the positions of dean and superintendent. On the same day, the regents also approved a recommendation that a personnel program be activated as of July 1, at the School of Medicine and its hospitals, and that a booklet be published for employees describing the conditions of employment. Retirement for all administrative officers at the age of 65 years was established on October 1.

New faculty appointments for 1950–51 were as follows:

Max Niel Huffman, Ph.D.
    research professor of biochemistry

Edward C. Reifenstein, Jr., M.D.
    professor of research medicine

James P. Dewar, Jr., M.D.
  associate professor of pathology
Dale Allen Clark, Ph.D.
  assistant professor of biochemistry
Roy Cobb Lytle, L.L.B.
  assistant professor of medical
  jurisprudence
Norman J. Robinson, M.D.
  assistant professor of pediatrics
Lawrence Vernon Scott, D.Sc.
  assistant professor of bacteriology
Charles David Bodine, M.D.
  instructor in obstetrics
Edward William Cubler, M.D.
  instructor in anesthesiology
Samuel M. Glasser, M.D.
  instructor in radiology
Alfred Allen Hellams, M.D.
  instructor in psychiatry and
  neurology
R. Gibson Parrish, M.D.
  instructor in anesthesiology
Frank L. Adelman, M.D.
  clinical assistant in psychiatry and
  neurology

Nello Brown, M.D.
  clinical assistant in medicine
John J. Coyle, M.D.
  clinical assistant in gynecology
Charles Earl Delhotal, M.D.
  clinical assistant in pediatrics
Charles Louis Freede, M.D.
  clinical assistant in pediatrics
John Francis Head, M.D.
  research fellow in medicine
Edmond H. Kalmon, Jr., M.D.
  clinical assistant in radiology
Neil B. Kimerer, M.D.
  clinical assistant in psychiatry and
  neurology
Dick Moss Lowry, M.D.
  clinical assistant in
  otorhinolaryngology
Dean Robertson, D.D.S.
  clinical assistant in dental surgery
Sumner Russman, D.D.S.
  clinical assistant in dental surgery
Douglas A. Yeager, D.D.S.
  clinical assistant in dental surgery

Teaching in the clinical years continued to assume new dimensions with the innovation of a streamlined curriculum. Nine months of uninterrupted work, without trimester or semester, was recommended in the third year, with the didactic work continuing on the semester basis. The entire fourth year was spent in the outpatient clinics, as steps were taken to strengthen weak spots in the efficacy of the expanded activities.

Because of the confusion resulting from the designation of a dental clinic in the outpatient department of University Hospital (where no general dentistry was ever performed) Doctors Reichmann and Hirschi requested that this outpatient clinic and the offices in which the work of the department was done be designated as the Oral Surgery Clinic, though they thought the work might be best designated by the term "Exodontia and Dental Surgery." By the same token, the doctors asked that the dental clinic in Children's Hospital be designated "Children's Dental Clinic," since most of the work done was orthodontia, pedodontia, and the necessary amount of oral surgery.

The Department of Radiology asked to have its training program for students in x-ray technology changed from a one-year to a two-year course as of September 1, 1950. Under the new plan, the first year was without pay and the second year at a salary of about $150 per month, after which time students would be eligible to take the examination for the American Registry of X-ray Technicians. In this connection, Dr. Russo, chairman of the Department of

Radiology, requested that, after completion of the two-year course, a certificate be issued to show that the training had been satisfactorily completed at the School of Medicine of the University of Oklahoma.

Since 1948 the board of directors of the Urban League of Oklahoma City had corresponded with Dean Everett relative to the expansion program for the School of Medicine and University Hospitals, hoping that—if and when facilities were adequate—a "transfer of Negro children would be made to Crippled Children's Hospital." And on June 7, 1950, Negro children under 14 years of age were transferred from the main University Hospital to the Crippled Children's Hospital where a number of additional beds had been made available for these children. Besides, the transfer made possible the addition of six more beds for adult Negro patients at the main hospital.

In reply to Dean Everett's letter, in which he informed Cernoria D. Johnson, executive secretary, Urban League of Oklahoma City, that he was happy to relay the good news to the league, Mrs. Johnson stated: "The Urban League Board of Directors and its membership wish to express appreciation for the excellent manner in which you provided more adequate care for Negro crippled children. It is gratifying to know that with your many, many responsibilities *you did remember our request* and continued to correct the situation. By this very deed, you have further strengthened our confidence. . . ."

In the same vein, W. L. Haywood, chief of staff on the Negro ward in University Hospital, complimented Robert C. Lowe, medical director, on the far-reaching effect of activities which were "gradually opening the door to a helpless minority group, plaintively pleading for an opportunity to train and educate our race, so we can better fit into human relationships, and keep pace with this progressive American civilization."

Another time, on the occasion of receiving new furnishings for his office, Dr. Haywood expressed his surprise and pleasure—"so I could hardly speak"—after the furniture had been put in place. "Not only is it serviceable, it is exquisitely beautiful. . . . one should be able to make tangible progress in the ultimate aim of helping minority people."

During a faculty meeting in late November, Dean Everett drew attention to a five-year report recently completed on University Hospitals, which revealed tremendous increases in many hospital services during the period. Even so, the per diem cost of the University Hospitals was at least 25 per cent less than any other teaching hospital in the United States. And increased medical care continued to be provided in 1950–51, as evidenced by a record 160,693 inpatient days and 112,087 outpatient treatments in the hospitals.

An annual report showed that the University and Crippled Children's hospitals, with hardly any increase in available beds, accommodated 40 per cent more patients in 1950–51 than they did 10 years earlier. In the 12 months preceding July 1, 1951, the hospitals discharged 10,555 patients, compared to 6,394 in 1941–42. The average patient at the University Hospital spent three and one-half days less time in the hospital and, in Crippled Children's Hospital five days less than previously.

There were 3,137 admissions to Crippled Children's Hospital, with average stay of 21.4 days. Although the number of patients who visited the outpatient department was about the same (16,000 in 1941 and 1951), the number of treatments more than doubled. Moreover, there was an enormous increase in laboratory examinations and tests made in the hospitals. In 1941 there were 112,000 laboratory examinations, whereas the total came to 216,000 in 1950–51. There were 185 employees of the hospitals working a 48-hour week at a maximum salary of $100 per month or less, with 90 per cent receiving *less* than $100 per month!

The total income for the university at Norman for 1950–51 was $5,069,046, of which $3,500,574 was appropriated by the state; for the School of Medicine $408,722 was appropriated out of a total income of $511,775, plus a capital fund of $604,319; for University Hospitals, $920,170 was appropriated out of a total income of $1,968,703, plus a capital fund of $844,181.

There were 280 students enrolled in the School of Medicine for 1950–51 and 149 in the School of Nursing. The M. D. degree was awarded to 74 graduates in 1950, and certificates of nursing were received by 27 graduates.

The cost of educating a medical student, exclusive of providing suitable hospital facilities, was carefully figured at $3,339 per student, according to a survey in 1950 by the National Fund for Medical Education. A general fee of $175 per semester was required of all medical students who were residents in Oklahoma. Nonresidents were required to pay $350 per semester.

The School of Medicine had a series of contracts with the United States Army to provide resident training to selected personnel beginning in May, 1950, because the Medical Reserve Officers Training Corps (established at the School of Medicine in 1947) had steadily increased its enrollment to include approximately 60 per cent of the medical students by 1950.

A first-year class of 80 students was admitted to the School of Medicine in the fall—all bona fide residents of the state of Oklahoma since applications of nonresidents were not accepted. All students were governed by the principle of the honor system.

There were 2,703 doctors of medicine in Oklahoma in 1909 (an average of 587 persons per doctor), but when the population stood at 2,233,351 in 1950, the number of physicians in the state was only 2,164.[3] In 1909 there were fifteen counties having no town with as many as 2,500 inhabitants, yet these same counties had a total of 278 doctors when Oklahoma was a new state, but *only 78 doctors* in 1950!

The inauguration of the preceptorship program for fourth-year medical students in 1949, in an attempt to promote special interest in the practice of medicine in the more rural areas of the state, exceeded all expectations by the end of the year, with tremendous possibilities for the betterment of medical practice in Oklahoma. Even the "Voice of America," in a discussion of the

[3.] In 1950, Oklahoma City had a population of 243,504, Tulsa, 182,740, and Norman, 27,006.

preceptorship plan at the School of Medicine, was telling people in Europe, Asia, and Africa how the University of Oklahoma "put the finishing touches on its medical students."

Introduction of the two-year general practice internship promised to be an important step in the development of graduate training too, and representatives from other medical schools began visiting the medical center in regard to all aspects of our developing postgraduate education system and the creation of our Medical Research Foundation.

During the first year of the general practice postgraduate program, Dr. Beller had effected some very excellent organizational work, which resulted in an active program in the various clinical specialties and in the basic sciences. One graduate, who returned for a two-day course in abdominal surgery, lost no time in saying that he thought the "old school" had "made many advancements within the past two years," and that he was ready and happy to do anything he could to help get adequate appropriations for the school through the senators and representatives in his geographical area.

In an effort to encourage physicians to start premature nurseries in hospitals in their home towns, the University Hospitals offered a series of short post-graduate courses to doctors and nurses on modern care for premature babies. The new premature nursery at the Crippled Children's Hospital comprised four rooms with an operational cost of $15,000 per year.[4]

In April the university regents approved a general budget for postgraduate instruction for 1950–51, which was generously supported by a second allotment from the five-year commitment of $130,000 by the W. K. Kellogg Foundation to assist the School of Medicine in developing decentralization of medical education. The total budget amounted to $71,180: $37,000 from the Kellogg Foundation, $12,180 from the School of Medicine, and $16,000 from the State Department of Health (for assistant directors in obstetrics and pediatrics) leaving a balance of $6,000 for operational expenses.

The number of full-time graduate students in the School of Medicine and affiliated hospitals on July 1, 1950, was 132: 47 interns, 66 residents, 8 fellows, and 11 graduate students. Sister Mary Agnes, administrator of St. Anthony Hospital, wrote Dean Everett in December that approval of their three residency programs in general surgery by the Conference Committee on Graduate Training in Surgery, was "due to your personal efforts and our affiliation with the University Hospitals."

In trying to systematize the budgets and expenditures of the School of Medicine and the University Hospitals (in accordance with recognized business practice), the administration was confronted with the fact that the expenses of the School of Nursing were not shown as a systematized unit. So the administration submitted an auxiliary or separate budget for the School of Nursing for 1950–51, which was approved by the president of the university in October.

---

4. See the *Daily Oklahoman*, February 5, 1950.

This was essential for accreditation by nursing agencies. A program that would lead to the degree of Bachelor of Science in Nursing was also approved.

According to a United States Supreme Court ruling, June 5, 1950, there was "no alternative but to provide housing and other facilities for Negroes on the same basis as for other students" on the campus of the medical school, according to the attorney general of the state of Oklahoma. And on December 14, 1950, Oklahoma City newspapers announced that Negro girls would be accepted for admission to the University of Oklahoma School of Nursing for the first time in February, 1951. The office of George Cross, as president of the university, informed the press that girls would be permitted to enroll if they could pass the entrance examinations and physicals set up for other students, and that they would live in nurses' dormitories without discrimination.

Budgets were a bugaboo, no matter which way the administration looked, and in November, Kenneth Wallace, the business administrator, advised Dean Everett that the Crippled Children's Commission was approximately $185,000 in arrears for the current year's services, and that, unless a considerable portion of that amount was paid by early in December, the University Hospitals would be unable to meet their payroll.

On December 9, Dean Everett informed President Cross that the administration had prepared a revised biennial budget for the School of Medicine and University Hospitals, as instructed, but that, in order to keep individual items within the totals approved by the State Regents for Higher Education, it had been necessary to delete all necessary operating expenses for the neuropsychiatric addition to University Hospital (then under construction) and for isotope services rendered by the School of Medicine to cancer patients in the hospital.

"I consider it my duty," wrote the dean, "to recommend for your consideration that a statement be made to the governing boards that unless funds are provided for the above functions, they cannot be operated during the next biennium; and that a statement should again be made, that unless new legislation is secured, the University Hospitals can realize only a fraction of the estimated income designated in the request as 'other funds,' and large sections of the University Hospitals will have to close."

But the building program continued, even if there were insufficient funds in the crystal ball of the immediate future to operate the growing physical plant. On December 13, Hudgins, Thompson, Ball and Associates, architects, presented preliminary plans to the university regents for an addition to Crippled Children's Hospital, at an estimated cost of $670,400. It would include a one-story addition for a physical therapy department. The legislature and governing boards had cut the original request for $640,000 by 50 per cent, making only $320,000 available for this addition in anticipation of aid from the Hill-Burton Fund of the federal government.

The short warm days of late December brought a glimmer of hope for some financial aid when the American Medical Association launched a multimillion-dollar campaign to help the medical schools train future doctors, and trustees of the association appropriated $500,000 to give immediate assistance to 79 approved schools of medicine in the United States.

The jolliest surprise of 1950, however, had nothing to do with either budgets or building contracts or even Christmas bonuses, but with medical science and an unscientific proof which startled a district judge, a jury, and a courtroom full of spectators. For Homer Marsh, professor of bacteriology in the School of Medicine, took a dare by the lawyer for a complainant and drank from a pop bottle containing a dead mouse—to prove that no one would suffer harmful effects from a mouse drink! "It's all in the mind," Dr. Marsh said blithely, as the visibly shocked lawyer who issued the challenge had his case thrown out of court by a chuckling judge.

Chapter XV.
The Cabal Overplays
Its Hand: 1951–52

 The eyes of medical educators in America were watching the University of Oklahoma School of Medicine and its alumni association (probably the most active in the nation) by 1951—from Arkansas, California, Chicago, Colorado, Connecticut, Georgia, New York, and Omaha—"because of the remarkable number of advances in the last two years" and "the leadership . . . given this school at an important period in its development."[1]

Active and intense programs, having to do with building funds and operation and maintenance of the School of Medicine and University Hospitals, had indeed proved effective in less than two years time. "When we started planning for the Medical Center," Dean Everett said, "I was not sure that the construction goals could really be achieved, but this happy result has actually come to pass."

However, the medical center had gone about as far as it could go with the tools at hand, and additional provisions, which only the state legislature could provide, were needed to develop its potentialities, inasmuch as the major unsolved problem was financing the care of indigent patients in Oklahoma. While physicians had always donated their services to these unfortunate citizens, there was no way they could resolve the cost of hospitalization for them. This was a problem which related to all citizens in the counties and communities of the state, to the legislators, and to the Oklahoma State Regents for Higher Education, who controlled the destiny of the taxpayer's hard-earned dollar for operation of the system of higher education.

Johnston Murray, an attorney and son of former Governor William Murray, was the fourteenth governor of Oklahoma. He and Boyd Cowden, president pro tempore of the senate, and James M. Bullard, speaker of the house, were immediately faced with the challenge of making sufficient operational funds available to the School of Medicine or of insuring that a portion of the expanded facilities for instruction of medical students remain idle during the next two

---

[1] Donald G. Anderson, secretary, Council on Medical Education and Hospitals, American Medical Association, in a letter to Mark R. Everett, February 10, 1950; and Dean F. Smiley, secretary, Association of American Medical Colleges, in a letter to Mark R. Everett, February 13, 1950, respectively.

185

years—an unpalatable alternative. The twenty-second legislature had purposely appropriated funds for expansion of facilities to make possible a class of 100 first-year medical students, largely because the shortage of doctors in the state was so deplorable.

Governor Murray was in favor of operating the medical school at full capacity, and the house advanced a $1,950,000 supplementary appropriation for institutions of higher education in February, "after blistering oratory, charging the state regents with mismanagement," according to a local press release on February 21. Sponsors of the measure said the appropriation was necessary because the twenty-second legislature had reduced allowances for the second year of the biennium by more than $1,000,000.

Governor Murray signed the bill on March 24, and the State Regents for Higher Education made the supplemental apportionments on March 26, with allotments listed as follows: University of Oklahoma School of Medicine, $27,375 and University Hospitals, $183,772. The final appropriation bill for higher education for the next biennium (passed by the twenty-third legislature) stated that enough money should be set aside by the State Regents for Higher Education to make possible an entering class of 100 students for the next academic year.

Although the legislature had no power to specifically earmark funds for any institution of higher education under the jurisdiction of the state regents, it had for some time followed this practice of making recommendations in order to show intent. Its intent in 1951 was obviously favorable to the School of Medicine, for $320,000 was reappropriated,[2] and an additional appropriation of $350,000 was allocated to the State Regents for Higher Education for a new wing on the Crippled Children's Hospital (House Joint Resolution No. 11). An additional $300,000 was appropriated to put the new psychiatric wards into operation at University Hospital.

On March 22 a news item reported that House Bill No. 241, making impounded animals available to stated institutions for essential research, was advanced to final passage in the house of representatives "despite barks, growls, whistles, and typical legislative humor." This bill, subsequently passed by the senate, was signed by Governor Murray on April 26, 1951.

Following adjournment of the twenty-third legislative session, the administration of the School of Medicine and University Hospitals was confronted once more with the beds and budget dilemma, for the Oklahoma State Regents for Higher Education allocated only $780,000 in state funds for the operation of the University Hospitals—the lowest allocation since 1947–48—making the budget for operating University Hospital for the current fiscal year approximately $204,000 short of the income needed. Compounding the difficulty further, the state regents advised the university regents that they would not ask for any supplementary funds for the hospitals. Whereupon President Cross recommended to the university regents on September 12 that the hospital

---

[2.] This amount had actually been appropriated two years previously but had lapsed because of failure to receive expected federal funds.

administration be authorized to convert 50 charity beds to private pay beds, as an alternative to closing beds, since a class of 100 medical students was scheduled to enter the School of Medicine momentarily. "While this is not desirable," President Cross said, "It is the only solution to the problem." (Small wonder that the temperature was "91° at 8 a.m. and 100°from noon on" in the dean's office during September!)

Since only practicing physicians could advise patients to use private bed facilities, there was no chance that the University Hospitals could guarantee that additional private beds would be filled, and therefore it was impossible for the administration to be at all certain that any set income could be derived from private beds. Furthermore, Dean Everett advised President Cross that it would be necessary to convert 102 beds (all that were available in small rooms) to private pay status and to close an additional 70 beds in order to balance the budget under this catastrophic plan; and that such a conversion of beds would only reduce the number of dependable teaching cases and interfere drastically with the choice of cases for a balanced teaching program.

The executive committee of the faculty board endorsed the dean's policy of "keeping the beds open at any price," but the University of Oklahoma's Board of Regents, in session on December 3, still hoped that, by putting one-fourth of the total number of hospital beds on a paying basis, the financial crisis would be averted and the University School of Medicine relieved of its terrific load of charity patients to boot.

A principal factor in attaining acceptable accreditation of the School of Medicine in 1948 was the reopening of 100 previously closed beds in the University Hospitals, and obtaining teaching privileges in local affiliated hospitals for 260 additional beds not financed by state funds. Therefore, Dean Everett found himself in an untenable position since the reduction of teaching cases either directly or indirectly would be, in his opinion, a violation of the dean's duty to provide adequate professional instruction for students in the School of Medicine of the University of Oklahoma. On this basis, Dean Everett submitted his resignation, as dean of the School of Medicine and superintendent of the University Hospitals, to President Cross on December 3, 1951, "to become effective as soon as events beyond this administration's control make it impossible to maintain the present number of teaching cases."

President Cross replied on December 5 that he could appreciate Dean Everett's concern about the possibility that the School of Medicine's professional status might be jeopardized by a change in the number of teaching beds available, but that he had confidence in the dean's "ability to meet this crisis in the same successful way that you have met the many other serious problems that have arisen during your term of office."

On December 13 a communication from T. G. Sexton, administrative assistant for the state regents, was submitted to the university regents, which stated that, inasmuch as efforts to get laws passed to force counties to pay for their respective patients had failed, "the Oklahoma State Regents for Higher Education hereby authorize and strongly recommend that the University Hospitals accept additional private patients, as directed by law, to the extent deemed necessary and practicable by the governing board of the institution, in order that adequate teaching facilities may be maintained.''

Finally, the university regents approved a motion (initiated by Regent Benedum) that the university regents request the state regents to confer with Governor Murray in an attempt to induce him to cover the $125,000 deficiency from his contingency and emergency fund, in order to complete operation of University Hospitals for the current fiscal year ending June 30, 1951.

Dean Everett, who was invited to be present at this meeting, emphasized his conviction that closing 70 additional charity beds would only further reduce clinical facilities without balancing the budget. Whereupon, President Cross stated that there was no authority for creating obligations in excess of anticipated revenue (in fact, there was a penalty for such action), and that he would not be a party to creating a deficit.

In a current news story on the imbroglio, Chancellor Nash was quoted as saying that only a small part (about 20 percent of operating expenses for University Hospitals should be charged to the teaching program in the first place, and that the remainder should be derived from public service rendered to indigents of the state.

In spite of all the clamor about lack of funds to operate existing facilities, the physical plant continued to expand under the momentum of the drive for educating more doctors and nurses in Oklahoma. The $255,000 wing for the School of Nursing building was completed in June, making it possible for the first time for the entire school to be housed under one roof. The new section, which was built with 60 per cent federal monies under the Hill-Burton Construction Law had 42 units bringing the housing capacity to 172 students.

Construction of the addition to the School of Medicine building was progressing on schedule, and diagonally across Thirteenth Street and to the east, the nine-story neuropsychiatric hospital and outpatient department was mushrooming.[3]

According to a report of the federal hospital construction program on July 1, 1951, a total of $1,092,779 in federal aid had been given to the University of Oklahoma School of Medicine and University Hospitals in the past three fiscal years: $35,087 for equipment for the addition to University Hospital; $897,358 for construction and equipment of the neuropsychiatric and outpatient wing; $7,480 for remodeling Crippled Children's Hospital kitchen; and $152,853 for construction of the wing for the School of Nursing building.

Elmer T. Peterson commented in an editorial in the *Daily Oklahoman* that a double-edged sword hung over the whole system of medical education, ''with one edge cutting down available private beneficence, by reason of extremely high income taxes, and the other producing inflation and insidiously inviting all institutions to come under the federal wing.''

On November 14 the university regents accepted a bid for construction of the

---

[3.] For an illustrated progress report, see the brochure by the University of Oklahoma School of Medicine Alumni Association, April 9, 1951.

addition to Crippled Children's Hospital and awarded a contract to the Secor Building Company, Inc. Specifications were for a three-story building with a basement, at a cost of $559,990. This construction expanded the hospital's outpatient and X-ray departments, included two wards with a capacity of approximately 60 beds, and permitted enlargement of the physiotherapy section. Construction financed and in progress for affiliated institutions included the Oklahoma Medical Research Institute and Hospital (at construction costs of $900,000 and $250,000, respectively) and the $8,000,000 veterans' hospital.

Faculty and staff continued to come and go in the various buildings—some receiving appointments and others resigning from the faculty, as in all years. On July 11, Joseph M. Thuringer, professor and chairman of the Department of Histology-Embryology resigned.[4] Cyril E. Clymer was promoted to the rank of professor emeritus, Department of Surgery, and George Winn succeeded Cleve Beller as director of the office of postgraduate instruction. Initial appointments were as follows:

George M. Brother, M.D.
  professor of preventive medicine
  and public health
Charles D. Kochakian, Ph.D.
  professor of research
  biochemistry
Kirk Thornton Mosley, M.D.,
  D.P.H.
  professor of epidemiology and
  consulting professor of preventive
  medicine and public health
Leonard P. Eliel, M.D.
  associate professor of research
  medicine
R. Palmer Howard, M.D.
  associate professor of research
  medicine
Shirley L. Wells, M.S.
  associate research professor of
  nutrition
Betty Jane Bamforth, M.D.
  assistant professor of
  anesthesiology
Norma J. Collins, B.S.
  assistant professor of nutrition
John Francis Lhotka, Jr., M.D.,
  Ph.D.
  assistant professor of anatomy
  and histology

William Taylor Newsom, M.D.
  assistant professor of pediatrics
Henry Louis Schmidt, Jr., M.D.,
  assistant professor of medicine
James William Hickman Smith,
  M.D.
  assistant professor of physiology
Paul Paine Webb, M.D.
  assistant professor of physiology
John Ahrens Blaschke, M.D.
  instructor in pharmacology
David Jackson Geigerman, M.D.
  instructor in anesthesiology
Sister Mary Bonaventure Hirner,
  M.S.
  instructor in nutrition
David Charles Lowry, M.D.
  instructor in radiology
Paul Michael Obert, M.D.
  instructor in pathology
Donald D. Albers, M.D.
  clinical assistant in urology
Ruth Vivian Annadown, M.D.
  clinical assistant in medicine
William Lawrence Bond, M.D.
  clinical assistant in obstetrics
Beverly Colvin Chatham, M.D.
  visiting lecturer in obstetrics
John Hatchett Clymer, M.D.
  clinical assistant in surgery

[4.] The Department of Histology and Embryology was made part of the Department of Anatomy in 1951.

Charles Riley Cochrane, M.D.
clinical assistant in obstetrics
Everett Ellis Cooke, M.D.
clinical assistant in surgery
Earl Richard Cunningham, D.D.S.
clinical assistant in dental surgery
James Burnett Eskridge, III, M.D.
clinical assistant in obstetrics
William Nason Flesher, D.D.S.
clinical assistant in dental surgery
John Florence, M.D.
clinical assistant in orthopedic
and fracture surgery
Russell D. Harris, M.D.
clinical assistant in orthopedic
and fracture surgery

Katherine Kaufman Hudson, M.S.
assistant in psychosomatic
teaching
John Daniel Ingle, M.D.
clinical assistant in surgery
Ray Ulman Northrip, M.D.
visiting lecturer in pathology
George Edward Reynolds, Jr.,
D.D.S.
clinical assistant in dental surgery
S. Fulton Tompkins, M.D.
clinical assistant in orthopedic
and fracture surgery
A. Ray Wiley, M.D.
visiting lecturer in surgery

O. Alton Watson was made chairman of the Department of Otorhinolaryngology, replacing Dr. McHenry, Neil B. Kimerer became a full-time psychiatrist on the psychosomatic teaching program, and H. G. Bennett became coordinator of the cancer teaching program. The Department of Histology and Embryology was made part of the basic science Department of Anatomy.

During recent years a number of progressive actions had been taken by the faculty to expedite instructional programs in accordance with recommendations by national medical agencies. Any problems arising were not unique to our institution, however. They were nationwide and were caused by changing concepts of the organized medical profession. To cope with these ensuing clinical instruction problems and to devise improved arrangements wherever needed, in cooperation with the chairmen and vice-chairmen of clinical departments, S. N. Stone, a visiting doctor in the Department of Surgery, was appointed as part-time associate dean of the school, July 11, 1951.[5]

In the broader perspective of efficient administration of the School of Medicine, standing boards and committees, as here listed, played a very large part in the various administrative divisions of the institution: advisory board to the dean, dean's committee for the Veterans Administration Hospital, faculty board (chairmen of departments), research, library, preceptorship, planning, supervisory for the affiliated hospitals, cancer teaching, cardiovascular teaching, admissions, coordinating, curriculum, honors, postgraduate advisory board, executive committee of the hospital board, and committee on the outpatient department.

[5.] Dr. Stone received his B.A. degree from the University of Oklahoma in 1929 and his B.S. degree in 1930, going on to study medicine at the University of Pennsylvania, where he received his M.D. degree in 1932. Following graduation, Dr. Stone interned for two years at Philadelphia General Hospital and then accepted a four-year fellowship in surgery at the Mayo Foundation. He practiced medicine for one year in Ardmore, Oklahoma, and served in the United States Navy before entering private practice in Oklahoma City in 1945.

The relationship between the Oklahoma Medical Research Foundation and the School of Medicine continued to be mutually advantageous, with each giving cordial support to the other. Both institutions had physical facilities for conducting additional research programs to an extent approximately twice the number in progress at the time. Fifty investigative research projects were going on in eighteen departments of the school and the affiliated research institute, all in the basic and clinical sciences. Hugh Payne, general manager of the research foundation, was a member of the National Advisory Cancer Council, one of the top advisory groups in the United States Public Health Service.

The medical school one of the first schools to have its plan for use of grants accepted by the National Cancer Institute in 1948, received a third grant of $25,000 in 1951; and the first check in the amount of $15,000 was received from the National Fund for Medical Education of the American Medical Association. In addition, the twenty-third legislature appropriated $40,000 to the Oklahoma State Regents for Higher Education for each of the fiscal years ending June 30, 1952, and June 30, 1953, with the intention that the appropriation be allocated to the University of Oklahoma School of Medicine for the purpose of conducting research in heart disease and cancer control. As director of the isotope clinic at the Medical Center, Peter Russo was in charge of this research, with a budget of $12,400 for salaries, maintenance, equipment, and travel.

Remodeling of an entire wing on the fourth floor of the University Hospital afforded the Department of Obstetrics and Gynecology much needed space and by the end of the year provided ten teaching beds in addition to an anticipated 50 beds in the Crippled Children's new wing and 60 in the neuropsychiatric addition.

Clerkship teaching in the hospitals (outpatient as well as inpatient) received considerable emphasis with the appointment of Dr. Stone as associate dean of clinical instruction. Doctors working on the clerkship program (September 1, 1951, to June 1, 1952) included Sterling Crawford, Edward Farris, W. C. McClure, William Reiff, M. J. Serwer, H. B. Strenge, George L. Winn, and Fred A. Quenzer, the clerkship coordinator at the Veterans Hospital. The instruction in the outpatient division was not up to that on the inpatient services in 1951, making improvement of outpatient teaching relative to the clinical years one of the most urgent problems facing the medical school in 1951.

During the year 1951–52, 9,880 persons received inpatient care in the University Hospitals (an average of 383 per day) with an average stay of 13.5 days for adults and 23.1 for children; occupancy was 81 per cent. There were 16,839 individuals who made a total of 69,496 visits to the outpatient department, and the laboratories performed 192,204 clinical examinations.

According to the comptroller's office, the state appropriation for the University of Oklahoma for 1951–52 was $3,543,051 out of a total income of $5,016,668; for the medical school, $565,259 out of a total income of $687,078, with a capital fund of $217,097; for the University Hospitals, $780,000 out of a total of $1,775,522, with a capital fund of $333,155.

Sixty-five graduates of the School of Medicine received the M.D. degree at the end of the 1950–51 academic year, and 318 students were enrolled in the school in 1951–52. There were 100 students in the entering class, one of whom was Daniel Webster Lee, Jr., the first Negro medical student to be trained in the state of Oklahoma. At Langston University, where he was graduated the previous May, he won the alumni scholarship award every semester for four years and made a record of only two subjects lower than an A while a college student. Studying medicine in a nonsegregated school was the fulfillment of a life-long dream for Daniel Webster Lee, Jr.

Approximately 132 full-time graduate students (interns, residents, and fellows) were enrolled in the postgraduate program of the School of Medicine during the year, and 32 candidates for the Ph.D. degree were enrolled in the medical sciences, an expanded program approved by the State Regents for Higher Education. With the cooperation of the Oklahoma State Medical Association, 19 symposia were presented in nine centers throughout the state, with interest in such gatherings growing steadily; and a program in the basic sciences for the residents of the affiliated hospitals was held during alternate weeks, with topics divided into two groups—medical and surgical. The Bone and Joint Hospital in Oklahoma City was affiliated with the School of Medicine for the purpose of graduate training for a resident in orthopedic surgery and fractures. Western State Hospital in Clinton and Hillcrest Hospital in Tulsa were also approved for affiliation in 1951.

On February 7, 1951, 40 years after the school had come into existence, two Negro girls—pioneers in their own right in the state nursing field—enrolled in the School of Nursing. According to a survey in June, 838 persons had completed the nursing program during those 40 years, with many of the graduates continuing their education elsewhere—later holding responsible positions in large general hospitals, in public health nursing, in nursing schools, and as examiners on state boards.

Forty-three certificates of nursing were issued in 1951 and the School of Nursing provided affiliations in pediatric nursing for six of the nine other nursing schools in the state. During the summer the State Regents for Higher Education approved a program in the School of Nursing leading toward a degree of Bachelor of Science in Nursing, to be granted by the College of Arts and Sciences of the university at Norman. In order to received the Bachelor of Science degree in Nursing, the student was required to complete one year and one summer of general college work, followed by thirty months of nursing training and a final year of college, either at the University of Oklahoma or at some other college meeting the university's requirements.

On September 12 the university regents appointed Ada Hawkins to succeed Mrs. Caron as director of the School of Nursing on the Oklahoma City campus at a salary of $5,200 effective September 1.[6]

[6.] During her three-year tenure as director of the School of Nursing, Mary Caron had devoted herself to the school with a great deal of enthusiasm and loyalty, but she felt that her lack of experience in administering a degree program loomed as a handicap for her, causing her to submit her resignation in July.

Miss Hawkins had earned her master's degree in nursing education at the University of Chicago, and since 1943 had been assistant director at the University of Michigan School of Nursing, where diploma and certificate nurse students were about evenly divided. To assist Miss Hawkins, Helen Patterson, director of nursing services at University Hospital, and Evelyn Hamil, assistant director at Children's Hospital, were recommended for promotions to assistant professors. With the return of all faculty members from vacation on September 1, the following major committees were activated in view of the degree program: curriculum, library resources, faculty regulations, research and promotion of studies and publication, public relations, student health and welfare, and admissions, promotions, scholarships, loans, and awards.

On December 13 the university regents voted to request the State Regents for Higher Education to change the name of the School of Nursing to the University of Oklahoma School of Nursing, retroactive to November, 1947, when the university regents had approved administrative reorganization which made the director of the school responsible to the dean of the School of Medicine and the president of the university for all educational activities.

The dietetic internship in the University Hospitals was approved by the Hospital Approval Committee of the American Dietetic Association on January 19, making it one of sixty-five approved dietetic internships in the United States. And, on September 7, the dietary staff was increased from eight to twelve members allowing the staff dietitians to accept the responsibility of "in service" training for dietetic interns, nurses, student nurses, medical students, and house staff. As an added bonus for the year, the dietetic internship was approved by the University of Oklahoma for five graduate credits in advanced diet theory. This was at a time when the University Hospitals and St. Anthony Hospital were the only civilian dietetic internships in the Southwest. These were not being offered in Texas, Arkansas, New Mexico, or Arizona.

The Crippled Children's Hospital was again beseiged with requests for beds for poliomyelitis patients in the summer of 1951, with concurrent arguments over a shortage of beds and talk of closing beds (for budgetary reasons) in the face of a legitimate emergency. Dr. Everett had no recourse but to ask President Cross for authorization to open additional beds as needed on an emergency basis; and this authorization was granted on July 30 because there was no humane alternative. So, August 7, opening of additional beds in emergency buildings was authorized in an effort to cope with the summer nightmare.

Since the Oklahoma supreme court had held that Section 13 of the 1949 Crippled Children's Act (requiring counties to make a tax levy for hospitalization of crippled children) was unconstitutional, it did seem that some state appropriated and federal funds would have to be diverted to other hospitals within the state for the care of crippled children.

Children's Convalescent Hospital, Inc., Bethany, Oklahoma—a 3-unit modern hospital building begun in 1947—was completed in 1951 and dedicated on June 14. Soon thereafter, this building was licensed, by the State Department of Health, as a specialized hospital and utilized for convalescent patients by the administrators of Crippled Children's Hospital.

A potential national scandal was averted in 1951 when Senator Hubert Humphrey, chairman of a subcommittee of the Committee on Labor and Public Welfare of the United States, ordered an inquiry to be held in executive session regarding the departure of Paul B. Magnuson from his post as medical director of the Veterans Administration.

One of the chief difficulties appeared to be that some medical schools were receiving mass resignations of the professional personnel in their affiliated veterans' hospitals because of the "firing" of Dr. Magnuson as a result of his long-time differences with Major General Carl R. Gray, Jr., veterans' administrator, "over whether doctors of politically inspired meddlers were to run medical services for veterans."[7]

Dr. Magnuson had inherited "an administrators' nightmare" six years previously but in four years had built medical care for veterans "from a fourth-rate bureaucracy-ridden service into the best available anywhere," principally by locating hospitals near medical schools and resisting all attempts of members of Congress and others "to determine hospital sites by considerations of patronage." General Gray had not only refused to make hospitals responsible to the medical director, but had gone so far as to appoint a three-man board for the selection of hospital managers without even consulting Dr. Magnuson.

The report of the senate group of inquiry was released on July 10.[8] Aside from various recommendations for procedural reforms within the Veterans Administration and changes in the organic law to protect the veterans from the destruction of the relationship of the chief medical officer with outside medical schools and private physicians (on which the senators agreed the high quality of the program depended), the committee submitted evidence that General Gray had "most decidedly administered, directly and indirectly, Veterans Administration Hospitals . . . and had given coeval assistants the authority to move in on the individual manager and to exercise influence over his decisions."

The senators' censure of Major General Gray for his administrative interferences was such as to "deter any head of the agency henceforth from repeating the acts which culminated in the protest of Dr. Magnuson. . . . In declining to resign and insisting on being discharged, Dr. Magnuson had exposed administrative corruption in time for it to be eliminated."

[7] The *Washington Post* editorial page, January 17, 1951.
[8] See "Salvaging the Medical Care of the Veterans," *New York Times*, July 11, 1951.

Chapter XVI.
The Raison d'Être:
1952–53

Steel and concrete structures going up on the campus of the School of Medicine in January, 1952, showed tangible evidence of efforts to meet the requirements of national accrediting agencies. However, growth in physical size was not in itself commensurate with the creation of a better medical school. Professional services in matters related to the school's primary purpose—medical education—were an essential ingredient, including sufficient funds to support at least a nucleus of full-time instructors and to maintain a physical plant. This made the School of Medicine unique from a budgetary standpoint, compared with other institutions of higher education in the state.

Early in January authorization for hospitalization of patients at Crippled Children's Hospital was curtailed, and on February 12 the census in the hospital totaled only 136 patients, with 92 beds unoccupied, in spite of vigorous efforts by the admissions department. These unprecedented vacancies were due to the recent supreme court decision upholding the Muskogee county commissioners in their fight against a 1/5 mill levy from each county for hospitalization of indigent children at the University and private hospitals, a decision which deprived Children's Hospital of an anticipated $290,000.

Meanwhile, the operating costs remained rather stationary while loss of revenue from empty beds mounted daily for Crippled Children's Hospital, increasing the deficit at the rate of $1,000 a day. Some help finally came on March 10 when the United States Children's Bureau allocated $30,000 to help pay hospitalization for children on the waiting list "for beds standing empty at Children's and other hospitals"—90 in Children's out of a total of 220—and two wards in Children's Convalescent Hospital in Bethany, making the patient count there 45 against a normal capacity of 65. This was an ironic situation at a time when the Crippled Children's Commission had a list of 77 top priority cases waiting to get into hospitals.

Nevertheless, the survey committee[1] from the accrediting agencies was not dismayed during its inspection of the medical school, March 17–20, as evi-

---

[1.] Doctors Donald Anderson, Dean Smiley, and John Youmans, respectively, for the Council on Medical Education and Hospitals, the Association of American Medical Colleges, and the American Medical Association's accrediting agency.

denced by a comment from Donald Anderson to the effect that the School of Medicine had actually made "outstanding progress," and that there was "no question that the rehabilitation of the medical school in the last few years is one of the major contributions to medical education in the postwar period." Continuing, he said, "I hope that our report, when it comes out, will repay you for your effort on our behalf by providing substantial support for your plans for the future development of the school."[2]

Conversion of 42 general charity beds at University Hospital to private status (by order of the State Regents for Higher Education the previous December) cut that hospital's medical service to Oklahoma indigents by at least 20 per cent by April, 1952, placing about 1,260 indigent patients per year on the hospital's already burdensome waiting list. The private beds measure, originally instituted as a partial stopgap against the growing operations deficit for the ensuing year, was unworkable, because admission of patients had to be controlled on a dual basis—medical needs of patients and teaching requirements of the University of Oklahoma School of Medicine.

Late in May the state regents ate crow and appealed for help for University Hospitals to Governor Murray from his contingency fund. Prompted by a financial crisis which presaged the University Hospitals operating on a seven-month budget and unable to open the nine-story neuropsychiatric ward and outpatient department, Governor Murray (at the instigation of the alumni of the School of Medicine) called a committee meeting on June 10. This was a thirty-member committee composed of five subcommittees, with Glen E. Leslie, a Tulsa banker, as chairman. The purpose of this committee was to make an extensive study of the financial problems at University Hospitals "in an attempt to end the almost annual series of requests for emergency funds to finance the University Hospitals, . . . to overhaul the state welfare policies providing hospital care for indigent patients in Oklahoma," and to report its recommendations to the governor in December.

According to a news release in the local press on July 31, a seven-month budget for the University Hospitals was passed by the State Regents for Higher Education and approved by the budget officer, who said that these regents had also signed a resolution approving operation of the hospitals for seven months at their present level of operation. "There will be no money after February 1," retiring budget officer Don Blundell said, "unless the legislature meets the crisis when it convenes in January." And he warned that a supplemental appropriation of $600,000 would need to be made by the legislature within 30 days of the opening session, or the hospitals would be closed. Asked how the regents could anticipate that appropriation in advance of the legislative session, Blundell replied, "They can't but they asked the 1951 session to pull them out of a hole and they are counting on the same thing this session."

All of this maneuvering was a source of irritation to the chief executive, since he was not allowed to control funds that went to the state regents and had no administrative power over the hospitals. So many a bow and arrow was trained

2. Letter to Dean Mark R. Everett under date of March 21, 1952.

on the State Regents for Higher Education, who constantly padded the budget for University Hospitals with income that could not be realized, knowing full well that public sympathy would force supplemental funds from the next legislature. For, to even the most myopic observer, it was obvious that the new nine-story addition at the old University Hospital—completed in May—was not built to be ornamental, even though it had not opened as scheduled on July 1.[3]

Upon his return on August 5, Dean Everett softened some of the criticism directed at the state regents by conceding that they had thought for some time—"and perhaps rightly so"—that they were being compelled to use educational funds to pay for indigent care.

A major change in administration during the year was the appointment on April 9 of Arthur L. McElmurry as new business administrator of the University Hospitals, following the resignation of Kenneth Wallace, who had served as business administrator for the past four years.[4] McElmurray, who held a bachelors degree in business administration from the University of Oklahoma, became chief accountant of the University Hospitals in June, 1948, and assistant business administrator in July, 1951.

Mark Johnson, a graduate of the School of Medicine in 1946, became assistant director in charge of the admitting and outpatient departments of the University Hospitals in 1952. Cleve Beller terminated his services in the office of postgraduate medical instruction on July 1, after developing the initial phase of postgraduate training. Irwin H. Brown, instructor in surgery, was then appointed director of the office of postgraduate instruction at a salary of $9,000 annually, succeeding George L. Winn. Florene Kelly, associate professor of bacteriology, was appointed acting chairman of that department, effective August 1, following the resignation of Homer Marsh to become acting dean of the University of Miami's new School of Medicine, the first medical school in the state of Florida. A. N. Taylor, chairman of the Department of Physiology, was appointed associate dean of student affairs at the School of Medicine effective August 1, replacing Dr. Marsh. Kirk T. Mosley was transferred from the Norman campus to become professor of preventive medicine and public health and chairman of the department, following the resignation of George M. Brother. Charles F. Obermann resigned as state mental health director, though not from the faculty; Robert L. Schreiber became public relations assistant on

[3.] Dean Everett missed two months of the hospital budget squabble while he sailed as an official representative of the University of Oklahoma with *Naval Cruise Abel* leaving Norfolk on June 8, 1952. But in reply to a report from S. N. Stone, acting dean, Dr. Everett wrote from London on July 13, "Your report sounded like the same old tactics by our bosses, but, once we get a decent budget adopted, it is possible we can lead a more peaceful life."

[4.] Kenneth Wallace, during his tenure of office, had established a new departmental budget accounting system to tie in with the entire university system of accounting. He had served very effectively as the first adequately trained business administrator of the medical center.

December 1, at an annual salary of $3,600, paid from the National Fund for Medical Education grant.

The number of salaried faculty members in the School of Medicine totaled 59 in 1952, including those named in the list of new appointees which follows:

Stewart George Wolf, M.D.
    professor of medicine
Carl Rupp Doering, M.D., D.Sc.
    consulting professor of preventive
    medicine and public health
Robert Montgomery Bird, M.D.
    associate professor of medicine
Robert Howard Furman, M.D.
    associate professor of research
    medicine
John Milton Hale, Ph.D.
    associate professor of
    bacteriology
John M. Cairns, Ph.D.
    assistant professor of histology
    and embryology
John P. Colmore, M.D.
    assistant professor of medicine
Simon Dolin, M.D.
    assistant professor of radiology
Hal Harrison Ramsey, II, Ph.D.
    assistant professor of bacteriology
Robert A. Schneider, M.D.
    assistant professor of medicine
Philip Edward Smith, D.Sc.
    assistant professor of preventive
    medicine and public health
Leroy William Steinmann, M.D.
    assistant professor of preventive
    medicine and public health
Irwin H. Brown, M.D.
    instructor in surgery
Elias Cohen, Ph.D.
    instructor in pathology
Winfield W. Evans, M.S.
    instructor in radiology
Muriel Hall Hyroop, M.D.
    instructor in psychiatry and
    neurology
Mark Royal Johnson, M.D.
    instructor in medicine
Carl Krieger, Jr., M.D.
    instructor in anesthesiology
George Townley Price, D.V.M.
    instructor in pathology

James Samuel Binkley, M.D.
    clinical assistant in surgery
Clifford Blair, M.D.
    clinical assistant in
    ophthalmology
John Louis Boland, Jr., M.D.
    consultant in otorhinolaryngology
Robert Lawrence Casebeer, M.D.
    clinical assistant in
    otorhinolaryngology
William S. Croom, M.D.
    clinical assistant in medicine
Arthur Furman Elliott, M.D.
    clinical assistant in medicine
Virgil Ray Forester, M.D.
    clinical assistant in medicine
Allen E. Greer, M.D.
    clinical assistant in surgery
Thomas Jefferson Huff, Jr., M.D.
    clinical assistant in surgery
Dave Bernard Lhevine, M.D.
    visiting lecturer in radiology
James E. Loucks, M.D.
    clinical assistant in gynecology
Robert P. Messinger, M.D.
    clinical assistant in medicine
Thomas Harvey Miley, D.D.S.
    clinical assistant in dental surgery
William R. Paschal, M.D.
    clinical assistant in medicine
Ira O. Pollock, M.D.
    clinical assistant in surgery
Frank William Stewart, D.M.D.
    clinical assistant in dental surgery
William Best Thompson, M.D.
    clinical assistant in medicine
Ethan Allen Walker, Jr., M.D.
    clinical assistant in
    otorhinolaryngology
Kelly McGuffin West, M.D.
    clinical assistant in medicine
Richard Wyrick, M.D.
    clinical assistant in
    ophthalmology

A significant step forward in improving the clinical departments of the School of Medicine in 1952 was the employment, as of April 15, of a full-time head of the Department of Medicine, Stewart G. Wolf, Jr., associate professor of medicine at Cornell University Medical School, at an annual salary of $12,000 and "with freedom to come and go whenever I see fit, always with the broadest interests of the department and the University in mind." Dr. Wolf's appointment also designated him as consultant in internal medicine at the veterans' hospital on the Oklahoma City campus and as head of the neuroscience section of the Oklahoma Medical Research Institute.[5] The services of R. Q. Goodwin, retiring chairman of the Department of Medicine, were many. He was a valuable member of the faculty who was called upon for many assignments, including service on the very search committee which unanimously recommended Stewart Wolf as his successor.

Grants and gifts to the University of Oklahoma School of Medicine in 1952 included the following: extension of an undergraduate cardiovascular training grant for another year, $14,000; renewal of an undergraduate training grant in psychiatry with Neil Kimerer as salaried director; $15,000 from the Medical Education Fund of the American Medical Association; $20,000 from the W. K. Kellogg Foundation for the postgraduate program at the University of Oklahoma School of Medicine for the year beginning July 1, 1952; a $6,416 emergency grant from the Commonwealth Foundation to supplement the comprehensive care and teaching program; a $28,000 grant from the National Foundation for Infantile Paralysis to buy physical therapy equipment and operate a rehabilitation program for polio patients in anticipation of a physical therapy school in the new wing of Crippled Children's Hospital; $20,614 from the National Foundation for Medical Education; and $7,000 from the Junior League of Oklahoma City, for construction of a glass-enclosed playroom on the third floor of the Crippled Children's Hospital.

The Arthritis and Rheumatism Foundation of the United Fund allotted the sum of $4,800 to a local group, to be used in basic research in the field of arthritis. This program was originally set up by W. K. Ishmael who had worked with the indigent arthritic clinic at the University Hospital for 16 years. And J. E. Heatley, professor emeritus in the Department of Radiology, bequeathed $25,000 to that department on July 26, with the stipulation that, until the time of his death, the interest was to be put into a special fund for the advancement and improvement of the Department of Radiology.

While the purposes of the affiliated hospitals of the School of Medicine of the University of Oklahoma (to unify the standards of graduate training in Oklahoma City and to increase clinical cases for the medical school) had remained the same since 1948, differences in administrative structure, size, location, and types of services of the individual hospitals had made accomplishment of these purposes variant. By 1952 the affiliated hospitals seemed to have fallen into

---

[5.] Dr. Wolf received his primary education at the Friends' School in his native city, Baltimore, Maryland, and his secondary schooling at Phillips Academy in Andover, Massachusetts. In 1938 he received his M.D. degree from Johns Hopkins University.

three groups: (1) those under the direct control of the School of Medicine, such as the University Hospitals and Veterans Administration Hospital; (2) those hospitals recognized by the accrediting agency of the American Medical Association for full intern training (and in most cases resident training) but not under the direct control of the School of Medicine for any function (Hillcrest Memorial and St. John's Hospitals in Tulsa, and Mercy, St. Anthony, and Wesley Hospitals in Oklahoma City); and (3) those hospitals of a specialized type whose relations involved only the training of residents or interns in a specialty for a short period of time, such as, the Bone and Joint Hospital in Oklahoma City, for orthopedic surgery, and Valley View Hospital, Ada, and Western State Hospital, Clinton, for rotation of general practice residents.

Recognizing these actualities the administration of the School of Medicine dissolved the supervisory committee for the affiliated hospitals on July 1, 1952, and suggested that each of the above groups be designated (1) affiliated hospitals (with administrative control by the School of Medicine implied by the term "affiliated"); (2) associated hospitals; and (3) special affiliated hospitals.

The committee for intern and resident training at the associated hospitals replaced the supervisory committee of the affiliated hospitals, with the University of Oklahoma having no jurisdiction over the residents or interns in the associated hospitals, except those in rotation from the University Hospitals or the veterans' hospital in Oklahoma City.

The state appropriations for the University of Oklahoma for 1952–53 were as follows: Norman campus, $3,346,911 out of a total income of $4,810,641; School of Medicine, $565,259 out of a total income of $687,071; and University Hospitals, $1,345,000 out of a total income of $2,422,299, plus $90,000 in capital funds. The University Hospitals provided 131,189 days of inpatient care and 77,994 outpatient treatments in 1952–53.

The total enrollment in the School of Medicine, 1952–53, was 368 students, 9 of whom were women, 100 first-year students, and 156 veterans.[6] In the School of Nursing there were 65 first-year students out of a total enrollment of 168. Fifty-four graduates received M.D. degrees, and 36 graduates received the certificate of nursing in 1952.

Nine young women were graduated from the University Hospital dietetic internship program on August 28, 1952, at a time when the course was one of 65 dietetic internships in the nation approved by the American Dietetic Association.

Graduate students for 1952–53 numbered 27 in the medical sciences—9 women and 18 men, 12 of whom were veterans, and 10 fellows, 6 of whom were veterans. Seven women and five men were in training as x-ray technologists and four women and one man as medical technologists. There were 24 interns and 35 residents on duty in the hospitals.

The value of the preceptorship plan for students in the senior year continued

---

[6.] It is of interest to note that in 1977 there was an entering class of 176 medical students.

to be demonstrated, principally in the contact the student had with the patient, on a level with a practicing physician. As one student who was in the first class to participate in the program said, "They told me I was going to learn about small town practice of medicine, but I found it 'big town medicine' practiced in a small town." His only problem, he confessed, was that he sometimes lacked a sense of correlation of the vast amount of medical knowledge he had acquired.[7]

On September 12, 1952, according to the *Norman Transcript*, the university regents approved a new research achievement award plan for students in the School of Medicine, which called for presentation of a certificate of achievement in research in the form of a special citation to be conferred along with the M.D. degree. To receive such an award, a student was required to perform original research successfully in one of the departments of the School of Medicine and to prepare an acceptable thesis, in addition to passing an examination in the department chosen for his or her research.

On November 20 the highest possible ranking in the nation was received by the School of Nursing of the University of Oklahoma, when the basic diploma program of the school was approved for full accreditation by the National League of Nursing. The league further commended the faculty of the school for marked improvement in almost every area during the year.

Testimony at a meeting on December 3 of the governor's committee on hospital care for the indigent revealed that approximately half of the employees of the University Hospitals were paid less than $100 a month, and that the turnover was unusually high because personnel, barely trained, would leave for higher paying positions. These facts were brought out during an interchange between Dean Mark Everett of the School of Medicine and John Rogers of Tulsa, member of the State Board of Regents for Higher Education and head of a submcommittee of the governor's hospital study committee.[8]

Rogers charged that the chief complaint against the University Hospitals had always been "inefficient operation." After listening to about ten minutes of hints concerning "improper, inefficient management," Dean Everett arose to correct what he termed "some misstatements by my good friend, John Rogers. I have never wanted this job and I don't want it now. My attitude has been one of trying to help, and I have spent five years endeavoring to clarify a lot of rumors of inefficiency. To that end, a skilled business manager was employed . . . and placed solely in charge of the spending of every cent of the hospitals' appropriations, and during the past five years no budget has ever been exceeded. This deficit was not caused by inefficient operation. It was caused by lack of income . . . estimated each year by our governing boards at more than the traffic would bear."

Although Dean Everett expressed opposition to dual control of the School of Medicine and the University Hospitals, a proposal for the separation of the

---

[7.] The beloved preceptor at Sentinel, Oklahoma, James F. McMurry, passed away during the summer of 1952.

[8.] *Oklahoma City Times*, December 4, 1951.

duties of the dean and administrator, submitted by John Rogers, was passed unanimously by the governor's committee.[9]

Mr. Leslie, chairman of the committee, said that he and other committeemen believed that doctors could not run hospitals—that a medical man's job was *to teach*. In all fairness, however, Mr. Leslie recognized the real problem, saying that the University Hospitals had been underfinanced by about $250,000 each year and that emergency appropriations had had to be made to keep the hospitals open.

Nearly everyone on the committee had something to say. Carl K. Stewart, editor of the *Oklahoma City Times*, said that the medical school needed a friend in court just as much as the Norman campus did, and that the subcommittee on which he was serving wanted the legislature to make direct appropriations to the medical institutions rather than through the state regents; Senator James Nance of Purcell felt that the dean of the medical school should be relieved of running a charity hospital; and Rabbi Levenson, chairman of another subcommittee, warned that division of authority might endanger the accreditation of the University Hospitals.[10] He pointed out that the dean's job was medical education and asked provocatively whether the hospital was or was not a teaching facility.

The governor's committee finally recommended that nothing be deleted from the hospital and medical school programs, and that enough money be made available—between three and four million dollars per year—to make possible operation of the new facilities. In addition, the committee proposed a school of medical librarians, strengthening of the School of Nursing, and expansion of the physical occupational therapy and radiological technician staffs—extras which would cost approximately another $84,000 per year.

James Nance, speaker designate of the house of representatives, said on December 29 that the dean of the medical school and the administrator of the hospitals should hold equal administrative powers, both directly responsible to the University of Oklahoma Board of Regents through the president of the university. But he also said that Governor Murray's hospital committee would meet in a few days to take a new look at controversial recommendations made earlier in the month.

There seemed to be a conspiracy of grievances against the School of Medicine in 1952. As if the State Regents for Higher Education were not enough of an aggravation all along, the case of the two sisters of one William Albert Teague, deceased, surfaced on September 2, when "Dean Mark R. Everett, Dr. Ernest Lachman, and Dr. Leo J. Starry, members of the Anatomical Commission, and the Perrine Funeral Home in Oklahoma City," were named defendants in a $20,000 damage suit filed in district court. The sisters'

[9.] This political action touched off speculation in the press that Mark Everett would resign as dean and superintendent of the School of Medicine and University Hospitals, but the dean himself dampened the speculations, saying that the question of his resignation was not brought up except by reporters.

[10.] Issue of October 6, 1951.

petition stated they were never notified of their brother's death, and that his body was turned over to the University of Oklahoma School of Medicine where it was "dissected and mutilated and cut up by medical students."

The women asked $10,000 exemplary and punitive damages and $10,000 actual damages. Happily, the case was dismissed by the judge for lack of sufficient evidence, inasmuch as the body was still intact—actually quite unwanted for burial by his concerned relatives.

The relation of the dean to the University Hospitals and School of Medicine at the close of this controversial year was as an executive assistant to the president of the university, under the Board of Regents of the University of Oklahoma, with a medical director (Robert C. Lowe) responsible to the dean, and a business administrator (Raymond Crews) responsible not only to the dean but to the vice-president in charge of finances on the Norman campus.

Dual control of the School of Medicine and University Hospitals had not been successful during the regime of Lewis J. Moorman, when contrived division of authority had led to chaos and a senate investigation. Dean Everett maintained in 1952 that dual control would still be inadvisable, because separation of the duties of the dean and administrator would put two persons in charge (responsible to the president) and make the president of the university assume the duties of the director of the Medical Center.

In its origin, the University Hospital was never set up as a service institution, but for the purpose of training doctors, nurses, residents, interns, and auxiliary personnel, and with no other objective. Since it was the main teaching hospital of the School of Medicine, within this teaching program many of the sick and indigent of the state of Oklahoma were gradually admitted to the hospital for medical care and treatment. However, in order to maintain the accepted student-case ratio and essential safeguards against loss of our hard-won compliance with teaching standards, controlled admission of patients became a necessity, as well as operation of an adequate number of teaching beds. In other words, medical education was the raison d'être.

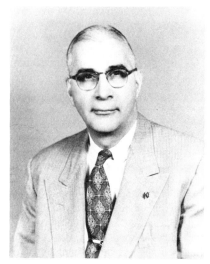

John H. Lamb, M.D., head of the
Department of Dermatology, 1956–61.

Courtesy University of Oklahoma
Medical Center

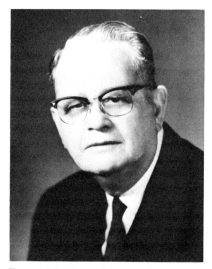

Forrest M. Lingenfelter, M.D., chairman of the Department of Surgery,
1952–56.

Courtesy University of Oklahoma
Medical Center

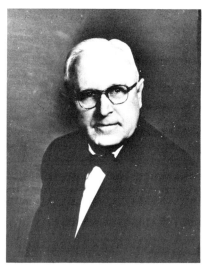

James P. McGee, M.D., chairman of
the Department of Ophthalmology,
1945–52.

Courtesy University of Oklahoma
Medical Center

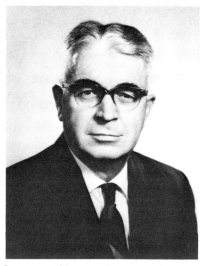

Lawrence Chester McHenry, M.D.,
chairman of the Department of
Otorhinolaryngology, 1948–51.

Courtesy University of Oklahoma
Medical Center

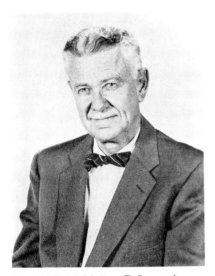

Donald B. McMullen, D.Sc., acting
chairman of the Department of
Preventive Medicine and Public
Health, 1940–43.

*Courtesy University of Oklahoma
Medical Center*

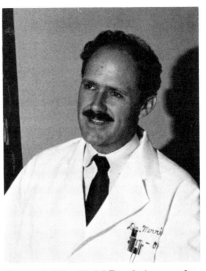

James A. Merrill, M.D., chairman of
the Department of Obstetrics and
Gynecology, 1961–(64).

Courtesy Sooner Medic

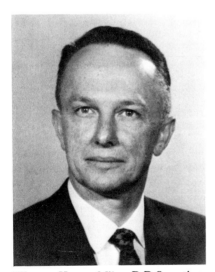

Thomas Harvey Miley, D.D.S., acting
director of the Department of Oral
Surgery, 1961.

*Courtesy Oklahoma State Dental
Association*

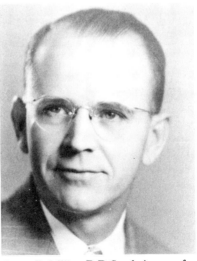

James R. Miller, D.D.S., chairman of
the Department of Oral Surgery,
1954–55.

Courtesy Dr. James R. Miller

205

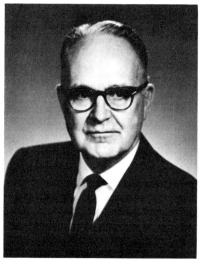

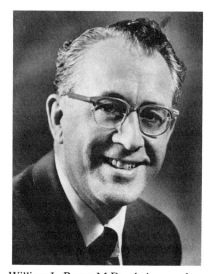

Don H. O'Donoghue, M.D., chairman of the Department of Orthopedic and Fracture Surgery, 1948–(64).

Courtesy Sooncr Mcdic

William L. Parry, M.D., chairman of the Department of Urology, 1962–(64).

Courtesy University of Oklahoma Medical Center

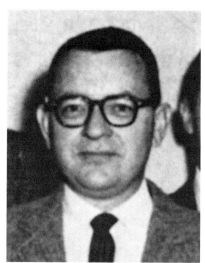

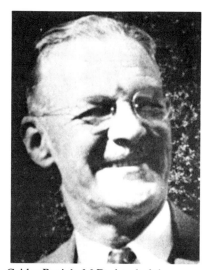

Richard W. Payne, M.D., chairman of the Department of Pharmacology, 1961.

Courtesy Sooner Medic

Grider Penick, M.D., head of the Department of Gynecology, 1940–50.

Courtesy Sooner Medic

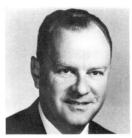

Theodore Robert
Pfundt, M.D., acting
head of the Department
of Pediatrics, 1957–58.

*Courtesy Oklahoma
State Board of
Medical Examiners*

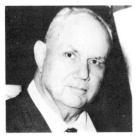

Charles Ralph Rayburn,
M.D., chairman of the
Department of Psychi-
atry and Neurology,
1940–48.

*Courtesy Dr. Hayden
H. Donohue*

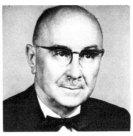

James R. Reed, M.D.,
chairman of the Depart-
ment of Ophthalmology,
1952–62.

Courtesy Commentary

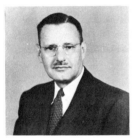

Francis J. Reichmann,
D.D.S., chairman of the
Department of Oral
Surgery, 1935–41,
1946–51.

*Courtesy University
of Oklahoma Medical
Center*

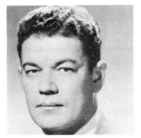

Gus Ray Ridings, M.D.,
chairman of the Depart-
ment of Radiology,
1957–62.

*Courtesy Oklahoma
State Board of
Medical Examiners*

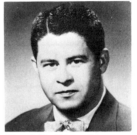

Harris D. Riley, Jr.,
M.D., chairman of the
Department of Pedi-
atrics, 1958–(64).

*Courtesy University
of Oklahoma Medical
Center*

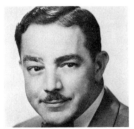

J. Millard Robertson,
D.D.S., chairman of the
Department of Oral
Surgery, 1951–54.

*Courtesy Oklahoma
State Dental
Association*

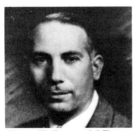

Peter E. Russo, M.D.,
chairman of the Depart-
ment of Radiology,
1948–57.

Courtesy Sooner Medic

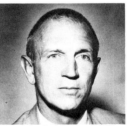

John A. Schilling, M.D.,
chairman of the Depart-
ment of Surgery, 1956–
(64).

*Courtesy University
of Oklahoma Medical
Center*

207

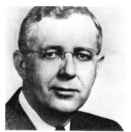

William W. Schottstaedt, M.D., chairman of the Department of Preventive Medicine and Public Health, 1960–(64).

Courtesy Madelon B. Katigan

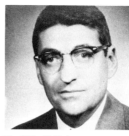

Carl Emil Schow, D.D.S., chairman of the Department of Oral Surgery, 1961–62.

Courtesy Oklahoma State Dental Association

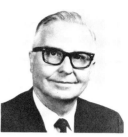

Lawrence Vernon Scott, D.Sc., chairman of the Department of Bacteriology, 1961–(64).

Courtesy University of Oklahoma Medical Center

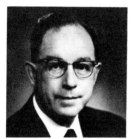

Milton J. Serwer, M.D., chairman of the Department of Obstetrics, 1954–61.

Courtesy University of Oklahoma Medical Center

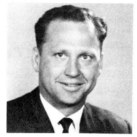

Kenneth W. Shons, D.D.S., M.S.D., chairman of the Department of Oral Surgery, 1962–(64).

Courtesy Oklahoma State Dental Association

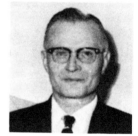

Paul W. Smith, Ph.D., chairman of the Department of Pharmacology, 1957–61.

Courtesy Sooner Medic

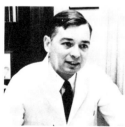

James B. Snow, Jr., M.D., chairman of the Department of Otorhinolaryngology, (1964).

Courtesy University of Oklahoma Medical Center

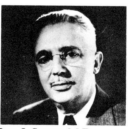

Leo J. Starry, M.D., chairman of the Department of Surgery, 1948–52.

Courtesy University of Oklahoma Medical Center

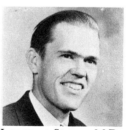

Lawrence Stream, M.D., acting chairman of the Department of Anesthesiology, 1955–56.

Courtesy Oklahoma State Board of Medical Examiners

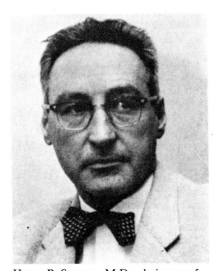

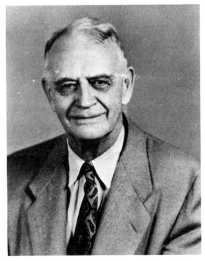

Henry B. Strenge, M.D., chairman of
the Department of Pediatrics, 1955–57.

Courtesy Sooner Medic

Charles B. Taylor, M.D., acting chairman of the Department of Urology,
1943–44.

*Courtesy University of Oklahoma
Medical Center*

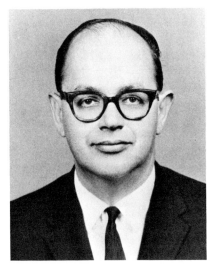

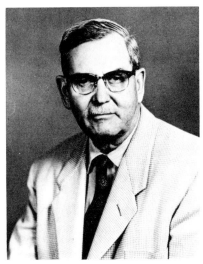

Sidney P. Traub., M.D., chairman of
the Department of Radiology, 1963–
(64).

*Courtesy University of Oklahoma
Medical Center*

Theodore G. Wails, M.D., chairman
of the Department of Otorhinolaryngology, 1936–48.

*Courtesy University of Oklahoma
Medical Center*

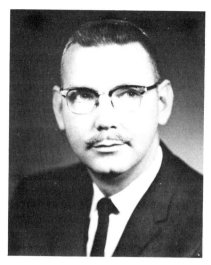

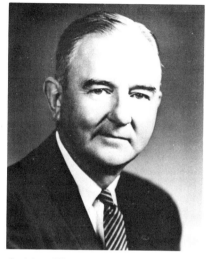

Ethan A. Walker, Jr., M.D., chairman
of the Department of Otorhinolaryngology, 1962–64.

*Courtesy University of Oklahoma
Medical Center*

O. Alton Watson, M.D., chairman of
the Department of Otorhinolaryngology, 1951–59.

*Courtesy University of Oklahoma
Medical Center*

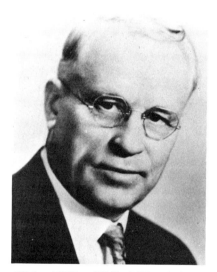

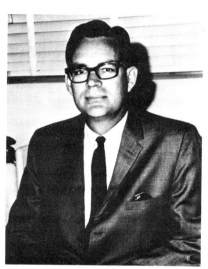

Walter William Wells, M.D., chairman
of the Department of Obstetrics,
1933–45.

*Courtesy University of Oklahoma
Medical Center*

Kelly M. West, M.D., head of the
Department of Continuing Education,
1963–(64).

Courtesy Sooner Medic

210

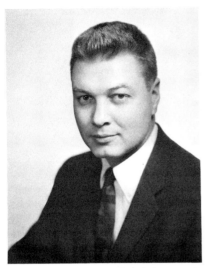

Louis Jolyon West, M.D., chairman of the Department of Psychiatry, Neurology, and Behavioral Sciences, 1954–(64).

Courtesy Sooner Medic

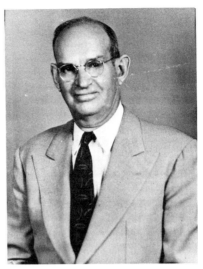

Willis K. West, M.D., chairman of the Department of Orthopedic and Fracture Surgery, 1936–37, 1943–48.

Courtesy University of Oklahoma Medical Center

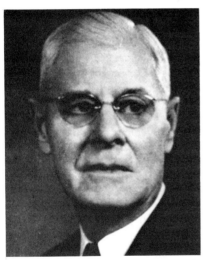

Leslie M. Westfall, M.D., chairman of the Department of Ophthalmology, 1938–45.

Courtesy Mrs. Max Morgan, daughter

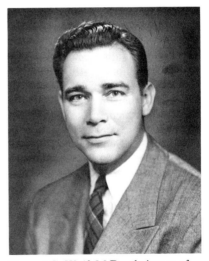

Stewart G. Wolf, M.D., chairman of the Department of Medicine, 1952–(64).

Courtesy University of Oklahoma Medical Center

211

Chapter XVII.
Progression Perseveres:
1953–54

On January 1, 1953, a fiscal budget request for 1953–54 was proposed for University Hospitals, totaling $3,255,134, that would balance the ledgers and provide the twenty-fourth legislature with a guide for tagging appropriations for institutions of higher learning. The medical center did not receive the requested $630,000 supplemental appropriation, but the legislature did appropriate $565,000 for operation of the University Hospitals for the remainder of the 1952–53 fiscal year and included an additional $20,000 for urgently needed repairs. In any event, spirits were soaring by February 8, Medical Sciences Day, on the occasion of the dedication of the expanded School of Medicine building at 800 N.E. Thirteenth Street.

Governor Johnston Murray, principal speaker at the formal opening of the enlarged School of Medicine building, was introduced by Mark R. Everett, who mentioned that the addition, completed in 1951, had doubled the floor space of the building, and that the total number of medical students enrolled at the medical school for 1953–54 would be at least 361 as contrasted with 280 in the year 1950–51. Others participating in the ceremony were George L. Cross, president of the University of Oklahoma, John Carson, Shawnee, president of the School of Medcine's alumni association, Alfred R. Sugg, Ada, president of the Oklahoma State Medical Association, and Reverend Frank Dudley, president of the Oklahoma City Council of Churches.

The medical school library, situated in new quarters in a new wing of the building, was a showplace in its day, occupying nearly four times its former area, with a reading room almost as large as the previous total floor space. Downstairs, stacks housed volumes of periodicals and books published prior to 1932, inasmuch as the library was receiving 800 periodicals annually, in addition to its collection of more than 32,000 volumes. On the lower level luxury features were the study cubicles for more private study or research.

Opening of the new $1,264,000 outpatient and neuropsychiatric addition to the University Hospitals (standing idle for nearly a year) was tentatively scheduled for March 5, but only the outpatient clinics on the lower floors of the eight-story wing actually opened on March 16. The official opening of the total structure was almost two months later, on May 10, and then without the neuropsychiatric floors in operation.

On May 10 an appropriation of $3,000,000 was made to the State Regents for Higher Education (committee substitute for Engrossed Senate Bill No. 36), with *legislative intent* that it be used for operation and maintenance of the University Hospitals for the biennium ending June 30, 1955, and that it provide "an outstanding full-time professor as head of each of the separate clinical services in the hospital." The house of representatives substitute bill also delineated intent regarding private patients and reasonable limits on the earnings of the full-time clinical professors.

The University Hospital Psychiatry and Neurology Service Act (House Bill No. 585) passed the house of representatives and the senate on June 5 and was signed by Governor Murray on June 15, 1953. This was an act relating to the School of Medicine of the University of Oklahoma, establishing a psychiatry and neurology service and facilities.

Under this act, authority was provided for the transfer of any patient of the psychiatry and neurology facilities and services of the University Hospital to a component facility of the State Department of Mental Health, and vice versa. A full-time chief of psychiatry and neurology was to be appointed by the university regents as a member of the faculty of the School of Medicine.

One week later, on June 22, the State Regents for Higher Education lowered the boom again, creating a barrier that made it absolutely impossible to open the psychiatry and neurology unit. The only *intent* of the house of representatives that was observed by the regents was the allocation of the separate appropriation of $3,000,000 to the University Hospitals for the biennium. Not one red cent was allocated from the total appropriation to the regents to $22,253,800 in operational funds for institutions of higher learning. So the psychiatry and neurology unit was forced to continue awaiting future appropriations before going into operation. The state regents had reneged again, foreclosing wards built for psychiatric patients in the new wing of University Hospital, even though the final payment on the building contract had been made by the university regents on May 14, 1952.

At a meeting of the university regents on July 9, President Cross called attention to a resolution adopted by the faculty of the School of Medicine calling for a realistic fiscal policy for the University Hospitals in place of the recurring need for deficit financing. The resolution stated that it had been agreed in a meeting of the governor's committee, and acknowledged by representatives of the state regents present at the time, that 20 per cent of the total cost of operatigng the University Hospitals was an equitable financial obligation to be assumed by the State Regents for Higher Education in view of the educational role of the hospitals.

The university regents were in complete sympathy with the faculty resolutions, expressing disappointment not only with the failure of the state regents to provide adequate funds for operation of the University Hospitals, but in their provision year after year of an even smaller percentage increase than to most other institutions.

The university regents were disappointed, but the faculty, alumni, and executive committees of the School of Medicine and the professional organizations were incensed, realizing that Dean Everett might feel bound to resign because of his inability to meet the expectations of the Council on Medical Education solely as a result of inadequate allocations from the State Regents for Higher Education. Complete confidence in Dean Everett's academic aims and administrative capabilities was expressed openly and personally, as evidenced by resolutions and personal letters in the files of the office of the dean.[1]

Meanwhile, it was learned that the nonpaid faculty of the School of Medicine had scheduled a meeting to plan some action on their charge that the hospitals were shortchanged by the state regents, as they pointed out in the recent faculty resolution sent to President Cross and Governor Murray, emphasizing their lack of faith in this board.

Governor Murray acknowledged that he had received two petitions from the faculty of the medical school and that one resolution was about the possible resignation of Dean Mark R. Everett over the financial situation. "I hope he doesn't," the governor said, "for he has been of tremendous value."[2]

About the same time, Representative Robert OL Cunningham, Oklahoma City, revealed that he was studying tape recordings of testimony given during the last legislative session, to determine just what it was that the State Regents for Higher Education promised to do for the University Hospitals; and there is ample evidence in current newspaper clippings that Cunningham was actively engaged in trying to get suitable funds for the hospitals.

On July 12 the *Daily Oklahoman* ran an editorial entitled "Why This Continued Crisis?" It said in part that men whose opinions were entitled to the very highest respect bore testimony that the work done at the medical center was excellent and "earning its way admirably in giving the taxpayer value received." The editorial went on to assert that there seemed to be no lack of money when the late legislature was in session, that money was "appropriated by the tens of millions," and that ample funds were found for causes far less worthwhile than the education of doctors. "No Legislature in our history ever spent so much money," the editor said, "yet the medical school is facing another crisis only two months after the adjournment of the legislature. . . . Something is wrong somewhere, and that wrong, whatever it is, should be ascertained by our governing authority as speedily as possible and corrected without unnecessary delay. We refuse to believe that Oklahoma is too poor to support a first-rate medical school adequately."

Apparently the State Regents for Higher Education and the faculty of the School of Medicine resolved some differences in a joint session on July 19, for President Cross announced that money would be available "to open new beds standing empty at the University of Oklahoma Hospitals as rapidly as possible," and that every effort would be made to secure additional money from state and private agencies and foundations. Guy H. James, a member of the state

---

[1] The salary of Dean Everett was "fixed at $13,000 annually" by the university regents.

[2] *Oklahoma City Times*, July 9, 1953.

regents, even stated that there was a strong possibility that funds would be made available from the Department of Public Welfare.[3]

President Cross went so far as to say that the hospitals would be financed ''by money borrowed from the next year's budget in the belief that new sources of income could be tapped before 1954–55.'' Under ths proposed plan the hospitals were to receive a total of $1,800,000 from the $3,000,000 appropriation for the biennium, leaving a balance of $1,200,000 for 1954–55, a true case of deficit financing. Notwithstanding, the new wing of Children's Hospital (two floors of beds) and the neuropsychiatric unit were assured of being put into operation at long last.

Expressing complete confidence with the administration of the School of Medicine and its hospitals, Governor Murray vetoed a legislative plan for a commercial efficiency study of the medical center, saying that he was fairly well satisfied with operations there, so far as he was able to know, and that an efficiency study was a legislative function which should have been attended to when the hospitals' appropriations were being considered. ''I think they are doing the best they can with the money allotted them,'' the governor added.

Time and misfortune reaped their toll from the faculty relentlessly in 1953: D. W. Griffin, professor emeritus of psychiatry and neurology, superintendent of Central State Hospital for more than 50 years, and for thirty-seven years a member of the faculty, died on January 1; Louis A. Turley, professor emeritus of pathology, who played an important role early in the century in shaping the growth of the University of Oklahoma School of Medicine, died on July 27;[4] Horace Reed, professor of surgery, 1910–36, died October 7; William C. McClure, assistant professor of medicine, met an untimely death by accident on September 24; and Oscar Clarence Newman, renowned pioneer physician of Shattuck, Oklahoma, and a past preceptor, died on March 14.

The faculty, alumni, and administration of the School of Medicine remained determined that current financial difficulties should not interrupt the continued academic growth of our school. And new personnel continued to be attracted to the medical center, in part because of the enthusiasm of the new head of the Department of Medicine, Stewart Wolf.

Changes in faculty appointments during the year were as follows: Donald Branham, vice-chairman of the Department of Urology, became chief of the urology clinical service in the veterans' hospital; Ella Mary George was appointed a full-time faculty member at the Veterans Administration Hospital; Joseph Kelso assumed the chairmanship of the gynecology department and was also named secretary of the faculty; Milton J. Serwer succeeded J. B. Eskridge, Jr., as head of the obstetrics department (at the request of Dr. Eskridge, who wished to be relieved of those duties but to remain on the faculty), and John W. Records became vice-chairman of the department. O. A. Watson became head

[3.] Imogene Patrick, the *Daily Oklahoman*, July 20, 1953.

[4.] Dr. Turley had the distinction of having been one of the first preclinical teachers in the School of Medicine in 1908, and of being elected to the Oklahoma Hall of Fame in 1950.

of the Department of Otorhinolaryngology. Marie Cecelia McKnight Mink was appointed teaching assistant in the School of Nursing on January 15, 1953, the first Negro faculty member at the University of Oklahoma Medical Center.

New appointments to the faculty of the School of Medicine are listed as follows:

Jean Spencer Felton, M.D.
associate professor of medicine and preventive medicine and public health

Ranwel Caputto, M.D.
assistant professor of research biochemistry

Vincent Paul Cirillo, Ph.D.
assistant professor of preventive medicine and public health

Richard G. Hahn, M.D., M.P.H.
assistant professor of medicine and assistant professor of preventive medicine and public health

William W. Schottstaedt, M.D.
assistant professor of preventive medicine and public health

Vivian Sweibel Smith, Ph.D.
consultant assistant professor of preventive medicine and public health

Annice Florine Bettis, M.A.
instructor in nutrition

Paul William Goaz, D.D.S.
instructor in research dental surgery

Ruben Hilton Mayberry, M.D.
instructor in anesthesiology

William S. Pugsley, M.D.
instructor in medicine

Edward Martin Schneider, M.D.
instructor in medicine

Samuel Sepkowitz, M.D.
instructor in pediatrics

William Thomas Snoddy, M.D.
instructor in pathology

Marcus S. Barker, M.D.
visiting lecturer in psychiatry and neurology

James M. Behrman, M.D.
visiting lecturer in psychiatry and neurology

Berget H. Blocksom, Jr., M.D.
visiting lecturer in urology

Paul B. Champlin, M.D.
visiting lecturer in surgery

Howard Murdock Cohenour, M.D.
visiting lecturer in urology

Frank E. Darrow, M.D.
clinical assistant in surgery

Marvin Bryant Hays, M.D.
clinical assistant in orthopedic and fracture surgery

Gilbert Louis Hyroop, M.D.
clinical assistant in surgery

Richard B. Lincoln, M.D.
clinical assistant in medicine and consulting clinical assistant in psychiatry and neurology

Emanuel Nathan Lubin, M.D.
visiting lecturer in urology

Sam N. Musallam, M.D.
clinical assistant in medicine

Gebert Rebell, B.S.
associate in research bacteriology and dermatology

Carl Emil Schow, D.D.S.
clinical assistant in dental surgery

Alfred R. Sugg M.D.
visiting lecturer in urology

Jean Spencer Felton, who was appointed assistant professor of preventive medicine and public health on July 9, had previously served for eight years as medical director of the Oak Ridge National Laboratory. Upon assuming his new duties at the School of Medicine in Oklahoma City, he became interested in developing a modern health service for employees, students, and faculty; and he set up a consultant health service to deal with employee health problems in state industries, becoming the first physician on the faculty to be an industrial consultant to the state health department.

The position of chief resident and clinical assistant was effected November 1 in the Departments of Medicine, Obstetrics-Gynecology, Orthopedics, Pediatrics, and Surgery in order to provide these departments with an opportunity to improve the house staff group and to develop responsibility and academic interest. Candidates were required to be recommended through a department and for the last year only of their residency in the hospitals.

For the furtherance of research, the School of Medicine received a five-year grant of $122,500 from the W. K. Kellogg Foundation, commencing on July 1, 1953, with specified yearly allocations as follows: $25,100, $36,200, $32,000, $18,000, and $11,000. This grant provided a unique opportunity to develop teaching and research in preventive medicine as an important aspect of the medical curriculum. President Cross, noting "the progress of the medical school in the last six years," said that recognition of our School of Medicine through such grants as this was a source of great satisfaction.

In the year 1953–54 the cost of research projects being conducted in the School of Medicine totaled $237,946, of which only $60,000 were appropriated by the legislature, with $177,946 coming from outside sources. The $60,000 appropriation was earmarked for heart disease and cancer research as in the past three years, and these monies were carefully parcelled out for promising beginnings of research in the control of heart disease and cancer in order to secure financial support available from national fund-raising agencies. Investigators seeking such support from the National Institutes of Health and from the armed forces had to show evidence of preliminary pilot studies.

It is of note that research grants to the School of Medicine from outside sources grew in four years from trifling sums to approximately $200,000 in 1953. So "pump priming" with state appropriated research funds was the effective trigger for a medical research program about ten times the size of that financed by the state, encouraging competent scientists and making possible more adequate general facilities. More than 30 faculty members were making separate investigations into the complexities of these diseases in 1953–54, and over a period of two years 4,000 cancer patients and more than 1,000 persons afflicted with heart disease were directed to the medical center, profiting from studies in the tumor clinic, the heart clinic, the isotope clinic, and from services of the Oklahoma Medical Research Institute.

The fact that the staff of the research foundation and the staff of the School of Medicine continued to work together "in a true medical partnership" was evidence that the change in command of the foundation in July had occurred without disruption, when Ed Reifenstein was succeeded by Charles D. Kochakian, who supported the consolidated programs in every respect.[5]

The $8,000,000 Veterans Administration Hospital was opened on September 24, 1953, with Clarence E. Bates as manager,[6] and was officially

[5] Dr. Reifenstein resigned as director of the foundation because of apparent incompatibility with the foundation's planned program of cooperation with the University of Oklahoma School of Medicine.

[6] Dr. Bates, a graduate of the University of Oklahoma School of Medicine, was a

dedicated in a short, stirring ceremony, arranged by the Oklahoma City Chamber of Commerce on October 4, when about 1,000 persons turned out for the program, held on the lawn at the front of the building. The dedication address was delivered by Harvey V. Highley, administrator of Veterans Affairs, with Dr. Bates giving the response. Vice Admiral Joel T. Boone, chief medical director for the Veterans Administration, outlined the care of veterans and voiced praise for the nearby University of Oklahoma School of Medicine. The Veterans Administration's new ten-story, 496 bed hospital—though completedly appointed and well adequate in itself—was set up as a working unit of the whole medical center complex. Not only was its function to "provide the best possible care to the disabled men and women who had served our country in time of need," Admiral Boone said, "but also to work closely with the university to make this a great treatment and teaching center."

The appointment of James F. Hammarsten as the chief of medical service in this new hospital on the medical center campus was announced in the local press the following day.[7]

The state-wide hospital advisory board, created in 1948 in connection with the administration of the University Hospitals "for the purpose of improving public relations," was terminated by action of the university regents in September, 1953, bedause the board was handicapped in its purpose by lack of authority and by limited acquaintance with the urgent problems of the hospitals. By further action, the executive committee of the hospital board was renamed the executive committee of the clinical faculty.

State appropriations for the University of Oklahoma for 1953–54 were as follows: Norman campus, $4,195,550 out of a total income of $5,932,348; School of Medicine, $636,512 out of a total income of $794,200; University Hospitals, $1,800,000 out of a total income of $2,913,721.

The total number of patients admitted to University Hospitals, July 1, 1953, to June 30, 1954, was 10,890 (main 8,263; Children's 2,627). The total number of days of hospital care was 135,274 (main, 80,429; Children's 54,845), with the average number of days of hospital stay per patient 11.3 at main and 20.3 at Children's. Four thousand seventy operations were performed, including 24 cardiac catheterizations; 197,762 laboratory examinations and 8,521 cytology studies were executed. Treatments totaling 81,321 were given to 18,798 individuals making 63,335 visits to the outpatient departments.

During the second biennium the occupancy of the 60 private beds approximately doubled over the previous year. However, the number of children referred to the hospitals by agencies declined, and the income available to the hospitals was insufficient to maintain the number of patients.

Veterans Administration physician with 27 years of service. He came from Muskogee, where he had been chief medical officer for two years, to open the original hospital for veterans in Oklahoma City in the buildings at Will Rogers Field in July, 1946.

[7.] Dr. Hammarsten was formerly connected with the School of Aviation Medicine at Randolph Air Force Base, Texas.

The University Hospitals provided training during the year for approximately 80 interns and residents, for one of the largest groups of nursing students ever trained in the state, and for students in a number of technical schools and internships, making a grand total of 1,320 persons receiving training at the medical center during the year. There were 380 students enrolled in the School of Medicine and 178 in the School of Nursing in 1953–54. Seventy-eight graduates received the M.D. degree in June, 1953, and 25 graduates received the certificate of nursing. (According to national statistics, the average professional life of a nurse was under seven years at the time. The primary contributor to the nurse shortage was marriage; a low salary scale was a close second.)

The university regents raised the tuition fee for nonresident students in the School of Medicine from $350 to $400 per semester on September 10, 1953, and "hoped that the Admissions Committee would see fit to select at least a very few out-of-state students for the entering class . . . in the belief that such a policy would prevent our becoming a bit provincial."

The first issue of a University of Oklahoma medical center quarterly magazine, entitled *Commentary*, was published in September, 1953, containing information of interest to the alumni, faculty, and students of the School of Medicine. It reported items relating to the medical school proper and its affiliated hospitals, undergraduate student activities, and the tangible results of the efforts of highly motivated alumni and other professional friends of the medical school. Clifford A. Traverse, writing in the first issue said that engineers tell us that "the bee is so constructed that it cannot fly; but the bee not knowing this, keeps flying." This was the true spirit of the alumni—striving in every way to obtain appropriations and expanded facilities for their medical school.

J. William Finch (class of 1931), writing editorially in the December issue of the *Commentary,* spoke of the Alumni Association of the School of Medicine as being "solely responsible for the birth of the Oklahoma Medical Research Foundation," and of the sense of pride the originators derived from watching the foundation develop.

In regard to the postgraduate program at the School of Medicine, sixteen different courses were sponsored by the Division of Postgraduate Instruction in 1953–54, with anywhere from seven to 108 doctors attending these courses at any one time, making a total of 532 individual doctors in attendance during the year. The general practice training program was firmly established, its value becoming more and more apparent each year. The total postgraduate budget for the year was $33,308 derived from the W. K. Kellogg Foundation and School of Medicine funds.

The year ended on a cardiac note, with "medical students wearing deep sea diving masks being dunked periodically, to establish the true mathematical potential of the heart's electric field." The props for the scenario were a large steel submerging tank and a hugh spherical copper diving bell, built to specifications of Robert H. Bayley, professor of medicine and head of the cardiac clinic in University Hospital, whose inventive mind had added many refinements to the art of heart testing.[8] In this unique experiment to prove a scientific theory, a volunteer medical student, wearing a diving mask for his oxygen supply, sat in the center of the copper bell, submerged in water, with electrodes fastened to his body and to the copper bell. Dr. Bayley said that he did not expect to find any marked improvement on what was already known, but that "with vector cardiology the coming heart science, it was important to try to make previous theories absolute."

The administration of the School of Medicine tried desperatedly in 1953 to make some "previous theories absolute" too concerning an orderly expansion of personnel and physical facilities to meet the need for increasing the number of physicians graduating from the University of Oklahoma School of Medicine. Since a commensurate increase in financial support was an essential element of this equation, the continuing failure of the State Regents for Higher Education to provide that support posed an uphill struggle. However, with vigorous moral support from friends of the School of Medicine in many walks of life and from the accrediting agencies, progress though slow was eventual. The new wing of the School of Medicine building was officially opened, and the new wing of Children's Hospital and the Neuropsychiatric unit were assured of opening. With a total investment of $17,877,000 in the medical center, some form of financial security educationally and economically sound became an obvious requisite to the most casual observer.

The faculty put its house in order on November 14, 1953, by adopting a workable set of bylaws (as requested by a survey team as early as 1948). All 119 members of the faculty present at the meeting voted favorably for adoption; and an additional 203 voted by mail, without one vote being cast against acceptance. This was a real tribute to the committee appointed to make the compilation, after studying carefully all past faculty minutes for previous actions by the faculty and reviewing all actions per se taken by the regents of the university. Charles DeGaris, chairman of the committee, was ably assisted by Harold Shoemaker and A. N. Taylor.

Installation of the honor medical fraternity, Alpha Omega Alpha, at the University of Oklahoma School of Medicine on May 1, 1953, was one more cog in the wheel of recognition and progress. Walter L. Bierring, national president, presented the charter, and Josiah M. Moore, national secretary-treasurer, presented keys and certificates to 26 physicians who were inducted as charter members. Mark R. Everett accepted the charter for the School of Medicine, and George L. Cross and Thomas R. Benedum, respectively, accepted for the university and the university regents. Peter Russo, who had been instrumental in getting a charter established here, gave the response for Alpha Omega Alpha members in Oklahoma.

[8.] Illustrated story in the *Daily Oklahoman*, December 29, 1953.

Chapter XVIII.
An Emerging Road of
Progress: 1954–55

 A group of Oklahoma dentists was granted a hearing before the University of Oklahoma regents on January 14, 1954, regarding establishment of a School of Dentistry in Oklahoma. Rolla Calkin of Guthrie, president of the Oklahoma Dental Association, reported that their executive council favored founding a grade A School of Dentistry, in conjunction with the School of Medicine, that could accommodate approximately 150 students with classes of 35 members, and that the estimated building cost would be around $1,375,000, with an annual operating budget of $400,000.

President Cross said that the problem was not whether Oklahoma needed a dental school so much as it was a question of finding the finances to operate one; and he suggested that the taxpayers would be confronted with no small dental bill if such a dental school as recommended was established. However, Dr. Cross was cognizant that many of those who went out of the state to study dentistry did not come back—the upshot being that many towns and areas in Oklahoma were without dentists—and that those we did have were getting older as a group. (There were fewer than 700 practicing dentists in the state, although some 1,034 were licensed, according to the *Norman Transcript*, January 16, 1954.)

On January 22, Dr. Calkin was advised that the university regents had voted unanimously to approve the recommendation that every possible means of establishing a highly accredited dental school in Oklahoma be pursued, but they suggested further conferences to formulate plans to get the matter before the proper authorities.

Twelve members of the dental school committee of the Oklahoma Dental Association[1] met on March 4 and adopted a motion to secure a survey study by disinterested parties,[2] to determine the advisability of establishing a dental

[1] Doctors Max Armstrong, Rolla Calkin, John Cole, A. R. Drescher, A. L. Frew, R. P. Keidel, D. M. Matteson, Joe Osmun, Fred Pitney, F. J. Reichmann, T. J. Richardson, Dean Robertson, J. M. Robertson, C. A. Sebert, Ward L. Shaffer, and L. D. Wright.

[2] See Walter J. Pelton, D.D.S., M.S.P.H., Division of Dental Resources, *A Study of Oklahoma's Dental Manpower Requirements*, United States Department of Health, Education and Welfare, (1954).

school in Oklahoma, although several hundred dentists in the state were opposed to the idea at the time. The opposition (perhaps erroneously) maintained that the University of Kansas City and Baylor University in Texas were taking all available applicants from Oklahoma with the proper credentials. A total of 146 students left the state to study dentistry elsewhere in 1952–53, according to a statistical census.

The conclusions and recommendations of the survey study were that a dental school with facilities for at least 200 undergraduate dental students be established in Oklahoma; that facilities be provided to accommodate a dental hygiene school with a minimum enrollment of 40 students; that the dental school provide opportunities for postgraduate training; and that, if there was to be a dental school, it should be located at the medical center in Oklahoma City.

Meanwhile the president's long-range planning committee for the School of Medicine and University Hospitals, headed by Stewart Wolf, was getting off to an enthusiastic start, only to run smack into some adverse publicity for the medical center, resulting from an audit of the hospitals by Paul Cooke for the legislative council. Though it was ultimately established, to the satisfaction of the legislative council, that Mr. Cooke had misinterpreted the duties of the hospital employees and that his findings did not constitute an indictment of the hospitals' administration, the planning committee felt that an appraisal of efficiency of the operation of the hospitals by a completely impartial agency was essential ''to effectively erase any lingering impressions in the mind of the public and its servants.''

Subsequently, a report from Dr. Wolf and his committee,[3] presented to the university regents on May 13, called attention to a recently published official report by the Commission on the Cost of Hospital Care, emphasizing that the School of Medicine had not only gained substantially in scholastic standing and national prestige since 1948 but that it had been operating at a per diem cost actually lower than hospitals of comparable size and scope in the nation.

President Cross called attention to two recommendations made by the planning committee: (1) that it be the policy of the university to provide full-time department heads and a teaching nucleus of other full-time teachers for each of the major clinical departments—pediatrics, psychiatry, obstetrics, and general surgery—responsible for the planning and supervision of the department's educational program and the conduct of research; (2) that well-authenticated data be presented to the physicians of the state, to the legislature, and to the general public, as soon as possible, ''so that they may have a clear picture of the purposes of the medical center, its limitations with reference to indigent care, its growing scholastic standing and national prominence, its relatively economical operation, and its needs with reference to maintaining standards for accreditation in view of the currently larger classes.''

The two recommendations were approved by the university regents, who

[3.] Vice-president Pete Kyle McCarter, Matt H. Connell from Picher, Jess D. Hermann, Ernest Lachman, R. Q. Goodwin, Dean Mark R. Everett, Raymond Crews, and Dean Laurence Snyder from Norman.

also voted accolades to Dr. Wolf and his committee for their fine work, which was most helpful in understanding the progress as well as the problems of the School of Medicine.

In view of the fact that the proposed budget request for University Hospitals (1953–54) exceeded the available income by $227,831, the State Regents for Higher Education, the University of Oklahoma Board of Regents, hospital authorities, and the appropriations and budget committee of the legislative council, meeting on May 26, reached the decision to operate the University Hospital on its present basis for the first three quarters of the next fiscal year, with the legislature again being asked to provide funds to complete the final quarter.[4] This decision was compatible with a recommendation by Governor Murray that the next legislature make a $227,000 supplemental appropriation rather than reduce the enrollment in the School of Medicine by 40 students. For approximately twenty years the administration of the School of Medicine had gone through the same predicament with its biennial budget requests, and for the past several years the deficit figure had ranged around the $220,000 mark.

Dial Curran, chairman of the State Regents for Higher Education, expressed appreciation to all connected with the operation of the hospitals, saying that he felt that they were sincerely attempting to provide the highest type of service with the available funds. And Herbert Hope of Maysville, chairman of the Senate Appropriations Committee, said the legislature specifically appropriated $3,000,000 for the hospital in 1953, because the hospital officials feared that the State Regents for Higher Education would not give it to the hospitals unless it was in a separate bill. The governor concurred in this opinion, but the chairman of the House Appropriations Committee, Representative W. H. Langley, did not acquiesce. As a matter of fact, he called for the resignation of Mark R. Everett as dean of the University of Oklahoma Medical School, according to an article by Hugh Hall in the *Oklahoma City Times* on June 8, saying, ''As long as they have Dean Everett over there, they will have to have a supplemental appropriation every time the legislature meets. In my opinion, they should fire him and get someone who knows how to run a medical school.'' Mr. Langley added that the theory of writing the separate appropriation bill for $3,000,000 was to take University Hospital out from under ''the domination of a little medical clique in Oklahoma City'' and that, until they straightened out ''that place'' and put it on a business basis, there would continue to be trouble.

George Short, president of the university regents, recalled that he was one member of that board who had voted to curtail University Hospital operations making it imperative to run on available funds; but President Cross reminded the regents that many of the improvements at the medical school were due to the efforts of Dr. Everett; that, when he became dean in 1947, the school was on probation with the American Medical Association but was now rated within the upper 5 to 10 per cent of all accredited medical schools in the country.

There is little doubt but that establishment of imposed operational deficits

4. *Daily Oklahoman*, May 27, 1954.

unjustly injured the name and reputation of the University of Oklahoma School of Medicine. Therefore, the goal of all interested parties was adequate financing of the medical school and its hospitals in order to maintain an entering class of 100 medical students. To this end, the alumni association printed a brochure, entitled *Lifesavers Need Help Too*, in an effort to sharpen the focus on why medical training was expensive, why 150 hospital beds were empty, how a teaching hospital differed from a general hospital, how our budget compared with those of neighboring schools, and the fate of the School of Medicine under a financial policy of deficit spending.

On August 30 the president's Committee on Future Plans for the Medical Center recommended that the administration of the medical center remain centralized in one person responsible to the president. The committee expressed the feeling that an organization which was based on divided administrative responsibilities was not conducive to efficiency of operation and good morale; and that, since the purpose of the center was education, the educational officer, namely the dean, should be in charge.

This approach, together with other recommendations, made a favorable impression on the university regents, and George F. Short, president, informed Dean Everett that he had taken the liberty of writing personally to Dr. Wolf, saying that he did not know whether he was "a qualified M.D. or D.D.S. but that he was a master salesman."

In a summary of objectives of the medical center prepared for the legislative council, September 14, 1954, the educational program of the School of Medicine was defined in reference to the more than 1,300 students who took part in the various programs in 1953, in reference to the affiliated Oklahoma Medical Research Foundation, the Veterans Administration Hospital, and the approximately forty outpatient clinics currently being operated for the medical school training program.

So far, full-time leadership and teaching in the clinical years had been established only in the Department of Medicine, where it worked well, in no way jeopardizing the participation in teaching of part-time clinical faculty members. Soon the Departments of Obstetrics and Psychiatry voted in favor of full-time heads for their departments, carrying out one of the three purposes for which the president's planning committee was formed—to improve the quality of teaching in the School of Medicine, to assist in solving the recurring financial deficiencies, and to combat unfair criticisms of the dean and the faculty.

Two members of the faculty brought special honors to the medical center during the year: Harry E. Wilkins, neurosurgeon and professor of surgery at the School of Medicine, was elected president of the Harvey Cushing Society, the largest neurosurgical society in the world; and William T. Newsom, a young assistant professor of pediatrics, became the first Markle Scholar within our medical center, when he received a $6,000 fellowship from the John and Mary R. Markle Foundation in New York. The chief purpose of the Markle Scholar awards was to encourage promising young men to remain in academic work.

Henry B. Strenge was advanced to head of the Department of Pediatrics on

July 1, 1954, succeeding Clark Hall, who was cited for exceptional service to the University of Oklahoma School of Medicine (continuing to serve on a part-time basis).[5] Jenell Hubbard was promoted to the position of acting director of the nursing services on October 1, and Marie Mink became an instructor in nursing.

Lewis J. Moorman, professor emeritus of medicine and former dean of the School of Medicine (1931–1935) died on August 2, 1954, in Oklahoma City. He was secretary-editor of the *Journal of the Oklahoma State Medical Association* for 15 years and a past president of the association.

New appointments to the faculty for 1954–55 are listed below:

Shelby G. Gamble, M.D.
 professor of physical medicine
Louis Jolyon West, M.D.
 professor of psychiatry and
 neurology
Robert Leverne Cranny, M.D.
 assistant professor of pediatrics
Hayden Hackney Donahue, M.D.
 consultant assistant professor of
 psychiatry and neurology
John F. Dunkel, M.D.
 assistant professor of pathology
Walter F. Edmundson, M.D.
 assistant professor of preventive
 medicine and public health
Mary Googe, M.D.
 assistant professor of
 anesthesiology
Thomas Hulen Haight, M.D.
 assistant professor of medicine
 and of preventive medicine and
 public health
Thelma Pedersen, M.A.
 assistant professor of physical
 therapy
Alfred Max Shideler, M.D.
 assistant professor of pathology
Lawrence Stream, M.D.
 assistant professor of
 anesthesiology

Jenner G. Coil, M.D.
 instructor in otorhinolaryngology
Kenneth Keith Faulkner, M.S.
 instructor in anatomy
Eugene Richard Flock, M.D.
 instructor in preventive medicine
 and public health
Leon C. Freed, M.D.
 instructor in medicine
Joseph W. Funnell, M.D.
 instructor in gynecology
William Clark Galegar, M.S.
 instructor in preventive medicine
 and public health
Margaret E. Gwinn, M.S.
 instructor in preventive medicine
 and public health
Robert Proulx Heaney, M.D.
 instructor in medicine
Philip E. Morgan, M.D.
 instructor in preventive medicine
 and public health
James Burton Pitts, Jr., M.D.
 instructor in gynecology
Arthur Schmidt, M.D.
 instructor in medicine
Robert Sukman, M.D.
 instructor in radiology
Robert Cecil Troop, Ph.D.
 instructor in physiology

[5.] Dr. Hall was also presented an appreciation scroll by the members of the board of the Children's Convalescent Hospital in Bethany in November, 1953, as an expression of thanks to the pediatrician who had served as chief of staff there for 13 years without pay.

Professor Strenge, a graduate of Yale Medical School, had interned at Johns Hopkins Hospital and was chief resident in pediatrics at the Strong Memorial Hospital in Rochester, New York. He had served four years in the U.S. Army.

C. Jack Young, M.D.
instructor in dermatology and syphilology
Byron Lewis Bailey, M.D.
clinical assistant in medicine
James Stanton Boyle, M.D.
clinical assistant in urology
Forest Reed Brown, M.D.
visiting lecturer in preventive medicine and public health
Thomas Merwin Buxton, M.D.
clinical assistant in medicine
John Merwin Carey, M.D.
clinical assistant in surgery
Mervin Leslie Clark, M.D.
clinical assistant in medicine
William Jackson Dowling, M.D.
clinical assistant in surgery
Paul D. Erwin, M.D.
clinical assistant in surgery
Emil P. Farris, M.D.
clinical assistant in ophthalmology
William Hampton Garnier, M.D.
clinical assistant in ophthalmology
Orion Russell Gregg, M.D.
visiting lecturer in preventive medicine and public health
Taswell Paul Haney, Jr., M.D., D.P.H.
visiting lecturer in preventive medicine and public health
Charles M. Harvey, M.D.
clinical assistant in medicine
Rosemary Boles Harvey, M.D.
visiting lecturer in preventive medicine and public health
Lynn E. Hollis, M.D.
visiting lecturer in preventive medicine and public health
Robert Wallace King, M.D.
clinical assistant in ophthalmology

John Emmett Lewis, D.D.S.
clinical assistant in dental surgery
Clair Liebrand, M.D.
clinical assistant in medicine
Robert Harold Mayes, M.D.
visiting lecturer in preventive medicine and public health
John Meyer, M.D.
consultant clinical assistant in psychiatry and neurology
Clifford W. Moore, M.D.
visiting lecturer in preventive medicine and public health
Ralph William Murphy, M.D.
visiting lecturer in pediatrics
E. Cotter Murray, M.D.
visiting lecturer in preventive medicine and public health
Frank Harrison McGregor, M.D.
clinical assistant in surgery
Kenneth W. Navin, M.D., M.P.H.
visiting lecturer in preventive medicine and public health
Don L. Oesterreicher, M.D.
clinical assistant in surgery
Maurice L. Peter, M.P.H., M.D.
visiting lecturer in preventive medicine and public health
Ralph R. Robinson, M.D.
clinical assistant in obstetrics and gynecology
Henry Thomas Russell, M.D.
visiting lecturer in pathology
Bob Jack Rutledge, M.D.
clinical assistant in surgery
Loraine Schmidt, M.D.
visiting lecturer in preventive medicine and public health
Mary Frances Schottstaedt, M.D.
clinical assistant in medicine
Harry Fields Singleton, M.D.
clinical assistant in medicine
James Barrett Thompson, M.D.
visiting lecturer in surgery

W. K. West, Department of Orthopedics, was very helpful in making the School of Physical Therapy a possibility by 1954, having worked with the American Physical Therapy Association, the American Medical Association, and the National Foundation for Infantile Paralysis in paving the way for a four-year course for physical therapists, which would lead to a bachelor of arts degree. The initial financing for the new school was made possible by a total grant of $25,504 from the National Foundation for Infantile Paralysis, including $19,000 to aid in purchasing equipment for the recently expanded Crippled Children's Hospital, where the department was to be housed, and $5,800 for the salary of the director, Thelma Pedersen.[6]

From 1952 to 1954 there was a steady growth in psychiatry teaching, proceeding from activities covered by a teaching grant from the National Institutes of Health. These activities necessitated changes in curriculum, and Robert A. Schneider, assistant professor in both psychiatry and medicine, effected innovations in the diagnosis and care of both outpatients and inpatients. For instance, the physical diagnosis course in the second year was completely revamped, placing special emphasis on talking with the patient and on history taking as groundwork for the inpatient clerkship in the third year. Furthermore, demonstrations in interviewing patients were conducted before the entire class.

Opening of psychiatry wards in the new addition to University Hospital raised the question of a full-time head of psychiatry as early as April, and in September the university regents appointed Lewis Jolyon West to the chairmanship.[7] Dr. West's appointment was aimed at strengthening the teaching program in psychiatry and neurology for the School of Medicine and reinforcing the quality of instruction in such mental hospitals as the Central State Hospital in Norman and the Veterans Administration Hospital in Oklahoma City.

The appointment of Dr. West brought the number of full-time faculty in the School of Medicine to 62, with an additional 11 full-time teachers in the School of Nursing, and 77 consulting and attending physcians at the veterans' hospital who were chiefly from the volunteer staff of the School of Medicine. Approximately 90 per cent of the 550 physicians and medical scientists were serving on the School of Medicine faculty on a voluntary basis and as consultants to numerous health agencies, hospitals, and organizations. In other words, the School of Medicine was a central agency for numerous interests—frequently

---

[6.] Miss Pedersen received her graduate training in physical therapy at Stanford University and came to Oklahoma from Mt. Sinai Hospital, Chicago, to start a physical therapy program with only three students. She had helped to train and graduate 398 physical therapists and said, upon retiring in 1975, that retirement did not mean that she planned "to ride out into the sunset."

Miss Pedersen became a member of the newly established Department of Physical Medicine, of which Shelby G. Gamble was chairman and Ella Mary George a member. Dr. Gamble served besides as medical director of the rehabilitation center in Okmulgee under a cooperative plan worked out between the center there and the University of Oklahoma School of Medicine.

[7.] Dr. West, age 30, was a graduate of the University of Minnesota School of Medicine, resident in psychiatry at the Payne-Whitney Clinic in New York City, and currently chief of the psychiatry section of the United States Air Force Hospital in San Antonio.

cooperative in character—sponsored by national and state agencies and foundations.

On December 30, 1954, John Colmore, newly appointed chief of the outpatient department and director of a pioneer program begun two years previously, announced that the Commonwealth Fund, over a period of two years, had appropriated $51,750 to the University of Oklahoma School of Medicine in support of the "communications project" for the salaries and overhead expenses for a public health nurse, a pediatrician, a psychiatry social worker, and a secretary. This personnel group was added to the comprehensive care and teaching program in the medical and pediatric outpatient departments, in accordance with the initial request for the grant.

An effort to maintain continuity of medical care for indigent patients in the University Hospitals had been made possible by an emergency grant from the Commonwealth Fund in August, 1952, whereby open communication was established between the hospitals and the referring doctors in distant communities, so that a patient could be properly cared for after discharge from the hospital, thus avoiding needless complications and recurrences.

Operation of the program was made easier by a complete reorganization of the outpatient department and of the fourth-year teaching curriculum, which made it possible for every patient to be first carefully evaluated in the medical clinic by a student who would continue to care for the patient throughout the year. This meant that when a student referred an outpatient from the medical clinic to another clinic, he referred the patient to himself on a day when he would be in the other clinic. And when the patient was discharged from the hospital, a channel of communication was set up between the University Hospitals and the home community of the patient, making it possible for the treatment of an individual to be carried out in an appropriate manner by the local physician with the help of county health facilities.

In discussing changes in administration of the outpatient department, it should be noted that the psychiatry clinic, which was professionally a part of the Department of Psychiatry and Neurology, was supervised by Dr. Colmore, director of the outpatient department, but that the treatment of patients was conducted by the staff of the Department of Psychiatry and Neurology in accordance with the best medical and psychiatric practice without regard for the financial status of the patient. Necessarily, admission of patients to the hospitals was on a basis of teaching needs and requirements of the School of Medicine and in conformity with the Oklahoma Mental Health Law.

Integration of the Department of Preventive Medicine with other divisions of the medical center, participating actively in the program outlined above, was another extension of services for indigent patients. And the development of an oral surgery division within the Department of Surgery was yet another innovation during this period of development.[8] The first application for a residency in oral surgery was in July, 1954.

[8.] J. M. Robertson was the first chairman of the division, succeeded by James R. Miller, who later requested military leave, at which time Albert Drescher became the chairman.

Support from the W. K. Kellogg Foundation came at a very opportune time for the School of Medicine to stimulate progressive interest in judicious medical practices. And the effectiveness of $59,000 in grants made by the National Fund for Medical Education over a period of three years was similarily helpful, due entirely to the fact that the money was unrestricted.

Marvin Shetlar, who became chief of the reserach laboratory at the veterans' hospital in 1954, personally received a grant from the American Cancer Society for investigation of serum polysaccharide in cancer patients following treatment.[9] The local cancer society was helping to support the tumor clinic at University Hospital, and the isotope laboratory was funded with $21,190 for the year, chiefly from the legislative appropriation for heart disease and cancer study.

The Department of Medicine was fortunate, too, in receiving a contribution of $1,850 from the American College of Physicians toward its postgraduate program for residents in medicine. And Robert Bayley, professor of medicine, received a grant of $5,000 from the National Institutes of Health in support of his electrographic counting project.

State appropriations for the University of Oklahoma and the School of Medicine and University Hospitals for 1954–55 were as follows: Norman campus, $4,195,550 out of a total income of $6,245,803; School of Medicine, $636,512 out of a total income of $804,533; University Hospitals, $1,444,000 out of a total income of $2,636,157.

The number of patients admitted to University Hospitals, July 1, 1954, to July 1, 1955, was 11,291 (8,529 to the main hospital and 2,762 to Children's Hospital); days of hospital care were 133,346 (79,355 at main and 53,991 at Children's); and the average number of hospital days per patient, 10.8 at main and 18.6 at Children's. A total of 4,171 operations were performed in both hospitals, including 34 heart catheterizations. There were 23,708 physiotherapy treatments, 33,634 x-ray examinations, 220,452 examinations in the clinical laboratories, 3,034 ECG examinations at the heart station, and a total of 9,525 studies in the cytology laboratories. In the outpatient department 18,946 individuals (12,159 adults and 6,787 children) received a total of 85,993 treatments.

Seventeen interns, 64 residents, and one fellow were training in the University Hospitals (1954–55), with a new residency in neurological surgery approved on June 10.[10]

There were 388 students enrolled in the School of Medicine during the same period: 154 in the School of Nursing and 54 in the Graduate College, 25 of whom were studying toward Ph.D. or M.Sc. degrees in one of the basic sciences.

A highlight of the year for members of Alpha Omega Alpha, honorary

[9] Concurrently, the American Cancer Society was making block grants to the Oklahoma Medical Research Foundation.

[10] During this period of expansion, Raymond Crews was promoted to the position of administrator of University Hospitals at a salary of $8,000, following the resignation of Arthur McElmurry.

medical fraternity, was a lecture by Sir Alexander Fleming on the use of antibiotics, at the groups' first annual lecture and initiation on April 22. The formal program for the banquet carried the names of Sir Alexander Fleming, London University, and Dean Mark R. Everett, Harvard University, as honorary initiates.

The preceptorship for senior medical students continued to be a success—a laboratory for the practice of medicine, under the guidelines set out for preceptors by the administration of the medical school in suggested "do's" and "don't's."

An official estimate of the number of medical students required to meet Oklahoma's need for medical services, based on a statewide survey made in 1954, revealed certain facts: the number of licensed physicians in Oklahoma in 1952 was 2,257 and the ratio of aged physicians unusually high—the median age being 50 years as compared with 47 for the entire United States. Only two other states had a higher median age. Moreover, Oklahoma had an average of only one physician to 985 persons, whereas the average in the entire United States was one physician to 725 persons. Since many medical doctors filled positions in which they were not available to the public, this further reduced the average of actively practicing physicians to one doctor for every 1,407 persons compared with one to 1,029 in the entire United States.

On the other side of the coin, during the period of 1949–53 the average age of students entering the School of Medicine was 22 years, and the average age for the beginning of medical practice was 28 years, with an attrition average of 2 per cent of the student body. Based on these data, it was estimated that enrollment of 115 first-year students and graduation of 111 doctors per year would be necessary to bring the ratio into the national average within 35 years.

Lilah B. Heck, head librarian of the School of Medicine, was given faculty standing with the title of assistant professor of medical library science by the university regents in June. During the ten-year span, December, 1943, to January, 1953, the total number of volumes in the library increased from 18,697 to 34,376, which was an increase of nearly 80 per cent; and subscriptions to journals increased from 295 to 851. Happily, circulation also increased, from 16,863 volumes in 1951–52 to 24,537 in 1952–53, indicating a marked step-up in the use of library services.[11]

Enthusiasm continued to be apparent for courses offered by the Division of Postgraduate Instruction of the School of Medicine, under the direction of Irwin Brown,[12] with a remarkable increase in attendance during the few preceding years. The primary intent of these programs had always been to provide a review of a given area of medicine for the general practitioner, and all courses,

[11.] Gifts totaling thousands of items were made during the ten-year period noted; funds were made available for purchases in the field of dentistry by a research group of the Oklahoma County Dental Society; and the use of the interlibrary loan service, between Norman and Stillwater, increased by 60 per cent.

[12.] Dr. Brown, assistant professor of surgery as well as director of the postgraduate office, received a salary of $11,500 as of July 1, 1954.

of which there were 12 in 1954–55, were approved by the Oklahoma Academy of General Practice for credit toward postgraduate training requirements. Anywhere from 12 to 152 physicians were enrolled in the different courses, with a total of 792 individuals attending, and the number of physicians from surrounding states—Kansas, Missouri, Texas, and New Mexico—was more than double the turnout for the previous year.[13]

A marked drop in the average daily occupancy in Crippled Children's Hospital (from 197 in 1950–51 to 155 in 1952–53) was the result of the Crippled Children's Commission's denial of county funds to University Hospitals, pursuant to a state supreme court decision on the matter in 1951. The regents of the university, therefore, requested the commission to prepare a workable plan of operation whereby payments to the University Hospitals would be stabilized. As a result, an agreement was consummated on July 1, 1954, obligating the commission (insofar as practicable) to use the facilities of the Oklahoma Hospital for Crippled Children "to a degree that will enable the University of Oklahoma School of Medicine to maintain its proper patient ratio for accreditation." And the commission agreed also to reimburse the outpatient clinic services in the amount of $50,000 per year and to furnish a variety of consultation services through its own staff.

By virtue of a recreational program, under the auspices of the Society of the Oklahoma Hospital for Crippled Children, little patients in the hospital were made definitely happier too. From May 1, 1949 to May 1, 1954, a total of 713 sewing clubs provided 19,345 garments for the children; 773 Red Cross volunteers donated 10,145 hours of service; and 1,691 other volunteers devoted 10,145 hours to recreational activities. In addition, movies were shown on Saturdays to a total of 11,465 patients, and operators from beauty salons contributed their services on 7,554 occasions.

The Junior League of Oklahoma City was responsible for the only building project on the School of Medicine campus in 1954—a new home for the University of Oklahoma Speech and Hearing Clinic, currently housed in a tiny annex of the Crippled Children's Hospital.

According to Mrs. Dick Lowry, vice-president of the league, proceeds from the 1953 annual charity horse show in Oklahoma City had been set aside for this project in a charitable building corporation—the School of Speech and Hearing, Inc.—and all proceeds from the 1954 event (May 19–22) were added to the amount already contributed toward a construction goal of approximately $80,000.[14] Ground-breaking ceremonies were held on Thursday morning, May 20, at a building site directly north of the Medical Research Foundation

---

13. James R. Reed, chairman of the Department of Ophthalmology, reported that 88 doctors had attended the first annual convention of the Oklahoma City Academy of Ophthalmology and Otolaryngology, held on March 26 under the auspices of the postgraduate division of the School of Medicine, and that this result was "remarkable."

14. The Junior League of Oklahoma City had previously given $11,757 for recreational facilities at the Crippled Children's Hospital, in addition to $7,000 for a playroom in 1952.

building, on land donated by the University of Oklahoma. Adding glamour to the occasion were Roy Rogers, King of the Cowboys, and Dale Evans, Queen of the West, who were celebrities at the current charity horse show. Mark Alford, a little student at the Speech and Hearing Clinic—decked out in cowboy regalia—helped Roy Rogers break ground with a golden shovel.

Continual progress in the postwar years was much in evidence in 1954 in the size and quality of the faculty, the enlarged student body, and the expanding physical plant—with the School of Medicine the nucleus of medical education and good medical care for the indigent patient in the state of Oklahoma.

The free interchange of knowledge and skills, which had long been the cornerstone of progress in the medical world, had developed to a high degree on the medical campus in only a few years, not just within the parent organization, the School of Medicine, but within the Oklahoma Medical Research Institute and the Veterans Administration Hospital, as well as augmenting the broad education of the medical student.

Hill-Burton matching funds, granted to the University of Oklahoma School of Medicine and University Hospitals (1948–52), were of tremendous aid to the building program at a time when financial security was educationally and economically unsound, contributing a total of $1,142,775 to construction projects: 1948–49, $35,087 for equipment for the main hospital addition; 1949–50, $7,480 to remodel the Crippled Children's Hospital kitchen; and $152,851 for the nurses' home addition; 1950–51, $897,357 toward the outpatient and neuropsychiatric addition; and 1951–52, $50,000 for equipment for the Crippled Children's Hospital addition.[15]

In its attempt to meet the increased teaching commitment imposed by the university regents—on a deficit budget allocated by the State Regents for Higher Education—the administration was untiringly supported by the governor of Oklahoma, as the state's period of political evolution and Governor Johnston Murray's term of office came to a close. It was as though a bridge between frontier politics and an emerging broad road of progress had finally been traversed precariously.

[15.] Records of the state health department, 1948–52.

Chapter XIX.
One Hundred Graduates
in Medicine: 1955–56

Raymond Gary was elected governor of the state of Oklahoma in November, 1954, and, when his first legislative session commenced on January 25, 1955, the financial fate of the School of Medicine of the University of Oklahoma was, as expected, hanging in the balance—the inevitable result of deficit financing. As usual, the State Regents for Higher Education were requesting the legislature for an immediate supplemental appropriation. After 12 years of similar requests ranging from $100,000 to $683,736, the "rerun" sounded rather irksome to legislators.

Ray Parr, writing in the January 26 issue of the *Daily Oklahoman*, reported that the state house of representatives had staged a two-hour fight over supplemental appropriations, including those to keep the University Hospitals open, and had issued stern warnings to all departments and institutional heads that the legislature was "not going to tolerate deficit budgeting." Some members, "in righteous indignation," even criticized the University Hospitals for difficulties encountered in getting patients admitted for treatment. However, when their spleen was spent, they approved two supplemental appropriations, as nearly everyone had taken for granted anyway. The irony of the farce was that the floor leader had to tell the "watch dogs" that the legislature had overspent its own appropriations, and that a supplemental appropriation of $330,000 was necessary to keep the legislature operating the rest of the fiscal year!

Surprisingly enough, one of the two representatives who voted against the additional appropriations for the University Hospitals was Cleeta John Rogers of Oklahoma City, who led a fight to send the hospital bill back to committee for a public hearing. While Rogers deplored the fact that University Hospitals came to the legislature every two years for supplemental appropriations, the State Regents for Higher Education also drew some fire for forcing the hospitals to run short of funds year after year while increasing the teaching load. Solely as a result of unrealistic financing, 150 beds were standing empty and unused, raising havoc with the teaching program.

Representative Glen Ham from Pauls Valley appreciated the fact that the University Hospitals were primarily teaching hospitals and he said that the legislative council, after a full investigation in the summer of 1954, had urged

233

officials of the medical center not to curtail operations in order to bring expenditures within the budget because the people of Oklahoma were demanding more doctors, and the school's accreditation was being jeopardized.

When Governor Gary learned that it would cost $1,400,000 a year to competently carry out the program of training doctors and treating patients for the state, he appointed a committee of senators[1] to study the needs for appropriations for the medical school and hospitals above those requested by the regents of the university.

The actual state of affairs at the medical center was that the University Hospitals, owing to insufficient funding, had fewer teaching beds in operation in 1955, with a graduating class of 100 medical students, than in 1952, with a graduating class of 58, and without any substantial increase in the budget allotment for the faculty.[2] The state appropriation figure was little more than half the national average figure and the budget substantially below the national average for state schools, with $1,040,000 for 100 students per class. There were 1/7 as many "indigent beds" per unit of population as Louisiana, 4/5 as many as Kansas, and 7/10 as many as Colorado.

The estimated per diem costs for caring for the indigent patient in University Hospitals in 1955 was $19.91—considerably below the cost at that time for similar services at the University of Kansas Medical Center ($22.58) and the University of Colorado Medical Center ($23.50).

The president's Committee on Future Plans for the Medical Center pointed out that presently the University Hospitals provided only 50 percent of the teaching hospital facilities used by the School of Medicine, the other 50 per cent being furnished by the Veterans Administration Hospital, St. Anthony Hospital, Mercy Hospital, and Wesley Hospital, without any cost to the state.

In spite of the fact that the University Hospital was obviously vastly inadequate as a facility for caring for the indigent sick of Oklahoma, it did provide valuable and unparalleled services in caring for the number of indigent patients who were admitted to the hospital—clearly a public welfare service. Therefore, the planning committee reached the decision that the cost of caring for patients should be stably provided for by appropriate legislation, rather than by charging the whole cost to higher education.

Doubt concerning the economy of operation of University Hospitals— frequently an excuse for questioning appropriations, with the administration being subjected to innuendo and implication that the enterprise was not providently managed—was entirely unsubstantiated as exemplified by the above analysis.

The consensus of the faculty board on January 18 was that no group (or person) other than the faculty could judge the adequacy of teaching facilities for training classes of 100 medical students; and that it was the duty of the faculty to

---

[1] The committee was composed of James M. Bullard of Duncan, chairman, Oliver Walker of Dale, Herbert Hope of Maysville, and Glenn C. Collins of Konawa.

[2] The minimum requirement for accreditation of the School of Medicine was three new patients per week per student; the ideal was five.

make its judgment known. The board further expressed the opinion that satisfactory instruction of 100 medical students was impossible at the time, according to all current standards of medical education, because of a lack of patients for teaching and inability to employ sufficient faculty personnel. So the faculty board recommended that only 70 students be admitted to the medical school in the fall of 1955, and that the faculty communicate its grave concern to the governor of the state of Oklahoma and to the president of the university.

The alumni of the School of Medicine were so concerned about the status of their alma mater by February 15 that 173 doctors pledged $6,801 for an educational campaign to get the neuropsychiatric wards open at University Hospital. Special teams, composed of trustees of the alumni association and members of the faculty, visited personally with most of the State Regents for Higher Education in their home bivouacs, and President Cross reported that he had received requests for additional funds for the School of Medicine from several county medical societies.

On April 25 the secretary of the university regents released the statement that the regents were fully appreciative of the financial problems of the School of Medicine and expected to do everything possible to help solve those problems. But they were emphatic in their decision that there would be no reduction in the size of the entering class in the fall, and that all commitments to applicants must be honored. However, the admission of a firstyear class of 100 after the fall of 1955 was considered debatable unless more adequate financing of University Hospitals was forthcoming.

On July 14 the university regents approved a budget and operating procedure for the Department of Psychiatry and Neurology of the School of Medicine and University Hospitals, with monies sufficient to permit expansion of the outpatient psychiatric clinic and the opening of one 20-bed floor for emotionally disturbed patients in the new addition to University Hospital, at a cost of $250,000 a year. Two other floors totaling 40 beds remained unopened, pending future allocation of sufficient funds for their operation.

The operating procedure approved by the regents complied with Section 53 of the Oklahoma Mental Health Law, for, while patients were not to be committed by the courts directly to University Hospitals, those already committed to other state institutions might, by special arrangement, be transferred to the University Hospitals for purposes of teaching, research, or special studies.[3]

The first physicians ever to receive specialist training in psychiatry at the University Hospitals began their residencies on July 1. They were James A. Cox, who had had one year of previous training in the United States Army, Wayne J. Boyd, Charles E. Smith, and Boyd K. Lester. The first three patients admitted to the neuropsychiatric unit were assigned to their rooms on Monday morning, August 8.[4]

[3.] All practices and policies of the Department of Psychiatry and Neurology in its operation of the new facilities were to be in accordance with provisions of House Bill No. 585 passed by the 1953 legislature.

[4.] Full-time faculty physicians engaged in teaching psychiatry were as follows: Louis

An amendment to the bylaws of the faculty of the School of Medicine, dealing with departmental advisory committees, was adopted by the faculty on September 29, 1955, as follows: At specific intervals of every two years each clinical department shall recommend names of its faculty members to the dean as suggested candidates for membership on the departmental advisory committee, which shall consist of a minimum of three members. From these recommendations, appointments shall be made by the dean, after consultation with the chairman or head of the department. Eligibility for these nominees shall be limited to those department members having the rank of assistant professor or above.

In order that full-time faculty members should not become too prominent on the faculty board, a second amendment to the bylaws was also adopted by the faculty, to wit: that the faculty board should consist of the chairmen or heads of academic departments, and in addition one part-time faculty members from each of the major clinical departments (medicine, surgery, obstetrics, pediatrics, and neuropsychiatry) should be appointed by the dean at two-year intervals from the membership of the respective departmental advisory committees. Both amendments were passed by the faculty 214 to 26 and approved by the university regents on March 8, 1956.

Shelby Gamble, professor of physical medicine, was given the additional title of medical director of the School of Physical Therapy on July 1; and the Council on Medical Education and Hospitals voted to extend approval to that school on June 4. The fee per semester was $125.

Joseph M. White became chairman of the Department of Anesthesiology, following the resignation of Howard A. Bennett on August 1; Jenell Hubbard replaced Helen Patterson as director of the nursing service; and Edith Schroeder was appointed acting director of the medical social service department in August, replacing Elizabeth Walton, a very constructive director of the Department of Social Service since 1950, who resigned to become associate professor of social casework at Western Reserve University.

New appointments to the faculty are listed below, raising the total number of persons on the faculty (including preceptors) to approximately 490:

Joseph M. White, M.D.
  professor of anesthesiology
Donald C. Greaves, M.D.
  associate professor of psychiatry,
  neurology, and behavioral sciences

Herbert L. Kent, L.R.C.P.
  associate professor of physical
  medicine

Jolyon West, professor and head of the department, Donald C. Greaves, associate professor, John Gussen, assistant professor, and Robert A. Schneider, associate professor; also Harold Witten, associate professor, Tracey H. McCarley, assistant, and Joe Yamamoto, assistant professor at the Veterans Administration Hospital. Coyne H. Campbell, professor and former chairman of the department, remained as a part-time teacher.

William Seeman, Ph.D.
associate professor of medical
psychology in psychiatry,
neurology, and behavioral
sciences
Paul C. Benton, M.D.
assistant professor of psychiatry,
neurology, and behavioral sciences
Arley Tunis Bever, Jr., Ph.D.
assistant professor of biochemistry
John Gussen, M.D.
assistant professor of psychiatry,
neurology, and behavioral sciences
James A. Hagans, M.D., Ph.D.
assistant professor of medicine
Philip Carl Johnson, M.D.
assistant professor of medicine
Jerome J. Landy, M.D.
assistant professor of surgery
Earl G. Larsen, Ph.D.
assistant professor of biochemistry
Tracey H. McCarley, Jr., M.D.
assistant professor of psychiatry,
neurology, and behavioral sciences
Theodore Robert Pfundt, M.D.
assistant professor of pediatrics
Joe Yamamoto, M.D.
assistant professor of psychiatry,
neurology, and behavioral sciences
James Thomas Boggs, M.D.
instructor in radiology
Vernon W. Corder, M.D.
instructor in anesthesiology
Sarah Gruss, B.A.
instructor in physical therapy
Ruth R. Gussen, M.D.
instructor in pathology
Rex E. Kenyon, M.D.
instructor in pathology
Paul Baker McCay, Ph.D.
instructor in physiology
Leonard N. Norcia, Ph.D.
instructor in research biochemistry
William Branch Renfrow, M.D.
instructor in anesthesiology
Robert L. Anderson, M.D.
visiting lecturer in surgery
Harle Virgil Barrett, M.D.
visiting lecturer in preventive
medicine and public health

Mildred M. Benjegerdes, M.D.
clinical assistant in anesthesiology
Robert Victor Bolene, M.D.
clinical assistant in obstetrics and
gynecology
Carl G. Coin, M.D.
clinical assistant in radiology
James K. Devore, M.D.
clinical assistant in medicine
Roy W. Donaghe, M.D.
clinical assistant in pediatrics
Ancel Earp, M.D.
clinical assistant in surgery
David Gold, M.D.
clinical assistant in medicine
Harry G. Hightower, M.D.
clinical assistant in psychiatry,
neurology, and behavioral sciences
Thomas Oran Hodges, M.D.
clinical assistant in surgery
James F. Hohl, M.D.
clinical assistant in medicine
Lillian M. Hoke, M.D.
clinical assistant in pediatrics
Mary Duffy Honick, M.D.
clinical assistant in medicine
Fred G. Hudson, M.D.
clinical assistant in medicine
Marvin K. Margo, M.D.
clinical assistant in orthopedic and
fracture surgery
Frank John Martin, M.D.
clinical assistant in medicine
Robert Charles Mayfield, M.D.
clinical assistant in surgery
Eric B. Meador, Jr., M.D.
clinical assistant in pediatrics
Charles Henderson Miller, M.D.
visiting lecturer in preventive
medicine and public health
Harold R. Pollock, D.D.S.
clinical assistant in oral surgery
Jack Lee Riggall, M.D.
clinical assistant in medicine
James R. Riggall, M.D.
clinical assistant in surgery
Richard G. Shifrin, M.D.
clinical assistant in anesthesiology
William O. Smith, M.D.
clinical assistant in medicine

Robert W. Spencer, M.D., M.Sc.
clinical assistant in ophthalmology
Albert C. Tipton, D.D.S.
clinical assistant in dental surgery

Rolf J. Ullestad, D.D.S.
clinical assistant in oral surgery
Carryle W. Wiggins, M.D.
clinical assistant in medicine

The Oklahoma State Regents for Higher Education allocated to the School of Medicine $40,000 for research in heart disease and cancer control from a separate appropriation by the twenty-fifth Oklahoma legislature. This was for the year ending June 30, 1956, when approximately 60 individual research projects had already been initiated through funds provided by the heart disease and cancer research appropriation of $60,000 for the current biennium. One of the accomplishments of such individual studies, in addition to helping patients receive the benefits of new methods and medical agents such as radioisotopes, was to stimulate research, thus producing results far beyond the state's dollar investment. One eager investigator developed a $450 allotment into a national grant of $9,000!

On the administrative side, Dean Everett was an ardent supporter of research, lending encouragement where indicated and breaking fetters of red tape wherever possible, in an effort to secure research monies for programs conducted by faculty of the medical school and allied institutions.[5]

Relationships between the Veterans Administration and the medical school continued at a high level. A new radioisotope research laboratory, under the direction of Philip C. Johnson, opened on the third floor of the veteran's hospital on January 12, 1955. Dr. Johnson came to the center from the University of Michigan, where he was assistant coordinator of the radioisotope laboratory at the University Hospital. He was very interested in the use of irradiated iodine to study thyroid diseases and in the use of phosphorus 32 as a convenient way to treat certain cases of chronic leukemia.

Kenneth Richter, Department of Anatomy, who was also interested in leukemia, received a $16,524 grant from the cancer institute for a study of leukemic cells; and two alumni, Robert H. Akin and Meredith M. Appleton, specified that their original contributions to the Akin and Appleton Medical Research Fund[6] be used to give financial backing to tissue work under the

---

[5.] An interesting sidelight on research was gleaned from Jajaval Osathanondh, assistant dean of the School of Medicine in Bangkok, who was studying in the United States in 1955 on a public health service fellowship. When he and Dean Everett were conferring on mutual problems regarding medical education, Dr. Osathanondh said that Crown Prince Mahidol, one of the sons of King Chulalongkorn (the romantic monarch in the motion picture, *Anna and the King of Siam*), had been educated as a physician in Harvard University. Upon returning to his native Thailand, he devoted his life and his fortune to teaching medicine to native doctors—a fascinating sequel to the story of the humanitarian king, who sought to apply techniques of western civilization to his tiny country.

[6.] Dr. Akin and Dr. Appleton, two Oklahoma City urologists, established the Akin and Appleton Medical Research Fund as a memorial to their pioneer mothers, with an original contribution of $1,500 by Dr. Akin.

direction of Dr. Richter. To this purpose, they donated an electron microscope to the University of Oklahoma School of Medicine. This is believed to have been the only such instrument used in basic research in the state at the time.

The opening of the 20-bed floor in the neuropsychiatric wing in July guaranteed a supplement of $15,000 as a graduate teaching grant from the National Institute of Neurological Diseases and Blindness; and the Junior Hospitality Club of Oklahoma City pledged $10,000 to the Oklahoma Medical Research Foundation for neuropsychiatric research in the field of pediatrics.

Since the services of the clinical pathology laboratories (as opposed to tissue pathology) had been under fire from involved faculty members for the better part of thirty years, Dean Everett tackled the problem by appointing an advisory committee in January to seek a plausible solution to the relative ineffectiveness of the clinical laboratories. The committee was composed of the two full-time faculty members directing the laboratories, plus six other pathologists and representatives of large clinical departments.

In its report, the committee agreed that all the ills could not be cured with money alone, but that money would be a great help, because salaries were too low to attract and hold competent technicians. The committee recommended that salaries of the head technologists in the individual sections should run up to $400 per month—an increase which would call for a salary budget of $130,000. However, the committee felt that this increase could be offset by a commensurable increase in the gross income from laboratory services; from July, 1953, to June, 1954, the income from 201,425 examinations totaled $629,883.

The recommendation of the committee, relative to the more serious problems in the operation of the laboratories, was establishment of a Department of Clinical Pathology separate from tissue pathology. This recommendation was unanimously endorsed by the faculty board and forwarded to President Cross in March, for approval by the regents of the university as soon as funds could be made available. When seven months had elapsed without any word of approval, Dean Everett again requested authority to establish a Department of Clinicial Pathology in University Hospitals, and authorization was granted.

According to a memorandum from the office of the medical director on December 12, the accrediting agencies, upon recommendation of the individual specialty boards and their residency review committees, had approved the following residencies in University Hospitals: anesthesiology, general practice, dermatology and syphilology, internal medicine, neurological surgery, obstetrics and gynecology, ophthalmology, pathology, pediatrics, surgery, urology, plastic surgery, otolaryngology, and radiology—a record warranting a true badge of progress.

State appropriations for the University of Oklahoma and the School of Medicine and University Hospitals for 1955–56 were as follows: Norman campus, $4,281,674 out of a total income of $6,619,418; School of Medicine, $675,406 out of a total income of $866,494; University Hospitals, $2,014,200 out of a total income of $3,373,212.

The total number of admissions to University Hospital from July 1, 1955, to

July 1, 1956, was 8,535 and to Children's Hospital 3,437. The total number of x-ray treatments in both hospitals was 35,558, and of clinical laboratory examinations, 229,898. (In the short span of eight years the work load had almost doubled.) The total number of case visits to the outpatient department of both hospitals was 76,305.

There were 377 students enrolled in the School of Medicine in 1955–56 and 122 students in the School of Nursing. Medical students who were nonresidents of the state were required to pay a nonresident tuition fee of $400 per semester ($800 per year) while the resident tuition was $450 per year.

On June 5, 1955, the University of Oklahoma conferred M.D. degrees upon 100 graduates of the School of Medicine for the first time in the history of the school. A very real contributory factor in achieving this goal, which represented a service of no mean proportion in the interest of the state, was the strenuous work and day-to-day diligence on the part of members of the faculty. Worthy of note, too, on this date, was the fact that a total of 97 women had now received the degree of Doctor of Medicine, creditable members of the medical profession in their own right.

Another distinctive feature feature of the commencement exercises was that it was the first time in the history of medical education in Oklahoma that the degree of Doctor of Philosophy in Medical Sciences was conferred on a graduate student.

At the same commencement three young women had the distinction of being the first graduates to receive the new degree of Bachelor of Science in Nursing from the University of Oklahoma, and 44 graduates received the certificate of nursing. For the year 1955–56 the degree program for nurses, which was established in 1951, claimed approximately 50 enrollees, and 47 students graduating in 1955 pushed the total number of nurses who had received training at the University Hospitals past the 1,000 milestone.

The number of patient days in Crippled Children's Hospital paid by the Oklahoma Commission for Crippled Children had decreased steadily from 62,898 in 1950–51 to 42,237 in 1953–54, which was one of the factors contributing to the perennial financial problems of University Hospitals. During the ensuing fiscal years difficulties developed on a number of occasions, because payments received from the commission were insufficient to reimburse services rendered by University Hospitals, necessitating appeals to the legislature for deficiency appropriations.

The obvious solution seemed to be budgeting of some definite portion of the commission's funds solely for services rendered, especially since it was the general understanding, when the new act was being formulated by the legislature in 1949, that appropriations made to the University Hospitals for care of crippled children to that date were being transferred to the commission with the intent that payment for services in Crippled Children's Hospital be continued.

As early as April, 1952, the Board of Regents of the University of Oklahoma, with whom the commission had a contract for hospital services for children, requested the commission to use all available funds to increase the census in Crippled Children's Hospital to a level which would maintain the accreditation of the School of Medicine. On several occasions during 1954 the dean of the medical school conferred informally with the director of the commission, Ira McConnell, requesting a statement of commitment from the commission.

Finally, on January 26, 1955, Raymond Crews, business administrator of University Hospitals (in accordance with his strict duty), requested the commission for a statement of a minimal sum that would be available during the current fiscal year, in order to provide the president and regents of the university with an estimate of hospital income—essential in preparing the official budget for the hospitals. But since this request was to no avail, Dean Everett informed President Cross on May 5 that all attempts to secure fiscal information from the director of the Commission for Crippled Children having failed, University Hospitals had no exact estimate of expected income for 1955–56. As a matter of fact, the estimated payments as of June 30, 1955, had amounted to $520,000, but there was an outstanding unpaid balance of $317,000 for services rendered.

By June 14, with budget time limits running out, the Oklahoma Commission for Crippled Children took steps to remove Ira E. McConnell as director of the Crippled Children's Commission; and a letter terminating his employment as director was delivered to McConnell by Paul Harkey, attorney for Governor Gary.[7] The letter stated that after careful consideration the Crippled Children's Commission (consisting of Grady Matthews, chairman, Mark R. Everett, Oliver Hodge, and Lloyd E. Rader) had regretfully come to the conclusion that the operation of the commission and its program did not, under McConnell's direction, comply with the Crippled Children's Act and the instructions of the commission. Governor Gary seemed to feel that the commission was sincere in its efforts to carry out recommended policies, and that a new director was essential to that purpose, for two days later in a news release the governor was quoted as saying that he intended ''to make the firing of Ira McConnell stick; that he had been charged to a certain extent with running the government as chief executive, and that he intended to do it to the best of his ability.'' He revealed that, out of $1,350,000 in state and county funds available to the commission the past year, only $500,000 had been apportioned to the Crippled Children's Hospital; he felt funds for Children's Hospital should be increased to $800,000 for the next fiscal year, and that less money should be spent for the care of children in private hospitals.

The upshot of all this activity was that Ira McConnell announced that he would fight his dismissal; and leaders of the Oklahoma State Hospital Association (in special session) went on record as opposing the governor's ''one hospital program for indigent children,'' and they made plans to resist the move.

When Dean Everett was asked to comment on statements by Mr. McConnell that the dean had sought to have larger sums of money earmarked for Children's Hospital, he declared that he had no personal plan and no personal role in the impasse. ''I am enmeshed in it only because I am a member of the commission,'' the dean said, ''and requests for funds for Crippled Children's Hospital

---

[7.] *Daily Oklahoman*, June 15, 1955.

are requests from our university regents. The financing of the University of Oklahoma Hospitals is not a problem for the dean. I sit as a member of the commission and whatever relationship the commission has with the hospitals in regard to contracts is through the regents.'' After Judge Clarence Mills upheld that the director might be removed ''only for cause,'' the Crippled Children's Commission rescinded its order to dismiss Ira McConnell, on motion by Mark R. Everett and seconded by Lloyd E. Rader, June 29, 1955.

Governor Gary asserted that the administrative costs of the department were the most extravagant in the state government, and that he was of the opinion that the Crippled Children's Commission was right in the first place in wanting another director. In an effort to untangle the controversy between the commission and the University Hospitals, he designated James Bullard, veteran Duncan legislator, chairman of a special committee[8] to make an overall study of the state's crippled children program and to devise a workable formula for the next legislature to follow.

The formulated policy of earmarking $800,000 from the commission's funds for Crippled Children's Hospital (favored by Governor Gary and a majority of the commissioners) ran into opposition from the State Hospital Association which favored continuing a program wherein 75 private hospitals throughout the state participated in services to crippled children, rather than channeling them to the Children's Hospital in Oklahoma City. The admitting department of Children's Hospital was even accused of refusing to admit children who were not ''teaching cases,'' or whenever a service quota was filled. This was a gross misrepresentation, and so was the charge that services rendered by Children's Hospital were twice as expensive as similar services in private hospitals.

The term ''teaching case'' was bandied about to a rather ridiculous degree because any human being in need of medical help presents a learning situation for the student of medicine, the resident house staff, or the student of nursing. There is really no such thing as a ''teaching case'' or a ''nonteaching case.'' A patient may be admitted to the hospital who is not a good teaching case, but because he needs admission, he will not be turned down. The provision of the Crippled Children's Act calls for caring for crippled children in such a way as to maintain a proper student-patient ratio for accreditation of the School of Medicine and stipulates that this exception shall not cause undue hardship to the patient—an obligation imposed by law on the commission.[9]

Financing of University Hospitals, always a problem because the State

[8] Dean Everett, Mr. Rader, Dr. Henson of Enid, past president of the Oklahoma Medical Association, Dr. Wadsworth, chairman of the association's public health committee, and state senator John Russell of Okmulgee were members of the study committee.

[9] Ira McConnell was quoted as saying—at a meeting of the Crippled Children's Commission in September—''I think this accreditation thing should be thrown out the window''; to which Dr. Everett replied, ''It is more crucial than your remarks would imply.'' *Journal of the Oklahoma State Medical Association*, Vol. XLVIII (October, 1955), 331.

Regents for Higher Education never apportioned the necessary money, became an even larger problem in 1955 when the unused beds in Crippled Children's Hospital developed into a two-pronged concern for the administrators of the hospital, jeopardizing the care of indigent children and the accredited teaching program of the School of Medicine. Crippled Children's Hospital versus private hospitals and state funds versus Crippled Children's accounts in the various counties became penetrating issues, especially when it was reported that there was an unspent balance in the Crippled Children's county accounts of some $159,000 for the fiscal year 1954–55.

The Crippled Children's Commission, headed by Grady Matthews as chairman, pointed out that the Crippled Children's Act made it mandatory that county funds be levied for the purpose of caring for indigent children, and that in many instances hospitalization for needy children could have been financed with this money instead of using state funds.

The State Medical Association and the Oklahoma State Hospital Association leveled some pretty heavy criticisms at the commission for recommending diversion of indigent children and county funds to Oklahoma City in order to occupy beds in Crippled Children's Hospital, "invading the realm of socialized medicine" so to speak—all of which smacked of political high jinks. However, it is regrettable that any hospital association would have taken a position on a question without first checking into the facts and determining the consequences of dissemination of false information.

On the more optimistic side, constructive undertones were projecting into the future; Ollie McBride, of the class of 1937, said that he did not believe the School of Medicine would ever have adequate financial provision until the hospitals were separated from the School of Medicine and operated on funds secured elsewhere than from the State Regents for Higher Education.

Further signs of depth perception became evident on October 25 when a master plan drafted by members of two planning and zoning commissions—set up by the twenty-fourth legislature—was adopted after public hearings. These plans called for eventual development of a thirty-five-block campus for the Medical Center and a major face-lifting for areas surrounding the state capitol building.

The medical center master plan envisioned a concentration of private and public hospitals, doctors offices and clinic buildings, and other related institutions in areas south, east, and west of the University of Oklahoma medical center. Relocation of the state health department into the area of the School of Medicine and construction of possible privately financed hospitals were also included in the eventual extension—a mighty progression from "the act authorizing construction of a hospital and buildings for the medical department of the University of Oklahoma," with an appropriation of $200,000 by the Oklahoma sixth legislature in 1917.

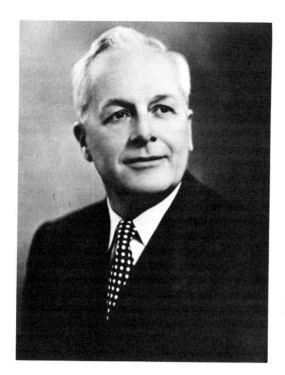

Hugh G. Jeter, M.D.,
director of University
Hospitals, 1935.

*Courtesy University
of Oklahoma Medical
Center*

Egil Thorbjorn Olsen,
M.D., medical director of
University Hospitals, 1935–
40; acting chairman of the
Department of Preventive
Medicine and Public
Health, 1938–40.

*Courtesy University
of Oklahoma Medical
Center*

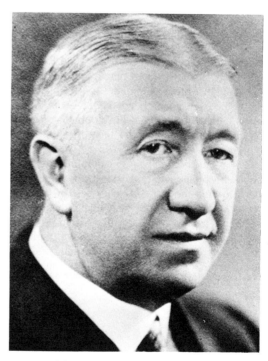

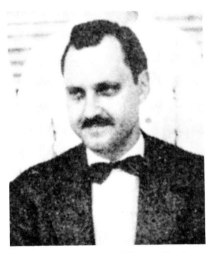

Lewis Labon Reese, M.D., medical
director of University Hospitals,
1940–41.

*Courtesy University of Oklahoma
Medical Center*

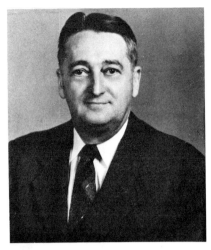

George N. Barry, M.D., director of
Outpatient Department, 1937–40,
1941–42; acting medical director of
University Hospitals, 1941–44; medical
director, 1944–45.

*Courtesy University of Oklahoma
Medical Center*

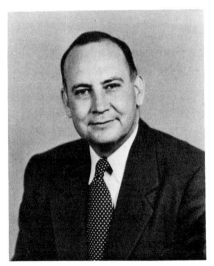

Vernon D. Cushing, M.D., medical
director of University Hospitals,
1948–49.

*Courtesy University of Oklahoma
Medical Center*

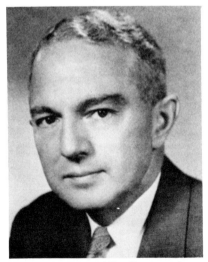

Robert C. Lowe, M.D., director of
Outpatient Department, 1946–49;
medical director of University Hospitals, 1949–56; superintendent, 1957–58.

Courtesy Sooner Medic

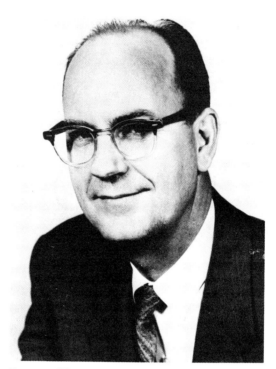

Raymond Drake Crews, LL.B., superintendent of
University Hospitals, 1959–(64).
Courtesy University of Oklahoma Medical Center

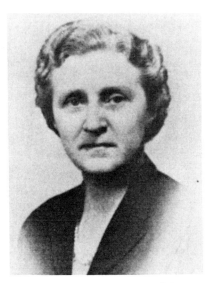

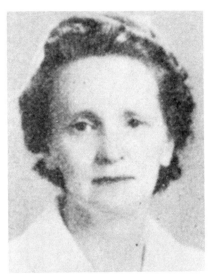

Ada Reitz Crocker, director of the School of Nursing, 1924–27, acting director, 1947–48.

Courtesy Helen Patterson Chapman

Edythe Stith Triplett, director of the School of Nursing, 1937–41.

Courtesy Helen Patterson Chapman

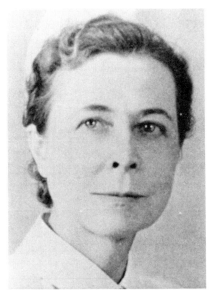

Clara Wolfe Jones, R.N., acting director of the School of Nursing, 1944–45.

Courtesy Tequoyah

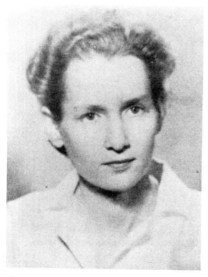

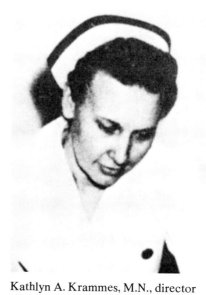

Clare Marie Jackson Wangen, M.A., director of the School of Nursing, 1941–43.

Courtesy Helen Patterson Chapman

Kathlyn A. Krammes, M.N., director of the School of Nursing, 1943–47.

Courtesy Helen Patterson Chapman

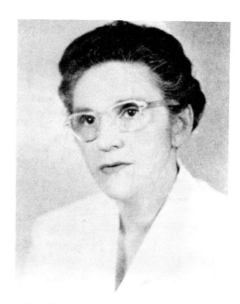

Mary Rosch Caron, R.N., M.A., director of the School of Nursing, 1948–51.

Courtesy Helen Patterson Chapman

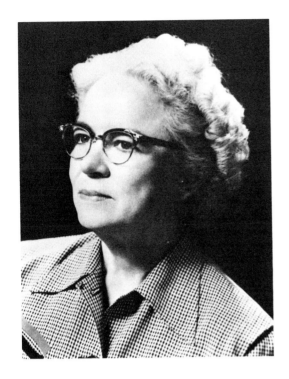

Ada Hawkins, R.N., M.S.,
director of the School of
Nursing, 1951–60.

Courtesy Sooner Medic

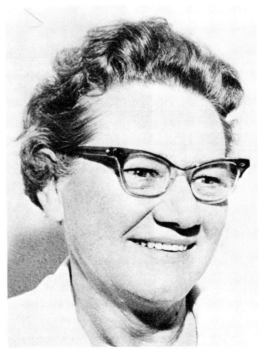

Helen Patterson, R.N.,
M.A., dean of the School
of Nursing, 1960–(64).

*Courtesy Helen Patterson
Chapman*

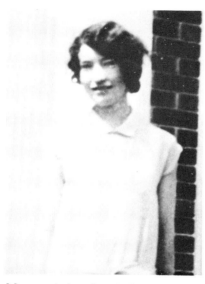

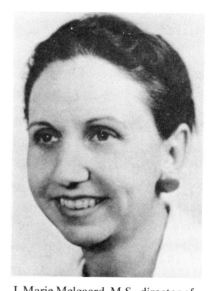

Margery Ardrey Sewell, B.S., director
of Dietetic Internship, 1932–36.

*Courtesy University of Oklahoma
Medical Center*

J. Marie Melgaard, M.S., director of
Dietetic Internship, 1936–45.

Courtesy Tequoyah

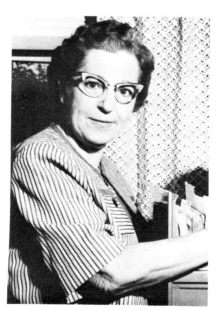

Vera Parman Peters, M.S., director
of Dietetic Internship, 1945–48.

Courtesy Commentary

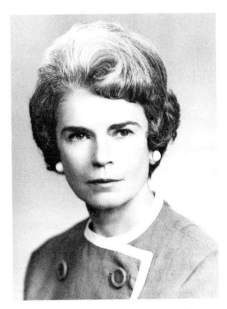

Mary C. Zahasky, B.S., director of
Dietetic Internship, 1948–(64).
Courtesy University of Oklahoma
Medical Center

Chapter XX.
The University of
Oklahoma Medical Center:
1956–57

The report of Governor Gary's committee to study the crippled children's program in Oklahoma— including finance, allocation of patients, and the needs of the University Hospitals—recommended

that the Legislature appropriate sufficient funds, with all due safeguards, for financing and operation of the University Hospitals; that it appropriate a sufficient sum of money for the Crippled Children's Commission to carry out its program throughout the state; that a codification be made of all laws pertaining to medical care of all crippled children; and that a careful study be made by the Legislature (through the Legislative Council and proper committees) of submitting a proposal for an amendment to the constitution to provide that all counties should pay to the University Hospitals, on the same basis that they paid individual hospitals, for the care of indigent patients.[1]

Governor Gary further aided the School of Medicine and its hospitals by appointing another committee, chaired by Stewart Wolf, Jr., to make a study of the specific needs of the school and hospitals and to recommend legislation for consideration by the twenty-sixth legislature.[2] "Oklahoma's School of Medicine is on the verge of greatness," the governor said. "Its graduates are sought for internships by hospitals throughout the nation because of their qualifications. It is the responsibility of the people as well as the legislators, governing bodies, and the executive department to see that progress is continued."

The official name for the grouping of the School of Medicine, the University Hospitals, and the School of Nursing, on N.E. Thirteenth Street, became

[1.] Minutes of the Board of Regents of the University of Oklahoma, January 12, 1956.

[2.] Members of the committee were Carl Bailey, Stroud, M. A. Connell, Picher, Senator Roy E. Grantham, Ponca City, Representative James Bullard, Duncan, and Hugh G. Payne, secretary of the Oklahoma Medical Research Foundation.

"University of Oklahoma Medical Center" by action of the regents on March 8, 1956. At the same time, Mark R. Everett, who had held the title of medical school dean and Superintendent of hospitals, was designated director of the Medical Center and dean of the School of Medicine; and by this change in title Dr. Everett became the chief administrative officer of the Medical Center, responsible for integration and general management of all its units.[3]

Dean Everett, as ex officio chairman, also became head of a new Medical Center executive committee set up to deal with matters of major policy on the Medical Center campus (negating the former hospital review board). The new committee was composed of the dean, the associate dean of clinical instruction, the business administrator of the Medical Center, a representative from the preclinical faculty and from the clinical faculty, the director of the School of Nursing, plus the vice-president and business vice-president of the University of Oklahoma as nonvoting members.

Construction of a Speech and Hearing Clinic center on the Oklahoma City campus was assured in January, 1956, by a $93,000 federal grant-in-aid. With a balance of $87,000 held in escrow for this building by the Oklahoma City Junior League, the university regents were able to award a construction contract for the clinic building for $176,440 on June 4—three years after League members first started working toward that goal.

A fifth annual grant from the National Fund for Medical Education for support of instructional salaries in the School of Medicine amounted to $29,098, making a five-year total of $114,460 in grants from this source.

Louis J. West, head of the University of Oklahoma School of Medicine's Department of Psychiatry, reported for full-time duty in July—after nearly two years of commuting between here and San Antonio—bringing with him an air force grant of $35,000 in support of prisoner-of-war research, cosponsored by the Oklahoma Medical Research Institute. And within a month Dr. West requested that the name of the psychiatry department be changed to Department of Psychiatry, Neurology, and Behavioral Sciences, thus establishing a precedent which, in time, was adopted by many medical schools. Other name changes combined the Departments of Obstetrics and Gynecology and designated the Department of Bacteriology as the Department of Microbiology.

The position of professor and head of the Department of Otorhinolaryngology was approved by President Cross, effective on July 1, 1957, carrying an annual salary of $12,000, with $10,000 coming from the National Fund for Medical Education trust fund and an additional $2,000 a year from the Veterans Administration Hospital for services as a consulting or attending physician.

A committee from the Department of Radiology also requested a full-time head of that department to relieve Dr. Russo who had given a tremendous amount of time and effort over a period of years in behalf of numberless patients. But the x-ray service had become so extensive and the Department of

---

[3.] The regents set the salary of Dean Everett at $13,000, that of Robert Lowe, superintendent of the hospitals, at $11,600, and that of Raymond Crews, business administrator of the Medical Center, at $8,900.

Radiology so large that part-time radiologists without full-time leadership could no longer do justice to the heavy work load.

The appointment of John A. Schilling, of the University of Rochester School of Medicine, to the newly created post of full-time head of the Department of Surgery at the University of Oklahoma School of Medicine was announced by the university regents on June 14. Dr. Schilling received his M.D. degree from Harvard University and was a resident at Roosevelt Hospital in New York City.

On July 1, Basil Hayes was given the title of professor emeritus of urology, and J. P. McGee (a member of the faculty since 1928) was given the title of professor emeritus of ophthalmology. Phil E. Smith, associate professor of preventive medicine and public health, was given the additional title of associate dean of the graduate school; the rank of J. S. Felton was raised to professor of preventive medicine, Peter Russo, to professor of radiology, and Milton J. Serwer, to professor of obstetrics. Helen Kendall retired, after serving the School of Medicine as registrar for approximately 17 years.

A list of new appointees to the faculty follows:

John Albert Schilling, M.D.
  professor of surgery
Muzafer Sherif, Ph.D.
  consultant professor of social
  psychology in psychiatry,
  neurology, and behavioral
  sciences
Raymond Drake Crews, A.B.,
  LL.B.
  assistant professor of
  administrative medicine in
  preventive medicine and public
  health
Chesterfield Garvin Gunn, Jr.,
  M.D.
  assistant professor of preventive
  medicine and public health
Michael T. Lategola, Ph.D.
  assistant professor of physiology
Dale W. Peters, M.D.
  assistant professor of psychiatry
  and neurology
George Barnes, M.S.
  instructor in preventive medicine
  and public health
Leonard Harold Brown, M.D.
  instructor in surgery
Phillip LaTorre, M.S.
  instructor in preventive medicine
  and public health
Edward Robert Munnell, M.D.
  instructor in surgery

Joe O. Rogers, M.D.
  instructor in preventive medicine
  and public health
Karl Kenneth Boatman, M.D.
  clinical assistant in surgery
Charles M. Brake, M.D.
  clinical assistant in medicine
Claude H. Brown, M.D.
  clinical assistant in pediatrics
David Randolph Brown, M.D.
  clinical assistant in orthopedic
  and fracture surgery
Farris Webb Coggins, M.D.
  clinical assistant in gynecology
Joe Ed. Collins, M.D.
  clinical assistant in urology
Marion Joe Crosthwait, M.D.
  clinical assistant in medicine
Kieffer D. Davis, M.D.
  visiting lecturer in preventive
  medicine and public health
William F. Denny, M.D.
  clinical assistant in medicine
Guy Wesley Fuller, M.D.
  clinical assistant in medicine
William Norris Harsha, M.D.
  clinical assistant in orthopedic
  and fracture surgery
Robert Eugene Herndon, M.D.
  clinical assistant in pediatrics
Davis T. Hunt, M.D.
  clinical assistant in obstetrics

George Harry Jennings, M.D.
clinical assistant in gynecology
David I. Kraft, M.D.
clinical assistant in medicine
George Ignatius Lythcott, M.D.
clinical assistant in pediatrics
Haven Winslow Mankin, M.D.
clinical assistant in radiology
Robert D. Mercer, M.D.
clinical assistant in anesthesiology
David Clinton Mock, M.D.
clinical assistant in medicine

John Fay Montroy, M.D.
clinical assistant in anesthesiology
Roy Laurence Neel, M.D.
clinical assistant in radiology
Pamela Prentice Parrish, M.D.
clinical assistant in medicine
Able Jay Sands, M.D.
clinical assistant in medicine
Louis Elliott Speed, M.D.
clinical assistant in surgery
Walter H. Whitcomb, M.D.
clinical assistant in medicine

Since the introduction of the Ph.D. program in the School of Medicine in 1951, graduate training had expanded measurably in the preclinical departments of the school; for example, biochemistry was no longer an isolated division, with the responsibility of teaching all medical biochemistry, as was the case in 1925 when the department attracted its first graduate student. On the contrary, seven students were enrolled in the graduate program of the Department of Biochemistry in 1956, out of a total of 50 graduate students in the entire medical school. Master's degree programs were offered at the time in anatomy, bacteriology, biochemistry, medical illustration, pathology, pharmacology, physiology, and preventive medicine and public health.

A new poison information center was instituted and developed on the Medical Center campus during the year by Harold A. Shoemaker, Department of Pharmacology, whereby any physician or hospital in the state of Oklahoma could call the center, describe the toxic agent swallowed by a patient, and get an immediate suggestion as to the best possible treatment. No financial commitment on the part of the university was involved, since the Children's Bureau of the federal government provided the financial support. However, the university did provide two small offices in the annex to the School of Medicine building, where telephones were installed and approximately 50,000 informational cards were on file as sources for saving hundreds of lives in Oklahoma.

The second-year physical diagnosis course in the Department of Medicine retained its name but altered its aims in 1956; for it was held that physical diagnosis should involve not only the elicitation of sights, sounds, and sensations from various parts of the body, but also an opportunity to appraise evidence obtained by talking with patients as well as examining them. The pathological basis for abnormal signs was discussed with the entire class, and later small supervised groups of students practiced the technique of examination by conversing with patients.

Another major curricular change was implemented in the fourth year, where a longitudinal curriculum for the student outpatient clerkship replaced the old block system of assigning students to clinics. Under the new plan each student was assigned to various clinics on different days of the week throughout the entire year; and a checkup at the close of the year showed that, in approximately 75 per cent of the cases, the change permitted single students to follow their patients from clinic to clinic, week after week. This method afforded the student experience in handling cases he might be expected to encounter in his future practice and in selecting patients for referral who required expert psychiatric help.

The ablest and most experienced teachers were assigned to the outpatient department, where opportunities for the richest teaching prevailed, but because the material was often difficult to present effectively, junior members of the staff, who were attempting to qualify for inpatient attending status, were not assigned there.

These innovative curricular changes attracted visits of a goodly number of teachers from other schools of medicine, as informed observers became convinced that a renowned medical center was developing in our rapidly growing and increasingly important region of the country—with 75 reserach teaching grants, providing nearly $600,000, in operation at the University of Oklahoma School of Medicine in 1956. Faculty members received research monies amounting to $225,000 during the year, and a rather large grant was received from the National Heart Institute—$26,620 for each of two years, ending December 31, 1958—"for research in any aspect of the cardiovascular field." An institutional grant of $32,100 for combined cancer research in the School of Medicine and the Oklahoma Medical Research Institute was received from the American Cancer Society; and a grant of $25,000 from the Oklahoma Epileptic League (through the National League) made possible the study of some 14,000 epilepsy patients in Oklahoma, under the guidance of Jean Felton.

Marvin Shetlar, associate professor of biochemistry, was one of 44 recipients in the nation of a five-year research fellowship from the public health service, which carried a cash grant of $10,000 and an additional $2,000 for research expense yearly; and Harold Muchmore, physician at the Veterans Administration Hospital, was appointed to one of the thirty newly created research posts in the nation, described as "clinical investigators," with the opportunity to devote most of his time to research over a three-year period.

In cooperation with the Vocational Rehabilitation Division of the State Board of Vocational Education, a sum of $20,490 of surplus federal funds was made available for the fiscal year 1956–57 as a planning grant to organize a cardiac evaluation unit of University Hospital staff physicians. The proposal, which also included a pledge of an additional operating sum not to exceed $15,690 for the fiscal year 1956–57, depended on approval by the university regents of a contract for purchase of modern angiocardiographic equipment (before the close of the fiscal year on June 30, 1956) for $27,320–with $6,830 of the purchase price coming from another trust fund under the direction of Stewart Wolf.

A safer and more efficient system of providing oxygen for patients in University Hospitals was completed in the fall of 1956, whereby a liquid oxygen unit—the first in use in the Okalhoma City area—fed a pipeline that served both hospitals, making life-saving gas immediately available at 218 different wall outlets in hospital rooms; and the operating rooms were completely piped, too, not only with oxygen but with the most commonly used anesthetic gases.

Seventy-nine doctors were listed in the residency programs of 16 departments of the University of Oklahoma Medical Center, including those on affiliated programs at the Veterans Administration Hospital in 1956–57. The Department of Orthopedic and fracture Surgery, alone, received thirty-five applications for three appointments for the full four years of training in orthopedic surgery.

State appropriations for the University of Oklahoma and the School of Medicine and University Hospitals for 1956–57 were as follows: Norman campus, $4,395,851 out of a total income of $6,912,208; School of Medicine, $692,350 out of a total income of $860,606; and University Hospitals, $2,061,246 out of a total of $3,496,519. Additional funds were made available by the Crippled Children's Commission which made it possible, for the first time since 1950, for the director of the commission to pay contract costs for all of the children whose hospitalization was approved by the commission. This in turn enabled University Hospitals to end the fiscal year without the usual deficit. During 1956–57 there were 12,229 patients admitted to the hospitals—8,789 at the University Hospital and 3,440 at Children's Hospital. Some 18,694 outpatients were treated in the outpatient department. Laboratory examinations in the two hospitals totaled 240,577.

A new orthoptic clinic was opened in Crippled Children's Hospital under the auspices of the ophthalmology department and direction of James P. Luton; and Alpha Iota Chapter, of Delta Gamma sorority, made a donation for eye exercise equipment, as well as contributing toward a sophisticated instrument (used mostly in advance of surgery) to determine whether proper function in both eyes simultaneously would be assured by surgery. Purchase of an iron lung and a hydraulic lift was made possible by a generous gift of $2,500 from the estate of Cora Velva Duncan.[4]

In the interest of increased educational experience, the School of Medicine embarked on the quarterly system in June, 1956, for the third-year class. Under this arrangement, the faculty instructed this class for eleven months of the year instead of nine, and vacations were rotated. Students were permitted vacations during any of the four quarters. With the new calendar each individual student was assigned approximately 25 per cent more patients without adding to the financial costs. Furthermore, patients in the hospitals during the summer period, who had been drawn upon reluctantly before this time, became a valuable source of teaching cases.

Three hundred and seventy-four students were enrolled in the School of Medicine and 129 in the School of Nursing. Ninety-six graduates received the

---

[4] Carl H. Bailey and his wife, Gladys, made a gift of the Stroud General Hospital, valued at $157,000, to the Oklahoma Medical Research Foundation, which Dr. Bailey continued to operate under a contract with the foundation.

M.D. degree in 1956, thirty nurses received certificates in nursing, and one received a Bachelor of Science in Nursing.[5]

Charles Pfizer and Company set up a $1,000 fund for a scholarship for a medical student in each medical school in the United States in 1956; and 16 medical students were the recipients of fellowships totaling $6,500 for vacation reserach studies and training. These were made available for the most part in amounts of $400 for two months by the National Institutes of Health, the National Foundation for Infantile Paralysis, and the Lederle Laboratories. A research achievement committee of the medical school made the selections.

Unfortunately, a strained atmosphere developed between the dean's committee of the University of Oklahoma Medical Center and the management of the veterans' hospital in the spring of 1956, and, in spite of the efforts of Dean Everett and his committee to solve the conflicts, a feeling of distrust prevailed, creating a demoralizing state of affairs. This was largely due to the fact that Dr. Bates, manager of the Oklahoma City Veterans Administration Hospital, became antagonistic to some progressive ideas proffered by the staff members; for example, Dr. Bates quibbled about paying Dr. West the fee that had been promised to him for two visits per week as a consultant in psychiatry—a formal agreement that should have been fulfilled. Then he altered the structure of the residency program in psychiatry, effective in November, without affording Dr. West the opportunity to review the matter or even consult with the dean's committee, maintaining that he was carrying out the instructions of the central office in Washington, although the claim could not be sustained.[6]

So it came as no surprise when Dr. Bates tendered his resignation as manager of the Veterans Administration Hospital effective March 1, 1957. However, Dr. Bates stated that his resignation had nothing to do with the current medical controversy about the administration of the hospital, saying that he had reached retirement age after having been a Veterans Administration physician for over 34 years.

There were 2,542 residents in the Veterans Administration national hospital system in 1956–57—12 per cent of the total on duty in the entire United States. Five hundred and eighty-five of these (approximately 30 per cent) were conducted on an integrated basis, and some 50 per cent were maintained through a collaborative plan. Seven per cent represented affiliations, where the Veterans Administration Hospital itself had no approval for a given residency, participating through the approved hospital of the community. Twenty per cent of all residencies in psychiatry in the United States were in Veterans Administration hospitals.

There were 241 career residents in the fields of anesthesiology, neurology, pathology, physical medicine, psychiatry, and radiology. This coordinated

---

[5.] The budget for the School of Nursing was separated from that of the University Hospitals in 1956.

[6.] Whether initiated by the Veterans Administration or the medical school, the nomination of residents was ultimately cleared by the dean's committee and then recommended to the manager through the director of professional services.

relationship was further fortified by mutual participation in research projects, since the field for the study of disease was very fertile in the far-flung Veterans Administration hospitals.[7]

The greatest expansion in Oklahoma's medical education to date occurred during the ten years following World War II, as a result of challenges which arose. The citizens of Oklahoma voiced an increased demand for more physicians throughout the counties of the state, and an increased number of students sought admission to the School of Medicine. As a consequence, the size of the student body was nearly doubled by 1951, and an unprecedented building program had commenced to take shape: a School of Nursing building in 1947; an independent Oklahoma Medical Research Institute and hospital in 1950; two new wings on the basic science building of the School of Medicine in 1951; outpatient wings at University Hospital and Crippled Children's Hospital in 1952; a 496-bed Veterans Administration Hospital in 1953; and a Speech and Hearing Clinic building and radiology wing (under construction) in 1956.

Much of the inspiration for attempting progressive improvements on our campus was due to reforms instituted by the Flexner Report which strengthened medical education inestimably. Dean Everett had the privilege of attending a dinner honoring Abraham Flexner at the Waldorf Astoria Hotel in New York City on April 23, 1956—the outstanding event of Medical Education Week. Dr. Flexner, "a hearty 89," received the third annual Frank H. Lehey Memorial Award for his contribution to medical education, an award jointly sponsored by the Association of American Medical Colleges, the American Medical Association, and the National Fund for Medical Education.

[7.] William S. Middleton, Department of Medicine and Surgery, Washington, D.C., "The Significance of Medical Education in the Veterans Administration," an administrative paper, 1956.

Chapter XXI.
Golden Anniversary of
Statehood: 1957–58

Governor Gary's Committee on the Needs of the Medical Center, chaired by Stewart Wolf, recommended to the twenty-sixth legislature: (1) that appropriate legislation be enacted to enforce payment for hospital services by the counties; (2) that, until a constitutional amendment providing for payment by the counties could be voted on and put into effect, a special annual appropriation of $1,200,000 be made to the University Hospitals: (3) that a direct appropriation of $850,000 be made to the University Hospitals each year from funds allocated to the Crippled Children's Commission, the precise amount to be adjusted later each year to cover the actual number of patients treated; (4) that a direct appropriation of $500,000 be made to the University Hospital from the state welfare agency to cover the medical care of a reasonable quota of patients; (5) that an appropriation amounting to $2,595,476 annually be made from the general revenue fund to the State Regents for Higher Education with a statement of legislative intent that the entire amount be assigned to the Medical Center—total annual budget for the Medical Center to be $5,841,476 and (6) that a new building be erected to connect Crippled Children's and main hospitals to consolidate the services and to provide the required facilities, at an estimated cost of approximately eight million dollars. However, when the legislative session adjourned, the same old cracked record made it known that the Medical Center had been neglected once more "at the appropriation table," in spite of the fact that, when the figures were carefully analyzed, there was no more meritorious presentation of a tense financial condition than that for University and Crippled Children's Hospitals. The common school block, the pensioners, the highways, and over 100 local bills fared much better than the state's health services.

The twenty-sixth legislature appropriated $4,877,805 to the University of Oklahoma at Norman, which had a total income of $7,517,083 for 1957–58, $785,995 to the School of Medicine out of a total income of $1,007,687, and $2,277,358 to the University Hospitals out of a total income of $3,753,674. Actually, this was far below what was needed and much less than the funds made available to comparable neighboring medical schools. Furthermore, the legislature failed to make the usual appropriation for heart and cancer research or to provide matching funds for a $400,000 federal grant, which was due to expire December 31, for a research building—a provocation which caused many headaches for the governing bodies of the Medical Center, especially since the School of Medicine was the only facility for medical education in the state. In the face of the dereliction of the legislature, help and advice were sorely needed to prevent the state of Oklahoma from being marked with a national stamp of inferiority as a result of allowing this grant to go by default to some other state.

The alumni of the school mailed letters to 5,000 prominent citizens of the state in an effort to enlist assistance in reaching a subscription goal of $400,000 to match the federal grant. After all, the citizens of Oklahoma had contributed approximately $1,000,000 in taxes to the $90,000,000 appropriated for such construction purposes by Congress; and the year of the golden anniversary of statehood seemed hardly the time to take a negative attitude regarding an extremely important aspect of the state's institutional chores. Happily, with the help of Governor Raymond Gary, a six-month extension for the grant was negotiated in November.

The legislature did pass House Bill No. 634, which committed all state penal, reformatory, and elemosynary institutions to submit their unclaimed bodies to the anatomy department of the School of Medicine, a session law which in no way created any financial burden for the state; and House Bill No. 772—to change the name of the Oklahoma Hospital for Crippled Children (1945) to the Oklahoma Children's Memorial Hospital—was passed on May 31, 1957. However, changing the name did not change the austere circumstances at the hospital, and by October 17 the official allocation of beds at University Hospitals was 265 at main and 174 at Children's; unused beds at main equaled 40 and at Children's 82, making a total of only 317 occupied beds in the two hospitals.

Financial support of a stipend amounting to $4,200 per year for the director of the tumor clinic at the University Hospital was discontinued on June 30, 1957, because of a decrease of over 60 per cent in federal funds for cancer control and the increasing needs in other phases of the cancer program. (It should be recorded that the State Department of Health generously supported the tumor clinic for ten years, following an agreement made with the University of Oklahoma School of Medicine.)

A gift of special note was made to the library of the School of Medicine by Curt Von Wedel in 1957—1,500 bound volumes of medical journals valued at approximately $8,000, some dating back to 1826. The number of journals owned by the medical school at the time, either in whole or in part, comprised around 2,000 titles. By the close of the year 1957–58 the total library collection amounted to 44,424 volumes.

A check from the estate of Gearlean Shipman in the amount of $5,000 was forwarded by the executor on February 15, to be deposited to the Gearlean Shipman Heart Research Fund and to remain intact until a director for this fund was appointed; also a gift of $1,000 for scholarships for each of two deserving students in training at the School of Medicine was made in May, resulting in the establishment of the Mrs. Carl Owens Scholarship Trust Fund.

A grant of $82,321 was made to the School of Medicine by the W. K. Kellogg Foundation in September, and there was a grant of $39,180 from the National Fund for Medical Education in support of instruction at the medical school. In the seven-year interval, 1951–57, the National Fund for Medical Education contributed a total of $135,403 to the medical school, which was expended, for the most part, to improve medical education per se, in accordance with the ideal of the fund.

Probably very few people realized that the state of Oklahoma was appropriating less money for its School of Medicine than a number of private medical schools were receiving from their respective states. Without grants-in-aid, the Oklahoma Medical Center would have been very limited in its objectives, for no medical center can long operate without gifts and grants. In fact, the administration of grants and gifts gradually became a serious question for consideration by the university regents, who eventually authorized the director of the Medical Center to receive and accept gifts and grants on behalf of the center ''with the understanding that each such item be reported promptly to the President's Office for presentation to the Regents.''

New projection equipment for motion pictures was given to Children's Memorial Hospital at Christmastime by the local moving picture machine operators association, whose members had been showing pictures to the children weekly for 28 years. The operators were instrumental, too, in interesting 25 businessmen and firms to contribute materials and supplies for the projection project; and 60 union men donated their time and labor to the cause. The value of the completed installation was estimated at $12,000.

The new $200,000 Speech and Hearing Clinic building, which provided modern facilities for the school for the deaf and for pathology and audiology, was dedicated on May 26, 1957, and the entire clinic was moved from Children's Memorial Hospital into the new quarters. Fourteen full-time persons comprised the staff—a clinical supervisor of speech therapy and two therapists; a supervisor of teacher training in the school for the deaf and six teachers of the deaf; two clinical audiologists, a social worker, and the director. In addition, nearly forty university students were majoring in speech and hearing, doing their course work and most of their practice work in the clinic—all candidates for either bachelors, masters, or doctor of philosophy degrees. Because of its proximity to other medical facilities, the Speech and Hearing Clinic afforded a close integration of its medical, psychological, and vocational evaluation and services (for patients with speech and hearing limitations), with the services of the School of Medicine and its vocational rehabilitation division.

Writing in the *Journal of the Oklahoma State Medical Association* in September, 1957, John W. Keys, director of the clinic, predicted that approximately 1,100 outpatients would have been seen in the Crippled Children's Hospital clinic during the year, and that, in addition, 80 to 100 children would have received training of an educational or therapeutic nature in the clinic each week, notwithstanding the fact that the cost of educating a deaf child for one year was five times the expense of education for a child of normal hearing.

On June 19 the Department of Health, Education and Welfare gave preliminary approval to a Hill-Burton grant-in-aid of $250,000 to the Medical Center for construction of a radiology addition to the outpatient wing of the University Hospital to accommodate the powerful Van de Graaf x-ray therapy unit (donated by the Donner Foundation), and to permit centralization of other x-ray equipment in one location. The University of Oklahoma Medical Center was one of 12 institutions around the country to receive an x-ray generator of this magnitude for the treatment of deepseated cancer—the first installation of its kind in Oklahoma. Whereas conventional radiotherapy machines generated 250,000 volt X rays, the Van de Graaf generator produced 2,000,000 volt X rays, comparable to the energy emitted by radium.

The twenty-sixth legislature appropriated $100,000 toward the housing of the radiology construction project, and this amount, plus a $150,000 balance in the University Hospitals capital outlay fund, made a total of $250,000 in matching monies to meet the estimated $500,000 cost of the addition to the main hospital building. The $250,000 from Hill-Burton funds was the seventh federal grant[1] for University Hospital construction programs since 1947; and where only one building (the original University Hospital) had stood the campus of the School of Medicine in 1919, there was a physical plant valued at $16,000,000 by 1957. However, without a concurrent orderly organization of faculty and departments and the dvelopment of modern academic and patient care programs there would have been only very limited progress in medical education, health services, and medical research.

There were five deaths among the faculty in 1957; John Mosby Alford, associate professor emeritus of medicine, who had joined the faculty in 1911; Charles Bondurant, professor of dermatology and head of the department; Coyne H. Campbell, professor of psychiatry and neurology; Edward C. Mason, professor of physiology and head of the department; and William M. Taylor, professor emeritus of pediatrics.

Charles DeGaris became professor emeritus of anatomy with retirement on July 1; Theodore Pfundt was appointed temporary head of the Department of Pediatrics, following the resignation of Henry B. Strenge, head of the department since 1948 and a pioneer in cardiac diagnostic work, particularly heart catheterization; and Robert H. Bayley, full-time professor of medicine, was inducted into the Oklahoma Hall of Fame.

Fifty-five new names were added to the faculty roster:

William E. Jaques, M.D.
  professor of pathology
William R. Richardson, M.D.
  professor of pediatric surgery
Gus Ray Ridings, M.D.
  professor of radiology

Jay Talmadge Shurley, M.D.
  professor of psychiatry,
  neurology, and behavioral
  sciences

[1.] This grant-in-aid and the one for the Speech and Hearing Clinic building in 1956 were in addition to five federal grants for the University Hospitals construction program made previously.

George Adams, M.D.
 associate professor of preventive
 medicine and public health
John E. Allison, M.D.
 associate professor of anatomy
Merlin K. Duval, Jr., M.D.
 associate professor of surgery
Rudolph Emil Eyerer, M.D.
 assistant professor of pathology
Laurence Gable Gumbreck, Ph.D.
 assistant professor of anatomy
Irvin Glenn Hamburger, M.D.
 assistant professor of
 anesthesiology
M. Jack Keyl, Ph.D.
 assistant professor of physiology
Rene Menguy, M.D., Ph.D.
 assistant professor of surgery
Lawrence E. McClure, Ph.D.
 assistant professor of research
 biochemistry
Hugh Barrett O'Neil, M.D.
 assistant professor of medicine
 and psychiatry and neurology
Oren T. Skouge, M.D.
 assistant professor of medicine
Raul Esteban Trucco, Ph.D.
 assistant professor of research
 biochemistry
McWilson Warren, Ph.D.
 assistant professor of preventive
 medicine and public health
Margaret Doepfner Wettstein,
 Ph.D., M.D.
 assistant professor of psychiatry
 and neurology
Thomas Edward Wilson, Ph.D.
 assistant professor of research
 microbiology
Basilus Zaricznyj, M.D.
 assistant professor of orthopedic
 and fracture surgery
James Walter Coin, M.D.
 instructor in radiology
Odis A. Cook, M.D.
 instructor in preventive medicine
 and public health
James W. Kelley, M.D.
 instructor in surgery

Lloyd A. Owens, M.D.
 instructor in dermatology
Edna Schmidt, M.Ed.
 instructor in physical therapy
Roy W. Teed, M.D.
 instructor in ophthalmology
Harry Wallace Vandever, M.D.
 instructor in pediatrics
Charles Ernest Baker, M.D.
 visiting lecturer in preventive
 medicine and public health
Stanley E. Berger, M.D.
 clinical assistant in medicine
Gladys Berry, Ph.D.
 research associate in medicine
Karl Austin Bolten, M.D.
 research associate in pathology
Raymond Kenneth Bower, Ph.D.
 research associate in
 microbiology
George M. Brown, Jr., M.D.
 visiting lecturer in surgery
William Omer Coleman, M.D.
 clinical assistant in surgery
James Paul Costeloe, M.D.
 research associate in medicine,
 psychiatry, neurology, and
 behavioral sciences, and
 preventive medicine and public
 health
Donald Counihan, Ph.D.
 consultant in otorhinolaryngology
Nancy Ryan Craig, M.D.
 clinical assistant in anesthesiology
Robert Smith Ellis, M.D.
 clinical assistant in medicine
William Finis Ewing, Jr., M.D.
 clinical assistant in medicine
Thomas C. Finn, M.D.
 clinical assistant in pediatrics
Harold Roy Gravelle, D.D.S.
 clinical assistant in oral surgery
Joseph Reid Henke, M.D.
 clinical assistant in
 ophthalmology
James R. Lowell, M.D.
 clinical assistant in medicine
Walter H. Massion, M.D.
 research associate in
 anesthesiology

Samuel M. Meyers, M.A.
  research associate in psychiatry
  and neurology
Herman C. Moody, M.D.
  clinical assistant in surgery
Stanley R. McCampbell, M.D.
  clinical assistant in medicine
Robert A. McLaughlin, M.D.
  clinical assistant in surgery
Bascum C. Pippin, D.D.S.
  clinical assistant in dental surgery
C. B. Ramana, Diplomate
research associate in psychology,
  department of psychiatry,
  neurology, and behavioral
  sciences

Thomas S. Ray, Ph.D.
  research associate in psychiatry,
  neurology, and behavioral
  sciences
Sidney E. Schnitz, M.D.
  clinical assistant in pediatrics
Phillip B. Smith, M.D.
  clinical assistant in psychiatry,
  neurology, and behavioral
  sciences
Lowell F. Thornton, M.D.
  visiting lecturer in pathology
Charles Albert Tollett, M.D.
  clinical assistant in surgery

Dr. Ridings, formerly of the University of Mississippi Medical Center, became head of the Department of Radiology on March 1, bringing to six the number of full-time chairmen of clinical departments in the College of Medicine; and on that same date Peter Russo, the first resident to complete training in the Department of Radiology and formerly head of the department, assumed a part-time position as professor of radiology at a salary of $4,200 per annum.

Almost immediately after taking office, Dr. Ridings recommended budgetary and equipment needs totaling $385,740 and asked for a clear definition of intent on the part of the Medical Center regarding a Department of Radiology. He also requested support in the form of expenditures for budget, equipment, and space. He found that the task of maintaining departmental functions while reorganizing the department—in the face of shortages in all areas—was indeed a mammoth one.

William E. Jaques was appointed full-time head of the Department of Pathology, effective June 1, to succeed Howard C. Hopps who had resigned on January 1, because he could not foresee adequate financing for the Medical Center here in the near future, and he felt that the University of Texas School of Medicine offered greater opportunities.[2]

J. T. Shurley, who was appointed professor of psychiatry, neurology, and behavioral sciences, was also named chief of the psychiatric service in the Veterans Administration Hospital.[3]

The university regents approved a recommendation by the administration in November that salaries of faculty members in the Departments of Anesthesiol-

[2] Dr. Jaques served his residency in pathology at Massachusetts Memorial Hospital and Children's Medical Center in Boston. He had taught at Harvard Medical School and Boston University and in 1953 joined the faculty of the Louisiana State University Medical School in New Orleans.

[3] Dr. Shurley served his residency at the Pennsylvania Hospital in Philadelphia as a Rockefeller Fellow in psychiatry, following an internship in Indianapolis.

ogy, Pathology, and Radiology could be supplemented from University Hospital funds. Supplementation of the salaries of full-time clinical professors across the board through acceptance of private patients for consultation was not an isolated problem in Oklahoma City but was a troublesome situation throughout the country. Fortunately, a truly unhealthy attitude between "town and gown" never did develop in Oklahoma, although there were occasional rumblings and grumblings. However, good will prevailed for the most part, no doubt because the full-time "gown men" were essentially teachers, devoted to the task of building a first-class medical center, not merely interested in supplementing their own incomes.[4]

A newly established National Institutes of Health senior research fellowship was granted to Marvin Shetlar, Department of Biochemistry in 1957, on the basis of his studies over eleven years in the field of glycoproteins; and David Mock, research fellow and instructor in the Department of Medicine, was the first recipient of a newly created $6,000 annual fellowship in the experimental therapeutic unit, contributed by the Upjohn Pharmaceutical Company in Kalamazoo, Michigan, home of Lawrence N. Upjohn, the first dean of the University of Oklahoma School of Medicine (organized in Oklahoma Territory).[5]

Under the sponsorship of Don O'Donoghue, head of the Department of Orthopedic Surgery, the second reunion of the Orthopedic Residents Club was held in Oklahoma City in 1957, thirty years after the initiation of the orthopedic residency program in the School of Medicine in July, 1927. The membership included 87 orthopedic surgeons who had gone into practice since that time, and the scope of the graduate training had broadened considerably. Four years of residency training were being offered in 1957, leading to full qualification for the national specialty board examination; and the only means of maintaining such an ambitious program was to arrange for admission of increased numbers of patients to the orthopedic service through the Crippled Children's Commission, inasmuch as its director had restricted admission of patients to the Children's Hospital.

The Department of Preventive Medicine and Public Health was awarded a $184,000 National Institute of Mental Health grant to develop a training program in medical statistics over a period of five years, to be directed by Carl R. Doering. Louis Jolyon West received both graduate and undergraduate training grants from the same institute. One hundred physicians (compared with eight the previous year) made application to take advanced training in

[4] Some of these professors were instrumental in organizing a faculty association and in creating a trust fund which eventually made it possible to purchase and operate the Faculty House, at the corner of N.E. Fourteenth Street and Lincoln Boulevard (only two blocks from the Medical Center campus). The house provided facilities for social as well as professional gatherings and accommodations for houseguests.

[5] Dr. Upjohn was appointed "Head of the Premedical Department and Director of Physical Culture at $1,000 a year "on October 2, 1900, by the Territorial Board of Regents. Mark R. Everett, *Medical Education in Oklahoma*, (Norman, University of Oklahoma Press, 1972), I, 9; II, 102.

psychiatry at the Medical Center in 1957, but only six were accepted because of a limited budget and insufficient facilities.

By October the residency program in neurology at the veteran's hospital was well integrated with that of University Hospital, under the aegis of Oren T. Skouge, newly appointed manager of the Veterans Administration Hospital in Oklahoma City.[6]

The National Cancer Institute gave a grant of $224,000 to Leonard Eliel and the Oklahoma Medical Research Institute for a four-year research program on cancer; and Ranwel Caputto, a biochemist of international stature, became chief of the biochemistry division of the institute, following the resignation of Charles Kochakian on July 1.

The Department of Surgery was branching out in several new endeavors as the year closed. Open-heart surgery was on the brink of reality as part of a new cardiac surgery program supported by the State Heart Association and financed, in part, by grants from the United States Public Health Service and the State Department of Public Health. Together, these agencies contributed $13,000 to the program. A type of heart-lung apparatus developed at the University of Minnesota, which was capable of taking over the functions of the heart and lungs during surgery to repair defects in the heart, had been secured, and preliminary studies were under way. An agreement with the State Heart Association to operate an artery bank (a depository of blood vessels) at the University Hospital, with the head of the department as director, was also consummated in 1957.

On Thursday, December 12, the university regents approved the appointment of William Robert Richardson as professor of pediatric surgery and head of a new service at the Medical Center devoted exclusively to surgical problems of children.[7] This appointment carried the additional designation of medical consultant to the Oklahoma Commission for Crippled Children, which had combined efforts with the School of Medicine to establish a pediatric surgical service. With the help of the United States Children's Bureau, the commission had pledged $34,000 to help develop the service over a period of two years; and a volunteer organization, Oklahoma Society for Crippled Children, voted to contribute $8,000 to the project.

Another innovation was the establishment of an eye bank at the University Hospital under the sponsorship of the State Lions Clubs, with Charles Royer, professor of ophthalmology, formulating preliminary plans. Under these plans the School of Medicine provided space at the University Hospital for the bank and furnished staff to supervise the technical aspects of the program, and the Lions Clubs employed a secretary responsible for getting corneas donated to the

[6.] Dr. Skouge, obtained his M.D. degree from the university of Iowa in 1941 and subsequently served four years in the army, two of which were spent overseas as a battalion surgeon with the Quartermaster Corps in England, France, Germany, and Luxembourg.

[7.] Dr. Richardson, was a graduate of Harvard Medical School and trained as a resident in surgery at Children's Hospital and at Massachusetts General Hospital in Boston.

eye bank from all areas of the state. Governor Raymond Gary signed the first donor card to give sight back to some blind person; and Dr. Royer estimated that as many as 1,000 persons in Oklahoma could experience restoration of some degree of sight by corneal grafts.

A description of the Oklahoma Poison Information Center by Imogene Patrick may be found in the *Daily Oklahoman* for November 12, 1957, wherein it is stated that letters had been sent to 4,000 manufacturers and distributors for details regarding the composition of their products. Under the direction of Harold Shoemaker, an index file of approximately 6,000 cards was being assembled, giving the composition of certain preparations. Together with other assembled sources, this material made it possible for the staff to give information on practically 25,000 preparations, a tremendous public health service.

The total number of students enrolled in the School of Medicine for 1957–58 was 371 and in the School of Nursing, 131. Eighty-eight graduates received the M.D. degree in 1957, and four graduate students at the College of Medicine received the Ph.D. in Medical Sciences, making a total of 17 persons who had completed the requirements for the degree since the Ph.D. program was commenced in 1951.

There were 30 interns and 113 residents in training at University Hospitals during the year, with an annual compensation of $338,900—$1,800 for an intern and $2,700 to $3,600 for a resident. The scholarship fund for residents in surgery amounted to approximately $11,940. Nine graduates received the bachelor of science degree in the School of Nursing, and twenty-four received the certificate of nursing.

Mark R. Everett was appointed to the executive council of the American Association of Medical Colleges in 1957—the tenth year of his administration as dean of the University of Oklahoma School of Medicine. "It has been a very heavy year for the dean's office," he said, "with an increasing number of problems requiring attention, but we have had more help from the faculty and the profession than ever before."

Of considerable effectiveness in making the people of Oklahoma aware of their Medical Center, during the year, was a series of articles in the *Daily Oklahoman* by Imogene Patrick, entitled "Medical Safari."[8] Accompanying the announcement of the series in May was a statement that medical research had become more than a million-and-a-half-dollar enterprise at the University of Oklahoma Medical Center, "home of one of the state's newest and fastest developing industries—a frontier of medical science." Whereas there had been only 20 research projects in the area in 1949 (supported by a microscopic total of $6,600), researchers, by 1957, were attracting $930,712 in research grants yearly, with which to purchase equipment and engage research assistants. More

---

[8.] Dean Everett extended the sincere appreciation of the faculty board to Miss Patrick on October 11 for her "remarkably fine series of special articles in the *Daily Oklahoman*," complimenting her on her clarity of expression and masterful grasp of technical matters.

than half of the research funds were coming from the federal government—primarily from the National Institutes of Health; and, according to the business administrator, it was taking almost the full-time services of two office employees to process the grant accounts.

Members of the Oklahoma State Medical Association became greatly interested in the progress of the school about this time, increasing their participation measurably in the hopes and dreams of its leaders because of the inclusive, intensive programs being developed at the Medical Center. Of particular note was the growing friendly relationship of the visiting staff with the full-time staff on the campus. "The faculty is one of the best in any school of medicine," the dean said, "a most democratic School of Medicine with a nonautocratic faculty board."

It was phenomenal that Oklahoma, in its fiftieth year of statehood, had a School of Medicine that could produce approximately 100 new physicians a year, for the way to that frontier had been neither direct nor smooth. Yet, with all that the Medical Center represented, Dean Everett felt that a point had not been reached where medical science could pause in its efforts or be content.[9]

9. "In commemoration of and as a party helping in the celebration of the Golden Anniversary of the great State of Oklahoma," the Oklahoma State Dental Association awarded a citation to Mark R. Everett in 1957, in recognition of his many activities in social welfare.

Chapter XXII.
Priceless Grants-in-aid:
1958–59

 The National Institutes of Health, which provided matching monies for construction of the radiology addition to the outpatient wing of the University Hospital,[1] had been for some time one of the few rays of sunshine in the discouraging financial picture of the School of Medicine. Only by supplementing meager state appropriations with funds from outside the state was it possible to develop what was primarily a mediocre college of medicine ten years previously into a healthy, growing educational institution of great potential by 1958. And for five years the spirit and drive of the bright, young, full-time clinicians, who wanted to make their school prominent in research and teaching methods, had been boundless, in spite of the fact that the necessary nourishment from the legislatures (in the form of larger appropriations) had not materialized thus far.

Consequently, President Cross and Dean Everett were doubly dismayed in March, when Stewart Wolf, who had been most effective in securing thousands of dollars in grants, not only for the School of Medicine but for the Research Institute as well, was offered a professorship at Vanderbilt at a salary of $20,000, plus fringe benefits, compared with a salary of $12,000 per year at the Oklahoma Medical Center. Dr. Wolf, who once told Alice Everett that he did not come to Oklahoma "to look at the sunsets," was persuaded to remain here only after the Oklahoma Medical Research Foundation agreed to supplement his salary to the extent of $6,000 annually and to buy an endowment contract which would provide $1,500 per year in addition, thereby guaranteeing that our window would continue to open toward the *rising* sun.

Approximately a quarter of a million dollars in financial aid was developed through the initiative of faculty members responsible for conducting 85 grant-backed research projects in progress at the Medical Center in 1958, while only a total of $29,000 from state appropriations was budgeted for research for the same period. Other states, having more medical center facilities than this state, received grant monies from National Institutes of Health far in excess of

---

[1.] On January 9, 1958, the regents of the University of Oklahoma approved a contract for this building project in the amount of $454,600 with the Charles M. Tuttle Construction Company of Oklahoma City.

Oklahoma's $630,680. Kansas received $1,018,020; Utah, $1,318,746; Texas, $2,286,637; and Missouri, $2,539,422.

Fortunately, the federal government allowed Oklahoma a further extension of time (until February 28, 1959) in which to raise its share of $400,000 for a proposed $800,000 research building at the School of Medicine.

The school's teaching program was assisted further by training grants awarded by the Kellogg Foundation, the National Institutes of Health, and state agencies; for example, the Tulsa Heart Association gave $3,190 for support of research studies in circulatory dynamics, directed by Lee Conrad; and the board of directors of the Oklahoma State Heart Association approved grants of $500 and $2,000 to Allen E. Greer, R. Gibson Parrish, and John M. Carey for experimentation in improved efficiency of the heart-lung machine.

The largest sum to date received by the School of Medicine for support of a single program was from two grants totaling nearly $250,000 for the development of a unique residency training program for graduate physicians in public health under the direction of John Shackleford of the state health department and William Schottstaedt, associate professor of preventive medicine and public health at the School of Medicine. One grant, from the National Institutes of Health, was for $147,960 to be spread over a five-year period and the second grant, from the Commonwealth Fund, was for $95,127 over a three-year period. These grants were awarded on the basis of a new idea for a residency program in public health advanced by Dr. Schottstaedt, which was medical school centered as opposed to the current procedure over the nation, whereby health departments conducted public health residency programs without medical school participation.

Atomic science became an integral part of medical education, as isotopes invaded all branches of teaching in schools of medicine. The equipment of our medical school laboratory, which was housed in the Oklahoma Medical Research Institute, was valued at $50,000 according to Peter Russo, head of the committee on isotopes; and the cost of instruments and machines at the veterans' hospital laboratory exceeded that figure. These two laboratories were the only complete isotope laboratories in the state of Oklahoma equipped to measure activity of a wide range of isotopes.

As a joint venture of the medical service of the Veterans Administration Hospital and of the Department of Medicine and the biostatistical unit of the Department of Preventive Medicine and Public Health at the University of Oklahoma, a therapeutic unit was established in 1958 for the evaluation of agents as "therapeutic tools" before marketing in pharmacies. This research unit included metabolic beds, offices, and a laboratory located in the veterans' hospital and was supported entirely by grants. The staggering total of 42,000 different drugs, currently available in pharmacies, emphasized the need for a more scientific assessment of these remedies.

Rene Menguy, staff surgeon at the Veterans Administration Hospital, joined the ranks of our Markle Scholars when he was notified in March that the University of Oklahoma School of Medicine would receive $30,000 over a five-year period in support of his research; and in May Robert H. Bayley, professor of medicine, was awarded an honorary fellowship in the American College of Cardiology.

The faculty of the School of Medicine, during its annual spring meeting on May 28, gave a rising vote of thanks to two alumni, Carl Bailey and Wendal Smith for their untiring efforts to help the "Medical Center achieve a sound economic structure"; and each of these doctors was presented a certificate of merit, signed by the chairman of the faculty board and the secretary of the faculty.

In tribute to the memory of Onis Hazel, an alumnus who died on December 8, 1957, Lloyd A. Owens established the Onis George Hazel Memorial Trust Fund in February. Dr. Hazel had been a member of the faculty since 1933 and was clinical professor of dermatology and syphilology at the time of his death.

Robert L. Schreiber, director of public relations, who resigned as of July 1, was succeeded, at a salary of $7,000 per annum, by Imogene Patrick Taylor, who had been on the staff of the *Daily Oklahoman* for 12 years and was a special writer in the fields of education and medicine for the past few years.[2]

In approving the proposed budget for the Medical Center on June 11, the university regents approved raising Dean Everett's salary to $14,500 and that of Raymond Crews to $9,800. John Walker Morledge became professor emeritus of medicine, and Ray M. Balyeat was appointed associate professor emeritus of medicine.

The list of new appointees to the faculty brought the number of full-time members of the teaching staff to 68 in 1958 and the number of part-time teachers to 502, with an additional 100 preceptors.

Gilbert Sadler Campbell, M.D.
professor of surgery
Paul R. David, Ph.D.
professor of medical genetics
Carl E. Marshall, M.D.
consultant professor of biostatistics and preventive medicine and public health
Harris D. Riley, Jr., M.D.
professor of pediatrics
Floyd S. Cornelison, M.D.
associate professor of psychiatry and neurology
DeWitt T. Hunter, M.D.
associate professor of pathology
Herbert H. Janszen, M.D.
associate professor of psychiatry and neurology

Walter W. Melvin, Jr., M.D., D.Sc.
associate professor of preventive medicine and public health
Glen G. Caylor, M.D.
assistant professor of pediatrics
Norman Allee Chance, Ph.D.
consultant assistant professor of psychiatry, neurology, and behavioral sciences
Paul Taylor Condit, M.D.
assistant professor of research medicine and research biochemistry
Frances G. Felton, Ph.D.
assistant professor of research microbiology

[2.] Imogene Patrick was a graduate of the University of Arkansas and a reporter for the *Tulsa World* before coming to Oklahoma City.

John Harry Gogerty, Ph.D.
assistant professor of
pharmacology
Allen R. Hennes, M.D.
assistant professor of medicine
Doman K. Keele, M.D.
assistant professor of pediatrics
Boyd K. Lester, M.D.
assistant professor of psychiatry,
neurology, and behavioral
sciences
Robert Dean Morrison, Ph.D.
consultant assistant professor of
biostatistics in preventive
medicine and public health
Sylvia O. Richardson, M.D.
assistant professor of pediatrics
Jose Rafael Rigual, M.D.
assistant professor of
otorhinolaryngology
Carl W. Smith, M.D.
assistant professor of medicine
John R. Sokatch, M.D.
assistant professor of
microbiology
Arthur N. Springall, M.D.
assistant professor of preventive
medicine and public health
Lucius Waites, M.D.
assistant professor of pediatrics
and assistant professor of
psychiatry, neurology, and
behavioral sciences
Peter J. L. Welt, M.D.
assistant professor of
anesthesiology
G. Rainey Williams, M.D.
assistant professor of surgery
Shatteen Blalock, M.D.
instructor in preventive medicine
and public health
Ted Clemens, Jr., M.D.
instructor in medicine
Mark Allen Everett, M.D.
instructor in dermatology
Melvin Clause Hicks, M.D.
instructor in radiology
L. Virginia Hunter, M.D.
instructor in pediatrics

Margie C. Jones, M.S.
instructor in nutrition
Stanley M. Kemler, M.D.
instructor in psychiatry,
neurology, and behavioral
sciences
Vernon V. Sisney, Ph.D.
instructor in medical psychology
in psychiatry, neurology, and
behavioral sciences
Charles E. Smith, Jr., M.D.
instructor in psychiatry and
neurology
Albert B. Wade, M.A.
instructor in psychiatry,
neurology, and behavioral
sciences
Alexander H. Woods, M.D.
instructor in medicine
Earl M. Bricker, M.D.
clinical assistant in gynecology
Warren L. Felton, M.D.
clinical assistant in surgery
Elizabeth P. Fleming, M.D.
visiting lecturer in preventive
medicine and public health
Max A. Glaze, M.D.
clinical assistant in psychiatry,
neurology, and behavioral
sciences
Hollis E. Hampton, M.D.
clinical assistant in gynecology
Ralston Raymond Hannas, Jr.,
M.D.
clinical assistant in medicine
Sam W. Hendrix, M.D.
clinical assistant in obstetrics
Edwin R. Maier, M.D.
clinical assistant in orthopedic
surgery
Alfonso Paredes, M.D.
research associate in psychiatry,
neurology, and behavioral
sciences
Alvin W. Paulson, M.D.
clinical assistant in medicine
Paul E. Plowman, D.D.S.
clinical assistant in dental surgery

C. Herman Reece, D.D.S.
clinical assistant in dental surgery
George T. Russell, M.D.
visiting lecturer in pediatrics
Wayne H. Schultz, M.D.
clinical assistant in radiology
Anna T. Scruggs
research associate in pediatrics

Henry Ernest Spuehler, M.S.
consultant in otorhinolaryngology
Wilson David Steen, Ph.D.
research associate in preventive
medicine and public health
Kathryn L. West, B.A.
research associate in psychiatry,
neurology, and behavioral
sciences

Harris D. Riley, Jr. (formerly with Vanderbilt University School of Medicine) assumed his position as professor and head of the Department of Pediatrics in January, 1958, with his salary set at $12,000 per annum. One of Dr. Riley's primary interests was in establishing a study center for exceptional children here, with activities initially directed toward the problem of mental retardation in children at all levels (etiology, diagnosis, prevention, and management), which would combine the resources of the Medical Center, the State Department of Public Health, and other agencies. This unit of the Department of Pediatrics was conceived as a nucleus around which the problems of growth and development of exceptional children—both inpatients and outpatients—could be observed and evaluated by interested persons from the preclinical and clinical faculty as well as from the paramedical sciences.

Space for the facilities of the study center—six adjoining rooms in Children's Memorial Hospital—made it possible to get the organization under way early in February, and Teresa Costeloe, clinical psychologist, reported for work on Wednesday, February 12, to begin testing a backlog of mental retardation cases from the Children's Hospital clinics. James Paul Costeloe had been appointed a research associate in medicine, psychiatry, neurology, and behavioral sciences and in preventive medicine and public health in 1957. On September 10 the university regents appointed Sylvia Richardson assistant professor of pediatrics. She became director of the child study center here,[3] and her appointment brought to 38 the number on the teaching staff in the Department of Pediatrics in 1958–59.

The Department of Psychiatry, Neurology, and Behavioral Sciences numbered 46 staff members, and the Department of Surgery had 27 staff members. Gilbert S. Campbell, a chest surgeon from the University of Minnesota Medical School, was named chief of surgery at the Oklahoma City Veterans Administration Hospital in 1958 and professor of surgery at the University of Oklahoma School of Medicine.[4]

[3.] Dr. Richardson received her M.A. degree from Columbia University in 1942 and completed four years of graduate work in the education of the exceptional child before starting her training in medicine.
[4.] Dr. Campbell was engaged in experimental work at the medical center in Minneosta which had an international reputation for open-heart surgery. He held an M.D. degree from the University of Virginia and both an M.D. in physiology and a Ph.D. in surgery from the University of Minnesota.

Harry Wilkins, chairman of the section on neurosurgery of the Department of Surgery, resigned from that position in 1958 after 27 years as senior neurosurgeon and asked that Jess Herrmann be officially established as chairman of the section on neurosurgery.[5] Earlier in the year, Dr. Wilkins, Dr. Herrmann, and R. Alvin Rix, Jr., contributed $1,260 toward the support of the neurosurgical residencies in the University Hospitals.

On July 21, Dean Everett issued a memorandum on the unanimous advice of the executive committee of the faculty board of the School of Medicine, placing the following instruction into effect as an operating procedure for advisory committees within clinical departments: (1) The advisory or liaison committee was to be nominated by ballot of the members of a given department and appointed by the dean, who would also appoint a spokesman for the group. Its purpose was to advise the head or chairman of the particular department concerning the desires and viewpoints of members of that department. (2) If any major disagreement were to develop between the advisory committee and the head or chairman of the department, which could not be resolved satisfactorily to all concerned, then it became the duty of the advisory committee, through its spokesman, to inform the dean. (3) All administrative decisions were to be the sole responsibility of the department head or chairman, after free consultation with his advisory committee on all important changes in policy, before undertaking any major changes in departmental conduct.

The residency program of the University Hospitals came under the scrutiny of the State Board of Medical Examiners early in the year, since some residents who were not citizens had been granted educational contracts by the Medical Center, albeit in good faith, who were not licensed to practice medicine. The University of Oklahoma School of Medicine and the University Hospitals eventually agreed to attempt education of these individuals as graduate students or academic fellows, as recommended by the faculty board on May 14, with any training involving patients under the direct supervision of a licensed physician, relieving the noncitizen of any responsibilities which would violate the Medical Practice Act of the state of Oklahoma.

In a memorandum to chairmen and heads of all clinical departments on December 11, Dean Everett clarified the above recommendation as follows: foreign citizens were not eligible for licensure in Oklahoma, and under this circumstance the University of Oklahoma Medical Center was constrained to limit its appointment of a physician who was a foreign citizen to that of visiting fellow in the School of Medicine, which meant a graduate student not in the practice of medicine and not recompensed for hospital service. The dean called attention to the fact that the Educational Council for Foreign Medical Graduates conducted medical qualification examinations twice yearly to ascertain whether a foreign citizen had preparation equivalent to that expected of graduates of approved medical colleges in our country and also a reasonable facility with the

---

[5.] In answering Dr. Wilkins' letter, Dean Mark Everett said he had often thought how fortunate he had been to have had both Dr. Wilkins and Dr. Herrmann as students, and that his admiration for each of them was something he cherished very much.

English language. The clinical departments of our school were therefore urged to require such certification whenever possible, with the objective of employing it for all foreign medical graduate applicants as soon as practicable. The Council on Medical Education and Hospitals of the American Medical Association on December 3 approved the residency program of the University Hospitals and the Veterans Administration Hospital for three years training. Questions regarding an agreement between the two hospitals, concerning resident benefits, were to be referred to the hospital concerned.[6]

There were 131 residents and 19 interns training in the clinical departments of the Medical Center in 1958–59. Of $64,397 in stipends for 14 psychiatry residents, 28 per cent was provided by the University of Oklahoma, 22 per cent by the National Institute of Mental Health, and 50 per cent by the Veterans Administration and the air force.

The University of Oklahoma School of Medicine became a participating institution in the program of Medical Education for National Defense on January 1, 1958, together with nine schools additionally selected, making a total of 45 medical schools in the country taking part in the program, which was begun five years previously under the auspices of the Council of the Association of American Medical Colleges. Stanley W. Olson, Baylor University College of Medicine, was chairman of the committee organizing the program, and Dean Everett was one of its members. The program was sponsored by the defense department and supported by the armed forces. Participating institutions were disconnected from any federal orders and/or regimentation, and no new courses were added to the curriculum; but medical problems related to the jet age— national emergencies and mass casualties—were incorporated into the current curriculum. James P. Dewar, associate professor of pathology and director of the University Hospitals' laboratories, was named coordinator of the program, and the school was given an initial grant of $2,000 for the orientation period.

The fourth-year curriculum included 44 weeks of actual instruction, 36 weeks spent on campus or with an affiliated hospital and eight weeks serving a preceptorship.

John A. Schilling, head of the Department of Surgery, was chief of the medical staff of the University Hospitals in 1958. The allocation of beds, as of December, was as follows: surgical, 82 at the main hospital and 100 at Children's; medicine, 95 at main; psychiatry, 20 at main; pediatrics, 104 at Children's; obstetrics and gynecology, 59, including 15 in gynecology on pediatrics, and 9 on admitting, making a total of 469 allocated beds, plus an additional 35 bassinets. The Veterans Administration Hospital had a capacity of 492 beds, and the Oklahoma Medical Research Institute operated a 24-bed unit primarily for metabolic studies. The total number of patients to visit the outpatient departments of University Hospitals in 1958 was 69,647.

[6.] Because of the need for central records concerning residents at the medical center, a resident record office was established in May in the School of Medicine building, from which all questions concerning the function of the office were referred to Associate Dean S. N. Stone.

The state appropriations for the University of Oklahoma for 1958–59 were $5,099,893 out of a total income of $8,007,969; for the School of Medicine, $821,871 out of total income of $1,128,189; for the University Hospitals, $2,381,046 out of a total income of $4,031,552.

Sources of income for the School of Medicine and University Hospitals for the fiscal year ending June 30, 1959, were as follows: miscellaneous, 27.5 per cent; research grants, 17.5 per cent; state appropriations, 16.5 per cent; training grants, 10.2 per cent; Veterans Administration, 9.2 per cent; faculty contributions, 7.3 per cent; private foundations, 6.4 per cent; and teaching grants, 5.4 per cent.

The Crippled Children's Commission fell short of meeting its promised $700,000 payment to Children's Memorial Hospital for the fiscal year ending June 30, 1958, and Lloyd Rader, a member of the commission, said that only $580,000 out of $1,648,388 in available funds had been paid by the director of the commission to Children's Hospital; whereas the hospital had rendered $700,000 in services to crippled children. Other funds available to the commission were: $413,444 from the Department of Public Welfare; $313,685 in the County Crippled Children budget account; $256,964 from the Children's Bureau of the federal government; and $34,243 from other sources.[7]

Many crippled children, dependent upon the Crippled Children's Commission for stronger and straighter bodies, but seldom seen by the casual visitor, were listed in the active file of 3,250 youngsters who frequented the orthopedic appliance shop in the basement of Children's Memorial Hospital. There, according to doctors' prescriptions, all kinds of braces and orthopedic prostheses were created or assembled by skilled workmen to correct or support crippling disabilities. And shoes were reshaped, according to specification, to help little folk take their first steps. Fortunately, a cash bonus of $12,000 for an oil and gas lease on land in Custer County was willed to Crippled Children's Hospital by Rosalee Powell in this particular year and gratefully accepted by the University regents.

President Cross brought up the question of student admissions to the School of Medicine at a meeting of the regents on June 11 and stated that, while each class was limited to 100 students, during the last six years withdrawals had averaged four each year. The regents then authorized the board of admissions to admit as many as 104 to each first-year class in order to compensate for the withdrawals and thereby graduate more doctors. There were only 371 students enrolled in the School of Medicine for the year 1958–59.

Eighty-eight seniors received the Doctor of Medicine degree during commencement exercises held in Holmberg Hall, Norman, Oklahoma, on June 1, 1958. Over 100 faculty members of the School of Medicine, in academic attire, participated in the colorful ceremony. Each senior was hooded by Dean

---

[7.] Governor Gary was distressed by the deficit in payments by the Crippled Children's Commission and said that the next legislature would have to appropriate "at least $1,000,000 in order to take care of Crippled Children's Hospital and the needs of children in this state."

Everett, assisted by George Garrison, professor of pediatrics and chairman of the faculty board Committee on Undergraduate Education; and the graduates were led in public affirmation of the *Sponsio Academica* by Don O'Donoghue, chairman of the faculty board.

Fifty-nine graduate assistants were enrolled in the basic sciences graduate college program during the year, and seven Ph.D. degrees and five M.Sc. degrees were awarded at the 1958 graduation exercises. Florene Kelly, chairman of the Department of Microbiology, who was very interested in the graduate program and was herself conducting research on staphylococci—for characteristics associated with their disease-producing power—once said in an interview, "We think of our cultures as gardens."

All postgraduate courses were held in the School of Medicine, and the postgraduate office cooperated with the State Department of Public Health, the Oklahoma County and State Medical Associations, the Academy of General Practice, and other health-related agencies and organizations in developing the courses. The Oklahoma County Medical Society made a gift of $500 toward the purchase of a copying machine.

Nine postgraduate courses lasting from one to nine days were scheduled for the academic year to aid state physicians. Out-of-state lecturers from other medical centers (as well as members of the Oklahoma Medical School faculty) were booked as speakers. More than 1,400 physicians, including 167 from other states, registered for these courses, which was an increase of 8 per cent in attendance over the previous year. In addition, there were ten other short courses with four hours of informal instruction once a month.

Especially appreciated by our clinical house staff was a series of lectures every second and fourth Tuesday, given as part of the staff's postgraduate training by members of the faculty of the School of Medicine.

Jenell D. Hubbard, director of nursing service for the University of Oklahoma Hospitals, received the first Lottinville Award[8] for excellence in nursing, selected jointly by representatives of the Oklahoma State Medical Association and the University of Oklahoma School of Nursing. Mark R. Everett, director of the Medical Center made the presentation on September 3 at the finishing ceremonies for graduating nurses. At the same time twenty-four nurses received certificates in nursing and nine received the Bachelor of Science in Nursing degree. One hundred and fifty-two students were enrolled in the school for 1958–59.

The School of Nursing received a $70,000 grant from the Kellogg Founda-

---

[8.] The Lottinville Award was established by Savoie Lottinville, director of the University of Oklahoma Press, Norman, in an effort to stimulate interest in the nursing profession. The award consisted of a certificate in Latin and a Georgian Castle silver service. Adhering to the donor's wishes, the honorarium was to be made each year to the outstanding graduate of either the diploma or the degree nursing program of the University of Oklahoma, on the basis of excellence in class, ward, and laboratory work, personal character, standing among fellow students and teachers, and potential influence as an active worker and leader in nursing.

tion, effective July 1, 1958, to help raise the educational level of nursing and, at the same time, to retain nurses in their home state. The aim of the program was to offer a curriculum toward the bachelor of science degree for those nurses who held only three-year certificates or diplomas, thus making it possible for Oklahoma-trained nurses to take additional college work necessary to let them enter specialized fields without having to go out of the state. The program was really started in 1957, following approval by the university regents, but the Kellogg grant for a five-year period got the program off the ground. Helen Patterson, former nursing service director at the University of Oklahoma Medical Center, returned to the campus to develop the program, a long time dream of her profession.

The Alumni Association of the University of Oklahoma School of Medicine honored a number of Oklahomans with citations for singular contributions to the medical sciences in Oklahoma on April 11, 1958. Among those cited for extraordinary involvement were former Governor Roy Turner and Governor Raymond Gary. Governor Gary was cited presently "for championing funds to open psychiatry beds—the means of training psychiatrists at the University Hospitals—and for helping to make an emergency appropriation available to build a new radiology unit."

The fiscal year ending June 30, 1958, marked the conclusion of the five-year project supported by the W. K. Kellogg Foundation to develop a program of teaching and research in preventive medicine and public health at the School of Medicine. On September 10, 1958, Dean Everett commented, in a letter to Matthew R. Kinde, director, Division of Medicine and Public Health of the Kellogg Foundation, that the value of the foundation's support was only partly reflected in reports and documents; that its promotion of better medical teaching and medical care had permeated the Medical Center with significant benefits to the field of medicine.

The effects of research grants from the National Institutes of Health on research programs in the Oklahoma medical school (one of 20 reviewed) was studied by a team of representatives of the institutes on November 24 and 25, 1958. And on December 12, J. Franklin Yeager, chief of the Grants and Training Branch, National Heart Institute, wrote Dean Everett as follows: "Your Medical School is outstanding in the expeditious and complete way in which the desired information was provided. . . . I was particularly glad to have this opportunity to chat with you and members of your faculty with whom I have had such pleasant dealings in the past."

In the same mail Dr. Everett received a letter from Owen H. Wangensteen, chief of the Department of Surgery, University of Minnesota Medical School, who said that it had been "wonderful to have the opportunity of returning to your burgeoning institution (after a period of almost twenty years) and to note the progress your School is making. . . . The institution seems fairly bursting at the seams and there is no cure for it as far as I can see, other than to continue expanding. . . . The spirit of research which is irradiated from every department is a great tribute to you and your vision."

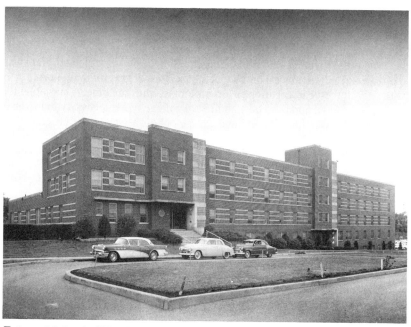

Enlarged School of Nursing building, 1951.

Courtesy Sooner Medic

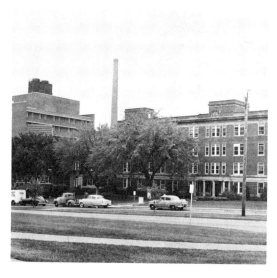

Outpatient building and
adjacent wing of University
Hospital, 1951.

Courtesy Sooner Medic

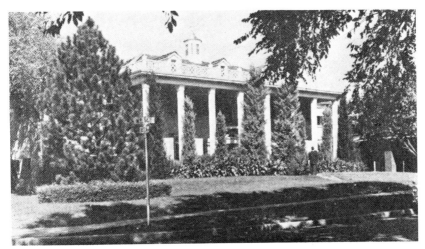

Faculty House.

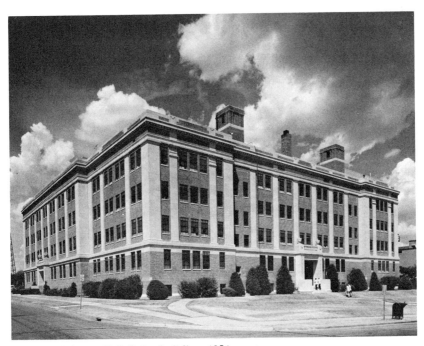

Enlarged School of Medicine building, 1951.

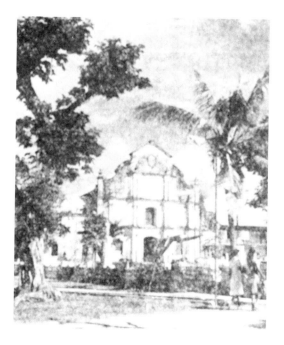

Evacuation Hospital No. 21 in Church of San Marcos, Philippines, 1945.

Courtesy Daily Oklahoman

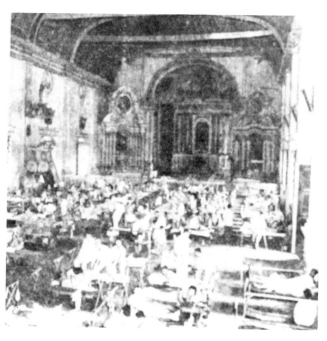

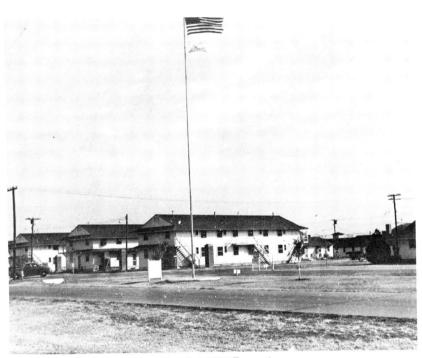

Old Veterans Administration Hospital (Will Rogers).

Courtesy University of Oklahoma Medical Center

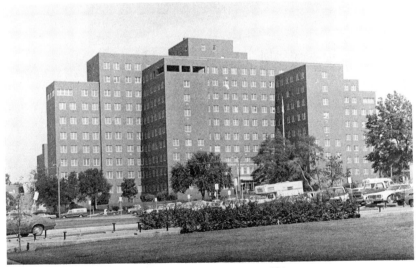

Oklahoma City Veterans Administration Hospital, 1953

Courtesy Veterans Administration

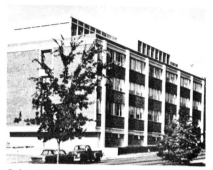

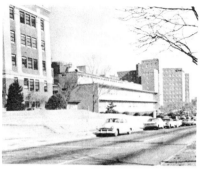

School of Medicine research building, 1961.

View of the north side of N.E. 13th Street, Oklahoma City.

Courtesy Sooner Medic

Courtesy Sooner Medic

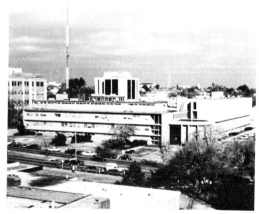

Enlarged Oklahoma Medical Research Foundation building, 1970.

Courtesy Oklahoma Medical Research Foundation

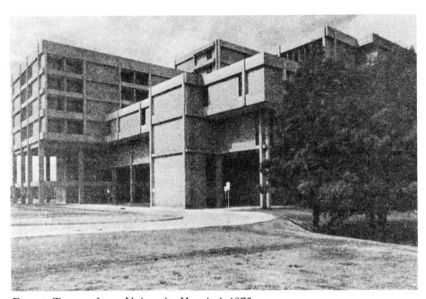

Everett Tower of new University Hospital, 1972.

Courtesy University of Oklahoma Medical Center

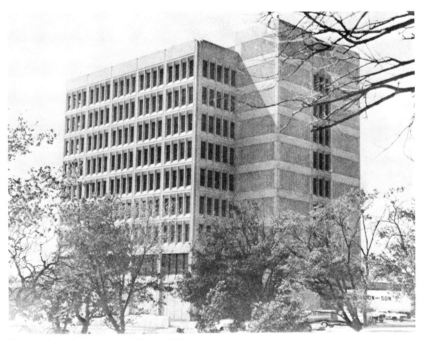

Biomedical Sciences building, 1976.

Courtesy University of Oklahoma Medical Center

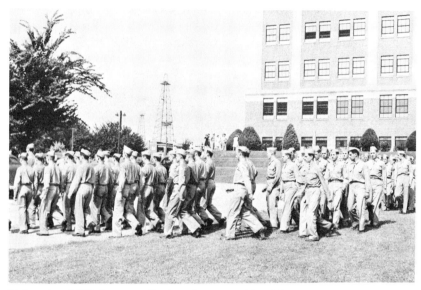

University of Oklahoma medical students marching, World War II, 1944.

Courtesy University of Oklahoma Medical Center

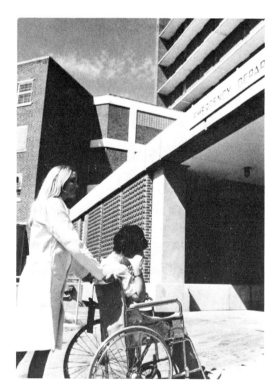

Entrance to Emergency,
University Hospital.

*Courtesy University
of Oklahoma
Medical Center*

286

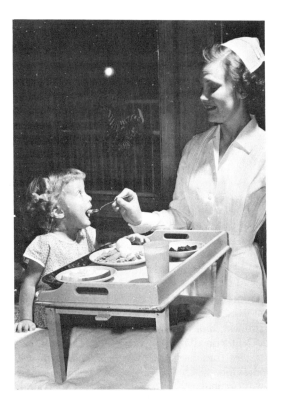

Dietetic intern feeding
child, University Hospital.

*Courtesy University
of Oklahoma
Medical Center*

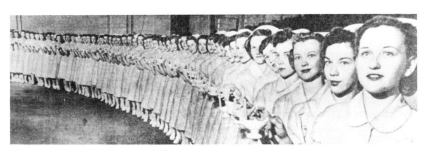

Nurses capping ceremony, 1949.

Courtesy Oklahoma City Times

Chapter XXIII.
Exodus of the Oklahoma Commission for Crippled Children: 1959–60

 J. Howard Edmondson, at age thirty-three, became the youngest governor ever elected in the state of Oklahoma, albeit by a small majority. His close advisers were vigorous, youthful men but new on the political scene, so the "old guard" dominated the twenty-seventh legislature.

Representative James Bullard was thoroughly committed to leading the legislative fight for the Medical Center on all phases of its programs, even over the opposition of the governor, but fortunately, Governor Edmondson was favorable to the objectives and sympathetic with the needs of the medical center. Mr. Bullard felt that it was particularly desirable to get the Chamber of Commerce active in support of the Medical Center "as an expanding industry of Oklahoma City."

In an effort to familiarize Oklahomans with the needs of their colleges and universities, the Alumni Association of the School of Medicine organized a citizens group on January 24, with Nolan J. Fuqua of Duncan, an industrial and civic leader of national repute, as chairman. Working with Mr. Fuqua, in an attempt to start a kind of grass roots movement to alleviate some of the financial woes of the state's institutions of higher learning, were forty-seven representative citizens from twenty-nine cities and towns in the state.

At the same time, the president's master plan committee (headed by Stewart Wolf) was looking to the future and recommended that appropriate state agencies initiate a land acquisition plan to provide adequate room for the expansion of the Medical Center southward from N.E. Thirteenth Street. And on April 1 the university regents appointed their own committee on the Medical Center, consisting of Regents Benedum and Savage, with a third member to be added later. This committee was delegated to work with Dr. Wolf and his planning committee and with Irwin Hurst, secretary of the capitol and Medical Center zoning committees, on long-range planning for the Medical Center campus.

Early in the twenty-seventh legislative session, Representative Bryce Baggett introduced House Bill No. 589 for an emergency appropriation of $400,000 in state funds to the University of Oklahoma Medical Center, to match the federal grant, which had undergone numerous "stays of execution" since 1957, for construction of a research facility on the campus. The bill, passed by both houses of the legislature without much opposition, was signed into law by Governor Edmondson; and at long last, on May 29, the State Regents for Higher Education authorized the stipulated amount ($400,000) to the School of Medicine for the purpose intended by the legislature.

Representative Frank Ogden, floor leader, led the fight in the house for Senate Bill No. 20 to transfer the financing of the state's crippled children's program to the welfare department, saying that every legislative session since 1954 had failed to finance the program adequately. On the other hand, opponents of the bill charged that use of welfare funds for crippled children would result in a reduction of old-age pension checks; and Ora Fox, vicariously concerned with "the old folks," headed a list of persons speaking against the bill. As a consequence, the dispute eventually turned into a kind of tug-of-war between crippled children and old-age pensioners. Ben Nicholson, a well-known pediatrician, said that he would like to represent the children, because "growing, developing children were allowed less money for food than needy old folks who should be watching their diets anyway"; and Dr. Nicholson further stated that he and other doctors "knew of no better way to make an incompetent, inadequate adult than to starve him during his years of growth."

Lloyd Rader,[1] public welfare commissioner, explained the bill at the outset of the hearings, saying that the welfare department was required to hold back a surplus of over $6,000,000 at any one time, and that there was almost twice as much as that in the current surplus fund. If the bill calling for the use of $1,250,000 a year in surplus funds were to pass, there would still be more than a $2,000,000 surplus above the holding amount required by federal regulation, and that such a surplus would be more than ample to finance the crippled children's program without cutting any welfare programs.

Dean Everett, commenting on the bill, said that it was evidently copied directly from the original Children's Act and that passage of the bill would make proper provision for Children's Memorial Hospital and a possible end to the fiscal chaos that had hounded the Oklahoma Commission for Crippled Children in recent years. "The sum of $1,250,000 coming from sales tax collections by the Department of Public Welfare," Dr. Everett said, "would more than double the amount of state appropriated funds going to the Oklahoma Commission for Crippled Children, and would allow the Children's Hospital to pay all of its bills for the first time ever."

Victory was finally assured for the proponents of Senate Bill No. 20 when it passed the upper house in May; and, when Governor Edmondson signed the bill into law on June 24, the scratch of his pen was music to the ears of many, for it sounded the death knell for the Oklahoma Commission for Crippled Children, which had made a less than equitable contribution to the Children's Hospital and to medical education in Oklahoma.

[1.] Governor Johnston Murray appointed Lloyd Rader director of the State Department of Public Welfare on November 12, 1952, following the resignation of Virgil L. Stokes.

Effective July 1, 1959, all properties, records, equipment, and supplies owned and in use by the Oklahoma Commission for Crippled Children were transferred to and became the property of the State Department of Public Welfare; and the entire staff of the Oklahoma Commission for Crippled Children was appointed to positions in the State Department of Public Welfare. Furthermore, all unexpended funds were transferred by the state treasurer to the State Department of Public Welfare and placed in a separate account with the state treasurer, known as the "State's Crippled Children's Fund."

Henceforth, the term "child" meant any person under twenty-one years of age whose parents or legal guardian were financially unable to provide essential medical care. The Children's Memorial Hospital, including its clinics and laboratories, was designated as a service institution for the physically handicapped children of this state. It also served as a teaching and training hospital for the School of Medicine of the University of Oklahoma. The Oklahoma Department of Public Welfare was obligated, insofar as practicable, to use the available facilities of the Children's Memorial Hospital to a degree that would enable the School of Medicine to maintain its proper patient ratio for accreditation, provided that this provision did not cause undue hardship to a patient.

Payments for services by the commission to the Children's Memorial Hospital were based on the actual per diem cost of patient care, exclusive of professional instructional expense. In the event the commission and the Board of Regents of the University of Oklahoma could not agree on a per diem charge for patients of the commission, the budget director, with the approval of the governor, was authorized to establish a rate of pay which would prevail. On the other hand, the commission was granted a priority in the assignment of hospital services (to Children's Memorial Hospital), to be distributed as equitably as possible among the counties of the state.

The twenty-seventh legislature made appropriations of approximately $2,500,000 to the State Regents for Higher Education for supplementary operating funds for various state colleges, and on May 25 the School of Medicine was allocated $74,900 and the University Hospitals, $217,019.

On July 8 the State Hospital Advisory Council earmarked Hill-Burton matching monies to assist two Medical Center building projects—$50,000 out of a total cost of $100,000 for radiology equipment[2] and $100,000 toward a Speech and Hearing Clinic addition, for which the State Regents of Higher Education had allocated $100,000 (Senate Bill No. 103). The total amount budgeted for this clinic for the fiscal year ending June 30, 1960, was $173,606, of which $76,770 was from the State's Crippled Children's Fund of the Department of Public Welfare, $32,471 from research and training grants, and $64,365 from the University of Oklahoma. One training grant from the Oklahoma Division of Vocational Rehabilitation amounted to $12,978, and there

---

[2] The new three-story addition to University Hospital was completed late in the year, providing laboratories for the Departments of Surgery, Medicine, and Anesthesiology on one floor, and diagnostic and treatment facilities of the Department of Radiology on the remaining floors.

were research grants from the same source, one for $13,660, and another through the State Office of Education.

The clinic initiated services for preschool cerebral palsy children, a cleft palata team was established, and classes had commenced for speech and auditory training at the adult level. Therapy for the laryngectomized was beginning to be offered and adult aphasics were receiving speech therapy. So far as was known at the time, the service program of the Oklahoma clinic was one of the largest of any university in the nation.

Before 1959, monies contributed to informal trust funds for the use and benefit of various departments of the University of Oklahoma Medical Center were expended for the benefit of the several departments and for their respective research and development programs. When it became apparent that a formal declaration of trust to provide uniformity and regularity to such funds should be declared, the faculty board appointed a temporary committee for departmental trusts, headed by Jess D. Herrmann. Meeting with the faculty board, Dean Everett explained that departmental trust funds were not funds of the school but of the departmental staffs, saying that the funds had been started more than six years previously, when a few faculty members chose to give some money to departments. ''The money does not go into the hands of the administration of the School of Medicine but is directly for departmental use,'' Dean Everett said; and he suggested that each department appoint a committee to draw up a plan for its own department as to how such funds should be used, for what purpose, and by whom. After rules and regulations for the governing of a department had been made, they should be submitted to the faculty board for approval through the trust fund committee.

In a memorandum to department heads and chairman on June 5, Dr. Kirk Mosley[3] reported that the trust fund committee appointed by the faculty board had obtained the advice of an attorney in regard to the establishment and management of trust funds being operated by departments in the School of Medicine. It was very important when tax deduction privileges were accorded to any donors to a trust fund, the attorney cautioned, that all legal provisions had been made to assure these donors that such deductions were valid. Therefore, the Medical Center was advised by the attorney to establish a formal trust fund for such funds and to draw up a document setting forth the stipulation of such a trust fund ''to be known and commonly described as the University of Oklahoma Medical Center Departmental Trust Fund,'' with trustees as outlined in the articles governing the trust.

In broad terms, the purpose of establishing the trust was ''to provide funds for the general welfare of the several departments with emphasis on assistance in teaching, research, and development,'' acknowledging, however, that expenditures for the use and benefit of individuals—particularly for those who might be residents—was a proper function of the trust. Funds other than Markle

[3.] Dr. Mosley, professor and chairman of the Department of Preventive Medicine and Public Health, was given the additional title of associate dean, in charge of research and special training programs, on January 14, 1959, at a total yearly salary of $12,000.

grants had been used to support the research activities of three Markle Scholars—Doctors Gilbert Campbell, Merlin DuVal, and Rene Menguy.[4]

Gilbert Campbell had succeeded in developing an active and creditable open-heart surgery program at Children's Memorial Hospital and had extended his research activities in the field of cardiovascular pulmonary physiology, while Dr. Menguy was carrying out his research and official functions at the Veterans Administration Hospital. An outstanding innovation at the Medical Center in 1959 was the open-heart surgery program initiated by a team of surgeons consisting of Doctors Campbell, Glenn Caylor, William Richardson, David Snyder, and Rainey Williams, with the first successful open-heart surgical procedure in the state of Oklahoma being performed on January 21 in Children's Memorial Hospital.[5] It is no exaggeration to say that the initial record of 12 consecutive patients with congenital heart disease being operated on successfully—without mortality and "under less than optimal physical conditions"—was unprecedented in the field of open-heart surgery; and much credit is due the physician-nurse teams which functioned as a unit during the long hazardous operations. Patients underwent surgery after the most painstaking diagnostic procedures which would give clues to the type of difficulty in respect to any particular case.

Five former members of the faculty passed away in 1959: George A. LaMotte, professor emeritus of medicine, on March 1; Charles B. Taylor, professor emeritus of urology, on April 7; Leander Armistead Riely, professor emeritus of medicine, on June 14 in Connecticut; Casriel J. Fishman, professor emeritus of medicine, on July 1 in Oklahoma City; and Joseph M. Thuringer on October 28 in Fayetteville, Arkansas. Doctors Clark H. Hall, Joseph C. MacDonald, Theodore G. Wails, and Carroll M. Pounders were respectively given the title of professor emeritus in 1959.

Robert C. Lowe, who resigned as superintendent of University of Oklahoma Hospitals on July 1, was made a research consultant in hospital organization and administration and given the title of associate professor of medicine and preventive medicine and public health. Dr. Lowe was succeeded as superintendent of the hospitals by Raymond D. Crews, business administrator of the Medical Center for a number of years. Mr. Crews was a graduate of the University of Oklahoma School of Law.

The highest salaries reported in the Medical Center in 1959 ranged from $18,000 to $24,000 for members of the staff designated as professors and heads of departments: Dr. Wolf, medicine, $24,000; Dr. Schilling, surgery, $24,000; Dr. West, psychiatry, $24,000; Dr. White, anesthesiology, $20,400; Dr. Ridings, radiology, $18,000; and Dr. Jaques, pathology, $18,000. The highest preclinical professorial salary was $13,000, and that of the director of the

[4] See the financial report to the executive director of the John R. Markle Foundation for the fiscal year 1958–59 by Dean Everett.

[5] The Veterans Administration Hospital afforded more than its share of financial and material support for this project, and $712 was contributed to aid the program by the United Fund of Perry, Oklahoma.

Medical Center and dean of the School of Medicine was $14,000. Dr. Eliel, scientific director of the Oklahoma Medical Research Foundation, received a salary of $20,000.

The full-time faculty members for the fiscal year 1959–60 totaled 94 in the School of Medicine and 16 in the School of Nursing. New appointees to the faculty for 1959–60 were as follows:

Martin M. Cummings, M.D.
  professor of microbiology
William B. Lemmon, Ph.D.
  consultant professor of psychiatry
  and neurology
Oscar Albert Parsons, Ph.D.
  professor of psychology in
  psychiatry, neurology, and
  behavioral sciences
Everett C. Bracken, Ph.D.
  assistant professor of pediatrics
Henry N. Kirkman, M.D.
  assistant professor of pediatrics
Frankie Nell Nations, M.D.
  assistant professor of
  anesthesiology
Jones Bautista Ballina, M.D.
  instructor in gynecology
Barbara F. Braden, M.D.
  instructor in preventive medicine
  and public health
Robert E. Campbell, M.D.
  instructor in ophthalmology
Walter Honska, M.D.
  instructor in medicine and
  preventive medicine and public
  health
Richard E. Johnston, M.S.
  instructor in radiological physics
  in radiology
Lucien C. Kavan, M.D.
  instructor in urology
Marjorie S. Keele, M.D.
  instructor in pediatrics
Norman K. Lee, M.D.
  instructor in pathology
Luiese Husen Lynch, B.S.
  instructor in physical therapy
Harry Martin, Ph.D.
  instructor in psychiatry,
  neurology, and behavioral
  sciences

Hideo Namiki, M.D.
  instructor in pathology
Loraine Neal, M.S.
  instructor in medical library
  science
Natoo C. Patel, M.D.
  instructor in medicine
Kenneth W. Shons, D.D.S.,
  M.S.D.
  instructor in dental surgery
Mary N. Sloan, M.S.S.
  instructor in psychiatry,
  neurology, and behavioral
  sciences
Stephen Wright Thompson, M.D.
  instructor in medicine
Jack Daryl Welsh, M.D.
  instructor in medicine
Nancy Leigh Adsett, M.A.
  clinical assistant in psychiatry
Julien W. Bahr, M.D.
  clinical assistant in medicine
George N. Bouthilet, Ph.D.
  research associate in pediatrics
Wayne J. Boyd, M.D.
  visiting lecturer in psychiatry,
  neurology, and behavioral
  sciences
Cecil C. Bridges, Ph.D.
  research associate in pediatrics
Walter R. Cooper, Jr., D.D.S.
  clinical assistant in dental surgery
James Alphonso Cox, M.D.
  clinical assistant in psychiatry and
  neurology
Roy E. Curle, M.D.
  clinical assistant in anesthesiology
Pearl D. Fisher, Ph.D.
  research associate in preventive
  medicine and public health
Frank G. Gatchell, M.D.
  clinical assistant in surgery

William S. Harrison, M.D.
  clinical assistant in medicine
Virgil Thomas Hill, Ph.D.
  visiting lecturer in psychiatry,
  neurology, and behavioral
  sciences
Everett Neal Holden, M.D.
  clinical assistant in preventive
  medicine and public health
William E. Hood, M.D.
  clinical assistant in obstetrics
Leon Horowitz, M.D.
  visiting lecturer in pediatrics
Herbert B. Hudnut, Jr., M.D.
  clinical assistant in preventive
  medicine and public health
Samuel B. Leslie, M.D.
  clinical assistant in
  ophthalmology
Thomas Neil Lynn, Jr., M.D.
  clinical assistant in medicine

Hugh Francis Maguire, D.D.S.
  clinical assistant in oral surgery
Joseph Louis Martin, M.D.
  clinical assistant in anesthesiology
George Fred McDonald, M.D.
  clinical assistant in surgery
Richard B. Price, M.D.
  clinical assistant in radiology
Galen Patchell Robbins, M.D.
  clinical assistant in medicine
Helen Hughes Schmidt, M.D.
  clinical assistant in radiology
Paul D. Shackelford, M.D.
  visiting lecturer in dermatology
Wilfred Erwin Wooldridge, M.D.
  visiting lecturer in dermatology
Bertrand Ray Worsham, M.D.
  clinical assistant in psychiatry and
  neurology

Martin M. Cummings[6] was named professor and chairman of the Department of Microbiology as of October 1, 1959, at a salary of $13,000 per annum, replacing Vernon Scott, professor of microbiology and temporary chairman of the department, following the resignation of Florene Kelly.

The State Regents for Higher Education approved the establishment of a School of Cytotechnology under the direction of the Department of Pathology in December, 1958, and as a result the first School of Cytotechnology in the Southwest was instituted at the Medical Center in April, 1959. The Oklahoma Division of the American Cancer Society and the Oklahoma State Department of Public Health supported the initial program with donations of $3,345 and $6,000, respectively.

Walter Hartford, the first resident in obstetrics and gynecology in 1947, was assistant professor of gynecology and pathology by 1959; and, after taking a two-week course in cytotechnology at the Dr. J. Ernst Ayers' laboratory in Montreal, Canada, Dr. Hartford started training cytology technologists in The Oklahoma Medical Center. The "school" was located on the sixth floor of the outpatient clinic wing of University Hospital. The physical facilities included one classroom, a laboratory, and a secretarial and storage room.

It was in such meager surroundings that the first students to take training in the technique of exfoliative cytology for detection of cancer spent their first six months. But as soon as accrediting groups had approved the curriculum of the new School of Cytotechnology, physicians in ever-increasing numbers began making a routine practice of taking vaginal smears, for, by then, trained

---

[6.] Dr. Cummings had been with the Veterans Administration in Washington, D.C., since 1949 and had been chief of the research service in the Department of Medicine and Surgery since 1953.

personnel had become available to handle the large volume of laboratory work.

Cytology, the study of the individual cell, was known to pathologists early in the middle of the nineteenth century, but it was not until 1939 that two scientists—George Papanicolaou and Herbert F. Traut—recognized hormonal changes on the individual cell and cellular changes related to neoplasia. Since that time it has become possible to make an early detection of cancer with a high incidence of accuracy.

All research programs, gifts, and grants from federal and voluntary agencies to the University of Oklahoma Medical Center for the fiscal year ending June 30, 1959, totaled $1,294,490. Approximately 14 per cent of this amount, which was $486,086 greater than the total figure for the previous year, was secured by the Department of Medicine, 14 per cent by the Department of Preventive Medicine and Public Health, 11.6 per cent by the Department of Psychiatry, and 11.5 per cent by the Department of Surgery. Thus for the second time grants brought into the state by teachers and researchers in the School of Medicine topped the appropriations allocated for operation of the school by the State Regents for Higher Education.

The research committee of the Medical Center, chaired by Richard W. Payne, did a great deal of detailed work to help develop research funds in 1959, and an estimated 120 faculty members were engaged in more than 100 research projects in clinical and basic science areas. Mention of only a few projects will suffice to illustrate the expansion of interests. J. R. Sokatch, assistant professor of microbiology, received a grant of $24,185 from the National Institutes of Health for research over a three-year period on pentose phosphate biosynthesis and a grant of $24,000 over the same period from the National Science Foundation in support of his work on oxidation of the branched chain amino acids.

The Department of Pediatrics received a grant of nearly $50,000 from the National Institute of Mental Health for its child study center to further enable the center to realize one of its chief aims—provision of cooperative, comprehensive care for mentally handicapped children. A surprisingly large number of children with specific reading disabilities resulted in the establishment of a developmental and remedial reading clinic, in cooperation with the city and state Departments of Special Education and the Children's Hospital school. The long range hope was that those many, many children, who would otherwise be advanced to high school or college without being able to read, might acquire this ability in a reading clinic.

At a departmental meeting on July 30, Harris D. Riley, chairman of the Department of Pediatrics, announced that financial aid of $147,479 was forthcoming from the National Institutes of Health to support some studies on the handicapped child, under the direction of Sylvia Richardson; $21,600 for training in pediatric neurology, directed by Lucius Waites; and $30,272 from the National Cancer Institutes for studies on leukemia, directed by Dr. Riley.

Kelly West, assistant professor of medicine, was the recipient of a $121,000 grant from the National Institute of Arthritis and Metabolic Diseases to train medical personnel in the field of diabetes, over a five-year period; and William

E. Jaques, head of the Department of Pathology, received a five-year grant of $150,000 from the National Heart Institute to support a program of advanced training for persons interested in academic and research pathology.

The National Heart Institute continued to support the research of Robert Bayley on the interpretation of electrocardiograms (with an electronic computer built to his own specifications) by awarding him a $125,866 grant. As director of the heart station at the University of Oklahoma Medical Center, Dr. Bayley earned an international reputation for his work on electrocardiography and was cited for "distinguished service to the research program of the American Heart Association." Along this same line, the Department of Physiology began developing a novel training program in 1959, under a five-year grant of $120,000 from the National Heart Institute, designed to bring undergraduate science teachers in state colleges and universities to the Medical Center for a summer course in cardiovascular physiology.

The Veterans Administration Hospital, the third major teaching hospital on the School of Medicine campus, was approved during the year for specialized treatment in cardiac surgery, corneal transplants, dermatology, medicine, neurology, radiation therapy, and thoracic surgery. More than 140 research projects were in progress there, with 75 papers being published in 1959.

Operation of the University Hospitals continued to present serious problems in the face of inadequate and unstable income, but Oklahoma was moving into the limelight anyway. In the fall of the year the Oklahoma Eye Bank became one of 15 eye banks over the nation to be affiliated with the Eye Bank for Sight Restoration in New York City. The State Lions Clubs, which sponsored the establishment of the bank here in 1957, continued to support the undertaking, which was housed in the annex to the School of Medicine building. The Oklahoma Lions Sight Conservation Foundation gave a complete set of surgical instruments for eye corneal transplant operations to the University Hospitals where much of the sight restoring surgery using live tissue was then being performed. In the first year and a half of operation the Oklahoma Eye Bank provided corneal material for 78 transplant procedures; and, after two years, 120 persons with practically no vision at all had received transplants of healthy corneas, donated to the eye bank from all areas in Oklahoma.

The postgraduate office conducted twenty courses for physicians on a variety of sbujects during the year, attended by 1,794 registrants at the Medical Center, 329 of whom were doctors from other states. This represented a 20 per cent increase in total registration over the previous year, much to the credit of Irwin H. Brown, director of postgraduate education, who was installed as president of the Oklahoma Chapter of the American College of Surgeons in 1959. Graduate training in the hospitals also increased both in quantity and quality, and needless to say, the awarding of a contract for architectural services on the medical research building by the university regents in June was a great stimulus to the training programs.

There were three visiting fellows, 19 interns, and 126 residents in University Hospitals commencing July 1, 1959. The total number of patients admitted to the hospitals in the ensuing year was 13,298 (3,830 at Children's Hospital and 9,468 at the main hospital). Total number of days of hospital care was 146,732 (63,990 at Children's and 82,733 at main) with the average number of patients per day (exclusive of newborns) 375.6, and the average number of days per patient (exclusive of newborns) was 12.6 (15.9 at Children's and 10.7 at main).

According to a report of the radiology department for the same period, 25,383 diagnostic x-ray examinations were made (9,907 at Children's and 15,476 at main); the clinical laboratories conducted 498,155 examinations. The heart station made 4,434 electrocradiograms, and the cytology laboratory carried out a grand total of 6,780 studies.

State appropriations for the University of Oklahoma for the year 1959–60 were $5,925,477 out of a total income of $8,653,566: for the School of Medicine, $1,003,754 out of a total income of $1,338,167; and for the University Hospitals, $2,646,705 out of a total income of $4,598,317. A long-range estimate of capital needs of the University of Oklahoma Medical Center (1959–69) for new construction or acquisitions reached an all time high of $12,385,000.

The total number of students enrolled in the School of Medicine for 1959–60 was 365, in the School of Nursing, 125. Ninety-two graduates received the M.D. degree in 1959. Thirteen nurses received the Bachelor of Science degree in Nursing and 31, the certificate of nursing. Seven medical students were awarded $600 special study fellowships financed with National Foundation for Infantile Paralysis monies.

On February 11 the university regents rescinded the requirement adopted November 13, 1952, that names of applicants for admission to the first-year class of the School of Medicine must be submitted to the regents for approval, returning the responsibility for acceptance of qualified applicants for admission to the freshman class to the School of Medicine. One hundred and four were selected to enroll on September 10, 1959. For the second successive year Mrs. Carl Owens of Chandler made a generous gift of $1,000 to finance two scholarships for students in the first-year class of the coming year.

In a report to President Cross on October 7, Dean Everett indicated that the faculty board of the School of Medicine believed the entering class could be increased to 120 admissions by 1963 with no loss of essential training of the students, provided some serious needs were fulfilled at the Medical Center by that time. The fact that the medical school rated in the upper half of all medical schools and, furthermore, of all state university medical schools, represented a major achievement, in the opinion of Dr. Everett, especially in view of the fact that our operating expenses were the fourth lowest of all state schools of medicine and the lowest of any medical school admitting 100 students in the first year.

Dean Everett also forwarded to Dr. Cross a resolution from the faculty board to the regents, requesting that the dean of the School of Medicine be authorized to permit the selection of ten additional students for the first-year class of medical school, with the proviso that they undertake a joint M.D.–Ph.D.

program, inasmuch as the National Institutes of Health were interested in developing such a combined endeavor. The plan called for fulfillment of all requirements of the university for both degrees over a period of six to seven calendar years, with no reduction of standards for either degree.

On the distaff side of "medical education in Oklahoma," Mrs. Mark R. Everett, wife of the dean of the School of Medicine, invited wives of full-time staff members of the school to attend a coffee at the Faculty House in March to stimulate interest in the organization of a volunteer service for University Hospitals. Special guests were Mrs. George L. Cross, wife of the president of the University of Oklahoma, Robert Lowe, superintendent of the University Hospitals, and Jennell Hubbard, director of nursing service. Subsequently, on April 14, officers were elected from the organizing nucleus, and a constitution and bylaws were approved for an auxiliary to the University Hospitals, with Mrs. James P. Dewar, president, Mrs. Carl W. Smith, vice-president, Mrs. Phillip E. Smith, secretary, Mrs. Floyd S. Cornelison, treasurer, and Mrs. Mark R. Everett, honorary chairman. Mrs. Louis J. West, Mrs. Vernon Scott, and Mrs. Paul Smith headed committees on initial projects in three fields: (1) information and guidance service for both patients and visitors; (2) sewing service offering at-home jobs for volunteers unable to do hospital duty; (3) a central supply service.

An embryonic corps of volunteers in red-and-white checked pinafores worked throughout the summer, and an expansion of services commenced in earnest in the fall, with the new Auxiliary to the University Hospitals recruiting and sponsoring volunteers from all walks of life, as part of a recently organized volunteer services division which coordinated the activities of all groups of individuals giving volunteer service in the hospitals.[7] Sixteen members of the University of Oklahoma Wives Club at Norman joined the auxiliary, seven of whom commuted regularly two days a month to serve in University Hospitals. Whatever the volunteer worker's skill or inclination, there was a task to match it.

The Oklahoma City Council of Jewish Women was the first civic group to join forces with the auxiliary to meet the needs for completion of a mobile food cart project, of which Mrs. Kenneth Richter was the able auxiliary chairwoman and Mrs. Edward S. Dauber chairwoman for the Council of Jewish Women. The council bought and equipped a food cart to service all clinic waiting rooms in University Hospital, and twenty-eight members of the council and the auxiliary staffed the cart five mornings a week for several years, selling food at cost.

[7.] In April, 1961, certificates of appreciation for assistance in the volunteer program at University Hospitals were presented to the following groups: Junior League, Junior Hospitality Club, Auxiliary to the University Hospitals, Junior Ready-to-Help Club, Village Lionesses, Del City Rebekah Lodge 151, University Women's Club of Norman, Council of Jewish Women, United Church Women, Tinker Officers Wives, Tinker NCO Wives, Barbers Union No. 743, Oklahoma Hospitality Club, International Association of Stage and Screen Employees, and the American Red Cross. Furthermore, 62 teenagers had assisted in hospital volunteer work.

Raymond Crews, superintendent of University Hospitals, in a letter to Mrs. James P. Dewar, president of the auxiliary, July 29, 1960, expressed sincere appreciation "for the wonderful service which your group has given," saying that the past year had been one of the best and most productive since the establishment of the hospitals in many ways, and that the auxiliary "had contributed in a major way to that success."

Mark R. Everett, director of the Medical Center and dean of the School of Medicine, wrote Mrs. L. M. Karchmer, president, Oklahoma City Council of Jewish Women, on October 22, 1962, saying that one of the major volunteer projects of the Auxiliary to the University Hospitals, for over three years, had been the mobile food cart in the waiting room of the outpatient clinics, with which the council was identified. "I cannot tell you how much we, the administration, and the patients appreciate the continued devotion and dependability of the members of your council who are giving their time and their energies to a most needed and rewarding volunteer service."

An indispensable function of the public relations office of the Medical Center in 1959 was a systematic release of news on a statewide basis, as a result of congenial working relationships with local newsmen—an ongoing cooperative effort in the preparation of a feature story or the release of information about patients to home papers.

Publications through which campus news and comment were regularly disseminated by the public relations office were the *Roundup*, a weekly with a circulation of 550, which included coverage of members of the part-time and full-time faculty; the *Commentary*, a quarterly with a circulation of 3,800, for alumni, faculty, and students of the School of Medicine; and the Medical Center section of the *Journal of the Oklahoma State Medical Association*. In addition to these sources of information, each employee and volunteer in the Medical Center was also a public relations person for the institution in his own right within his family and circle of friends and acquaintances.

Writing in the December, 1958, issue of the *Commentary* concerning graduates of foreign medical schools seeking further medical education in the United States, Dean Everett spoke of his recent visit to several European medical centers and of differences in temperament there and here.

We have a unique philosophy in America, not only in spirit of devotion to a profession but to its development and improvement. . . . Upon my return I observed faculty members with happy, alert faces—inspired tutors of our young men, devoted and dedicated beyond the ordinary call of duty, and enthusiastic with hopes, ideas, and plans that will lead to better instruction, research, and service.

I wish that you could share fully with me my strong conviction that an essential element of our progress is the freedom of all to voice opinions about our Medical Center's problems. To safeguard this precious heritage, each one has a duty to respect it, to uphold it and not abuse it. . . . Freedom to me is something precious that has to be protected continuously and utilized carefully through our lives and actions.

Chapter XXIV.
Reorganization of the
Alumni Association: 1960–61

Once more unto the breach they came—the alumni of the University of Oklahoma School of Medicine—with projected goals and enthusiasm for aiding the development of a medical center that would meet the state's long-range needs including support of the $35,500,000 bond issue for state institutional buildings, which was approved by the voters on July 5.

"As we have initiated and given influence to the development of the Oklahoma Medical Research Foundation, the alumni should foster the development of the School of Medicine," John R. Taylor, president of the alumni association, said, "the major plans to be worked out between the dean, members of the alumni assocation—and Mr. Hugh Payne in an advisory capacity—for its overall advancement and growth."

After Mr. Payne resigned as volunteer executive secretary of the alumni association in 1958, the alumni employed Lawrence W. Rember of Oklahoma City to fill the vacancy on a part-time basis until the university regents confirmed an appointment for Mr. Rember on a three-quarter-time basis as of July 1, 1960, at an annual salary of $6,000.[1]

One of Mr. Rember's first acts, upon receiving verification of his appointment, was to begin visiting the 37 trustees of the alumni association located throughout Oklahoma for the purpose of obtaining help and counsel—well aware that no matter how desperate the money requirements for developing the Medical Center might be, such requirements could not be realized "without the vehicle and channels to project the need to the proper sources."

In the reorganization of the alumni office, "Monte" DuVal was appointed as a liaison official between the faculty of the School of Medicine and its alumni for an exchange of ideas between the two groups and stimulation of every alumnus to work for the future progress of the Medical Center. About the same

[1] Mr. Rember, who received a Bachelor of Laws degree in May, 1960, at age 52, brought considerable medical and health experience to his new position, having served as nationwide field secretary of the American Medical Association for three years, as director of public relations for the American Hospital Association's Blue Cross Plans Commission for the United States and Canada for two years, and as director of public information for the American Red Cross for the seventeen-state midwestern area, including Oklahoma, for two years.

time, Governor Edmondson named Mark Johnson, a 1946 graduate of the School of Medicine, to the University of Oklahoma Board of Regents.

Adequate financing for development of the University of Oklahoma Medical Center for the next biennium—based on studies made by two committees appointed by former governors and by the university's Committee on Development of a Master Plan for the Medical Center—was as follows: for the School of Medicine, $1,440,000 each year; for the University Hospitals and the School of Nursing, $3,915,000; plus $2,970,000 as the biennial portion of a ten-year $14,850,000 construction fund. Other main goals were: (1) to encourage the medical postgraduate program, (2) to develop the alumni association into a more closely knit medical health unit, (3) to establish a beneficial liaison with students in the School of Medicine, and (4) to continue supporting further advancement of the Oklahoma Medical Research Foundation.

On October 23 a record 306 persons attended the banquet commemorating the fiftieth anniversary of the founding of the four-year School of Medicine and a half century of progress in medical education in Oklahoma. Robert Mayburn Howard, age 82, former chairman of the Department of Surgery, received the "Professor Emeritus of the Year" award presented annually by the alumni association.[2]

During the business session, W. F. Lewis, Lawton, was elected to succeed Dr. Taylor as president of the alumni association, and the alumni dedicated themselves "to such active support as may be required to guarantee implementation of the ten-year plan, recently approved by the regents of the University of Oklahoma for the development of the Medical Center; and to apprise the elected members of the legislature of Oklahoma, the executive divisions of the government of the state of Oklahoma, and its citizens of this goal—calling for an expenditure of $14,850,000 for land, buildings, and equipment, over the decade.''

Dean Everett concurred wholeheartedly in the aims and efforts of the alumni, for he felt that the Medical Center could not continue to go ahead for long with its programs without activation of the ten-year capital fund improvement program. "It is an unsound financial situation in which a faculty has to raise five dollars for every dollar allocated by the state,'' the dean said; and he reiterated that the size of our classes would have been curtailed long ago had it not been for the help of practicing physicians, the Oklahoma City veterans' hospital, private donors, and donations from federal and independent granting agencies. "Our school received $910,000 less budgeted university funds for basic operational needs, than the average American medical school for the fiscal year 1960–61,'' the dean said. "In 1958–59, the total operating cost of the University of Oklahoma School of Medicine was $4,504,100, of which

---

[2.] Dr. Howard had been in private practice in Oklahoma City from 1901, when he received his M.D. degree from the University of Michigan, until 1948. He had been a member of the Epworth faculty, when the clinical faculty of the four-year University of Oklahoma Medical School was formed in 1910, and had served as chief of staff of St. Anthony Hospital for 35 years.

only $32,000 was for general administration. During this same period, $742,241 of state of Oklahoma funds were allocated to the School of Medicine, and student fees provided $180,000, making a total of $922,241 compared with the $4,504,100 actual operating cost.''

While reviewing the contract for the proposed medical research building to be erected on the Medical Center campus in 1960 with Francis Schmehl, chief of the Health Sciences Research Facilities Branch, Washington, D.C., Dean Everett noted that several alternates had not been included in the contract; and in a letter to President Cross (presented to the university regents on January 6) he pointed out that ''all steps within our power'' should be taken to complete three floors of the building instead of just the one floor for which the present contract had provided, because we were technically in violation of our agreement with the granting agency of the federal government, if we did not intend to complete construction of the building according to original plans. Therefore, Dr. Everett requested that alternates be included in the contract at a total cost of $132,807 plus architect's fees in order to keep faith with the government agency which had originally extended the grant in 1957.

Fortunately, our additional financial commitments were eased when Mr. Schmehl approved transfer of federal grant funds available for purchase of mobile equipment to the government's share of funds for the construction project. Thus a three-year delay and an equivocal way to the realization of a goal was ended. The fact that the storm fiend of ancient mythology tried to foul up the ground-breaking exercises with an inclement snowstorm on January 5 merely forced the faithful into the auditorium of the School of Medicine building across the way for a mock ceremonial and a stirring talk by our guest speaker, Dr. Paul Weiss, head of the laboratory of developmental biology, Rockefeller Institute for Medical Research.

On January 13 the faculty board unanimously voted to petition the president and regents of the University of Oklahoma for designation of the new research building as the *Mark R. Everett Medical Research Laboratories*, saying that Dr. Everett has ''labored long and hard to make this new research building a reality, and that it seemed only fair to say that without his efforts it would never have come into being.'' And, in a letter addressed to Dr. Cross on February 9, Don H. O'Donoghue, chairman of the faculty board, wrote, ''This building was lost to us on two separate occasions and each time was rescued by the personal efforts of Dr. Everett.'' However, on February 17 the regents voted to reaffirm their previous policy of ''not naming buildings, financed wholly or in part by tax money, after people presently living.''

On June 9 the regents awarded a contract for construction of the addition to the Speech and Hearing Clinic to E. V. Cox Construction Company at a total cost of $172,936; and on June 27 the State Regents for Higher Education approved transfer of the administration and budget of the Speech and Hearing Clinic from the Norman campus to the Medical Center in Oklahoma City, with the name changed to the Speech and Hearing Division of the Medical Center and with qualified members of the department eligible for faculty appointments as of July 1, 1960.

Kirk Mosley became Oklahoma state health commissioner on July 1, following the resignation of Grady Matthews who had directed the Department of Public Health for the state of Oklahoma for 21 years.[3] William Schottstaedt, a member of the faculty since 1958, succeeded Dr. Mosely as chairman of the Department of Preventive Medicine and Public Health; and Hillard D. Estes, director of the Civil Aeromedical Research Institute in Oklahoma City, was appointed a consultant professor of research in the department. It was agreed that personnel of this institute were available to spend 25 per cent of their time for teaching purposes at the University of Oklahoma School of Medicine. Joseph White, professor of anesthesiology, replaced Dr. Mosley as associate dean in charge of special training and research programs.

Ben Nicholson relinquished his post as editor-in-chief of the *Journal of the Oklahoma State Medical Association* in February, after working six years to make it "second to none in its class." The June issue of the magazine carried a full page in tribute to the beloved pediatrician who not only edited a magazine but served as vice-president of Blue Cross and as clinical professor of pediatrics at the Medical Center, aside from his private practice.

The executive committee of the clinical faculty singled out Raymond Crews for commendation on June 11, upon the completion of his first year as superintendent of University Hospitals. On the same occasion John Schilling commented on the earmarks that were indicative of the effectiveness of administrative operations under Mr. Crews, and the university regents raised his salary to $12,000 per annum. Reginald Wilson, clinical professor of pediatrics at the University of British Columbia, Vancouver, who visited the Medical Center about this time, remarked that Raymond Crews was one of the most impressive hospital administrators he had ever met.

Harold A. Shoemaker, professor of pharmacology and toxicology and founder of the poison information center at the University of Oklahoma School of Medicine, died November 2, 1960, after 35 years of service to medical education. Singlehandedly, despite meager financing, he built the poison center (among the first ten in the nation) into an institution of considerable value to physicians in the state of Oklahoma. In addition to having been chairman of the Department of Pharmacology, Dr. Shoemaker was a former assistant dean and acting dean of the School of Medicine. Regrettably, within the year the poison information center—a service of the University of Oklahoma Medical Center—met its demise, at a time when there was no comparable service obtainable in the state.

Philip Johnson, chief of the radioisotope service at the Veterans Administration Hospital, resigned to become chief of a similar laboratory at Methodist Hospital in Houston, Texas, and associate in medicine at Baylor University. He was succeeded by Allen Hennes, assistant chief of the Veterans Administration medical service since 1958. Philip E. Smith was given the additional title of associate dean in charge of student affairs upon the resignation of A. N. Taylor.

[3.] Dr. Matthews moved into his new office in the School of Medicine building in August as professor of preventive medicine and public health.

Additions to the faculty roster in 1960 were as follows, making a total of 38 full-time faculty members in clinical departments:

Bruno Balke, M.D.
professor of research physiology
John Clark Brixey, Ph.D.
consultant professor of mathematical statistics in preventive medicine and public health
Robert T. Clark, Ph.D.
professor of research physiology
Hillard D. Estes, M.D., M.P.H.
consultant professor of research preventive medicine and public health
George Thomas Hauty, Ph.D.
professor of research physiology and psychiatry, neurology, and behavioral sciences
George J. Friou, M.D.
associate professor of medicine and research microbiology
James Albert Green, Ph.D.
associate professor of research biochemistry
Gunter R. Haase, M.D.
associate professor of neurology in medicine and associate professor of psychiatry, neurology, and behavioral sciences
Raymond F. Hain, M.D.
associate professor of pathology
Anton Lindner, M.D.
associate professor of pathology
Robert Arthur Patnode, Ph.D.
associate professor of microbiology
Pei Chin Tang, Ph.D.
associate professor of research physiology
David K. Trites, Ph.D.
associate professor of medical psychology in the department of psychiatry, neurology, and behavioral sciences
William Viavant, Ph.D.
consultant associate professor of computer science in the

department of preventive medicine and public health
Petar A. Alaupovic, Ph.D.
assistant professor of research biochemistry
Robert E. Coalson, Ph.D.
assistant professor of anatomy
Jennie Connery, M.S.
assistant professor of administrative medicine in preventive medicine and public health
Joe Mitchell Dabney, Ph.D.
assistant professor of physiology
Hazel I. McGaffey, M.D.
assistant professor of pathology
Jess Mack McKenzie, Ph.D.
assistant professor of research physiology
Chester M. Pierce, M.D.
assistant professor of psychiatry, neurology, and behavioral sciences
Howard B. Ruhm, Ph.D.
assistant professor of audiology in communication disorders
Olivia M. Smythe, M.A.
assistant professor of public health nursing in preventive medicine and public health
Edward Easton Soule, L.L.B.
assistant professor of medical jurisprudence in the department of medicine
William B. Stavinoha, Ph.D.
assistant professor of research pharmacology
Hooshang Taybi, M.D.
assistant professor of radiology
Helen Ross Walcher, M.A.
assistant professor of communication disorders
Paul W. Wigler, Ph.D.
assistant professor of research biochemistry

Mary Ida Abbott, M.D.
instructor in pediatrics
James Preston Bell, M.D.
instructor in orthopedic and
fracture surgery
Louis Joseph Bernard, M.D.
instructor in surgery
Charles M. Brodie, Ph.D.
instructor in medical psychology
in the department of psychiatry,
neurology, and behavioral
sciences
James Love Dunagin, M.D.
instructor in pediatrics
Ira Goldberg, Ph.D.
instructor in medical psychology
in the department of psychiatry,
neurology, and behavioral
sciences
Bernhard Horn, M.D.
instructor in anesthesiology
Jacob L. Kay, M.D.
instructor in pediatrics
Frank C. Knox, Jr., M.D.
instructor in psychiatry,
neurology, and behavioral
sciences
Robert Lewis Kramer, M.D.
instructor in ophthalmology
Joanne Marianos, M.S.
instructor in nutrition
Braxton Milburn, M.A.
instructor in communication
disorders
Robert Emmett Myers, M.D.
instructor in pediatrics
Franklin Nelson, Ph.D.
instructor in medical psychology
in psychiatry, neurology, and
behavioral sciences
Jimmy L. Simon, M.D.
instructor in pediatrics
Robert Edward Ashley, M.D.
clinical associate in psychiatry,
neurology, and behavioral
sciences

Ray Morton Balyeat, Jr., M.D.
clinical assistant in
ophthalmology
Carman E. Bloedow, M.D.
clinical assistant in medicine
David Childers, M.D.
visiting lecturer in pediatrics
William Robert Collins, M.D.
clinical assistant in
ophthalmology
William J. Craig, M.D.
clinical assistant in pediatrics
Ronald F. Crane, M.D.
clinical assistant in anesthesiology
Jere D. Guin, M.D.
visiting lecturer in dermatology
James W. Hampton, M.D.
clinical assistant in medicine
Gerald L. Honick, M.D.
clinical assistant in medicine
Larson Russell Keso, D.D.S.
clinical assistant in dental surgery
Adrian A. Kyriacopaulos, M.D.
clinical assistant in medicine
Robert D. Lindeman, M.D.
clinical assistant in medicine
James Ernest Mays, Jr., M.D.
clinical instructor in pediatrics
Dwane B. Minor, M.D.
visiting lecturer in dermatology
Riley W. Park, M.D.
clinical assistant in anesthesiology
Robert R. Phillips, M.D.
visiting lecturer in psychiatry
Lindberg J. Rahhal, M.D.
clinical assistant in radiology
Charles Lee Reynolds, Jr., M.D.
clinical assistant in urology
William Hale Simon, M.D.
visiting lecturer in pediatrics
Vernon G. Ward, M.D.
clinical assistant in medicine
Preston Wheeler, D.D.S.
clinical assistant in dental surgery
Johan Adolf Wulff, M.D.
clinical assistant in medicine

The 1959–60 report (in pamphlet form) of the Department of Surgery, University of Oklahoma Medical Center, outlined the scope and activities of the Department of Surgery and provided a source of valuable information regarding the department's teaching and training programs and its patient care; the total number of residents in training within the integrated four- and five-year general and thoracic surgical program at the time was 24. There were 305 surgical teaching beds available to the residency program, with only 5 per cent of the beds for private use. Resident stipends ranged from $2,400 for the first year to $5,600 for the fifth year.

Since the initiation of the open-heart surgery program in 1959, patients ranging in ages from two to fifty years came from all sections of Oklahoma to the Medical Center, where one or two such operations were performed weekly. Each surgery required a team of approximately twelve doctors, nurses, and technicians and lasted from two to four hours. With the aid of the Oklahoma Heart Association, a system of screening and obtaining blood donors in a patient's home community was developed, whereby donors were transported to the hospital on the morning of a scheduled operation. Successful results were realized in more than 80 per cent of the patients undergoing surgery.

Rainey Williams, assistant professor of surgery and a member of the open-heart surgery team, earned the distinction of becoming the School of Medicine's fourth Markle Scholar in 1960. And Monte DuVal, who was also a member of the surgery department and a member of Governor Edmondson's Committee on Higher Education, was appointed coordinator of the Medical Center development program.

A residency training program for dental surgeons was instituted in University Hospitals (the only place for dental training in the state) by the volunteer dental staff, and on October 12 the university regents formalized the status of the dental staff as a Division of Dental Surgery under the Department of Surgery, with the chairman, vice-chairman, and advisory committee of the new division to be chosen in accordance with bylaws applicable to departments of the School of Medicine.

Members of the ophthalmology department could not arrive at a formal majority decision to utilize the facilities of the Veterans Administration Hospital in their residency program because of some feeling that patient service as conducted by the veterans' hospital was against certain principles of private practice, which was an attitude reflecting opposition to "socialized medicine." However, when the Council on Medical Education notified Dean Everett that a three-year residency training program in ophthalmology had to be in operation by July 1, 1961, or the ophthalmology residency would be disapproved, the dean notified the department that it would need "every bit of help that the three teaching hospitals (main, Children's and veterans') can provide, in arranging to meet this requirement."

The Department of Orthopedic Surgery scored a first for the home front, according to an account in the June, 1960, issue of the *Commentary*, when the Orthopedic Letters Club, composed of about 75 orthopedists of the United States and several foreign countries (organized at the Medical Center ten years previously), initiated a program of orthopedic aid to Jordan, which would provide consultation services in the Middle East. Volunteers were asked to go to Jerusalem at their own expense and serve one month in rotation, at a time when the case load of patients was staggering, and there were no suitably qualified persons to do reconstructive orthopedic surgery in a country of two million inhabitants. Four doctors, former residents of Oklahoma, two of whom were then members of the faculty, went to the Middle East to participate in the program—Samuel T. Moore, Oklahoma City, John Jarrott, Hutchinson, Kansas, William Knight, Fort Smith, Arkansas, and William Harsha, Oklahoma City—earning jewels in their crowns for their humanitarian services.

The Department of Dermatology scored a first, too, for the Medical Center, when the American Board of Dermatologists accepted an invitation to give its annual examination west of the Mississippi, for the first time, during the week of January 11. Some twenty rooms in the radiology unit of University Hospital were readied for use, where a total of 116 candidates from 46 states were given their oral examinations.[4] And the University of Oklahoma Medical Center was selected as a site for an educational council examination for foreign medical graduates. Without having passed this examination, no foreign medical graduate was allowed to take further medical training in an accredited hospital in the United States.

Research and training grants rose to approximately $1,451,684 in 1960. Chase Mellon, Jr., executive vice-president of the National Fund for Medical Education, visited communities and key cities in the United States early in the year, in an effort to make the medical research program of the National Fund for Medical Education better understood, especially by United Fund committees.[5]

Doctors in the Department of Microbiology received some significant grants in 1960: Martin Cummings, chairman, received a $200,000 grant to support a training program in immunology for a five-year period from the National Institute of Allergy and Infectious Diseases, a training program designed for graduate and postdoctoral students; Everett Bracken, associate professor of microbiological research in pediatrics, received $32,300 from the National Science Foundation to support investigation over a two-year period of the mechanism of infection by viruses; and Vernon Scott, professor of microbiology, received two grants from the National Institutes of Health for continued support of two research projects. The National Institute of Neurological Diseases and Blindness awarded $48,710 to back his work for a five-year period on experimental herpes and simple infections in the fetus, and a grant of $29,517 for three years was awarded by the National Cancer Institute for studies on the nutrition and physiology of Rous sarcoma in vitro.

The National Cancer Institute also awarded $24,245 to the Cytotechnology

---

[4.] Under date of January 27, 1960, Beatrice Maher Kesten, secretary, American Board of Dermatology, wrote, "We have never experienced such genuine hospitality. . . . the new medical center, superbly arranged and equipped, was a revelation to us. . . . the kindly atmosphere which permeated the entire center was the most revealing aspect of all."

[5.] Dean and Mrs. Everett had the privilege and pleasure of accompanying Mr. Mellon during the Oklahoma and Arizona portions of his itinerary—a most rewarding personal experience, completely divorced from our gratitude for the monetary contribution in April of $37,260 from the National Fund for Medical Education.

School at the Medical Center to help support a cytoscreener training program for one year, making it possible to offer stipends to ten students, beginning in September, 1960.

L. J. West received $33,735 for continuation of his grant for graduate training and $7,222 toward undergraduate training in psychiatry; C. Herman Reece, instructor in dental surgery, was given a National Institutes of Health training grant in oral sciences, in the amount of $30,000 for the first year, with promise of four additional years of support; and William Schottstaedt, professor of preventive medicine and public health, received $85,450 in National Institutes funds for continued research training in biometry.

The Department of Pediatrics was awarded a four-year grant by the National Cancer Institute for studies on leukemia and solid tumors in infants and children; and Dr. Riley, chairman of the department, received a grant of $24,789 on June 30 from the National Foundation for Medical Scientific Research, Professional Education, and Medical Care to support the operation of a birth defects clinical study center.

Finally, the department of Health, Education and Welfare approved a supplemental application for a public health service grant from the fiscal year 1960 appropriation in an amount not to exceed $21,640 for movable scientific equipment.

The University of Oklahoma School of Medicine was one of twenty medical schools in the United States selected for study by the National Institutes of Health in 1960, in an effort to evaluate the effects of research grants to medical schools. And the Oklahoma school was one of six in the United States chosen for another study having to do with the evaluation of the effects of training grants.

In regard to the care of private patients in medical school hospitals by career teachers, the Liaison Committee on Medical Education (representing the executive council of the Association of American Medical Colleges) and the Council on Medical Service of the American Medical Association agreed that such private practice was proper and appropriate, provided: (a) that fees were established by the participating physician; (b) that the income from said fees was deposited in a separate fund of the University Medical School; and (c) that disbursements from the funds were made in accordance with a plan approved by the governing body of the faculty and by the University.

According to hospital statistics for 1959–60, the number of full-time hospital employees was 1,168, and the average patient stay in the hospital was only half as long as in the late thirties. The number of laboratory tests had increased eightfold in sixteen years, and the number of x-ray examinations was seven times the number made in 1944, with a similar rise in electrocardiogram readings. Estimated inpatient per diem cost, 1960–61, was $27. The outpatient clinics served 18,700 patients per year at this time at an estimated cost of $6 per diem—and the hospital was lucky if it collected. Representatives of 21 of the nation's medical schools had visited the Medical Center in recent years to study the unique patient care and teaching program of the outpatient department as instituted by Professor Wolf.

In the previous ten years clinical graduate training programs were initiated in the University Hospitals in cardiovascular diseases, diabetes, cancer, arthritis, psychiatry, pediatric neurology, infectious diseases, oral surgery, neurology, hematology, pathology, and other areas. In addition, ancillary teaching was instituted at the schools of physical therapy and cytotechnology, the degree program for the graduate nurse, vocational practical nurse training, courses for surgical technicians, and in-service instruction for other workers.

State appropriations for the University of Oklahoma for the year 1960–61 were $5,925,477 out of a total income of $8,895,551); for the School of Medicine, $1,003,754 from a total income of $1,232,320; and for the University Hospitals, $2,646,750 out of a total income of $4,436,300. The Oklahoma medical school was fourth lowest among state medical schools in operating income and eleventh lowest of all medical schools in the United States, Dean Everett advised the faculty on January 28. Nevertheless, a very influential visitor to the campus told the dean that this was one of two schools in the United States in which he had the greatest faith. "There are many people who have helped to build this school," the dean replied, and "there are many people who are helping to build it at present."

The total number of students enrolled in the School of Medicine in 1960–61 was 372; in the School of Nursing, 135. Eighty-five graduates received the M.D. degree in June, 1960, and three students received advanced degrees in medical science. Samih Y. Alami, Beirut, Lebanon, a graduate student here since 1957, became the thirty-first person to complete doctoral work at the Medical Center since the first group of graduate students received Ph.D. degrees in medical science in 1955. Eighty students were working toward graduate degrees in the Medical Center in 1960.

The W. K. Kellogg Foundation and Scholarship Fund, established in 1942 with money granted by the W. K. Kellogg Foundation, was available to worthy students in the School of Medicine up to $500 per year with a maximum of $1,000 during the four years; and Mrs. Carl Owens, Chandler, again made a gift of $1,000 to finance two scholarships for students in the entering class of the University of Oklahoma School of Medicine.

Twelve nurses received the Bachelor of Science in Nursing in 1960, and twenty-three received the certificate of nursing. The university regents appointed Helen Patterson, associate professor of nursing and director of the degree program, to the position of dean of the School of Nursing, effective November 15 at a salary of $8,500, and promoted her to the rank of professor. This action was in line with a recommendation of accrediting groups for schools of nursing, whose attitude represented preference for nursing instruction as a recognized university discipline.

Marie C. Mink, associate professor at the University of Oklahoma School of Nursing, was the 1960 winner of the Mary Mahoney Award for contributions to nursing. Mrs. Mink was cited for promoting minority group integration at the University of Oklahoma.

The fiscal year ending June 30, 1960, was the first year in the history of the University Hospitals that the university was reimbursed in full measure for medical care rendered to indigent children, and it was because a state agency, the Department of Public Welfare, under the direction of Lloyd Rader, had become responsible for the medical care of indigent children in the state of Oklahoma. "By accomplishing this," Dean Everett wrote Mr. Rader on June 27, 1960, "you have brought renewed opportunity and inspiration to the management of the University Hospitals, and you have helped insure the ability of the University Hospitals to render maximal care to its patients, especially to children.

"I know well that you recognize my personal gratitude and admiration for your honesty, intelligence, and industry, yet, I feel it is important for me to state this in writing. I will never forget this great friend and contributor to medical education."

Chapter XXV.
Promise of Fulfillment:
1961–62

 The Medical Center was slow in getting the legislative program off the ground for the biennium in
1961 but eventually made some significant gains,
largely because of the ceaseless efforts of alumni to present the center's needs to
officials of state government.

On March 22, with the blessing of House Speaker J. D. McCarty, George C.
Keys (Oklahoma County) authored and introduced House Bills No. 880 and
No. 881, to finance the first stages of the ten-year development plan for
expansion of the Medical Center. The two bills, cosponsored by the administration of the Medical Center and alumni association, called for an appropriation
of $950,000 for the purchase of real property, and $1,650,000 to finance the
first phase of construction of physical facilities and equipment.

On March 29, Robert Ellis, chairman of the legislative committee of the
alumni association, requested the trustees and officers and past presidents to go
into action. "This Friday, Saturday, and Sunday (March 30–April 2), while the
representatives and senators are at home," Dr. Ellis urged, "let's enlist
ourselves and any other physicians whom you know to let every one of the 165
legislators of Oklahoma know—by a personal visit, telephone call, or
telegram—just where we stand on House Bills No. 880 and No. 881. . . . If you
will do this, I think we"ll have it made." Numerous lawmakers, who had never
before heard from doctors in their districts, were favorably impressed with this
strategy, and they listened. However, a sales tax, called for by Governor
Edmondson and J. D. McCarty "to finance a decent program for the state of
Oklahoma during the next two years," failed of passage, and that spelled doom
for any appropriations to finance capital improvements. All other measures
suggested by the senate and house for raising revenue never even got off the
floor. But, in spite of the shortage of anticipated income, the legislators, on the
last day of the legislative session (July 28), did vote an appropriation of
$200,000 for purchase of real property for expansion of Medical Center
facilities—from monies in the general revenue fund for the fiscal year ending
June 30, 1962. And, in the eyes of the alumni of the School of Medicine, the
house and senate, in making such an appropriation, "had not only committed
themselves in a financial way to implementing the ten-year Medical Center
development plan, but had bound themselves to its fulfillment."

Because of their splendid relationship with legislators, there were still other accomplishments for which the alumni could legitimately take some credit in 1961: (1) activation by the legislature of the $30.5 million bond issue voted by the people of Oklahoma in July, 1960, to provide financial assistance to the institutions of higher education, including $1.1 million for the Medical Center; (2) establishment of a board of unexplained deaths (Senate Bill No. 81), which replaced the outmoded county coroner system; (3) an amendment modifying beneficially the Anatomical Board Act; and (4) a resolution of commendation for two full-blooded Osage Indians (Charles J. Shaw of Burbank and John Atkin of Grainola), who graduated from the University of Oklahoma School of Medicine on May 21, 1961.

Apropos of the new board of unexplained deaths, Oklahomans should be grateful to one alumnus in particular, the late W. Floyd Keller, clinical professor of pathology at the School of Medicine, who labored long and hard for passage of Senate Bill No. 81, only to learn that the legislature had overlooked making any specific appropriation for the services of personnel necessary for setting up the first State Medical Examiner System in Oklahoma. This was a great disappointment to Dr. Keller, and all effort seemed to have been in vain when the attorney general ruled that the medical school, itself, could not use any of its funds for the system. Then, once more up to the breach stepped two alumni—Dr. Keller himself as medical examiner on a temporary basis, to set up a state-wide system of medical examiners, and F. R. Hassler, director of the State Health Department Communicable Disease Control Laboratories, as deputy examiner. Serving on the three-member State Medical Examiner Commission, which officially appointed Doctors Keller and Hassler, were Mark R. Everett, dean of the School of Medicine, Kirk Mosley, state health commissioner, and Ralph Venamon, director of the State Crime Bureau.

Another legislative act, authorizing the creation of a School of Dentistry at the Medical Center—introduced in the house by Representative Bryce Baggett and enrolled as House Bill No. 829—received the blessing of the university regents on March 1 (a reaffirmation of the stand they had taken earlier, on January 14, 1954) and was signed by Governor Edmondson on July 21, 1961. But, unfortunately, this bill, too, carried no appropriation for implementing the provisions of the act, so was only a step in the right direction.[1]

Meanwhile, the State Regents for Higher Education had gone along with legislative intent in February, when they allocated $877,859 to the University

---

[1.] The act requested that a study report and comprehensive plan for initiation of the School of Dentistry be submitted by the State Regents for Higher Education to the twenty-ninth legislature. This report was received in January, 1963. It estimated the cost by the end of the fourth year as approximately $6 million for a facility for entering classes of 60 dental students and $895,000 as a yearly operating budget. This was the first positive step toward the development of a College of Dentistry in the Medical Center; the report was not activated until some years later. Francis J. Reichmann, a champion of dental education, devoted years of effort and patient endeavor to this project.

of Oklahoma, out of a $4,000,000 supplemental appropriation to state colleges: $148,706 to the School of Medicine and $392,109 to University Hospitals. And again on March 1 they were asked to seek an emergency appropriation of $75,000 toward underwriting losses due to severe flooding in the Department of Radiology in University Hospital.

On the night of February 17, following a cloudburst in the vicinity of the Medical Center, surface water rushed over the north portion of the campus, crossed Thirteenth Street, and inundated the lower floor of the radiology wing in University Hospital. This resulted in disastrous flooding despite attempts of hospital employees to stop it. Personnel from Oklahoma City's fire and engineering departments and personnel of the Medical Center worked tirelessly through the night, rescuing equipment and commencing the work of cleaning and decontaminating the area. Flood waters had mixed with sewage escaping from the sanitary sewer system, contributing to a serious health hazard. Effective work became practically hopeless and lives were endangered when a section of concrete flooring was blown up by the pressure of outside water.

It is to the credit of representatives of the legislature and the governing boards of the Medical Center that they visited the damaged quarters personally to witness the destruction—Governor Edmondson, House Speaker J. D. McCarty (donning boots and inspecting the havoc while the flood was in progress), President Cross, Tom Sexton (from the office of the State Regents for Higher Education), and the house appropriations committee led by Lou Allard of Drumright. House Bill No. 878, introduced by Representative Allard, appropriated $58,446 toward underwriting losses sustained during the flooding.

The University of Oklahoma Medical Center was unique in 1961 in that it combined a private, a state, and a federal institution on its campus, all dependent upon the federal government for matching monies and for many of their research grants (principally from the National Institutes of Health). True, $400,000 of the total construction cost of the new medical research building had been provided by a federal grant, but, since nothing had been appropriated by the state for conducting research there, all work carried on in the building had to be grant-supported; and the unfinished fifth floor had to be completed and equipped with grants-in-aid monies. This was an extraordinary bargain for the taxpayers of Oklahoma but a tall order for the administration and the faculty, since some medical schools were in a better position to lobby for federal assistance than others.

In any event, Dean Everett made a trip to Washington to discuss with Wilbur J. Cohen, undersecretary of Health, Education and Welfare the possibility of congressional action on behalf of medical education per se and financial operating assistance in particular for schools of medicine in need of such help.

The University of Oklahoma School of Medicine needed about $500,000 a year to stabilize its operation, according to Dr. Everett, ''which leaves much in the land of limbo,'' he said. In addition, there was the question of matching funds for modernization, expansion, and construction of medical and dental schools, to say nothing of the need to help the less fortunate schools into a status which would permit them to increase the size of their classes in the next few years.

Senator Robert Kerr, who was advised of Dean Everett's visit in Washington, pledged "to work to secure the passage of a bill in a mannre that will be of benefit to the University of Oklahoma Medical School"; and Senator Monroney, following his visit here for the dedication of the medical research building, wrote that no senator was more dedicated to the cause of better medical education than he, and that, as a member of the Subcommittee on Appropriations for the Department of Health, Education and Welfare, he would "work for the best possible bill."[2]

The medical research building was dedicated on March 11 in ceremonies presided over by Don H. O'Donoghue, chairman of the faculty board. Mark R. Everett, director and dean, introduced the guest speaker, Senator Mike Monroney, who said he was standing on a site where he "once rode a bicycle over a rutted country road." Referring to the construction as a partnership operation of federal and state governments, Senator Monroney asserted that "there is no investment so capable of eternal dividends as this building; the interest will be compounded through the remainder of time." Answering his own question, "Is it worth it?" ($800,000), the senator reminded his audience that the total yearly national cost for research support amounted to approximately $715 million, whereas the annual cost of disease was around $35 billion; "and another $5 billion is spent in the greeting card industry, which has a mainstay of get-well cards," the senator said.[3]

Major research programs were launched at the Medical Center in 1961, with two clinical research centers being established by means of grants totaling $4 million over a period of seven years.

A birth defects center was set up at Children's Memorial Hospital to serve the Southwest, with an initial $28,110 grant-in-aid from the March of Dimes to Harris D. Riley, Jr., chairmen of the Department of Pediatrics, as director of the new center. Basil O'Connor, president of the National Foundation, dedicated the center on January 25, preceding a symposium on congenital malformations.[4] Our local scientists and others of national repute reported their evaluations of research into the causes of birth defects that bring crippling or

---

[2] Letters in the dean's file dated respectively March 6 and March 8.

[3] "Now that our medical research building has been dedicated," Dean Everett wrote Bryce Baggett on March 15, "I would like to tell you how magnificent your help to us has been."

[4] Mr. O'Connor wrote Dean Everett from Washington on February 2 that he had come away thoroughly impressed by the presentations at the symposium and "with the feeling that the National Foundation could hardly have found a more felicitous locale and university medical school for collaboration on such a symposium, the first of its kind we have helped to sponsor." And Charles C. Bennett, science editor of the National Foundation, wrote Imogene Patrick, public relations director of the Medical Center, that she had "set a high precedent in friendly and result-getting cooperation for other university public relations departments to match."

disfigurement—or even early death—to children, with emphasis on ''better early diagnostic methods.''

Gifts and grants for research and special training programs reached an all time high of $3,411,288 during the fiscal year 1961–62. Dr. Riley and Sylvia O. Richardson, jointly, were awarded $48,052 by the National Institutes of Health for a project on collaborative management of mental retardation to run from September 1, 1961, to August 31, 1962. Dr. Riley was also awarded a $347,960 grant from the same source for the period December 1, 1961, through December 31, 1962, to establish a multicategorical clinical research center on the School of Medicine campus. This grant included remodeling a section of Children's Memorial Hospital into a research area, and Senator Monroney assured Dr. Riley that financial support would be continued for six additional years, up to a total of $2,000,000.

A second grant from the National Institutes of Health, promising two million dollars over a period of seven years, was for a neurological research center, with Stewart G. Wolf, Jr., head of the Department of Medicine, as the principal investigator. In the first stages of this research project, attention was focused on the relationship between the nervous system and arterial disease, branching out into the field of hypertension later on in the study. These two major grants to Dr. Riley and to Dr. Wolf gave the University Hospitals their first beds (14) maintained exclusively for research patients.

The National Institutes of Health awarded another grant over a period of five years to William Schottstaedt, head of the Department of Preventive Medicine and Public Health, to set up a medical research computer center on the School of Medicine campus. This grant of $124,399 was for the purpose of processing health research data at high speeds and training computer personnel to operate the scientific equipment essential to the purpose. The computer center became an arm of the biostatical unit directed by James A. Hagans, associate professor of medical biostatistics.

It is worthy of note that the National Institute of Dental Research awarded a $185,000 five-year training grant to the Medical Center on March 13 to develop a Master of Science degree program in dentistry in Oklahoma, with emphasis on oral surgery, anesthesiology, childrens dentistry, or dental research. This grant was a boon to the Division of Dental Surgery, Department of Surgery, since heretofore no opportunity for advanced training in dentistry in Oklahoma had been available, other than at the Medical Center. The first internship in dental surgery was initiated in 1923 in University Hospitals. By 1953 the Division of Dental Surgery was training two interns each year, and in 1957 the oral surgery residency program was approved by the American Dental Association. A restorative dentistry internship was started at Children's Memorial Hospital in 1959, and an important milestone was reached in June, 1960, when the first trainee to complete the full three years of training for certification by the American Board of Oral Surgery was awarded a Master of Science degree by the University of Oklahoma. Miraculously, through the years the part-time dental faculty had kept alive a spark for dental education in this state under the aegis of Francis J. Reichmann, while affording professional services for patients in the University Hospitals as well.

On October 7 the university regents appointed Carl E. Schow, oral surgeon of Lawton, as the first full-time chairman of the Division of Dental Surgery and director of the oral surgery training program, effective September 1 (succeeding A. R. Drescher).

Two powerful electron microscopes were acquired in 1961 through National Institutes of Health grants at a cost of about $31,000 apiece—one for the Departments of Pathology and Medicine, and one for use in research by William E. Jaques, head of the Department of Pathology; and, last but not least, the National Cancer Institute supported our cytotechnology training program for another year with a grant of $32,000 for ten training scholarships.

Federal appropriated research funds for the Veterans Administration Hospital for the period July 1, 1960, to June 30, 1961, amounted to $279,376 out of a total of $293,186 in research grants. The Oklahoma Medical Research Foundation received, for the same period, $381,412 in federal research grants and contracts, and $1,052,242 in nonfederal grants and contributions for programs of research conducted by faculty members of the School of Medicine.

The push to finish and equip the top floor shell space in the new medical research building as a research facility for environmental health got under way in Bethesda, Maryland, on February 2 (the day of the severe snowstorm in the Washington area), when Dean Everett and Raymond Crews visited with Francis Schmehl, Health Research Facilities Branch, Division of Research Grants, Department of Health, Education and Welfare. Subsequently, on February 20 application for a grant-in-aid award for health research facilities construction was made by the University of Oklahoma Medical Center to the above-mentioned agency of the federal government; and on March 21 a grant of funds was awarded, subject to certain limitations: expenditure of grant funds for construction and fixed equipment was not to exceed $75,000, and expenditure for movable equipment was not to exceed $7,689—all of which was subject to the raising of matching monies.

Carl Nau,[5] who had applied for the position of director of an institute of environmental health at the University of Oklahoma Medical Center, was subsequently appointed by the university regents on June 15, effective July 1, at a salary of $12,500, plus $4,500 from the state health department.

Dr. Nau, singlehandedly, raised $89,500 in contributions from industrial firms, in amounts ranging from $500 to $15,000, and the supplemental grant of $82,500 was approved by the surgeon general. On October 7 the regents awarded the contract for completion of the top floor of the medical research building on a bid of $157,344.

The School of Medicine received a $16,000 grant in August from the Avalon Foundation for student scholarships, which was the first gift by any foundation

[5.] Dr. Nau was head of the Department of Preventive Medicine and Public Health at the University of Texas medical branch in Galveston at the time and a member of the toxicology committee of the National Research Council.

for medical student scholarships across the board.[6] The sum, deposited in a fund known as the Avalon Trust Fund, was available until expended "for nonrefundable scholarships for deserving medical students to pursue their medical education." The only student scholarships available before this were the $1,000 per year awards made by Mrs. Carl Owens of Chandler, Oklahoma, to finance two students in the entering class of the School of Medicine.

State doctors voted to support a loan and scholarship fund for medical students in 1961 by increasing the Oklahoma State Medical Association dues by five dollars per year; and the constitution and bylaws of the association were amended in order to permanently establish the financial aid to education committee, and "The Oklahoma State Medical Association Loan and Scholarship Trust Fund."

According to the minutes of the university regents, April 13, 1961, George Ferguson deeded 160 acres of land in Texas County, Oklahoma, to the University of Oklahoma, income from same to go "for the use and benefit of the Crippled Children's Hospital." Also at a meeting of the regents on October 7, President Cross presented a schedule of cash and securities amounting to $79,861, willed to the University by Florence E. Daniel for the use and benefit of the Children's Memorial Hospital.[7]

Four members of the faculty departed this life in 1961: John Evans Heatley, professor emeritus of radiology, died on January 20; John Lamb, chairman of the Department of Dermatology and past president of the American Dermatological Association and the American Adacemy of Dermatology, died on February 23; Donald W. Branham, full-time chairman of the Department of Urology and chief of the urology service in the Veterans Administration Hospital, died on June 20; and Ray M. Balyeat, associate professor emeritus of medicine, died on July 2.[8] And, according to a news release in the *Daily Oklahoman*, October 21, 1961, Jacques P. Gray, former dean of the University of Oklahoma School of Medicine was reported to have died at Detroit, Michigan, at the age of 61.

The following changes in appointments were made during the year: Richard W. Payne was appointed chairman of the Department of Pharmacology on January 4 at an annual salary of $10,200, to succeed Paul Smith who resigned on January 1; Oren T. Skouge, associate professor of medicine, was given the additional title of consultant to the director of the Medical Center for interagency affairs, effective January 1; Regent Mark Johnson was appointed to the regents' committee on the medical school on January 4 and given a leave of

---

[6.] The Avalon Foundation had been created by Alisa Mellon Bruce of New York City some 20 years previously.

[7.] The bequest was accepted unanimously by the regents, on the condition that the total sum of $79,861 be invested, with only the income from the investment being used for the benefit of Children's Memorial Hospital.

[8.] By authorization of the faculty on January 27, a memorial fund was set up (through voluntary contributions) so that a memorial book might be purchased as an expression of respect for each past member of the faculty.

absence without pay as instructor in medicine, April 1, 1961, through March 31, 1964; Marion de Veaux Cotten was appointed professor and chairman of the Department of Pharmacology effective July 1 at a salary of $16,999; Phyllis E. Jones was appointed chairman of the Department of Dermatology, as of March 1, to succeed John Lamb, deceased; Kurt M. Dubowski was made director of the clinical chemistry and toxicology laboratories in the University Hospitals and associate professor of clinical biochemistry and toxicology at a salary of $16,000, effective September 15; and Francis J. Haddy was appointed head of the Department of Physiology and associate professor of medicine, as of the same date, at a yearly salary of $17,000.

Stewart G. Wolf's salary was increased from $13,000 to $20,000 annually, by virtue of a trust fund on August 3, and the salary of Ray Ridings, professor of radiology and director of the isotope laboratories and x-ray department, was raised to $19,000. Dr. Ridings was given the extra title of coordinator of cancer teaching.

Early in January the residency review committee for radiology, representing the American Board of Radiology and the Council on Medical Education and Hospitals, approved the radiology program at the University of Oklahoma Medical Center, to include University Hospitals, Veterans Administration Hospital, and Wesley Hospital for three years of resident training.

There were 130 faculty members in the Department of Medicine in 1961, and 63 in the Department of Psychiatry, Neurology, and Behavioral Sciences. New appointments to the faculty were as follows:

Marion de Veaux Cotten, Ph.D.
professor of pharmacology
Francis J. Haddy, Ph.D., M.D.
professor of physiology and
associate professor of medicine
James A. Merrill, M.D.
professor of gynecology and
obstetrics
James Arthur Cutter, M.D.
associate professor of
anesthesiology
Kurt M. Dubowski, Ph.D.
associate professor of clinical
chemistry and toxicology in
biochemistry and pathology
Marshall E. Groover, Jr., M.D.
associate professor of medicine
Lerner B. Hinshaw, Ph.D.
associate professor of research
physiology
John W. Kelly, Ph.D.
associate professor of pathology
Gaylord Shearer Knox, M.D.
associate professor of radiology

Carlton E. Melton, Jr., M.D.
associate professor of research
physiology
Stanley R. Mohler, M.D.
associate professor of research
preventive medicine and public
health
Larry J. O'Brien, Ph.D.
associate professor of research
physiology
P. F. Tampietro, Ph.D.
associate professor of research
physiology
Kurt A. Weiss, Ph.D.
associate professor of research
physiology
T. Glyne Williams, M.D.
associate professor of preventive
medicine and public health and
psychiatry, neurology, and
behavioral sciences
Margaret Lowe Bogle, M.S.
assistant professor of nutrition

Reagan Howard Bradford, M.D.
  assistant professor of research
  biochemistry
Lyle W. Burroughs, M.D.
  assistant professor of pediatrics
  and consultant in allergy,
  otorhinolaryngology
Marshall Edelson, Ph.D., M.D.
  assistant professor of psychiatry,
  neurology, and behavioral
  sciences
Wallace Friedberg, Ph.D.
  assistant professor of research
  biochemistry
J. T. Jabbour, M.D.
  assistant professor of neurology
  in psychiatry, neurology, and
  behavioral sciences and pediatrics
Joanne I. Moore, Ph.D.
  assistant professor of
  pharmacology
Jiro Nakano, M.D.
  assistant professor of
  pharmacology
Emogene Ogle, M.S.
  assistant professor of nutrition
Edward Newman Brandt, Jr.,
  Ph.D., M.D.
  instructor in medical
  biomathematics in preventive
  medicine and public health
Samuel Edward Dakil, M.D.
  instructor in otorhinolaryngology
Royal B. Dunkelberg, D.D.S.
  instructor in dental surgery
Robert W. Geyer, M.D.
  instructor in radiology
Theresa Brey Haddy, M.D.
  instructor in pediatrics
John D. Kyriacopaulos, M.D.
  instructor in medicine
John Barry Massey, M.D.
  instructor in psychiatry,
  neurology, and behavioral
  sciences

Orrin Walter Pearson, D.D.S.
  instructor in dental surgery
Bruce R. Pierce, M.A.
  instructor in communication
  disorders
Lou Ann Pilkington, Ph.D.
  instructor in physiology
Marilyn Porter, M.D.
  instructor in pediatrics
John Earl Ramsey, Jr., M.D.
  instructor in gynecology and
  obstetrics
Jack B. Austermann, D.D.S.
  clinical assistant in dental surgery
Richard Harold Bottomley, M.D.
  clinical assistant in medicine
Sylvia Stakle Bottomley, M.D.
  clinical assistant in medicine
Thomas Joseph Guthrie, D.D.S.
  clinical assistant in dental surgery
Phillip N. Hood, M.D.
  research associate in pediatrics
Jake Jones, Jr., M.D.
  visiting lecturer in pediatrics
John M. Kalbfleisch, M.D.
  clinical assistant in medicine
Ahmet L. Kutkam, M.D.
  research associate in pathology
John Patrick Naughton, M.D.
  clinical assistant in medicine
Ira Tom Parker, M.D.
  clinical assistant in medicine
George Victor Rohrer, M.D.
  clinical assistant in medicine
Jerry Benjamin Scott, Ph.D.
  research associate in physiology
Hilli Sevelius, M.D.
  clinical assistant in medicine
Ernest George Shadid, M.D.
  clinical assistant in psychiatry,
  neurology, and behavioral
  sciences
William F. Slagle, Jr., D.D.S.
  clinical assistant in dental surgery

The Departments of Gynecology and Obstetrics were combined into a single department by the university regents on April 13, 1961, to be known as the Department of Gynecology-Obstetrics; and James Merrill was appointed head of the new department, becoming the first full-time professor and chairman of the combined departments on May 1 at a salary of $13,000. Dr. Merrill was also named consultant to the state health department, with an additional stipend of $5,000.[9] A joint undertaking of the state health department and the Departments of Pediatrics, Gynecology-Obstetrics, and Preventive Medicine and Public Health—a perinatal project—combined research with teaching services to evaluate the relationships of obstetrical and neonatal factors to infants' need for special care. The subjects for the study comprised all patients admitted to University Hospital for delivery and their offspring.

Aversion of certain members of the Department of Ophthalmology to utilizing 20 beds available for teaching at the Veterans Administration Hospital reached major proportions during the year, and the administration was constrained to insist that the department accept the policy of the faculty, inasmuch as the veterans' hospital was an integral teaching unit of the medical school, both officially and by tradition, with every physician employed there a member of the faculty. In a letter on July 28 addressed to Doctor James P. Luton, chairman of the ophthalmology department advisory committee, Dean Everett spoke of the urgency of offering a third year residency or losing the ophthalmology residency program entirely; and he further stated that, as director of the Medical Center, it was his duty to see that "we grow in a forward manner, which necessarily means the utilization of existing facilities," asserting further that it was his desire to do everything possible to help without interfering. James R. Reed, chairman of the Department of Ophthalmology, informed Dr. Everett on September 9 that the ophthalmology residency program had been changed from two to three years, including training in the Veterans Administration Hospital.

During the year ending June 30, 1961, there were 3,366 referrals made to the social service department of University Hospital, an increase over the previous year but, more important, a continued increase in the number of referrals from the medical staff. This seemed to indicate that paramedical staffs were calling certain situations to the attention of the social service staff, while the patient was still in active medical treatment. Of 31,295 interviews and conferences held during the year, approximately 43 per cent or 13,465 were conducted with patients and their families.

University Hospitals were running at three dollars per diem less than the national average—$27.10 compared to $30.19—which could have been credited to underpaid employees who were subsidizing the costs; for, of 941 employees in the hospitals, 51.8 per cent were getting less than $200 per month. Even at that, the $27.10 patient cost per day was considerably over the 1954 cost of $17.47 per day, and laboratory tests over the same period doubled on nearly the same number of patients (18,000–19,000); the number of x-ray tests

[9] Dr. Merrill was formerly assistant professor of obstetrics and gynecology at the University of California Medical Center in San Francisco and had the distinction of being a Markle Scholar, the sixth member of the faculty of the University of Oklahoma School of Medicine to hold such a designation. Dr. Henry N. Kirkman, assistant professor of pediatrics, received the fifth Markle Scholarship in April.

increased from 33,000 to 81,800; and the number of physical therapy treatments from 23,908 to 41,617.

State appropriations for the University of Oklahoma for the year 1961–62 were $6,223,552 out of a total income of $9,854,478; for the School of Medicine, $1,067,277 out of a total income of $1,280,107; and for the University Hospitals, $2,646,705 out of a total income of $4,880,415.

The university regents authorized the School of Medicine to plan its commencement exercises "on a geographic basis" in 1961, because medical personnel favored a commencement separate from the one in Norman. Hence, 83 graduates of the University of Oklahoma School of Medicine received the M.D. degree in Oklahoma City University Auditorium on May 21, 1961, with Acting President Pete McCarter presiding.

Two recognition awards were established by the Mark Allen Everett Foundation, Oklahoma City, in 1961, for outstanding achievement in medical school—the Coyne H. Campbell Award to a junior student and the Mark R. Everett Award to a senior—each award carrying an honorarium of $50. Two other awards were set up to be given annually by doctors in recognition of outstanding work on the part of medical students: the Harry Wilkins Award in neuroanatomy and the Peter Russo Award in recognition of the highest scholastic record in radiologic anatomy.

On August 3, 1961, the regents rescinded action taken on May 3, 1937, which limited admissions to the entering class in the School of Medicine to not more than 20 per cent from any one county in the state. For the year 1961–62 there were 385 students (364 men and 21 women) enrolled in four classes.

Thirteen nurses received the Bachelor of Science degree and twenty-three received the certificate in nursing in 1961. Approximately 500 persons attended the fiftieth anniversary celebration of the University of Oklahoma School of Nursing, with Opal Filson, president of the alumni association, presiding. This was the School of Nursing's first homecoming and the principal speakers were Monte DuVal and Raymond Crews.

Under the direction of Irwin Brown, director of postgraduate education at the University of Oklahoma Medical Center, a special television series of postgraduate courses for Oklahoma physicians was inaugurated during the year through the combined efforts of the Medical Center, the Oklahoma State Medical Association, and the Oklahoma Educational Television Authority. One of the first television medical postgraduate series in the nation, the programs were televised "Always on Tuesday."

Interest in the long-range program for the Medical Center developed gradually during the twenty-eighth legislative session, and, in spite of difficulties, the house and senate passed a portion of Bill No. 880 ($200,000) for purchase of some additional land for the university, thus conceding token support, at least, for further changes in the landscape and physical profile of the Medical Center.

In the words of Dean Everett, "The success we enjoyed in getting funds from the legislature can be attributed to the untiring and dogged efforts of Monte

DuVal and Larry Rember, who afforded us liaison at the capitol of the sort we had never had before, and to the Trustees of the Alumni Association who contacted their legislators at home, urging them to support our cause.'' Reflecting on the triangle of governor, legislature, and State Regents for Higher Education, there was little doubt but that more progress had been made in getting recognition of the needs of the Medical Center with past governors and legislators than with the State Regents for Higher Education.

Opportunity for research was the lodestone that drew men to the University of Oklahoma School of Medicine from over the nation during these years—men who were willing to go to bat five to one for funds other than those appropriated by the state of Oklahoma. It was a gallant era, engendered by good will and noble purposes, well illustrated in an article by Imogene Patrick in the September issue of *Sooner Magazine*, entitled ''Hands to Mend the Heart—the Modern Miracle of Surgery.''

Chapter XXVI.
Esprit de Corps:
1962–63

The dean of the University of Oklahoma School of Medicine was back in Washington on January 24, 1962, where he was introduced to the House of Representatives Committee on Interstate and Foreign Commerce—holding hearings on House Resolution 4999, which was designed to furnish assistance to medical schools confronted with very serious problems.[1] In a statement filed with the committee, Dean Everett urged all who had the opportunity to take a position on the bill to "support it with conviction" and stated that the aid which the act proposed for medical schools demonstrated judicious interest by members of Congress in the future health status of the American community.

Two further statements were filed with the committee on February 9 through Representative John Jarman, one general and one stressing how much it would mean to Oklahoma if matching construction funds for teaching facilities under the ten-year development program at the University of Oklahoma Medical Center could be made available by Congress through H.R. 4999. Dean Everett again urged that "serious consideration be given to this bill and that all contentions not directly related to the problem be submerged in a desire to help medical schools of America surmount their difficult circumstances."

On October 2, 1962, the faculty of the University of Oklahoma School of Medicine urged that a night letter be sent to the Oklahoma members of the House of Representatives, urging "support in passage of amended H.R. 4999, soon to appear on the House floor"—legislation which would assist medical education in Oklahoma and the entire nation. This was about one year before the bill was finally passed.

The Liaison Committee on Medical Education, representing the American Medical Association and the Association of American Medical Colleges, made a survey of the University of Oklahoma School of Medicine from January 29 to February 1, 1962.[2] In the full report of the survey the members of the team

[1] Senate Bill No. 1072, of which Senator Robert S. Kerr was cosponsor, was identical with H.R. 4999.

[2] In a letter under date of February 7, Edward S. Peterson, expressed thanks for the team and for himself personally, to Dean Everett and his associates for "hospitality perfect in every way," and "special gratitude to Lora Johnson for her attentive concern for our welfare from the moment of arrival to the moment of departure."

extended their "congratulations to all associated with the School of Medicine of the University of Oklahoma for a decade of achievement and progress, the more remarkable in face of the limited financial resources made available." Later, full accreditation was unanimously voted by members of the Council on Medical Education and Hospitals, with extraordinary compliments to the medical school and to its dean.

Although the triangle determined the "limited resources" for the Medical Center each biennium, actually, state funds were supporting only 43 per cent of each professor's salary. While the administration and individual faculty members attempted to build the salaries up, chiefly through solicitation of training and research grants, it reached only to 77 per cent of the national average. At the same time, the average amount appropriated to medical schools per student by six adjoining states was twice what it was in Oklahoma; and some states were investing fourteen times as much as Oklahoma for capital construction.

The faculty, which had established a standard of excellence that was unbelievable, and employees, alike, had been living year to year on expectations that the triad responsible would solve the annoying financial problems harassing the School of Medicine and its teaching hospitals. But in that summer of discontent, 1961, disillusionment precipitated an exodus of fifteen members of the faculty for higher salaries elsewhere, in view of an appropriation to the School of Medicine of only $1,067,277 annually. Furthermore, out-of-state agencies, which had been underwriting a large share of the cost of medical education in Oklahoma, began to express concern over the state's lack of interest and responsibility to assume its own obligations to train *more rather than fewer doctors*. National standards called for 135 full-time faculty members in a school this size, whereas there were only 115, with salaries averaging approximately $12,000 when they should have been averaging $15,000 per year. So, there was only one answer to this dilemma; raise salaries or lose some of the most promising medical minds in the country, which had been recruited for the Medical Center with such pains.

As reported to the Oklahoma State Regents for Higher Education in 1960, the amount needed for buildings for the next ten years was $11,450,000: 1961–62, $1,450,000; 1963–64, $4,000,000; 1965–66, $4,000,000; and 1967–68, $2,000,000. The amount needed for other capital improvements, including equipment, repairs, and modernization, amounted to $3,234,000. In view of this projection, full-time student enrollment per class was expected to rise from 150 in 1961–62 to 190 in 1964–65, and to level off at 200 for the remaining five years.

Representative Lou Allard of Drumright, as chairman of the legislative council's appropriation and budget committee, recommended a hospital bill for consideration by the 1963 legislature that would call for a new 600-bed hospital to be erected between the University Hospital and Children's Memorial Hospital, in order to provide the University of Oklahoma School of Medicine with the facilities recommended for a teaching hospital. No sooner was the thought voiced than echoes were heard in the newspapers of Duncan, Shawnee, Miami,

Lawton, Pawhuska, Tulsa, Muskogee, and Guymon, under the dateline OK-LAHOMA CITY (AP or UPI), March 23. A committee to advise architects on construction of such a hospital, at a cost of approximately $20,000,000, was activated almost at once, with Robert Bird as chairman of long-range planning; and joy reigned when Representative Allard announced that the combined senate and house committee on appropriations and budget of the legislative council had recommended salary increases for the medical school faculty.

In order to keep pace with the increasing work load in the dean's office, Merlin K. DuVal was appointed assistant director of the Medical Center on May 1 at an annual salary of $16,000.[3] In this capacity, Dr. DuVal continued to be the Medical Center's liaison with the Alumni Association of the School of Medicine and other groups, at the same time coordinating the various phases of the Medical Center development program.

The alumni association, better organized than ever before, originated a board of councilors in 1962,[4] consisting of seven leaders in business and banking from various sections of Oklahoma, to assist in "getting the message" to the state regents and the legislators in anticipation of the twenty-ninth session of the legislature convening on January 8, 1963. In order to do this, any alumnus practicing in a senatorial or house district was urged to contact his legislators in support of a campaign for increased resources for the School of Medicine. Nominees for governor—W. P. Atkinson, Democrat, and Henry Bellmon, Republican—were also interviewed by alumni prior to the November elections. Active in this respect were President Samuel T. Moore, Oklahoma City, Vice-President Wayne Starkey, Altus, and Robert S. Ellis, Oklahoma City, who was chairman of the alumni legislative committee. Others in this group were Doctors Carl H. Bailey, Stroud, David B. Lhevine, Tulsa, O. L. Parsons, Oklahoma City, and James W. Wilson, Oklahoma City.

On October 12, E. T. Dunlap, chancellor of the State Regents for Higher Education, reported that the regents were recommending a 53.8 per cent raise in appropriations for operating the medical school for the next biennium, whereas the recommended increase for all colleges and universities was only 40 per cent. The recommended annual operating increase for the medical school, according to Chancellor Dunlap, amounted to $574,869.

It was good news that the Urban Renewal Authority authorized filing of an application for a $239,412 advance of federal funds for surveys and planning for a proposed urban renewal project south of the Medical Center. The area under consideration lay between Park Place and N.E. Fourth Street and between Stonewall Avenue and the future Lincoln Boulevard Expressway, which was included in State Highway Department plans.

While these topographical changes were being anticipated, inevitable

[3.] The university regents in September approved a salary raise to $17,100 for Dean Everett and $14,200 for Raymond Crews, business administrator and superintendent of University Hospitals.

[4.] Members of the board of councilors were Dean A. McGee, John E. Kirkpatrick, Donald S. Kennedy, Byron V. Boone, Ward Merrick, Henry Bass, and Russell Hunt.

changes in the lives of some members of the faculty were occurring inexorably. W. K. West, distinguished professor of orthopedic surgery since 1946, who gave liberally of his spirit, time, and talent to development of the Medical Center, suffered a heart attack and died on August 6 at the age of 71.[5]

Joseph Thomas Martin, retired city physician, died at the age of 79 on October 2. Dr. Martin, who was a member of a pioneer Martin family of Oklahoma, joined the faculty of the four-year University of Oklahoma School of Medicine in 1910, at its inception, and served actively for 37 years before becoming professor emeritus of medicine in 1947.

Two members of the faculty were given the title of professor emeritus of surgery in 1962—John Flack Burton and Leo J. Starry. Three faculty members resigned, including James F. Hammarsten, professor of medicine and chief of the medical service at the Veterans Administration Hospital, who was succeeded by W. O. Smith. Arthur N. Springall was the chief of that hospital staff. G. Ray Ridings, professor and head of radiology, director of X ray in the University Hospitals, and coordinator of cancer teaching and the isotope laboratories, resigned also; as well as Lilah B. Heck, after 23 years of service as librarian of the Medical Center. Miss Heck was succeeded by Leonard M. Eddy, assistant professor of medical library science, at a salary of $7,000 as of June 1, 1962.[6]

Our Markle scholars in 1962 were Monte DuVal, G. Rainey Williams, Henry N. Kirkman, and James Merrill, each receiving a $6,000 scholarship. G. H. Daron and Jimmy Simon were the first winners of Aesculapian Awards to be given annually by the student body of the School of Medicine in recognition of devotion to teaching and extraordinary contributions to teaching.

Harry Wilkins became president of the National Society of Neurological Surgeons in 1962; and Don O'Donoghue, professor of orthopedic surgery, was named president of the American Academy of Orthopedic Surgeons. An added feather in "Don's" cap was the fact that twenty-four orthopedic surgeons from Switzerland came to the campus during the year for a week of clinical presentations.

Samuel T. Moore, associate professor of orthopedic surgery and president of the alumni association, served for the second time on a tour of volunteer medical duty (this time in Saigon), under an overseas orthopedic aid program which he helped to launch in 1960 as a member of the Orthopedic Letters Club, a national society. The volunteer doctors not only treated patients during a

[5.] Dr. West earned his M.D. degree in 1915 and became a member of the faculty of his alma mater in 1919. He helped develop the center's internationally recognized residency program in orthopedic surgery and played a major role in the establishment of the first School of Physical Therapy in the state of Oklahoma. His father, A. K. West, was dean of the old Epworth Medical College which merged with the two-year University of Oklahoma School of Medicine in 1910 to become the present four-year medical school.

[6.] The library enrichment fund, commenced by Wann Langston with a personal check for $500 on July 19, 1962, totaled approximately $4,000 in gifts from members of the faculty by January 9, 1963. The school's library contained 46,000 volumes and 1,130 periodicals at that time.

two-month period but also trained native doctors in their specialty. The program was started in Jordan but soon expanded to South America and West Africa, as well as to South Vietnam. The most common orthopedic problems which Dr. Moore encountered in Saigon were "gunshot wounds, congenital malformations, poliomyelitis, and tuberculosis, which were rampant."

Additions to the roster of the faculty in 1962 were:

Jack Elwood Dodson, Ph.D.
professor of preventive medicine
and public health

Ernest Sydney Keeping, A.R.C.S.,
D.I.C.
consultant professor of preventive
medicine and public health

William L. Parry, M.D.
professor of urology

James T. Proctor, M.D.
clinical professor of child
psychology in psychiatry,
neurology, and behavioral
sciences

George Willard Reid, D.Eng.
consultant professor of preventive
medicine and public health

Patrick Romanell, Ph.D.
professor of medical philosophy

John Robert Dille, M.D.
associate professor of preventive
medicine and public health

John LeRoy Falks, Ph.D.
consultant associate professor of
preventive medicine and public
health

Vladimir Pishkin, Ph.D.
associate professor of medical
psychology in psychiatry,
neurology, and behavioral
sciences

Charles E. Shopfner, M.D.
associate professor of radiology

Coleman Taylor, M.D.
associate professor of
ophthalmology

Andre Muller Weitzenhoffer, Ph.D.
associate professor of psychiatry,
neurology, and behavioral sciences

Nicholas T. Werthessen, Ph.D.
associate research professor of
gynecology-obstetrics and
associate professor of physiology

Thomas Adams, Ph.D.
assistant professor of research
physiology

Genene Marie Baker, M.D.
assistant professor of radiology

John G. Bruhn, Ph.D.
assistant professor of medical
sociology in psychiatry,
neurology, and behavioral
sciences

Robert Lee Chester, M.D.
assistant professor of
anesthesiology

Leonard Eddy, M.L.S.
assistant professor of medical
library science

Gael Raymond Frank, M.D.
assistant professor of orthopedic
and fracture surgery

Earl H. Ginn, M.D.
assistant professor of medicine

Richard A. Marshall, M.D.
assistant professor of preventive
medicine and public health and
instructor in medicine

Clinton M. Miller III, Ph.D.
assistant professor of preventive
medicine and public health

Donald L. Mishler, M.D.
clinical assistant professor of
otorhinolaryngology

Alexander W. Pierce, Jr., M.D.
assistant professor of pediatrics

James Byron Snow, Jr., M.D.
assistant professor of
otorhinolaryngology

Gerald Arthur Studebaker, Ph.D.
assistant professor of
communication disorders

Robert A. Beargie, M.D.
instructor in pediatrics

Robert Leroy Carpenter, M.D.
instructor in medicine

Cecelia Agnes Coffey, M.S.
instructor in nutrition
William Alfred Cunningham, M.D.
instructor in ophthalmology
Gerald R. Dixon, M.D.
instructor in ophthalmology
Billy Richard Goetzinger, M.D.
instructor in anesthesiology
Joseph Ted Herbelin, M.D.
clinical instructor in
anesthesiology
Tom Lamar Johnson, M.D.
instructor in ophthalmology
Keith A. Klopfenstein, M.D.
instructor in medicine
Laurence Lyle Knight, M.D.
instructor in pathology
Yildiz Kutkam, M.D.
instructor in anesthesiology
Barney Joe Limes, M.D.
instructor in urology
David C. Lindsey, M.D.
clinical instructor in medicine
Thomas E. Nix, Jr., M.D.
instructor in dermatology
Robert J. Outlaw, M.D.
instructor in psychiatry,
neurology, and behavioral
sciences
Robert Rosenstein, Ph.D.
instructor in research
pharmacology
Gunnar George Sevelius, M.D.
instructor in medicine
Kenneth Lee Shewmaker, Ph.D.
instructor in medical psychology
in psychiatry, neurology, and
behavioral sciences
Jack D. Spencer, M.D.
instructor in orthopedic surgery
John B. Thompson, M.D.
instructor in medicine
George L. Tracewell, M.D.
instructor in otorhinolaryngology
Barnett R. Addis, B.S.
research associate in psychiatry,
neurology, and behavioral
sciences

James C. Beavers, M.D.
clinical assistant in gynecology-
obstetrics
Richard E. Bettigole, M.D.
clinical assistant in medicine
Salvadore Casals, M.D.
clinical assistant in medicine
Peter James Chandler, M.A.
research associate in psychiatry,
neurology, and behavioral
sciences
Quincy Edward Crider, Ph.D.
research associate in research
biochemistry
Gordon H. Deckert, M.D.
clinical assistant in psychiatry,
neurology, and behavioral
sciences
Johnny Bill Delashaw, M.D.
clinical assistant in medicine
John Whitfield Drake, M.D.
clinical assistant in medicine
Ralph Cameron Emmott, M.D.
visiting lecturer in urology
John Allan Foster, M.S.
visiting lecturer in engineering in
psychiatry, neurology, and
behavioral sciences
Wanda Gentry, M.S.W.
clinical assistant in psychiatry,
neurology, and behavioral
sciences
Alma C. Gideon, M.S.W.
clinical assistant in psychiatry,
neurology, and behavioral
sciences
Jan Owen Harris, M.S.W.
clinical assistant in psychiatry,
neurology, and behavioral
sciences
Thomas Hunter Henley, M.D.
clinical assistant in surgery
William Lyon Hughes, M.D.
clinical assistant in medicine
Eleanor S. Keeping, Ph.D.
research associate in
microbiology
Howard Barton Keith, M.D.
clinical assistant in surgery

Frederick D. Mannerberg, M.D.
clinical assistant in medicine
Leroy Lynn Myers, M.D.
clinical assistant in medicine
William Sylvester Myers, M.D.
clinical assistant in medicine
James D. Noble
research associate in radiology
Ralph E. Payne, M.D.
clinical assistant in orthopedic
and fracture surgery
William E. Price, M.D.
clinical assistant in surgery
Herbert P. Reinhardt, Jr., M.D.
visiting lecturer in preventive
medicine and public health and
clinical assistant in medicine
Raymond Edward Roth, M.S.
visiting professor of preventive
medicine and public health

William L. Savage, M.D.
clinical assistant in psychiatry,
neurology, and behavioral
sciences
George Edward Shissler, M.D.
clinical assistant in pediatrics
David Deal Snyder, M.D.
clinical assistant in surgery
Michael N. Spengos, D.D.S.
clinical assistant in dental surgery
Samir Talaat, M.B., D.S., M.Ch.
visiting lecturer in surgery
Jordan J. N. Tang, Ph.D.
research associate in research
biochemistry
Thomas Watson Thurston, M.D.
clinical assistant in pediatrics
Jack E. Tompkins, M.S.
research associate in medicine

The remarkable growth in gifts and grants for research and training programs over a period of approximately ten years reached an all time high of $3,960,556 for the fiscal year 1962–63, with the number of trust funds passing the 500 mark.[7] Federal funds were the largest contributory factor in this support, and nine departments of the School of Medicine (medicine, pediatrics, preventive medicine, psychiatry, microbiology, dermatology, pathology, communication disorders, and physiology), together with the dean's office, received the bulk of the restricted funds amounting to $3,317,875. One of the new grants ($107,835 for support of general research and related activities) proved very helpful to the administration in its management of numerous problems pertaining to the complicated research maze, the details of which are far too extensive in scope to be included in this volume. What needs to be emphasized here is that the prodigious growth of these allotments was due, almost solely, to individual faculty members—an unparalleled contribution to the life of any institution.

One career teaching award and three research career development awards were given respectively to Marshall Edelson (psychiatry), John Sokatch (microbiology), Everett Bracken (pediatrics), and Walter Massion (anesthesiology); while Robert H. Bayley (medicine) and J. Talmadge Shurley (psychiatry) received prestigious research career awards from the National Heart Institute and the Veterans Administration. Children's Memorial Hospital received a $10,000 radiology grant from the Junior Hospitality Club, as well as $10,345

[7.] Because of the increased financial dealings with the National Institutes of Health, the university regents appointed Ralph A. Stump, Jr., comptroller for the Medical Center in March, 1963, upon the recommendation of Raymond Crews, business administrator.

for support for the pediatric-endocrinology service from the Department of Public Welfare.

All of the wards in the Children's Hospital which had been previously closed because of lack of staff and funds for operation were reopened in 1962, and a member of our pediatric staff made ward rounds several times weekly at Children's Convalescent Hospital which, though not on the Medical Center campus, was closely allied with Children's Memorial Hospital for many years. Pediatric and other residents from University Hospitals served there on a rotating schedule, and patients were brought into the university outpatient clinics as often as indicated.

There were 36 members in the Division of Dental Surgery on April 10, and on July 1 two graduates of the Baylor University School of Dentistry reported to the Department of Pathology at the Medical Center in Oklahoma City for advanced degree study under the grant program sponsored by the National Institutes of Health.

As of August 31 a council of the medical staff of University Hospitals was established as an experiment to meet the need for adequate and effective day-to-day operation of the medical staff of University Hospitals and for speedy resolution of mutual problems of the staff and administration. The council (an advisory group) consisted of the assistant director of the Medical Center, the associate dean in charge of research affairs, the superintendent of the University Hospitals, and the business administrator, plus the heads of the following departments: gynecology-obstetrics, medicine, pediatrics, psychiatry, neurology, and behavioral sciences, and surgery. Any recommendations made by the council to the director and dean received prompt consideration, and the council was kept informed of ensuing decisions. John Schilling became chairman of this new council, and the former executive committee of the clinical faculty was now designated as the hospital board, with a chief of staff appointed for a two-year period by the director of the Medical Center from a list of three nominations from the board.

There were 1,254 full-time employees, 181 resident physicians and interns, 121 temporary full-time employees, and 193 part-time and student employees at the Medical Center, as of May 1, 1962.

State appropriations for the University of Oklahoma for the year 1962–63 were $6,223,552 out of a total income of $9,744,079, aside from gifts and grants; for the School of Medicine, $1,067,277 out of a total income of $1,434,529—with only overhead from grants included; for the University Hospitals, $2,646,705 out of a total income of $5,193,452.

During the 1962 calendar year 8,851 adults and 6,169 children visited the outpatient department of University Hospital; 8,674 patients were admitted to the main hospital and 3,843 to Children's Hospital. The average number of patients per day was 360. There were 369,326 examinations in the clinical laboratories and 75,199 in the chemistry-toxicology laboratories; 6,160 electrocardiograms and 13,759 cytology studies were made, plus 36,772 diagnostic x-ray examinations and 35,062 physical therapy treatments. Over the same period there were 15 residents in pediatrics at Children's Memorial Hospital.

One hundred and five students (97 males and 8 females) were selected for the class of 1967, entering in September, 1963—98 from within the state and 7 from out-of-state who were chosen from 140 applicants, an increase of 134 over out-of-state aspirants the previous year. This was due, at least in part, to the State Medical Association's recruiting program and its scholarship and loan plan. The total enrollment in the School of Medicine was 393, 25 of whom were women. Four students registered for a six-year joint M.D.–Ph.D. program, making 109 first-year students in all. Ninety graduates received the M.D. degree in 1962; 18 nursing graduates received the B.S.N. and 15 the certificate in nursing.

On August 2 the dean's office received a letter and resolution by the members and directors of the Shepherd Foundation, established by Lottie and Edith Shepherd of Oklahoma City, granting a sum of $25,000 to the University of Oklahoma Medical Center, to be known as the Shepherd Foundation Loan Fund. This was the largest grant for student aid the school had ever received from private individuals.

In accordance with action taken by the trustees of the Avalon Foundation, the School of Medicine received a second scholarship grant of $10,000 in 1962 as an unrestricted supplement to the scholarship funds of the medical school, "to be expended in conformity with the school's policy, and to be available until expended for nonrefundable grants to students."

Two men who had been closely associated with one another and with the development of the Medical Center since 1947 were Mark R. Everett and Hugh Payne, and special recognition came to each in turn in 1962.

Hugh Payne was given the title of executive secretary of the Alumni Association of the School of Medicine on February 25, 1947, and he assumed the responsibilities of that office, without salary, for thirteen ensuing years. At the end of his first year, 1948, he reported a paid regular membership in the association numbering 57 alumni, and also 138 life memberships. Thirteen years later, in 1960, Mr. Payne reported 664 regular members and 196 life members in the alumni association—an achievement record by any standard.

On February 13, 1962, Hugh Payne was notified that the board of trustees, the officers, and past presidents of the alumni association had voted a resolution, expressing their "gratefulness and heartfelt feelings of thanks for his abundant contributions while serving as their volunteer executive secretary—a central moving force in alumni association growth and accomplishment."

Some of the many accomplishments cited in the resolution in regard to Mr. Payne's executive secretaryship were the launching and initial financing of the Oklahoma Medical Research Foundation; helping to find ways and means to stabilize the biennium income of University Hospitals; enlarging the ten councilor districts in Oklahoma to twenty-nine trustee districts; participation in Governor Gary's Medical Center study committee; activities in aiding Dean Everett to raise $400,000 from the legislature to match federal funds in constructing the new research building on the campus; and conducting a citizens group campaign in 1959 for more adequate medical education and increased faculty salaries by obtaining increased appropriations for higher education.

On November 9, 1947, Mark R. Everett had been named dean of the University of Oklahoma School of Medicine by the university regents; and on November 9, 1962, the dean and director of the Medical Center was honored with a reception in the Faculty House, hosted by Don H. O'Donoghue, chairman of the faculty board. Two hundred and four members of the faculty came to say "thanks to the Dean" upon completion of fifteen years of devotion and service to the University of Oklahoma School of Medicine. "Under Dr. Everett's direction," Dr. O'Donoghue was quoted as saying, "the institution has developed into a comprehensive medical center complex and has gained national stature. . . . The national accreditation review team—which surveyed the school early in the year—was 'tremendously impressed by the esprit de corps and unique spirit of cooperation which Dr. Everett had engendered' . . . and felt it was the most important factor in the great progress of the medical school."

Chapter XXVII.
A Legacy: 1963–64

Very extensive and patient efforts over a period of years[1] to develop a modern medical center for Oklahoma culminated in 1963 in the greatest show of public support for medical education in the history of the state, with endorsement in April by the twenty-ninth legislature of a bond issue for capital improvements on the University of Oklahoma School of Medicine campus and passage of the bond issue on December 3, 1963, by the citizens of Oklahoma.

Henry Louis Bellmon,[2] the first Republican governor of Oklahoma, elected in November, 1962, assisted the Medical Center greatly in developing the plans necessary for its expansion and may justly be included in the company of those who were most effective in the development of medical education in Oklahoma. Governor Bellmon's Medical Center committee, appointed in September, recommended support of the bond issue by a vote of eight to one, with only Senator Ritzhaupt voting no.[3] And Governor Bellmon, having said earlier he would "stump the state for the capital improvement program," urged the citizens of Oklahoma to vote yes on the bond measure after he had received the report of his study committee.

Representative John McCune of Tulsa was the principal author of House Joint Resolution No. 535, calling for a December 3 ballot on State Question No. 411, which directed the secretary of state to refer to the people an ammendment to Article X of the Oklahoma Constitution, providing for capital improvements at the Medical Center. This bill authorized the legislature to enact laws whereby the state could become indebted to an amount not to exceed seven million dollars for the purpose of constructing new buildings and other capital improvements. "We are advised," Representative McCune reported to members of the house, "that the additional seven million dollars worth of bonds can be safely purchased out of the state depository account, without jeopardizing the

[1.] The transformation of the Medical Center began 15 years before the 1963 events, during which period ten construction projects were consummated.

[2.] Henry Bellmon was born in Tonkawa, Oklahoma, in 1921 and received the Bachelor of Science degree in Agriculture from Oklahoma State University. He was awarded the Silver Star for action on Saipan and the Legion of Merit for action on Iwo Jima. He was a member of the house of representatives during Oklahoma's twenty-first legislative session.

[3.] Other members of the governor's committee were Dick Huff, chairman, Henry Bennett, Allen Greer, Joe Duer, Arthur Hambrick, John Houchin, and W. T. Payne.

state's operation, and thus the bond issue will cost no interest. . . . The bonds would be state owned and paid out of the cigarette tax.''

The house of representatives, on April 8, 1963, passed the capital improvements bill for the Medical Center by a vote of 110 to 0; but it was held on the senate calendar for two weeks, on notice by Senator Ritzhaupt of Guthrie that he intended to move for reconsideration (a motion which failed 8 to 30). As a matter of fact, there was an outright attempt to prejudice the vote in the senate when a petition, signed by 116 doctors, was sent to a number of state senators. Senator Ritzhaupt refused to disclose any details of the petition, but in a letter to doctors over the state, Ritzhaupt said that he opposed the seven million dollar bond issue proposal in the house because it did not include a tax to retire the bonds.

Dean Everett said that the administration of the School of Medicine found it regrettable that this bill, currently being considered by the Oklahoma senate, would be so misrepresented by a small group of physicians in central Oklahoma, many of whom had given years of service to medical education.[4]

The Oklahoma State Medical Association decided to keep its hands off the controversial house joint resolution dealing with improvements at the University of Oklahoma Medical Center, after Dean Everett told the house of delegates (of which Marshall O. Hart of Tulsa was speaker) that many important businessmen had helped medical education in Oklahoma, and that they felt strongly that the medical profession should put its shoulder to the wheel. Henceforth, any attempt by the state association to delay action on House Bill No. 535 in the senate ran into rough sledding. As one physician said, ''We are attempting to bring up an issue which is being well resolved. Let us allow this question to lie and let the medical school get the first real boost it has ever received.''[5]

The School of Medicine finally ''crossed home plate'' on Monday, April 22, when the senate shook off all assaults on the bond issue and all attempts to defeat efforts to place it on the state ballot, thus leaving the question to a vote of the citizens of Oklahoma.

Meanwhile, there was accompanying action by the United States Congress to provide matching funds for new construction at medical and dental schools, as well as financial assistance for training additional students. House Resolution No. 12 of the Eighty-eighth Congress (identical with Senate Bill No. 911 and cited as the Health Professions Educational Assistance Act of 1963), which

---

[4] A few promoters of the abortive effort, most of whom were from Oklahoma City, wished to keep the names of signers secret, according to Senator Ritzhaupt, but after their names were listed in the local newspapers, some wrote or telephoned the dean that they had been misled into signing the petition; and a sizable number of other physicians sent a letter supporting the bond issue question, a list which was also published subsequently.

[5] Senator Glen Ham of Pauls Valley, the senate majority floor leader, pointed out that 31 of the 44 members of the senate were coauthors of the Medical Center bond issue proposal, and that its passage was practically a foregone conclusion.

spelled out the provisions of the act, was introduced in the House of Representatives in January and signed into law by President Kennedy in September, 1963, "with great satisfaction," according to a Washington, D.C., news release. The passage of this $236,400,000 bill, which was so essential to the University of Oklahoma Medical Center, in view of the proposed seven million dollar bond issue being submitted to the voters of Oklahoma in December, received the full support of Senators Dewey Bartlett and Ed Edmondson and Representatives Carl Albert and John Jarman.[6]

Regarding Oklahoma City's Urban Renewal Plan, the university regents, on February 13, 1963, furnished the renewal authority with a development plan for the use of land to be acquired for the expansion of the Medical Center, as well as a cooperating agreement between the regents and the renewal authority. This agreement, executed by the chairman of the university regents, stated that the regents were acquiring, and would hereafter acquire, land in Oklahoma City described within one-quarter of a mile of the boundary of the University of Oklahoma Medical Center; and they would (subject to the legislature) acquire the balance of land described south to Tenth Street and east to Stonewall Avenue over a period of three years from the date of undertaking. This resolution and agreement, on motion of Regent Mark Johnson, was unanimously approved by the university regents, who also authorized Raymond Crews to purchase land with the $200,000 appropriated by the twenty-ninth legislature; and shortly thereafter Mr. Crews reported that he had purchased nineteen parcels of land south of the Medical Center.

On May 15 the *Daily Oklahoman* announced that the Oklahoma City Urban Renewal Authority would receive a $206,804 federal grant to finance studies to develop a renewal plan, and that the area under consideration would include 209 acres in the vicinity of the Medical Center between Durland and Stonewall Avenues and extending from N.E. Thirteenth Street to N.E. Fourth Street. According to the Housing and Home Finance Agency in Washington, D.C., Oklahoma City would provide one-third of the cost of carrying out the project, and the federal government would provide the other two-thirds, or $1,837,237. A large part of the local share of the cost would be met by the proposed expansion progra for the Medical Center; that is for every dollar the center spent on land or clearance, the federal government would provide two dollars.

Given the green light by this windfall, no effort was spared to secure passage of State Question No. 411 in December. John Rogers, a Tulsa attorney and former member of the State Regents for Higher Education, accepted the chairmanship of a University of Oklahoma medical site development committee organized by the board of councillors of the School of Medicine alumni association, of which Dean A. McGee was chairman. And President Cross reported early in November that "over three hundred able, capable Oklahoma

6. Former Senators Robert S. Kerr and Mike Monroney had earlier given considerable support to legislation designed to furnish assistance to medical schools in 1961 and 1962.

business and professional men,'' representing practically every county in Oklahoma, had accepted membership on that committee.

The formation of the alumni board of councillors was one of the most effective accomplishments of the alumni association, and the willingness of Dean McGee, president of the Kerr-McGee Oil Company, to serve as chairman was one of our blessings. Dean McGee felt that a public relations program geared to assist Governor Bellmon, ''who had great respect for public relation specialists,'' called for writers, professional producers, television, radio, and donated time at a minimal cost of $5,000 to $10,000 and stated that the physicians of Oklahoma should be called upon to help the board underwrite this cost, as well as to make speeches, appear on television, and so on.

Support for the seven million dollar bond issue received an overwhelming vote at a Sunday night meeting of the alumni association on October 27, and according to a report in the *Daily Oklahoman*, October 28, 1963, ''the few no votes offered were drowned out in the applause and enthusiasm'' of the group as a whole.[7] The alumni organization, which had 900 active members and 286 life members, reached a peak of extraordinary effectiveness in soliciting support for capital improvements at the School of Medicine in 1963–64 under the tireless tutelage of Larry Rember, executive secretary of the association. Mr. Rember was ably assisted by Doctors Robert W. Lowrey of Poteau, president, James S. Petty of Guthrie, secretary, and Carl Bailey of Stroud, Johnny Blue of Oklahoma City, A. K. Cox of Watonga, Powell Fry of Stillwater, and Wendal Smith and Fred Woodson of Tulsa.

Robert S. Ellis, chairman of the alumni association's legislative committee, had said earlier that 74 trustees, officers, and past presidents of the association were active in emphasizing to their local legislators the need for a new, modern teaching hospital on the Medical Center campus; and on June 21 Dr. Ellis sent out a bulletin to alumni in which he said, ''The Oklahoma University Medical Center has the land, we have it within our power to obtain a modern, new building, and our operating monies are considerably improved. Our association has been successful in the past because it has taken no chances on resolution and bill passage; therefore, please contact your trustee district center this weekend. Our medical school and the University Hospitals would be in far worse shape than they are, were it not for your great help.''[8]

The Oklahoma Hospital Association, in convention in Tulsa, endorsed State Question No. 411, and such groups as the greater Oklahoma City League for Nursing, the Oklahoma City Clinical Society, and the Oklahoma Society for Crippled Children also backed the bond issue. Dr. Oliver Hodge, state superintendent of public instruction, issued a statement saying he was glad to lend what

[7.] Wayne A. Starkey of Altus was president of the association at the time.

[8.] On December 23, Dean Everett wrote Dr. Ellis, ''It is with kindest regard and deepest appreciation that I express my gratitude for your extraordinary aid to the Medical Center. You have achieved high honor in the hearts of alumni and faculty of the School of Medicine. Thank you for the many successful efforts you made during the legislative session and the bond issue campaign. It is given to few to become such great benefactors of medical education.''

support he could to the passage of Question 411, as did Mr. William Montin, president of the Oklahoma City Chamber of Commerce; and President Cross, on numerous occasions, reiterated his reasons for voting yes on the bond issue.

The news media gave full measure of support from the time the legislature convened in January until the votes were counted in December. A series of articles by Leonard Jackson may be read in the *Oklahoma City Times*, March 25 through April 10, 1963, covering the annual ten million dollar cost of operating "the sprawling medical School and its hospitals each year," the per cent of the operation supported by state appropriations and student fees (including patient care), the low third- or fourth-rung financial ranking of Oklahoma's School of Medicine among the 37 four-year state medical schools in the country, and the inpatient care cost at University Hospitals, which rose from $10.49 per day in 1948 to $28.66 in 1960, compared with the national average which went up from $13.09 to $32.23. Of the full-time faculty members (113 in the School of Medicine and 15 in the School of Nursing), 20 per cent were receiving their entire salary from federal grants at the time, and another 12 ½ per cent received half or more of their salary from the same source.

Two series of four articles by Claire Conley and Ray Parr appeared in the *Daily Oklahoman*, stressing support for the bond election; and several large, favorable political advertisements appeared in the Oklahoma City papers, financed by groups of citizens and physicians, including the Oklahoma County Medical Society.

The State Regents for Higher Education kept their counsel on the bond issue question until Chancellor Dunlap hinted to Claire Conley (*Daily Oklahoman*, October 11, 1963) that the state regents had been bypassed in a move to win the bond issue election, and that the proposal for a seven million dollar bond issue, as a necessity for federal matching funds, had never been brought before the state regents, although protocol called for application to them for funds. However, Dr. Dunlap conceded that this did not prevent individuals from going directly to the legislature, but that he did not see anything in the 1962 accreditation committee's report that had any bearing on loss of accreditation if expansion of medical school facilities failed to materialize. This was contrary to a statement in the report of the national accrediting committee that "immediate support should be given to permit realization of the ten-year development plan of the Medical Center"; and, when the chips were down, the state regents directed their chairman to take any steps necessary to help the cause.

On December 3, the day of the election, the *Daily Oklahoman* carried a banner headline recommending a yes vote on Question No. 411 and a no vote on the three other proposals; and on December 4 the same newspaper carried another banner headline: "Medical Bond Proposal Wins by Wide Margin." Ray Parr reported that the bond issue drew solid backing from voters throughout the state by an almost three-to-one margin, while the other long-term proposals drew statewide opposition. This was an astonishing victory for medical education, in view of the fact that some of the shrewdest political observers in Oklahoma, five days before the vote on the bond issue, had stated that they were of the opinion that the proposed seven million dollar question would go down to defeat. But it won! And the dean hailed the triumph with gratitude to the citizens of Oklahoma for authorizing funds to start updating and modernizing the University of Oklahoma Medical Center, thereby indicating a realization of the importance to the state of the work being done there. "This vote is a tribute to the many friends of medical education who have helped in the long effort to improve the Medical Center," the dean reasoned.[9]

Some of the forces working to obtain this convincing public endorsement of a strong medical institution in Oklahoma included the Oklahoma Medical Center development committee of 295 members, the sixty-six member doctors committee for a modern Oklahoma Medical Center, seventy-four member governing board of the alumni association, the nine member board of councillors to the alumni association, the seventy-eight presidents and secretaries of endorsing county medical societies, and the legislature and other supporters in government, including Governor Bellmon. Three hundred eighty-three physicians and members of the faculty contributed a total of $20,998 in funds to the University of Oklahoma Foundation Medical School Division, to be used in conducting the campaign favoring State Question No. 411, and contributions from businessmen provided an additional $14,000.

As early as 1962, when Dean Everett appointed a hospital construction committee, there were rumors that Wesley Hospital in Oklahoma City planned to move to the expanding Medical Center, so it became imperative to make definite plans for a brand new adjunct to University Hospital rather than to engage in some piecemeal building plan—something the legislature had deplored for years. Robert Bird was chairman of the committee, 1962–64, and during that period the committee assembled voluminous minutes and very lengthy dossiers as guidelines for the architect on construction of a 600-bed hospital, approved by the hospital board on March 18, 1963.

Minutes of the university regents show that Raymond Crews delivered the preliminary plans and specifications for such a teaching hospital—prepared by Benham Engineering Company and Bill J. Blair and Associates—to the regents in July; and that a motion by Regent Johnson was approved to employ Donald Hiscox, administrative assistant and resident architect for the Health Sciences Division of the University of Washington, as a special consultant to visit the Medical Center and give his recommendations regarding the preliminary plans and specifications, at a fee of $1,500 to be paid from the operating funds of University Hospitals.

---

[9] After the successful bond issue vote, Dean Everett wrote personal letters of appreciation to a large group of friends who had supported the bond issue, including Wendal Smith, Robert Lowry, Vernon Cushing, George H. Garrison, Hugh Payne, Lloyd E. Rader, Larry Rember, Senator Robert A. Trent, and E. K. Gaylord, publisher of the *Daily Oklahoman* and the *Oklahoma City Times*, whose journalists—Claire Conley, Leonard Jackson, and Ray Parr—kept the ball rolling right down to the goal line. "I will remember this major effort as the most significant in a long series of friendly actions by you and your associates to aid the University of Oklahoma Medical Center," the dean wrote in his letter to Mr. Gaylord.

In his report late in August Mr. Hiscox commended the planning committee for a "magnificent effort in attempting to pull together the hundreds of facets that must be considered in the design of such a complex and sophisticated building" and emphasized the concept that the function of the new hospital was teaching and not service, "which should be the prime criterion for use of space within the proposed hospital," but that service and research should surely be considered as additional phases of education.[10] The university regents later approved the plans with the transmittals from Mr. Hiscox.

At a regular session of the Thirtieth Oklahoma State Legislature in 1965 (the first annual session), House Bill No. 1032 was introduced by John McCune of Tulsa and J. D. McCarthy of Oklahoma City and, in the senate, by Senators Baggett, Rogers, Porter, and Smith. This act appropriated the seven million dollars to the Oklahoma State Regents for Higher Education—for the purchase of land, for construction and equipment of buildings, and for repairs to existing buildings at the Medical Center—from the proceeds of the sale of bonds voted by the citizens of Oklahoma on December 3, 1963.

Concurrently, President Cross reported to the university regents in February that an application to the Department of Health, Education and Welfare for two-to-one federal matching funds had been prepared for a joint construction grant to build a new hospital and outpatient quarters for clinical departments by expanding existing facilities. The total cost was estimated at approximately $14,000,000 from the federal government and $7,231,000 from the state of Oklahoma—a total of $21,231,500. The prepared application was approved by the university regents on the motion of Regent Mark Johnson, seconded by Regent Little.

A bill to create a medical research commission to supervise controversial research programs involving inmates in state institutions, which was introduced during the twenty-ninth legislative session by Senator Louis Ritzhaupt, had the full support of Governor Bellmon. This Senate Bill No. 103 gave the commission (composed of the dean of the School of Medicine as chairman, the executive vice-president of the Oklahoma Medical Research Foundation, the director of the Oklahoma Medical Research Institute, the state director of mental health, and the commissioner of public health—all serving without salary) supervisory jurisdiction and control over any proposed medical research wherein the facilities of prisoners of any penal institution or inmates of any other institution of the state of Oklahoma were involved.

The bill passed both houses and was signed by the governor in May, 1963; and in June the university regents adopted a resolution calling for a contractual agreement between the School of Medicine and the State Board of Affairs, under which the School of Medicine would conduct testing and experimentation in a research and biological production program in the McAlester State Penitentiary. Surplus funds above expenses were to be divided annually be-

[10.] Mr. Hiscox wrote subsequently, "I find that doing a critique on a 25 million dollar project of such complexity has turned out to be quite a job. I hope that you will agree that these transmittals will constitute the performance of my contract."

tween the State Board of Affairs and the regents of the university. At a September meeting of the university regents a proposed contract, which was presented by President Cross, was duly approved by the regents and forwarded to the State Regents for Higher Education.

John Colmore, associate professor of medicine and head of an experimental therapeutic unit in the School of Medicine, had the responsibility of developing any research projects in the penitentiary, which consisted mostly of testing and plasma production in 1963.

A three-story, $912,000 addition to the Oklahoma Medical Research Foundation Hospital, completed in 1963, provided 30 new laboratories. Of the building cost $348,000 was provided by individuals and organizations and the balance by the United States Public Health Service.

Hugh Payne, general manager of the Oklahoma Medical Research Foundation, died unexpectedly on May 25, 1964, at age 60, leaving a record of extraordinary achievement and a challenge to others to fulfill a program designed to benefit mankind.[11]

On June 6, 1963, members of the faculty passed resolutions bearing upon the deaths of several members of the faculty: Robert M. Howard, professor emeritus of surgery, who had served on the staff since 1910, died on February 22; Peter Russo, professor and former chairman of the Department of Radiology and president-elect of the Oklahoma State Medical Association, died on March 13; Grady Fred Matthews, professor of preventive medicine and public health, died on March 18; Charles Francis DeGaris, professor emeritus of anatomy and former chairman of the department, died on April 10; and Paul H. Fesler, former superintendent and administrator of the University Hospitals, died on April 4.

John M. Houchin of Bartlesville and Reuben Sparks of Woodward, appointees of Governor Bellmon, became members of the University of Oklahoma Board of Regents in April. At that same meeting the regents approved a recommendation by President Cross that Dean Everett be given the title of regents professor of medical sciences, effective in May, 1963.

Francis J. Reichmann was given the title of clinical professor emeritus in dental surgery, and John H. Robinson and Oscar R. White were each promoted to clinical professor emeritus of surgery.

Stewart G. Wolf, Jr., professor and head of the Department of Medicine, in 1963 was awarded a Commonwealth Fellowship amounting to $17,396 and was granted a leave of absence from the School of Medicine from July 1, 1963, to July 1, 1964, to spend a year in France—half-time as a consultant for the office of international research of the National Institutes of Health and part-time as a representative of the National Advisory Heart Council, of which he was a member. Robert Bird, professor of medicine and vice-chairman of the depart-

---

[11.] Hugh Payne's many talents were recognized by official resolutions from the faculty board of the School of Medicine, the National Institutes of Health, the advisory board of the National Cancer Council, and the research committee of the National Association of Mental Health.

ment, was made acting head by the university regents on July 1, 1963, for the duration of Dr. Wolf's leave of absence; and William S. Middleton became a visiting professor of medicine, as an internist and teacher.[12]

There were 702 faculty members in the School of Medicine in 1963–64, including 63 appointed in 1963:

Chester Stanley Clifton, Ph.D.
consultant professor of social work in psychiatry, neurology, and behavioral sciences

Robert Edelberg, Ph.D.
professor of psychophysiology in department of psychiatry, neurology, and behavioral sciences and of physiology

Ervin George Erdos, M.D.
professor of pharmacology

Albert Julius Glass, M.D.
clinical professor psychiatry, neurology, and behavioral sciences

Ben I. Heller, M.D.
professor of laboratory medicine

William S. Middleton, M.D.
visiting professor of medicine

Eugene Pumpian-Mindlin, M.D.
professor of psychiatry, neurology, and behavioral sciences

Sidney P. Traub, M.D.
professor of radiology

Seymour H. Levitt, M.D.
associate professor of radiology

J. Rodman Seeley, M.D.
associate professor of pediatrics

William R. Albers, M.D.
assistant professor of research preventive medicine and public health

J. Hill Anglin, Ph.D.
assistant professor of research dermatology and instructor in research biochemistry

Joseph R. Assenzo, Ph.D.
assistant professor of preventive medicine and public health

Glenn Stuart Bulmer, Ph.D.
assistant professor of microbiology

Raul Carubelli, Ph.D.
assistant professor of research biochemistry

Warren Melville Cosby, M.D.
assistant professor of gynecology-obstetrics

Floyd W. Emanuel, Ph.D.
assistant professor of communication disorders

Jess N. Hensley, M.D.
assistant professor of pathology

Eugene Oliver Mencke, Ph.D.
assistant professor of communication disorders

Peter Vincent Siegal, M.D.
assistant professor of research preventive medicine and public health

Landon Clarke Stout, Jr., M.D.
assistant professor of medicine

Charles Michael Van Duyne, M.D.
assistant professor of gynecology-obstetrics

Claude M. Bloss, M.D., M.P.H.
instructor in preventive medicine and public health

Gerald W. Boles, M.D.
instructor in radiology

Wilson J. Buvinger, M.D.
instructor in otorhinolaryngology

[12.] Dr. Middleton was connected with the University of Wisconsin Medical School for 43 years, including 20 years as dean of the school. He served with the British Expeditionary Force and the American Expeditionary Force in France in World War I; and in World War II he was chief consultant in medicine for the European theatre of operation. During eight years as medical director of the Veterans Administration in Washington, D.C., Dr. Middleton was an inspiration as a leader, counselor, and administrator.

Judith R. Cowan, M.D.
instructor in psychiatry,
neurology, and behavioral
sciences
Alice Frances Gamble, M.D.
instructor in anesthesiology
James Robert Geyer, M.D.
clinical instructor in urology
Frederick Redding Hood, Jr., M.D.
instructor in surgery
Wolfgang Karl Huber, M.D.
instructor in psychiatry,
neurology, and behavioral
sciences
Charles Dean Ingram, M.A.
instructor in medical library
science
David Edward Kemp, Ph.D.
instructor in psychiatry,
neurology, and behavioral
sciences
Barbara June Kersey, M.L.S.
instructor in medical library
science
Karl Guy Klinges, M.D.
clinical instructor in
gynecology-obstetrics
James Berry Mills, M.D.
instructor in ophthalmology
Catherine M. McCarty, M.S.
instructor in nutrition and in
preventive medicine and public
health
Virginia Newton Olds, R.N.,
M.S.W.
instructor in preventive medicine
and public health
Henry West Overbeck, M.D.
instructor in medicine
Jesse Eugene Pyeatte, M.D.
instructor in ophthalmology
Armond H. Start, M.D.
clinical instructor in pediatrics
Roger E. Wehrs, M.D.
instructor in otorhinolaryngology
George Dewey Wilbanks, Jr., M.D.
clinical instructor in
gynecology-obstetrics
Jones E. Witcher, M.D.
instructor in otorhinolaryngology

Morton H. Baxt, D.D.S.
clinical assistant in dental surgery
Jerry Lee Bressie, M.D.
clinical assistant in medicine
Joan L. Campbell, M.S.
clinical assistant in psychiatry,
neurology, and behavioral
sciences
Roy Barton Carl, M.D.
clinical assistant in surgery
Juan Francisca Correa, M.D.
clinical assistant in anesthesiology
Teresa M. Costilow, M.S.
research associate in pediatrics
Nancy Bess Farley, Ed.D.
research associate in pediatrics
Joseph M. Harroz, M.D.
clinical assistant in
gynecology-obstetrics
Paul Cullison Houk, M.D.
clinical assistant in medicine
Wayne B. Lockwood, M.D.
clinical assistant in orthopedic
and fracture surgery
LeRoy Long, M.D.
clinical assistant in surgery
Donald W. Marsh, M.D.
clinical assistant in
ophthalmology
Gerald W. McCullough, M.D.
clinical assistant in surgery
Herman Andrew Reisenberg, R.N.,
B.S.N.
clinical assistant in psychiatric
nursing, department of
psychiatry, neurology, and
behavioral sciences
Don Forrest Rhinehart, M.D.
clinical assistant in surgery
John Robert Scott, M.D.
visiting lecturer in preventive
medicine and public health
Russell Franklin Shaw, M.D.
clinical assistant in pediatrics
Carolyn W. Sherif, Ph.D.
consultant assistant of social
psychology in psychiatry,
neurology, and behavioral
sciences

Elizabeth M. Tackwell, M.A.
  clinical assistant (psychiatric
  social worker) in psychiatry,
  neurology, and behavioral
  sciences

Arthur Vega, Jr., M.A.
  research associate in psychiatry,
  neurology, and behavioral
  sciences

Eighty-seven new faculty members were appointed in 1964:

George A. Byran, Ph.D.
  consulting professor of
  communication disorders
James L. Dennis, M.D.
  professor of pediatrics
  dean of the School of Medicine
  and director of the Medical
  Center
Herman Floyd Flanigan, M.D.
  consulting professor of
  communication disorders
Marshall D. Schechter, M.D.
  professor of child psychiatry in
  psychiatry, neurology, and
  behavioral sciences and
  consultant professor of pediatrics
Harold L. Williams, Ph.D.
  research professor of psychology
  in psychiatry, neurology, and
  behavioral sciences
David William Bishop, M.D.
  associate professor of
  ophthalmology
George Clark, Ph.D.
  associate professor of research
  anatomy
Michael H. Ivey, Ph.D.
  associate professor of preventive
  medicine and public health
Betty Jane McClellan, M.D.
  associate professor of pathology
John Darrel Smith, M.D.
  associate professor of pediatrics
Charles Alexander Adsett, M.D.
  assistant professor of medicine,
  and psychiatry, neurology, and
  behavioral sciences, and
  preventive medicine and public
  health
Carl Robert Bogardus, Jr., M.D.
  assistant professor of radiology

Mary Frances Carpenter, Ph.D.
  assistant professor of research
  biochemistry
Ronald Leon Coleman, Ph.D.
  assistant professor of research
  biochemistry and preventive
  medicine and public health
William Allen Cooper, Jr., Ph.D.
  consulting assistant professor of
  communication disorders
Dick Herbert F. Helander, M.D.
  assistant professor of research
  medicine
Yu-Teh Li, Ph.D.
  assistant professor of research
  biochemistry
Robert Carroll MacKay, M.D.
  assistant professor of pathology
Arnold M. Mordkoff, Ph.D.
  assistant professor of psychiatry,
  neurology, and behavioral
  sciences
Norton Graham McDuffie, Ph.D.
  assistant professor of research
  biochemistry
Alvin Morton Revsin, Ph.D.
  assistant professor of research
  pharmacology
Guy Vivian Rice, M.D.
  assistant professor of preventive
  medicine and public health
Bobby Gene Smith, M.D.
  assistant professor of urology
Robert M. Wienecke, M.D.
  assistant professor of psychiatry,
  neurology, and behavioral
  sciences
James R. Beaty, M.D.
  clinical instructor in pediatrics
James Robert Carroll, M.D.
  clinical instructor in
  ophthalmology

Lawrence A. Chitwood, Ph.D.
instructor in pediatrics
George Robert Cornelius, M.D.
clinical instructor in
ophthalmology
James Dean Funnell, M.D.
clinical instructor in
gynecology-obstetrics
Donald Carroll Gilliland, M.D.
clinical instructor in
ophthalmology
Charles Hillman Lawrence, Ph.D.
instructor in preventive medicine
and public health
Jesse Samuel Little, M.D.
clinical instructor in radiology
Dan Mitchell, Jr., M.D.
clinical instructor in radiology
William Stanley Muenzler, M.D.
instructor in ophthalmology
Carl Behr Nagel, M.D.
instructor in surgery
O'Tar Norwood, M.D.
clinical instructor in dermatology
Robert Alan Nozik, M.D.
clinical instructor in
ophthalmology
Francis Willard Pruitt, M.D.
instructor in medicine
Charles W. Robinson, Jr., M.D.
instructor in medicine
Charles William Simcoe, M.D.
clinical instructor in
ophthalmology
Carl Ray Smith, M.D.
instructor in ophthalmology
Howard Smotherman, M.D.
clinical instructor in
gynecology-obstetrics
Richard Edward Sternlof, Ph.D.
research associate in preventive
medicine and public health;
instructor in medical psychology
in psychiatry, neurology, and
behavioral sciences
Kenneth Merlin Tucker, D.D.S.
instructor in dental surgery
Angelos P. Angelopoulos, D.D.S.
clinical assistant in dental surgery

Robert J. Boren, M.D.
visiting lecturer in dermatology
Donald K. Braden, M.D.
clinical assistant in surgery
Robert C. Brown, M.D.
clinical assistant in medicine
Robert B. Brownell, M.D.
clinical assistant in
otorhinolaryngology
Cosmelito Cagas, M.D.
clinical assistant in pediatrics
Raul Emir Chanes, M.D.
clinical assistant in medicine
Cecil Addison Childers, M.D.
visiting lecturer in psychiatry,
neurology, and behavioral
sciences
Clinton Maurice Coffey, M.D.
visiting lecturer in dermatology
Paul Avery Compton, M.D.
clinical assistant in medicine
William Floyd Crittendon, M.D.
clinical assistant in gynecology-
obstetrics
Richard Gene Dotter, M.D.
clinical assistant in medicine
Thomas F. Webb Dudley, D.D.S.
clinical assistant in the division of
dental surgery, department of
surgery
Bobby Gene Eaton, M.D.
clinical assistant in radiology
Marinus Flux, M.D.
clinical assistant in pediatrics
William J. Forrest, M.D.
clinical assistant in surgery
Delmar L. Gheen, Jr., M.D.
clinical assistant in pediatrics
Glen Dale Hallum, M.D.
clinical assistant in radiology
John E. Kauth, M.D.
visiting lecturer in radiology
Harry James Kearns, Jr., M.D.
clinical assistant in radiology
Ernest S. Kerekes, M.D.
visiting lecturer in radiology
Albert B. Kuritz, M.D.
clinical assistant in surgery

Takashi Kusakari, M.D.
    research associate in
    pharmacology
William Robert Loney, M.D.
    visiting lecturer in dermatology
Charles W. Macomber, M.D.
    clinical assistant in
    gynecology-obstetrics
Serge Bourgault Martel, M.D.
    clinical assistant in pediatrics
Donald Forsyth Mauritson, M.D.
    visiting lecturer in radiology
Julian Charles Monnet, M.D.
    clinical assistant in orthopedic
    and fracture surgery
Lloyd M. Mummer, M.D.
    clinical assistant in medicine
Robert L. Olson, M.D.
    clinical assistant in dermatology
Lucien Michele Pascucci, M.D.
    visiting lecturer in radiology
C. Dowell Patterson, M.D.
    clinical assistant in medicine

John Norman Penrod, M.D.
    visiting lecturer in dermatology
Jerry Lee Puls, M.D.
    clinical assistant in medicine
Mary E. Puntenney, M.D.
    clinical assistant in medicine
Thomas Rubio, M.D.
    clinical assistant in pediatrics
Robert H. Smiley, M.D.
    clinical assistant in surgery
Clyde Collins Snow, Ph.D.
    research associate in medicine
Jaime Tobias Tapuz, M.D.
    clinical assistant in anesthesiology
Milton Lee Wagner, M.D.
    clinical instructor in radiology
Sal Wilner, M.D.
    visiting lecturer in radiology
James Ward Wilson, M.D.
    clinical assistant in medicine
Hsiu-Ying Yang, Ph.D.
    research associate in
    pharmacology

In accordance with a recommendation by the committee on accreditation, which surveyed our institution in 1962, Dr. Everett asked to be relieved as chairman of the Department of Biochemistry on March 18, 1964, as soon as sufficient funds could be made available for more adequate facilities for teaching and research in biochemistry, including a considerable increase in salary for the head of the department. Members of a temporary committee[13] to recommend a new chairman were of the opinion that the resources in the biochemistry section of the Oklahoma Medical Research Institute should be combined with the resources in the School of Medicine, and that the School of Medicine should be prepared to increase the salary commitment to $21,000. That being the case, the research institute offered to contribute $12,000 a year for a period of two years toward the chairman's salary; and in June, 1964, Marvin R. Shetlar, chief of the research laboratories in the Veterans Administration Hospital from 1950 to 1957 and professor of biochemistry and senior research fellow of the National Institutes of Health until 1962, was named chairman of the Department of Biochemistry for the year July 1, 1964, to June 30, 1965.[14]

[13.] Members of the committee were Francis J. Haddy, head of the Department of Physiology, chairman, and Leonard Eliel, Robert Bird, Henry Kirkman, Wallace Friedburg, and Simon H. Wender.

[14.] Members of the Department of Biochemistry held a reception for Dr. and Mrs. Everett in the Faculty House on June 24 in honor of Dr. Everett's ''40 memorable years of service as head of the department.''

Kelly M. West, associate professor in the Department of Medicine (on leave of absence), was named professor and chairman of a new Department of Continuing Education by the university regents on June 7, 1963, effective July 1. Irwin Brown, director of postgraduate medical education, became associate professor in the new department.

Ben I. Heller, professor of medicine and director of the School of Medical Technology, was appointed head of a new Department of Laboratory Medicine in April, 1964, at a salary of $16,999 effective September 1. Dr. Heller's primary responsibility was to correlate the activities of the clinical laboratories with the various hospital services.[15]

Sidney P. Traub was appointed professor and head of the Department of Radiology and director of the x-ray department in University Hospitals at a salary of $18,000 supplemented by $3,000 annually from the Veterans Administration Hospital.

Seymour Levitt, a radiation therapist (badly needed in the University Hospitals), was appointed associate professor of radiology at a salary of $20,000 per year. And James B. Snow, Jr., assistant professor of otorhinolaryngology, became the first full-time head of that department.[16]

Mark Allen Everett, part-time member of the faculty as associate professor of dermatology, was named chairman of the department for the period 1964–66, succeeding Phyllis E. Jones, a 1940 graduate of the University of Oklahoma School of Medicine, who was the first woman to head a clinical department, when she succeeded John Lamb as chairman of the Department of Dermatology.[17]

The Department of Pediatrics joined with other teaching hospitals to form the Southwest Cancer Chemotherapy Study Group, after establishing a new outpatient tumor clinic. In November, 1963, a modern cardiopulmonary diagnostic laboratory was set up in Children's Memorial Hospital, under the direction of a pediatric cardiologist.

Gifts and grants to the faculty of the University of Oklahoma Medical Center for research and special training programs amounted to almost a million dollars more in 1963–64 than during the previous year; and the new total ($5,386,562) exceeded the state-appropriated funds for operation and maintenance of the entire Medical Center. Approximately 80 per cent of these funds came from federal agencies, and by October, 1964, the chief trust fund accountant had 799

[15] Dr. Heller was graduated from the University of Minnesota School of Medicine in 1942 and subsequently taught at Marquette University and served on the staff of Wood County, Wisconsin, Veterans Administration Center. Before coming to Oklahoma, he had spent five years as professor of medicine in the University of Arkansas Medical School.

[16] Dr. Snow received his premedical education at the University of Oklahoma and was graduated from Harvard Medical School in 1956, after which he was engaged in three years of residency training at the Massachusetts Eye and Ear Infirmary in Boston.

[17] Dr. Everett was graduated from the University of Oklahoma School of Medicine in 1951 and completed his training in dermatology in 1957 at the University of Michigan Hospitals in Ann Arbor.

separate trust funds to account for and some 600 detailed reports to prepare for the granting agencies, showing how their dollars had been spent. Seven hundred and fifty employees in the Medical Center were getting all or part of their salaries from these sources in 1963–64. Of the total grant income received, the Department of Medicine realized $1,300,000, the Department of Pediatrics, $628,000, and Preventive Medicine, $684,000. New gifts and grants to the Medical Center in 1963–64 totaled $4,875,222.

The School of Medicine was one of 31 institutions selected to participate in the evaluation of the National Institutes of Health extramural programs on May 21 and 22, 1964. The purpose of the study was to determine whether the grant-awarding mechanism and supervision of these institutes (which were supporting 40 per cent of the nation's medical research and contributing to colleges and universities 36 per cent of all federal funds available for research) were subsidizing the best scientific projects, and to what extent the fellowship and training programs were conducive to a healthy academic community.

Federal funds of $82,689, and $83,854 from industries, were used to modernize and equip the quarters of the Institute of Environmental Health, located on the top floor of the new research building of the School of Medicine, according to an initial financial resources report made on February 4, 1964, by Carl Nau, director of the institute. One of the major activities, involving nine persons, included the initiation of a training program in environmental factors, made possible by a grant from the United States Public Health Service.

The secretary of Health, Education and Welfare announced the appointment of a national advisory council on education for health professions, on March 3, 1964; and one of the members of the new council was Dean McGee, president of Kerr-McGee Oil Industries and a member of the board of councillors to the Alumni Association of the School of Medicine. The purpose of the advisory council was to advise the surgeon general of the U.S. Public Health Service on the administration of grants for the construction of new teaching facilities.

Harris D. Riley, Jr., a special consultant to the National Institute of Child Health and Development, received approval of a request for a grant of $50,000 in December, 1963, from the National Foundation to continue operation of the Birth Defect Clinical Study Center in Children's Memorial Hospital. The center, established in 1961, with a program of research training and patient care, admitted 87 patients during 1963; and 47 additional cases were examined in the center's weekly outpatient clinic. New information on genetic deficiency was revealed through researches by Henry Kirkman, associate professor of pediatrics.

Then there was the Oklahoma Child Study Center on management of mental retardation being operated by the Department of Pediatrics, which moved from quarters in Children's Memorial Hospital to 601 N.E. Eighteenth Street and Lincoln Boulevard in 1964—a move facilitated by a gift of $7,000 from the Junior League of Oklahoma City, which had maintained an active working interest in the center since 1958.[18]

[18.] This donation brought the league's contribution to approximately $15,000 since the study center was founded.

During 1963 new x-ray equipment was installed in Children's Memorial Hospital, partly through a gift of $10,000 from the Junior Hospitality Club. And three wards of the hospital were air-conditioned as a result of the efforts of groups and individuals in Oklahoma City; Charles Zlotogura headed a drive among businessmen, and B'nai B'rith and Emanuel Synagogue Men's Club, for funds for air conditioners. Simultaneously, another drive was begun by a group of individual artists, headed by Mr. and Mrs. Cliff Ward.

A grant of $14,036 from the American Medical Association Education and Research Foundation was presented in 1963 to the School of Medicine by Joe L. Duer, president of the Oklahoma State Medical Association; the East Central Oklahoma Medical Society gave to the medical school $2,500, derived from its polio immunization program; and the National Child Welfare Foundation of the American Legion gave a grant of $5,000 for research in cystic fibrosis at Children's Memorial Hospital.

In October, Dean Everett authorized the expenditure of $3,000 from the Herbert and Lela Berlin Trust Fund, to assist the Department of Radiology in securing special radiographic equipment necessary for research on the human spine. This trust fund was made possible in July, 1964, by the gift of $10,000 for general medical research, from the estate of Herbert and Lela Berlin.

The official budget of the University of Oklahoma Medical Center for 1963–64 was $10,344,699, of which $2,398,927 was from grants for purposes other than research. Total grants for sponsored teaching programs in that year were $1,438,289, and $1,835,782 for sponsored research programs. The total medical college cost—including sponsored programs but excluding grants for teaching hospitals and clinics—was $5,325,920. The state appropriation for the School of Medicine was $1,170,922 and for the University Hospitals, $2,800,450. In September, 1963, the university regents authorized a salary of $18,000 per annum for Dean Everett and $15,000 for Raymond Crews, business administrator.

By 1964 the University of Oklahoma Medical Center encompassed 23.38 acres. The operating income of the School of Medicine (including only the overhead from grants) was $1,693,830 and that of the University Hospitals was $5,941,286. In 1963–64, 12,253 patients were admitted to the hospitals (8,607 at main and 3,646 at Children's), and 20,008 persons needing medical attention visited the outpatient clinics during that period. Kenneth Babcock, after accrediting the hospitals in October, 1963, for three more years, commended Raymond Crews and the professional staff for the standards being maintained and the constant effort being made to improve the quality of patient care.

During the past 15 years the number of approved internships and residency positions had increased from 43 to 159; the house staff program for 1963 mentioned our three teaching hospitals (University, Children's Memorial, and Veterans Administration) with 947 teaching beds. There were 29 approved internships, 18 residencies accommodating 22 individual positions, and nine visiting fellows in 1963–64. Each resident was required to possess a temporary Oklahoma medical license.

As a matter of fact, the university's Medical Center had become big business, and in a letter to President Cross under the date of June 28, 1963, Dean Everett requested that the university regents appoint security officers and other individuals as campus police officers—by authority granted in Senate Bill No. 174 during the 1963 session of the legislature—in order to control certain undesirable occurrences on the campus and to protect employees and patients from outside criminal offenses.

An attack of a rather unjustified nature was leveled at the administration of the School of Medicine on February 4, 1964, by the Oklahoma Academy of General Practice because of the shortage of "family doctors" throughout the state. The administration sympathized with the general practice group's goal of encouraging more doctors to go into general practice—indeed, had continually made a special effort in this respect through establishment of the preceptorship program—but medical schools could not and cannot tell their graduates where to go or what type of practice to conduct. Commenting on the accusation the following day, Mark Johnson, a member of the university regents, said he was very sorry to see criticism of what he termed "a really tremendous and effective organization" because of somthing over which it had no control; and Regent James G. Davidson of Tulsa said he did not see what part the university could play in the matter—that it seemed to be "more of a problem for the medical profession than for the university."[19]

On January 8, 1964, the faculty board approved a recommendation by its curriculum committee that each medical student be required to take Part I and Part II of the National Board Examinations. James Merrill, who had required his students to take these examinations the previous year, was singled out by the students for outstanding teaching honors, together with William Jaques and Gunter Haase, when these three members of the faculty were given the second annual Aesculapian Awards.

The Shepherd Foundation increased its loan fund for medical students to $30,000 in June, 1963, and $4,065 in small loans were made to 44 students from the Wayman J. Thompson emergency loan fund. The Hughes-Seminole County Medical Society donated $4,500 for another student loan fund, and at the same time eighteen tuition scholarships were made available—two by the Oklahoma City Clinic, the Ray M. Balyeat Memorial scholarship by the Oklahoma City Allergy Clinic, a Mark R. Everett scholarship made possible by a group of Oklahoma City physicians, five Oklahoma State Medical Association scholarships, and ten Avalon Foundation scholarships.[20] Two new merit

---

[19] From 1960 through 1964 a number of issues of the *Oklahoma Family Doctor* had run editorials deploring the lack of sufficient general practitioners in the rural areas of the state. Robert T. Sturm and Marvin B. Glissman, respectively, presidents of the local section of the American Academy of General Practice, were very effective in arbitrating some of the recommendations of members of the academy.

[20] Other awards and honors listed on the 1964 commencement program for the School of Medicine were as follows: L. J. Moorman Award, Onis George Hazel Award, two research achievement awards, an Oklahoma City Surgical Society Award, Coyne H. Campbell Award, American Academy of Dental Medicine Certificate of Merit, two Merck Manual awards, Mrs. Eugene Faye Lester, Sr., Book Award, Mark R. Everett

awards were initiated—the Alexander D. Everett honorarium in biochemistry and the James G. Binkley memorial prize in obstetrics.

Ninety graduates of the School of Medicine received the M.D. degree in June, 1964, and 396 medical students were enrolled for the 1964–65 academic year. In addition, a total of 1,478 other students were enrolled on the Medical Center campus, including 169 in the graduate college, 150 in paramedical programs, 1,021 in postgraduate medical programs, and 138 in nursing.

For the first time since initiation of the collegiate four-year nursing program in 1951, the University of Oklahoma School of Nursing, late in 1963, was granted full accreditation for all three of its programs.[21] Thirty-one graduates of the School of Nursing received the degree of Bachelor of Science in Nursing in 1964, and 15 certificates of Graduate Nurse were issued. The Lottinville Award for excellence in nursing was given to Kathryn Nimmo, a degree graduate. The School of Nursing budget for the year 1963–64 was $144,416.

The extent to which the alumni rallied to the support of their school was a kindly benediction to Dr. Everett before his retirement as dean emeritus on June 30, 1964. The hard work of the alumni and Larry Rember, executive secretary of the alumni association, were important factors in the Medical Center bond issue election; and the tireless effort of Wayne Starkey of Altus, president of the association, was a badge of great loyalty. "The School of Medicine and Alumni Association have developed into most energetic and respected organizations, capable of providing leadership to the whole state, in regard to medical education," the dean wrote in the February, 1964, issue of the *Commentary*. And to members of the faculty, without whom there would be no medical education, he said:

> The present achievements must be maintained and extended by you, in order to further the growth and development of the Medical Center which, at this juncture, rests on the threshold of a great future. To translate the ten-year development plan of the University of Oklahoma Medical Center into reality will be a lengthy task, and will command strong and vigorous leadership.
>
> Universities should consider carefully the possible reorganization of medical center administration to keep pace with the day's greatly enlarged tasks and challenges, for director-deans or vice-presidents could not do proper planning when spending much of their time putting out small fires. One of the most difficult functions of medical center administration was to make decisions that recognized and supported the joint academic and patient-care responsibilities of a teaching hospital.

Award, Roche Award, Peter E. Russo prize in radiologic anatomy, Tom Lowry Award, LeRoy Long prize, and Harry Wilkins prize in neuroanatomy. Fifteen members of the class were admitted to Alpha Omega Alpha honor medical society.

[21.] The old three-year certificate program was terminated in 1965 by the State Regents for Higher Education.

Monte DuVal, who was named assistant director of the Medical Center in 1962, seemed the logical person to take on this task, for he believed there was "an unbeatable climate for progress in the Oklahoma City area and exciting developments in medicine in store for Oklahomans." He had been very active as a liaison with citizen groups and the medical school alumni, 1962–64, and the indefatigable energy with which he worked for passage of Senate Bill No. 411 in 1963 was a most significant element in the successful bond issue campaign. But fate sometimes laughs at probabilities, and Dr. DuVal, Markle Scholar and president of the Oklahoma Surgical Association, accepted the challenge to build a brand new medical school "from the ground up" in Tucson, Arizona—the University of Arizona's proposed College of Medicine.[22]

On June 11, 1964, the university regents appointed Joseph White, associate dean in charge of research programs and special training, as interim dean of the School of Medicine and director of the Medical Center from July 1 to September 1, when Dean Everett's successor, James L. Dennis, assumed the dual post at the University of Oklahoma School of Medicine, his alma mater. Dr. Dennis was professor of pediatrics and associate dean for clinical affairs at the University of Arkansas Medical Center in Little Rock, when he accepted the top administrative post in the University of Oklahoma Medical Center.

The end of an era in Oklahoma medical education was marked with a smile and a tear. One thousand three hundred and forty-one students had been graduated from the University of Oklahoma School of Medicine, since Mark R. Everett became dean in 1947, and on June 4, 500 alumni and friends attended an elaborate banquet in his honor, sponsored by the alumni association, in the Persian Room of the Skirvin Hotel in Oklahoma City. The feature of the occasion was the unveiling of a portrait of Dean Everett, which the association commissioned as a gift to the School of Medicine, to hang in the Medical Center library. The portrait was painted by the Hungarian artist, LeJos Markos, and unveiled by President George Lynn Cross.

Dr. Everett was rounding out 40 years of active association with the medical school, and he had weathered many a storm, especially while at the helm as dean. During his tenure the school was able to build an outstanding staff—with occasional differences of opinion, to be sure—and Mark Everett played a very valuable role in that he was able, somehow, to maintain harmony without stinting effort.

"If I may have been regarded in one sense," he said, "as head of this medical family for seventeen years, sharing its life and sustained by its affection, it constitutes a very full reward for my long and sometimes anxious labors."

[22.] In addition to Dr. DuVal, five other doctors, associated deans, and assistants who had worked with Dean Everett, became deans of medical or health schools: Homer F. Marsh, University of Miami, A. N. Taylor, Chicago Medical School, Joseph M. White, University of Texas, Edward N. Brandt, Jr., University of Texas, and Philip Smith, the University of Oklahoma College of Health.

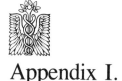

Appendix I.

West, Archa Kelly, M.D., *dean of Epworth College of Medicine*, 1904–1910

Upjohn, Lawrence Northcote, M.D., *administrator of the School of Medicine*, Oct. 2, 1900–1904

Stoops, Roy Philson, M.D., *director, head, then acting dean*, 1904–1908

Bobo, Charles Sharp, M.D., *dean*, Sept. 1, 1908 to Sept. 1, 1911

Williams, Robert Findlater, M.D., *dean*, Sept. 1, 1911 to Feb. 1, 1913

Jolly, William James, M.D., *acting dean*, Feb. 1, 1913 to Feb. 1, 1914

Day, Curtis Richard, M.D., *dean*, Sept. 1, 1915 to Aug. 8, 1931

Long, LeRoy, M.D., *dean*, Sept. 1, 1915 to Aug. 8, 1931

Moorman, Lewis Jefferson, M.D., *dean*, Sept. 1, 1931 to July 1, 1935

Turley, Louis Alvin, Ph.D., *acting dean*, July 1, 1935 to Sept. 1, 1935

Patterson, Robert Urie, M.D., *dean,* Sept. 1, 1935 to Nov. 15, 1942

Shoemaker, Harold Adam, Ph.D., *acting dean*, Nov. 15, 1942 to Oct. 15, 1943

Lowry, Thomas Claude, M.D., *dean*, Nov. 15, 1942 to Dec. 11, 1945

Langston, Wann, M.D., *dean*, Dec. 13, 1945 to Sept. 1, 1946

Gray, Jacques Pierce, M.D., *dean*, Sept. 1, 1946 to Nov. 7, 1947

Everett, Mark Reuben, Ph.D., *dean*, Nov. 10, 1947 to June 30, 1964

White, Joseph M., M.D., *acting dean*, July 1, 1964 to Aug. 31, 1964

Dennis, James Lowden, M.D., *dean*, Sept. 1, 1964

DuVal, Jr., Merlin K., M.D., *assistant director*, May 1, 1962 to Dec. 31, 1963

Everett, Mark R., Ph.D., *director*, Mar. 8, 1956 to June 30, 1964

White, Joseph M., M.D., *acting director*, July 1, 1964 to Aug. 1, 1964

Dennis, James Lowden, M.D., *director*, Aug. 1, 1964

Appendix II.
Associate Deans of the
School of Medicine,
1947–64

Marsh, Homer F., Ph.D., *associate dean of students*, 1947–52

Taylor, Ardell Nichols, Ph.D., *associate dean of student affairs*, 1952–60; *Chairman, physiology*

Smith, Philip E., D.Sc., *associate dean of student affairs*, 1960–to date

Turner, Henry H., M.D., *associate dean of clinical instruction*, 1947–50

Stone, Samuel Newton, M.D., *associate dean of clinical instruction*, 1951–to date

Hellbaum, Arthur A., Ph.D., M.D., *associate dean of graduate studies and research*, 1947–57; *chairman, pharmacology*

Smith, James W. H., M.D., *associate dean of graduate studies and research*, 1954–56

Mosley, Kirk T., M.D., D.P.H., *associate dean of special training and research programs*, 1956–60; *chairman, preventive medicine and public health*

White, Joseph M., M.D., *associate dean of special training and research programs*, 1960–64; *chairman, anesthesiology*

Appendix III.
Heads or Chairmen of
Academic Departments, 1900–64

ANATOMY

Upjohn, Lawrence Northcote, M.D., 1900–1904
Stoops, Roy Philson, M.D., 1904–1908
Capshaw, Walter Leander, M.D., 1908–15
Hargrove, Reuben Morgan, M.D., 1916–19
Stephenson, Joseph Clark, Ph.D., M.D., 1919–31
Salsbury, Carmen Russell, M.D., 1931–33
Emenhiser, Lee Kenneth, M.D., *acting head*, 1933–35
DeGaris, Charles Francis, M.D., Ph.D., 1936–45
Lachman, Ernest, M.D., 1945–64*

ANESTHESIOLOGY

Moffett, John Alfred, M.D., 1930–38
Bolend, Floyd Jackson, M.D., *emeritus head*, 1935–39
Doudna, Hubert Eugene, M.D., 1938–48
Bennett, Howard A., M.D., 1948–55
Stream, Lawrence, M.D., *acting chairman*, 1955–56
White, Joseph M., M.D., 1956–(64)

BACTERIOLOGY[1]

Ellison, Gayfree, M.D., 1912–28
Buice, William Alfred, B.S., *acting head*, 1928–29
Moor, Hiram Dunlap, M.D., 1929–51
Marsh, Homer Floyd, Ph.D., 1951–52
Kelly, Florene C., Ph.D., 1952–58
Cummings, Martin M., M.D., 1959–61
Scott, Lawrence Vernon, D.Sc., 1961–(64)

* When 1964 appears in parentheses, it indicates that this was not the final year of appointment.
[1.] Department of Bacteriology was established as Department of Bacteriology and Hygiene in 1912–18, then Department of Bacteriology, which became Department of Microbiology in 1956.

BIOCHEMISTRY

Everett, Mark Reuben, Ph.D., 1924–(64)

BIOLOGY

Van Vleet, Albert Heald, Ph.D., 1898–1909

CHEMISTRY

DeBarr, Edwin C., Ph.D., 1906–23

COMMUNICATION DISORDERS[2]

Keys, John Walter, Ph.D., 1960–(64)

CONTINUING EDUCATION[3]

West, Kelly McGuffin, M.D., 1963–(64)

DERMATOLOGY[4]

Lain, Everett S., M.D., 1916–42
Bondurant, Charles Palmer, M.D., 1942–56
Lamb, John H., M.D., 1956–61
Jones, Phyllis E., M.D., 1961–63
Everett, Mark Allen, M.D., (1964)

FORENSIC MEDICINE

Bobo, Charles Sharp, M.D., 1906–10

GYNECOLOGY[5]

Kuhn, John Frederick, Jr., M.D., 1924–39
Penick, Grider, M.D., 1940–50
Kelso, Joseph Willard, M.D., 1951–61
Merrill, James A., M.D., 1961–(64)

HISTOLOGY AND EMBRYOLOGY

Thuringer, Joseph Mario, M.D., 1920–50

[2] Department of Communication Disorders was established in 1960.
[3] Department of Continuing Education was established in 1963.
[4] Changes in Department of Dermatology title: 1913, Department of Dermatology, Electrotherapy, and Radiography; 1921, Department of Dermatology, Electrotherapy, and Radiology; 1935, Department of Dermatology, Radiology, and Roentgenology; 1935, Department of Dermatology and Syphilology; 1962, Department of Dermatology.
[5] Departments of Gynecology and Obstetrics were combined in 1961.

LABORATORY MEDICINE[6]

Heller, Ben I., M.D., (1964)

MEDICAL ILLUSTRATION

Hiser, Ernest Freeman, B.A., 1948–(64)

MEDICINE

West, Archa Kelly, M.D., 1912–25
LaMotte, George Althouse, M.D., 1926–44
Langston, Wann, M.D., 1944–47
Bayley, Robert H., M.D., 1947–48
Goodwin, Rufus Quitman, M.D., 1948–51
Wolf, Stewart G., M.D., 1952–(64)

NEUROLOGY[7]

Young, Antonio DeBord, M.D., 1916–30
Fishman, Casriel J., M.D., 1930–46

OBSTETRICS[8]

Hatchett, John Archer, M.D., 1912–33
Wells, Walter William, M.D., 1933–45
Allen, Edward Pennington, M.D., 1945–46
Eskridge, James B., Jr., M.D., 1946–54
Serwer, Milton John, M.D., 1954–61
Merrill, James A., M.D., 1961–(64)

OPHTHALMOLOGY[9]

Ferguson, Edmund Sheppard, M.D., 1916–38
Westfall, Leslie Marshall, M.D., 1938–45
McGee, James Patton, M.D., 1945–52
Reed, James Robert, M.D., 1952–1962
Coston, Tullos Oswell, M.D., 1962–(64)

ORTHOPEDIC AND FRACTURE SURGERY[10]

Cunningham, Samuel Robert, M.D., 1936

[6.] Department of Laboratory Medicine was established in 1964.
[7.] Department of Psychiatry and Neurology was established in 1946.
[8.] See note 5 above.
[9.] Department of Ophthalmology and Otorhinolaryngology combined temporarily from 1922 to 1924.
[10.] Department of Orthopedic Surgery was established in 1936; its title was changed to Department of Orthopedic and Fracture Surgery in 1948.

West, Willia Kelly, M.D., 1936–37
Colonna, Paul Crenshaw, M.D., 1937–43
West, Willis Kelly, M.D., 1943–48
O'Donoghue, Don Horatio, M.D., 1948–(64)

OTORHINOLARYNGOLOGY[11]

Buxton, Lauren Haynes, M.D., LL.D., 1916–22
Ferguson, Edmund Sheppard, M.D., 1922–24
Todd, H. Coulter, M.D., 1924–36
Wails, Theodore G., M.D., 1936–48
McHenry, Lawrence Chester, M.D., 1948–51
Watson, O. Alton, M.D., 1951–59
Emenhiser, Lee K., M.D., 1959–62
Walker, Ethan A., Jr., M.D., 1962–64
Snow, James Byron, Jr., M.D., (1964)

PATHOLOGY

Williams, Edward Marsh, B.S., 1906–08
Turley, Louis Alvin, Ph.D., 1909–44
Hopps, Howard C., M.D., 1944–56
Jaques, William E., M.D., 1957–(64)

PEDIATRICS

Taylor, William M., M.D., 1930–38
Hall, Clark Homer, M.D., 1938–55
Strenge, Henry Bonheyo, M.D., 1955–57
Pfundt, Theodore Robert, M.D., *acting head*, 1957–58
Riley, Harris D., Jr., M.D., 1958–(64)

PHARMACOLOGY

Everett, Mark Reuben, Ph.D., 1924–35
Shoemaker, Harold Adam, Ph.C., Ph.D., 1935–44
Hellbaum, Arthur Alfred, Ph.D., M.D., 1944–57
Smith, Paul Winston, Ph.D., 1957–61
Payne, Richard W., M.D., 1961
Cotten, Marion deVeaux, Ph.D., 1961–(64)

PHYSICAL MEDICINE

George, Ella Mary, M.D., 1952–54
Gamble, Shelby G., M.D., 1954–58
Advisory Committee, 1958–(64)

[11.] See note 9 above.

PHYSIOLOGY

Maclaren, John Dice, M.D., 1908–11
Hirshfield, Albert Clifford, M.D., 1911–12
Nice, Leonard Blain, Ph.D., 1913–27
Mason, Edward Charles, M.D., Ph.D., 1928–46
Hellbaum, Arthur Alfred, Ph.D., M.D., 1946–47
Taylor, Ardell Nichols, Ph.D., 1947–60
Keyl, M. Jack, Ph.D., 1960–61
Haddy, Francis J., Ph.D., M.D., 1961–(64)

PREVENTIVE MEDICINE AND PUBLIC HEALTH[12]

Ellison, Gayfree, M.D., 1912–32
Moor, Hiram Dunlap, M.D., 1934–35
Hazel, Onis George, M.D., *acting chairman*, 1936–37
Olsen, Egil Thorbjorn, M.D., *acting chairman*, 1938–40
McMullen, Donald Bard, D.Sc., *acting chairman*, 1940–43
Hackler, John Fielden, M.D., 1943–48
Goldsmith, Joseph Benjamin, Ph.D., *acting chairman*, 1948–51
Brother, George M., M.D., 1951–52
Mosley, Kirk Thornton, M.D., D.P.H., 1952–60
Schottstaedt, William W., M.D., 1960–(64)

PSYCHIATRY, NEUROLOGY, AND BEHAVIORAL SCIENCES[13]

Young, Antonio D., M.D., 1912–15
Duke, John Williams, M.D., 1916–19
Griffin, David Wilson, M.D., 1920–40
Rayburn, Charles Ralph, M.D., 1940–48
Campbell, Coyne H., M.D., 1948–54
West, Louis Jolyon, M.D., 1954–(64)

RADIOLOGY[14]

Heatley, John Evans, M.D., 1936–48
Russo, Peter Ernest, M.D., 1948–57

[12.] Changes in Department of Preventive Medicine and Public Health titles: for 1912 to 1918 see note 1 above; 1919, Hygiene and Preventive Medicine; 1929, Epidemiology and Public Health; 1936, Hygiene and Public Health; 1944, Preventive Medicine and Public Health.

[13.] Department of Psychiatry and Neurology established in 1946; titles include: 1916, Mental Diseases and Medical Jurisprudence; 1920, Mental Diseases; 1946, Psychiatry and Neurology; 1952, Psychiatry; 1957, Psychiatry, Neurology, and Behavioral Sciences.

[14.] Department of Radiology established in 1936; see also note 4 above.

Ridings, Gus Ray, M.D., 1957–62
Knox, Gaylord S., M.D., *acting chairman*, 1963
Traub, Sidney P., M.D., 1963–(64)

SURGERY

Jolly, William James, M.D., 1912–13
Riley, John William, M.D., 1913–15
Long, LeRoy, M.D., 1915–31
Howard, Robert Mayburn, M.D., 1931–43
Clymer, Cyril E., M.D., 1943–48
Starry, Leo Joseph, M.D., 1948–52
Lingenfelter, Forrest Merle, M.D., 1952–56
Schilling John A., M.D., 1956–(64)

ORAL SURGERY (DENTAL SURGERY)

Reichmann, Francis J., D.D.S., 1935–41
Bertram, Frank Pitkin, D.D.S., *acting director*, 1941–46
Reichmann, Francis J., D.D.S., 1946–51
Robertson, John Millard, D.D.S., 1951–54
Miller, James R., D.D.S., 1954–55
Drescher, Albert R., D.D.S., 1955–61
Miley, Thomas Harvey, D.D.S., *acting director*, 1961
Schow, Carl Emil, D.D.S., 1961–62
Shons, Kenneth W., D.D.S., M.S.D., 1962–(64)

UROLOGY[15]

Riley, John W., M.D., 1913–19
Wallace, William Jones, M.D., 1919–34
Bolend, Rex George, M.D., *acting head*, 1934–36
Bolend, Rex George, M.D., 1936–43[16]
Taylor, Charles B., M.D., *acting chairman*, 1943–44
Hayes, Basil Augustus, M.D., *acting head*, 1945–46
Hayes, Basil Augustus, M.D., 1946–54
Branham, Donald W., M.D., 1954–61
Parry, William L., M.D., 1962–(64)

[15.] This department's title was Department of Urology and Syphilology until 1935.
[16.] Rex George Bolend was on military leave of absence from September, 1940, to January, 1944.

Appendix IV.
Faculty of the University of Oklahoma School of Medicine, 1900–64[1]

Abbott, Mary Ida, M.D., *instructor in pediatrics*, 1960;[2] *clinical instructor*, (1964)[3]

Abreu, Benedict Ernest, Ph.D., *instructor in pharmacology*, 1939–41

Abshier, Alton Brooke, M.D., *assistant in dermatology and syphilology*, 1943; *associate professor*, 1959

Ackermann, Alfred Joseph, medical diploma, *instructor in radiology*, 1937; *associate in therapeutic radiology*, 1943

Adams, George, M.D., *associate professor of preventive medicine and public health*, 1957–58

Adams, Thomas, Ph.D., *assistant professor of research physiology*, 1962–(64)

Addis, Barnett R., B.S., *research associate in psychiatry, neurology, and behvioral sciences*, 1962–(64)

Adelman, Frank L., M.D., *clinical assistant in psychiatry and neurology*, 1950–51

Adsett, Charles Alexander, M.D., *assistant professor of medicine and public health*, (1964)

Adsett, Nancy Leigh, M.A., *clinical assistant in psychiatry*, 1959

Akin, Robert Howe, M.D., *instructor in urology*, 1930; *associate clinical professor*, (1964)

Alaupovic, Petar A., Ph.D., *assistant professor of research biochemistry*, 1960–; *associate professor*, (1964)

Albers, Donald D., M.D., *clinical assistant in urology*, 1951; *associate professor*, (1964)

Albers, William R., M.D., *assistant professor of research preventive medicine and public health*, 1963; *professor*, (1964)

Alford, John Mosby, M.D., *instructor in medicine*, 1911; *associate*

[1.] New faculty member appointments up to July 1, 1964, are included in this list.

[2.] When two titles are given, the first is that at time of appointment, and the second is the title at termination of employment at the medical school.

[3.] When 1964 appears in parentheses, it indicates that this was not the final year of employment.

professor emeritus, 1956

Allen, Edward Pennington, M.D., *instructor in medicine*, 1919; *professor emeritus of obstetrics*, 1949

Allen, George Thomas, M.D., *instructor in obstetrics*, 1934; *associate professor*, 1959

Allgood, J. M., *assistant in anatomy*, 1925–26

Allison, John E., M.D., *associate professor of antomy*, 1957–(64)

Ambrister, Joseph Campbell, M.D., *instructor in genitourinary, skin and venereal diseases*, 1911–12

Amspacher, James Charles, M.D., *clinical assistant in orthopedic surgery*, 1949; *associate professor of orthopedic and fracture surgery*, (1964)

Anderson, Hubert M., M.D., *clinical assistant in surgery*, 1949; *associate professor*, (1964)

Anderson, Robert L., M.D., *visiting lecturer in surgery*, 1955–(64)

Andreskowski, Wencelaus T., M.D., *assistant in pathology*, 1919

Andrews, Leila Edna, M.D., *instructor in pediatrics*, 1910; *assistant professor of medicine*, 1925

Angelopoulos, Angelos P., D.D.S., *clinical assistant in dental surgery*, (1964)

Anglin, J. Hill, Ph.D., *assistant professor of research dermatology and instructor in research biochemistry*, 1963; *assistant professor*, (1964)

Annadown, Ruth Vivian, M.D., *clinical assistant in medicine*, 1951; instructor, 1958

Anspaugh, Robert Douglas, M.D., *associate in obstetrics and gynecology*, 1946; *clinical professor*, (1964)

Appleton, Meredith Marcus, M.D., *assistant in urology*, 1940; *clinical professor*, (1964)

Archer, Homer V., M.D., *clinical assistant in obstetrics*, 1948; *instructor*, 1954

Ashley, Robert Edward, M.D., *clinical associate in psychiatry, neurology, and behavioral sciences*, 1960

Asling, Mary Lucille, B.A., *assistant in clinical pathology*, 1942

Assenzo, Joseph R., Ph.D., *assistant professor of preventive medicine and public health*, 1963–(64)

Atkins, William Howard, M.D., *clinical assistant in medicine*, 1946–48

Austermann, Jack B., D.D.S., *clinical assistant in dental surgery*, 1961–(64)

Avey, Harry Thompson, Jr., M.D., *assistant professor of medicine*, 1942; *associate clinical professor*, (1964); *director of outpatient department*, 1942–46

Aycock, Byron Wolverton, M.D., *instructor in otorhinolaryngology*, 1944–(64)

Bahr, Julien W., M.D., *clinical assistant in medicine*, 1959; *assistant professor*, (1964)

Bailey, Byron Lewis, M.D., *clinical assistant in medicine*, 1954;

instructor, 1961

Bailey, William Hotchkiss, M.D., *instructor in clinical pathology*, 1924; *professor of medical jurisprudence*, 1947

Baker, Charles Ernest, M.D., *visiting lecturer in preventive medicine and public health*, 1957–58

Baker, Genene Marie, M.D., *assistant professor of radiology*, 1962–(64)

Balke, Bruno, M.D., *professor of research physiology*, 1960–(64)

Ballina, Jones Bautista, M.D., *instructor in gynecology*, 1959; *clinical instructor*, (1964)

Balyeat, Ray Morton, M.D., *instructor in medicine*, 1920; *associate professor emeritus*, 1960

Balyeat, Ray Morton, Jr., M.D., *clinical assistant in ophthalmology*, 1960; *instructor*, 1963

Bamforth, Betty Jane, M.D., *assistant professor of anesthesiology*, 1951–54

Barker, Marcus S., M.D., *visiting lecturer in psychiatry and neurology*, 1953; *assistant professor of psychiatry, neurology, and behavioral sciences*, (1964)

Barkett, Nasry Fayad Vander, M.D., *assistant in surgery*, 1946; *clinical professor*, (1964)

Barnard, John Walter, Ph.D., *research fellow in anatomy*, 1943; *associate professor*, 1947

Barnes, George, M.S., *instructor in preventive medicine and public health*, 1956–58; *social service director*, 1956–58

Barrett, Harle Virgil, M.D., *visiting lecturer in preventive medicine and public health*, 1955–57

Barry, George Newton, M.D., *instructor in medicine*, 1937; *clinical professor*, (1964); *director of outpatient department*, 1937–40, 1941–42; *acting medical director of University Hospitals*, 1941–44; *medical director of University Hospitals*, 1944–45

Bates, Clarence Edgar, M.D., *instructor in medicine*, 1928; *associate professor*, 1957

Baxt, Morton H., D.D.S., *clinical assistant in dental surgery*, 1963–(64)

Bayles, Esther Grace, *instructor in dietetics*, 1920–23

Bayley, Robert Hebard, M.D., *professor of clinical medicine*, 1944; *professor of medicine*, (1964)

Beargie, Robert A., M.D., *instructor in pediatrics*, 1962–(64)

Beaty, James R., M.D., *clinical instructor in pediatrics*, (1964)

Beavers, James C., M.D., *clinical assistant in gynecology-obstetrics*, 1962; *clinical instructor*, (1964)

Behrman, James M., M.D., *visiting lecturer in psychiatry and neurology*, 1953; *assistant professor of psychiatry, neurology, and behavioral sciences*, (1964)

Bell, Austin Holloway, M.D., *lecturer in surgery*, 1937; *clinical professor*, (1964)

Bell, Ben, M.D., *clinical assistant in psychiatry and neurology*, 1946;

instructor, 1948

Bell, James Preston, M.D., *instructor in orthopedic and fracture surgery*, 1960–(64)

Beller, Cleve, M.D., *research fellow in endocrinology*, 1948; *assistant professor of medicine*, 1954

Benjegerdes, Mildred M., M.D., *clinical assistant in anesthesiology*, 1955–56

Bennett, Henry Garland, Jr., M.D., *assistant in gynecology*, 1941; *clinical professor*, (1964)

Bennett, Howard Allen, M.D., *professor of anesthesiology*, 1948; *clinical professor*, (1964)

Benton, Paul C., M.D., *assistant professor of psychiatry, neurology and behavioral sciences*, 1955; *associate professor*, (1964)

Berger, Stanley E., M.D., *clinical assistant in medicine*, 1957; *instructor*, (1964)

Berkenbile, Glen Lee, M.D., *graduate fellow in anatomy*, 1949–50

Bernard, Louis Joseph, M.D., *instructor in surgery*, 1960–(64)

Berry, Charles Nelson, M.D., *instructor in surgery*, 1920; *associate professor*, 1941

Berry, Gladys, Ph.D., *research associate in medicine*, 1957–58

Bertram, Frank Pitkin, D.D.S., *instructor in dental surgery*, 1935; *clinical professor (orthodontics)*, 1956

Bettigole, Richard E., M.D., *clinical assistant in medicine*, 1962–63

Bettis, Annice Florine, M.A., *instructor in nutrition*, 1953–56

Bevan, William Richard, M.D., *instructor in therapeutics*, 1910; *assistant professor of obstetrics*, 1914

Bever, Arley Tunis, Jr., Ph.D., *assistant professor of biochemistry*, 1955; *associate professor*, 1963

Bielstein, Charles Max, M.D., *clinical assistant in pediatrics*, 1946; *associate clinical professor*, (1964)

Binder, Harold Jacob, M.D., *associate in pediatrics*, 1942; *associate clinical professor and clinical professor of psychiatry, neurology, and behavioral sciences*, (1964)

Binkley, James Garfield, M.D., *instructor in obstetrics*, 1928; *professor emeritus*, (1964)

Binkley, James Samuel, M.D., *clinical assistant in surgery*, 1952; *associate professor*, (1964)

Bird, Robert Montgomery, M.D., *associate professor of medicine*, 1952; *professor of medicine and physiology*, (1964)

Birge, Jack Paul, M.D., *assistant in surgery*, 1938; *instructor*, 1948

Bisbee, Walter Griswold, M.D., *instructor in orthopedic surgery*, 1910–12

Bishop, David William, M.D., *associate professor of ophthalmology*, (1964)

Bjerregaard, Mathille Elizabeth, M.S., *assistant in bacteriology*, 1934; *associate in physiology*, 1939

Blachly, Lucile Spire, M.D., *clinical assitant in medicine*, 1943; *assistant professor emeritus*, 1958

Blair, Clifford J., M.D., *clinical assistant in ophthalmology*, 1952; *assistant professor*, (1964)

Blalock, Shatteen, M.D., *instructor in preventive medicine and public health*, 1958–60

Blaschke, John Ahrens, M.D., *instructor in pharmacology*, 1951; *assistant professor*, (1964)

Blatt, Adolph Ebner, M.D., *clinical assistant in medicine*, 1946

Blesh, Abraham Lincoln, M.D., *professor of surgery and clinical surgery*, 1910; *professor of clinical surgery*, 1934

Blocksom, Berget H., Jr., M.D., *visiting lecturer in urology*, 1953–60

Bloedow, Carman E., M.D., *clinical assistant in medicine*, 1960; *instructor*, (1964)

Bloss, Claude M., M.D., M.P.H., *instructor in preventive medicine and public health*, 1963–(64)

Blue, Johnny A., M.D., *clinical assistant in medicine*, 1945; *associate clinical professor*, (1964)

Boatman, Karl Kenneth, M.D., *clinical assistant in surgery*, 1956; *instructor*, (1964)

Bobo, Charles Sharp, M.D., *lecturer in forensic medicine*, 1906; *professor of forensic medicine and therapeutics*, 1911; *dean of the School of Medicine*, 1908–11

Bodine, Charles David, M.D., *instructor in obstetrics*, 1950; *associate clinical professor*, (1964)

Bogardus, Carl Robert, Jr., M.D., *assistant professor of radiology*, (1964)

Boggs, James Thomas, M.D., *instructor in radiology*, 1955; *assistant professor*, 1962

Bogle, Margaret Lowe, M.S., *assistant professor of nutrition*, 1961–(64)

Bohan, Kenneth Earl, M.D., *clinical assistant in pediatrics*, 1949; *assistant clinical professor of pediatrics*, (1964)

Boland, John Louis, Jr., M.D., *consultant in otorhinolaryngology*, 1952–(64)

Bolend, Floyd Jackson, M.D., *instructor in children's diseases*, 1912; *associate professor of medicine and head of department of anesthesiology emeritus*, 1939

Bolend, Rex George, M.D., *instructor in dermatology and genitourinary diseases*, 1912; *professor or urology*, 1948

Bolene, Robert Victor, M.D., *clinical assistant in obstetrics and gynecology*, 1955–56

Boles, Gerald W., M.D., *instructor in radiology*, 1963–(64)

Bolten, Karl Austin, M.D., *research associate in pathology*, 1957–60

Bond, William Lawrence, M.D., *clinical assistant in obstetrics*, 1951; *assistant clinical professor of gynecology-obstetrics*, 1962

Bondurant, Charles Palmer, M.D., *instructor in dermatology*, 1928; *professor of dermatology and syphilology*, 1956

Bonham, William Lawrence, M.D., *instructor in otology, rhinology, and laryngology*, 1931; *clinical professor of otorhinolaryngology*, 1960

Borecky, George Lumar, M.D., *instructor in genitourinary diseases*, 1927; *instructor in urology*, 1947

Boren, Robert J., M.D., *visiting lecturer in dermatology*, (1964)

Bottomley, Richard Harold, M.D., *clinical assistant in medicine*, 1961; *instructor*, (1964)

Bottomley, Sylvia Stakle, M.D., *clinical assistant in medicine*, 1961; *instructor*, (1964)

Bouthilet, George N., Ph.D., *research associate in pediatrics*, 1959; *instructor in preventive medicine and public health*, (1964)

Bowden, David Thomas, M.D., *assistant professor of epidemiology and public health*, 1929–30

Bowen, Ralph, M.D., *instructor in medicine*, 1933–39

Bower, Raymond Kenneth, Ph.D., *research associate in microbiology*, 1957–58

Boyd, Thomas Madison, M.D., *instructor in bacteriology*, 1917

Boyd, Wayne J., M.D., *visiting lecturer in psychiatry, neurology, and behavioral sciences*, 1959–63

Boyle, James Stanton, M.D., *clinical assistant in urology*, 1954; *assistant professor*, (1964)

Bozalis, George Sam, M.D., *clinical assistant in medicine*, 1946; *assistant professor*, (1964)

Bracken, Everett C., Ph.D., *assistant professor of microbiology research in pediatrics*, 1959; *associate professor (departments of pediatrics and microbiology)*, (1964)

Braden, Barbara F., M.D., *instructor in preventive medicine and public health*, 1959; *instructor in medicine*, (1964)

Braden, Donald K., M.D., *clinical assistant in surgery*, (1964)

Bradford, Reagan Howard, M.D., *assistant professor of research biochemistry*, 1961; *associate professor of biochemistry and instructor in medicine*, (1964)

Bradford, Vance Arthur, M.D., *clinical assistant in surgery*, 1948; *associate professor*, (1964)

Brake, Charles Arthur, M.D., *instructor in psychiatry*, 1935; *assistant professor of psychiatry and neurology*, 1947

Brake, Charles M., M.D., *clinical assistant in medicine*, 1956; *instructor*, (1964)

Brandt, Edward Newman, Jr., Ph.D., M.D., *instructor in medical biomathematics in preventive medicine and public health*, 1961–(64)

Branham, Donald Wilton, M.D., *instructor in genitourinary diseases and syphilology*, 1935; *professor of urology*, 1960

Bressie, Jerry Lee, M.D., *clinical assistant in medicine*, 1963–(64)

Brewer, Augustus Malone, M.D., *assistant in urology*, 1938; *instructor*, 1947

Bricker, Earl M., M.D., *clinical assistant in gynecology*, 1958; *clinical instructor in gynecology-obstetrics*, (1964)

Bridges, Cecil C., Ph.D., *research associate in pediatrics*, 1959–60

Brixey, John Clark, Ph.D., *consultant professor of mathematical statistics in preventive medicine and public health*, 1960–(64)

Brodie, Charles M., Ph.D., *instructor in medical psychology in the department of psychiatry, neurology, and behavioral sciences*, 1960; *assistant professor*, (1964)

Broeg, Charles Burton, M.S., *research fellow in biochemistry*, 1940–41

Brother, George M., M.D., *professor of preventive medicine and public health*, 1951–52

Browder, Sue Elizabeth, B.A., *graduate assistant in anatomy*, 1940; *instructor*, 1943

Brown, D. Alton, M.D., *clinical assistant in medicine*, 1940; *associate professor*, (1964)

Brown, Claude H., M.C., *clinical assistant in pediatrics*, 1956; *clinical instructor*, (1946)

Brown, David Randolph, M.D., *clinical assistant in orthopedic and fracture surgery*, 1956; *assistant professor*, (1964)

Brown, David Von, M.D., *assistant professor of pathology*, 1946–47

Brown, Forest Reed, M.D., *visiting lecturer in preventive medicine and public health*, 1954; *assistant professor*, (1964)

Brown, George M., Jr., M.D., *visiting lecturer in surgery*, 1957–(64)

Brown, Ida Lucile, B.A., *instructor in bacteriology*, 1929–41

Brown, Irwin H., M.D., *instructor in surgery*, 1952; *assistant professor of surgery and director of postgraduate medical education*, (1964)

Brown, Leonard Harold, M.D., *instructor in surgery*, 1956; *assistant professor*, (1964)

Brown, Nello, M.D., *clinical assistant in medicine*, 1950; *instructor*, 1959

Brown, Robert C., M.D., *clinical assistant in medicine*, (1964)

Browne, Howard Storm, M.S., *instructor in pharmacy*, 1912; *dean of the School of Pharmacy and assistant professor of materia medica*, 1918

Brownell, Robert B., M.D., *clinical assistant in otorhinolaryngology*, (1964)

Brues, Alice M., Ph.D., *assistant professor of anatomy*, 1946; *professor*, (1964)

Bruhn, John G., Ph.D., *assistant professor of medical sociology in psychiatry, neurology, and behavioral sciences*, 1962; *assistant professor of preventive medicine and public health*, (1964)

Brundage, Carl Langley, M.D., *instructor in dermatology*, 1930; *clinical professor of dermatology and syphilology*, 1950

Bryant, Homer LaFayette, M.A., *assistant professor of physiology*, 1924–25

Buchner, Harold W., M.D., *clinical assistant in pediatrics*, 1946; *associate professor*, (1964)

Buice, William Alfred, M.D., *assistant professor of bacteriology and hygiene*, 1926; *assistant professor of bacteriology*, 1929

Bulmer, Glenn Stuart, Ph.D., *assistant professor of microbiology*,

1963–(64)

Bunde, Carl Albert, Ph.D., *research fellow in physiology*, 1937; *assistant professor*, 1942

Burke, Richard Michael, M.D., *visiting lecturer in medicine*, 1940; *associate professor*, (1964)

Burnett, Hal A., M.D., *instructor in surgery*, 1949–51

Burns, Thomas Craig, M.D., *instructor in nervous and mental diseases*, 1910; *assistant professor of neurology*, 1919

Burroughs, Lyle W., M.D., *assistant professor of pediatrics and consultant in allergy, otorhinolaryngology*, 1961–(64)

Burton, John Flack, M.D., *instructor in surgery*, 1931; *professor*, (1964)

Butler, Hull Wesley, M.D., *assistant in histology, organology, and embryology*, 1931; *associate in histology and embryology and associate in medicine*, 1946

Buvinger, Wilson J., M.D., *instructor in otorhinolaryngology*, 1963–(64)

Buxton, Lauren Haynes, M.D., LL.D., *professor of ophthalmology*, 1910; *professor emeritus of otology, rhinology, and laryngology*, 1924

Buxton, Thomas Merwin, M.D., *clinical assistant in medicine*, 1954; *instructor*, (1964)

Bynum, William Turner, M.D., *visiting lecturer in medicine*, 1941; *assistant professor*, (1964)

Byran, George A., Ph.D., *consulting professor of communication disorders*, (1964)

Cagas, Cosmelito, M.D., *clinical assistant in pediatrics*, (1964)

Cailey, Leo F., M.D., *instructor in ophthalmology, otology, rhinology, and laryngology*, 1929; *associate professor of ophthalmology*, (1964)

Cairns, John M., Ph.D., *assistant professor of histology and embryology*, 1952; *assistant professor of anatomy*, 1956

Campbell, Berry, Ph.D., *assistant professor of anatomy*, 1937–42

Campbell, Coyne Herbert, M.D., *instructor in pathology and anatomy*, 1933; *professor of psychiatry, neurology, and behavioral sciences*, 1957

Campbell, Gilbert Sadler, M.D., *professor of surgery*, 1958–(64)

Campbell, James Franklin, M.D., *instructor in anatomy*, 1929–30

Campbell, Joan L., M.S., *clinical assistant in psychiatry, neurology, and behavioral sciences*, 1963–(64)

Campbell, John Moore, III, M.D., *instructor in surgery*, 1942; *clinical professor*, (1964)

Campbell, Robert E., M.D., *instructor in ophthalmology*, 1959–(64)

Canavan, William Paul Newell, Ph.D., *associate professor of bacteriology*, 1929–39

Capehart, Maurice Philip, M.D., *graduate fellow in neurosurgery*, 1949–50

Capshaw, Walter Leander, M.D., *professor of anatomy*, 1908–15

Caputto, Ranwel, M.D., *assistant professor of research biochemistry*, 1953; *professor*, 1963

Carey, John Merwin, M.D., *clinical assistant in surgery*, 1954; *assistant professor*, (1964)

Carl, Roy Barton, M.D., *clinical assistant in surgery*, 1963–(64)

Carpenter, Mary Frances, Ph.D., *assistant professor of research biochemistry*, (1964)

Carpenter, Richard Everett, M.D., *clinical assistant in medicine*, 1949; *associate professor of medicine and assistant professor of psychiatry, neurology, and behavioral sciences*, (1964)

Carpenter, Robert Leroy, M.D., *instructor in medicine*, 1962; *assistant professor of medicine and of preventive medicine and public health*, (1964)

Carr, Helen, B.A., *instructor in medical social work*, 1935–41; *social service director*, 1934–41

Carroll, James Robert, M.D., *clinical instructor in ophthalmology*, (1964)

Carroll, William Bradford, M.D., *instructor in neuropsychiatry*, 1944–45

Carubelli, Raul, Ph.D., *assistant professor of research biochemistry*, 1963–(64)

Casals, Salvadore, M.D., *clinical assistant in medicine*, 1962–(64)

Casebeer, Robert Lawrence, M.D., *clinical assistant in otorhinolaryngology*, 1952; *assistant professor*, (1964)

Cavanaugh, John William, M.D., *assistant professor of surgery*, 1943–45

Caviness, James Jackson, M.D., *instructor in ophthalmology, otology, rhinology, and laryngology*, 1926; *clinical professor emeritus of ophthalmology*, (1964)

Cayler, Glen G., M.D., *assistant professor of pediatrics*, 1958; *associate professor*, 1962

Champlin, Paul B., M.D., *visiting lecturer in surgery*, 1953–(64)

Chance, Norman Allee, Ph.D., *consultant assistant professor of psychiatry, neurology, and behavioral sciences*, 1958–61

Chandler, Peter James, M.A., *research associate in psychiatry, neurology, and behavioral sciences*, 1962–(64)

Chanes, Raul Emir, M.D., *clinical assistant in medicine*, (1964)

Charney, Louis Harry, M.D., *instructor in medicine*, 1931; *associate professor*, (1964)

Chase, Arthur Brown, M.D., *instructor in therapeutics*, 1917; *professor of clinical medicine and lecturer in medical ethics*, 1936

Chase, Ralph Edward, M.A., *assistant in physiology*, 1926; *instructor in anatomy*, 1954

Chatham, Beverly Colvin, M.D., *visiting lecturer in obstetrics*, 1951–55

Chester, Robert Lee, M.D., *assistant professor of anesthesiology*, 1962–(64)

Childers, Cecil Adison, M.D., *visiting lecturer in psychiatry, neurology, and behavioral sciences*, (1964)

Childers, David, M.D., *visiting lecturer in pediatrics*, 1960–(64)

Chitwood, Lawrence A., Ph.D., *instructor in pediatrics*, (1964)

Chont, Lasla Kendey, M.D., *assistant in therapeutic radiology*, 1942

Cirillo, Vincent Paul, Ph.D., *assistant professor of preventive medicine and public health*, 1953–55

Clark, Dale Allen, Ph.D., *assistant professor of biochemistry*, 1950; *associate professor*, 1954

Clark, George, Ph.D., *associate professor of research anatomy*, (1964)

Clark, Mervin Leslie, M.D., *clinical assistant in medicine*, 1954; *associate professor*, (1964)

Clark, Ralph Otis, M.D., *instructor in surgery*, 1943–53

Clark, Robert T., Ph.D., *professor of research physiology*, 1960–(64)

Clay, Richard Allen, M.D., *clinical assistant in ophthalmology*, 1948; *associate professor*, (1964)

Clemens, Ted, Jr., M.D., *instructor in medicine*, 1958–(64)

Clements, Donald Gene, M.D., *fellow in oncology*, 1949–50

Cleverdon, Margaret, B.S., *assistant in clinical pathology*, 1943

Clifton, Chester Stanley, Ph.D., *consultant professor of social work in psychiatry, neurology, and behavioral sciences*, 1963–(64)

Clymer, Cyril Ebert, M.D., *instructor in surgery*, 1913; *chief of dispensary staff*, 1917–24; *professor emeritus of surgery*, (1964)

Clymer, John Hatchett, M.D., *clinical assistant in surgery*, 1951; *assistant professor*, (1964)

Coalson, Robert E., Ph.D., *assistant professor of anatomy*, 1960–(64)

Cochrane, Charles Riley, M.D., *clinical assistant in obstetrics*, 1951; *instructor*, 1954

Coffey, Cecilia Agnes, M.S., *instructor in nutrition*, 1962; *assistant professor*, (1964)

Coffey, Clinton Maurice, M.D., *visiting lecturer in dermatology*, (1964)

Coggins, Farris Webb, M.D., *clinical assistant in gynecology*, 1956; *assistant clinical professor*, (1964)

Cohen, Elias, Ph.D., *instructor in pathology*, 1952; *research associate*, 1956

Cohenour, Howard Murdock, M.D., *visiting lecturer in urology*, 1953–60

Coil, Jenner G., M.D., *instructor in otorhinolaryngology*, 1954–60

Coin, Carl G., M.D., *clinical assitant in radiology*, 1955; *assistant professor*, (1964)

Coin, James Walter, M.D., *instructor in radiology*, 1957; *assistant professor*, (1964)

Coleman, Ronald Leon, Ph.D., *assistant professor of research biochemistry and of preventive medicine and public health*, (1964)

Coleman, William Omer, M.D., *clinical assistant in surgery*, 1957; *instructor*, (1964)

Coley, Joe Henry, M.D., *clinical assistant in obstetrics*, 1936; *assistant clinical professor*, (1964)

Collins, Herbert Dale, M.D., *instructor in gynecology*, 1928; *associate professor*, 1942

Collins, Joe Ed., M.D., *clinical assistant in urology*, 1956; *instructor*, (1964)

Collins, Norma J., B.S. (Mrs. Craig), *assistant professor of nutrition*,

1951–57
Collins, William Robert, M.D., *clinical assistant in ophthalmology*, 1960; *instructor*, (1964)
Colmore, John P., M.D., *assistant professor of medicine*, 1952; *associate professor*, (1964); *director of outpatient department*, 1952–61
Colonna, Paul Crenshaw, M.D., *professor of orthopedic surgery*, 1937–43
Colvert, James Robert, M.D., *clinical assistant in medicine*, 1949; *assistant professor*, (1964)
Colyar, Ardell Benton, M.D., *instructor in preventive medicine and public helath*, 1946–48
Compton, Paul Avery, M.D., *clinical assistant in medicine*, (1964)
Condit, Paul Taylor, M.D., *assistant professor of research medicine and research biochemistry*, 1958; *assistant professor of research biochemistry and associate professor of research medicine*, (1964)
Cone, Jess Donald, Jr., M.D., *graduate fellow in anatomy*, 1948
Connery, Jennie, M.S., *assistant professor of administrative medicine in preventive medicine and public health*, 1960; *social service director*, 1959–61
Conrad, Loyal Lee, M.D., *clinical assistant in medicine*, 1948; *associate professor*, (1964)
Cook, Odis A., M.D., *instructor in preventive medicine and public health*, 1957–59
Cooke, Everett Ellis, M.D., *clinical assistant in surgery*, 1951; *associate professor*, (1964)
Cooley, Ben Hunter, M.D., *instructor in minor surgery*, 1922–29
Cooper, Fay Maxey, M.D., *instructor in ophthalmology*, 1932; *clinical professor*, 1953
Cooper, Walter R., Jr., D.D.S., *clinical assistant in dental surgery*, 1959; *instructor*, (1964)
Cooper, William Allen, Jr., Ph.D., *consulting assistant professor of communication disorders*, (1964)
Cooper, Zola Katherine, Ph.D., *assistant professor of histology and embryology*, 1946; *associate professor of histology and embryology and consulting associate professor of dermatology and syphilology*, 1949
Copeland, Evan Leonard, M.S., *research fellow in physiology*, 1939–40
Corder, Vernon W., M.D., *instructor in anesthesiology*, 1955–61
Cornelison, Floyd S., M.D., *associate professor of psychiatry, neurology, and behavioral sciences*, 1958–63
Cornelius, George Robert, M.D., *clinical instructor in ophthalmology*, (1964)
Correa, Juan Francisca, M.D., *clinical assistant in anesthesiology*, 1963–(64)
Corson, Samuel Abraham, Ph.D., *assistant professor of physiology*, 1942–43
Cosby, Warren Melville, M.D., *assistant professor of gynecology-obstetrics*, 1963–(64)

Costeloe, James Paul, M.D., *research associate in medicine, in psychiatry, neurology, and behavioral sciences, and in preventive medicine and public health*, 1957–(64)

Costigan, Daniel Gilbert, M.D., *instructor in orthopedic and fracture surgery*, 1948–49

Costilow, Teresa M., M.S., *research associate in pediatrics*, 1963–(64)

Coston, Tullos Oswell, M.D., *instructor in ophthalmology*, 1936; *professor*, (1964)

Cotten, Daisy Van Hoesen, M.D., *clinical assistant in obstetrics*, 1949; *assistant professor*, 1957

Cotten, Marion deVeaux, Ph.D., *professor of pharmacology*, 1961–(64)

Cottle, Isaac Newton, M.D., *instructor in gynecology*, 1912–13

Counihan, Donald, Ph.D., *consultant in otorhinolaryngology*, 1957; *associate professor of communication disorders and consultant in otorhinolaryngology and in speech therapy of pediatrics*, (1964)

Cowan, Judith R., M.D., *instructor in psychiatry, neurology, and behavioral sciences*, 1963–(64)

Cox, James Alphonso, M.D., *clinical assistant in psychiatry, neurology, and behavioral sciences*, 1959; *assistant professor*, (1964)

Coyle, John J., M.D., *clinical assistant in gynecology*, 1950; *assistant professor*, 1961

Craig, Nancy Ryan, M.D., *clinical assistant in anesthesiology*, 1957; *assistant clinical professor*, (1964)

Craig, William J., M.D., *clinical assistant in pediatrics*, 1960; *instructor*, (1964)

Crane, Ronald F., M.D., *clinical assistant in anesthesiology*, 1960

Cranny, Robert Leverne, M.D., *assistant professor of pediatrics*, 1954–57

Crawford, Sterling Thomas, M.D., *clinical assistant in gynecology*, 1949; *assistant professor*, (1964)

Crews, Lowell Thomas, M.S., *research fellow in biochemistry*, 1939–40

Crews, Raymond Drake, B.A., LL.B., *assistant professor of administrative medicine in preventive medicine and public health*, 1956–(64)

Crider, Quincy Edward, Ph.D., *research associate in research biochemistry*, 1962–(64)

Crittendon, William Floyd, M.D., *clinical assistant in gynecology-obstetrics*, (1964)

Croom, William S., M.D., *clinical assistant in medicine*, 1952–54

Crosthwait, Marion Joe, M.D., *clinical assistant in medicine*, 1956–(64)

Cubler, Edward William, M.D., *instructor in anesthesiology*, 1950

Cummings, Martin M., M.D., *professor of microbiology*, 1959; *professor of microbiology and associate professor of medicine*, 1963

Cunningham, Earl Richard, D.D.S., *clinical assistant in dental surgery*, 1951; *associate professor*, (1964)

Cunningham, John Ashby, M.D., *assistant in surgery*, 1938; *associate professor*, 1962

Cunningham, Perry J., M.D., *instructor in anesthesiology*, 1947
Cunningham, Samuel Robert, M.D., *professor of gynecology*, 1910; *professor of orthopedic surgery*, 1936
Cunningham, William Alfred, M.D., *instructor in ophthalmology*, 1962–(64)
Curle, Roy E., M.D., *clinical assitant in anesthesiology*, 1959–61
Cushing, Vernon D., M.D., *instructor in medicine*, 1947; *associate professor*, (1964); *acting medical director of University Hospitals*, 1948; *medical director*, 1949
Cutter, James Arthur, M.D., *associate professor of anesthesiology*, 1961; *clinical professor*, (1964)
Dabney, Joe Mitchell, Ph.D., *assistant professor of phsyiology*, 1960–(64)
Dakil, Samuel Edward, M.D., *instructor in otorhinolaryngology*, 1961–(64)
Daniel, John Furman, M.D., *clinical assistant in gynecology*, 1949; *instructor*, 1954
Daniels, Harry Anthony, M.D., *assistant in medicine*, 1942; *associate professor*, (1964)
Danielson, Irvin S., Ph.D., *assistant professor of biochemistry*, 1937–42
Danstrom, John Richard, M.D., *clinical assistant in radiology*, 1946; *associate professor*, (1964)
Darcey, Henry Joseph, B.S., *lecturer on hygiene and public health*, 1936; *instructor in preventive medicine and public health*, 1951
Darden, Paul Martin, M.D., *graduate fellow in pharmacology*, 1946; *assistant professor*, 1948
Daril, Louis Najib, M.D., *assistant in medicine*, 1938–40
Darling, John Chester, M.D., *associate professor (physical director)*, 1908; *physical director*, 1913
Daron, Garmon Harlow, Ph.D., *associate professor of anatomy*, 1947; *professor*, (1964)
Darrow, Frank E., M.D., *clinical assistant in surgery*, 1953; *assistant professor*, (1964)
David, Paul R., Ph.D., *professor of medical gentics*, 1958–(64)
Davis, Edward Francis, M.D., *lecturer in clinical ophthalmology and otorhinolaryngology*, 1911; *associate professor of ophthalmology*, 1928
Davis, Kieffer D., M.D., *visiting lecturer in preventive medicine and public health*, 1956–(64)
Dawson, Clarence Benton, M.D., *clinical assistant in urology*, 1948; *associate professor*, (1964)
Day, Curtis Richard, M.D., *professor of genitourinary and veneral diseases*, 1910; *professor of pathology, serology, and clinical microscopy*, 1915; *dean of the School of Medicine*, 1914–15
Day, John Lewis, M.D., *instructor in physical diagnosis and minor surgery*, 1920–29
DeBarr, Edwin C., Ph.D., *professor of chemistry and physics*, 1892; *vice-president*, 1909; *professor of chemistry*, 1923

Deckert, Gordon H., M.D., *clinical assistant in psychiatry, neurology, and behavioral sciences*, 1962; *assistant professor*, (1964)

DeGaris, Charles Francis, M.D., Ph.D., *professor of anatomy*, 1936; *professor emeritus*, 1963

Delashaw, Johnny Bill, M.D., *clinical assistant in medicine*, 1962

Delhotal, Charles Earl, M.D., *clinical assistant in pediatrics*, 1950; *assistant clinical professor*, (1964)

DeMand, Francis Asbury, M.D., *instructor in obstetrics*, 1930; *associate professor*, 1943

Dennis, James L., M.D., *professor of pediatrics and dean of the School of Medicine and director of the Medical Center*, (1964)

Denny, Earl Rankin, M.D., *visiting lecturer in medicine*, 1941–49

Denny, William F., M.D., *clinical assistant in medicine*, 1956

Dersch, Walter Henry, M.D., *clinical assistant in medicine*, 1942; *assistant professor*, (1964)

Deupree, Harry Linnell, M.D., *assistant in medicine*, 1938; *clinical professor of obstetrics*, (1964)

Devanney, Louis Raynor, M.D., *clinical assistant in surgery*, 1946–47

Devore, James K., M.D., *clinical assistant in medicine*, 1955; *instructor*, 1963

Devore, John Woodrow, M.D. *graduate fellow in anatomy*, 1947; *instructor in medicine*, (1964)

Dewar, James P., Jr., M.D., *associate professor of pathology*, 1950; *associate clinical professor*, (1964)

Diamond, Louis Edward, M.S., *instructor in biochemistry*, 1941–51

Dickens, Karl Lavon, M.S., *instructor in anatomy*, 1929–31

Dickson, Green Knowlton, M.D., *instructor in medicine*, 1925; *instructor in surgery*, 1930

Dill, Francis Edward, M.D., *instructor in gynecology*, 1933–46

Dille, John Robert, M.D., *associate professor of research preventive medicine and public health*, 1962–(64)

Dixon, Gerald R., M.D., *instructor in ophthalmology*, 1962–(64)

Dixon, Winfield Eugene, M.D., *assistant professor of otology, rhinology, and laryngology*, 1915; *professor*, 1930

Dodson, Harrell Chandler, Jr., M.D., *assistant professor of surgery*, 1948; *associate professor*, (1964)

Dodson, Jack Elwood, Ph.D., *professor of preventive medicine and public health*, 1962

Doering, Carl Rupp, M.D., D.Sc., *consulting professor of preventive medicine and public health*, 1952; *professor*, 1963

Dolin, Simon, M.D., *assistant professor of radiology*, 1952; *associate professor*, 1956

Donaghe, Roy W., M.D., *clinical assistant in pediatrics*, 1955; *clinical instructor*, (1964)

Donahue, Hayden Hackney, M.D., *consultant assistant professor of psychiatry and neurology*, 1954; *associate professor of psychiatry*, neurology, and behavioral sciences, (1964)

Donnell, John J., M.D., *clinical assistant in medicine*, 1948; *associate professor*, (1964)

Dornfeld, Ernst John, Ph.D., *instructor in histology and embryology*, 1937–38

Dorwart, Frederic Griffin, M.D., *visiting lecturer in medicine*, 1941–51

Dotter, Richard Gene, M.D., *clinical assistant in medicine*, (1964)

Doudna, Hubert Eugene, M.D., *lecturer in anesthesiology*, 1938; *professor*, (1964)

Dougherty, Thomas Francis, Jr., M.A., *research fellow in pathology*, 1937–39

Dowling, William Jackson, M.D., *clinical assistant in surgery*, 1954; *instructor*, (1964)

Drake, John Whitfield, M.D., *clinical assistant in medicine*, 1962–(64)

Drescher, Albert R., D.D.S., *clinical assistant in dental surgery*, 1942; *clinical professor (prosthodontia)*, (1964)

Dubowski, Kurt M., Ph.D., *associate professor of clinical chemistry and toxicology in biochemistry and pathology*, 1961–(64)

Dudley, Alberta Webb, M.D., *assistant in medicine*, 1945; *instructor*, 1953

Dudley, Thomas F. Webb, D.D.S., *clinical assistant in the division of dental surgery, department of surgery*, (1964)

Duke, John Williams, M.D., *professor of nervous and mental diseases*, 1915; *professor of mental diseases and medical jurisprudence*, 1920

Dunagin, James Love, M.D., *instructor in pediatrics*, 1960; *assistant clinical professor*, (1964)

Duncan, Darrell Gordon, M.D., *instructor in dermatology*, 1930; *associate in therapeutic radiology*, 1940

Dunkel, John F., M.D., *assistant professor of pathology*, 1954; *visiting lecturer*, 1958

Dunkelberg, Royal B., D.D.S., *instructor in dental surgery*, 1961; *assistant professor*, (1964)

Dunn, John Hartwell, M.D., *clinical assistant in urology*, 1948; *associate professor*, (1964)

DuVal, Merlin K., Jr., M.D., *associate professor of surgery*, 1957; *professor of surgery and assistant director of the Medical Center*, (1964)

Earp, Ancel, M.D., *clinical assistant in surgery*, 1955; *assistant professor*, 1964

Eastland, William Edgar, M.D., *instructor in dermatology*, 1928; *professor of radiology*, (1964)

Eaton, Bobby Gene, M.D., *clinical assistant in radiology*, (1964)

Eddy, Leonard, M.L.S., *assistant professor of medical library science*, 1962–(64)

Edelberg, Robert, Ph.D., *professor of psychophysiology in department of psychiatry, neurology, and behavioral sciences and of physiology*, 1963–(64)

Edelson, Marshall, Ph.D., M.D., *assistant professor of psychiatry, neurology, and behavioral sciences*, 1961–(64)

Edmundson, Walter F., M.D., *assistant professor of preventive medicine and public health*, 1954–55

Edwards, Beatrice, M.A., *research associate in biochemistry*, 1934–36

Edwards, Reba Huff, M.D., *clinical assistant in medicine*, 1946; *instructor in psychiatry, neurology, and behavioral sciences*, (1964)

Eley, Norphleete Price, M.D., *instructor in medicine*, 1928; *associate clinical professor*, (1964)

Eliel, Leonard P., M.D., *associate professor of research medicine*, 1951; *professor*, (1964)

Elliott, Arthur Furman, M.D., *clinical assistant in medicine*, 1952; *assistant professor*, (1964)

Ellis, Robert Smith, M.D., *clinical assistant in medicine, 1957; assistant clinical professor*, (1964)

Ellison, Gayfree, M.D., *professor of bacteriology and instructor in anatomy*, 1910; *professor of bacteriology and epidemiology and public health*, 1932

Else, Frank Lester, B.S., *assistant professor of physiology*, 1929–30

Emanuel, Floyd W., Ph.D., *assistant professor of communication disorders*, 1963–(64)

Emenhiser, Lee Kenneth, M.D., *instructor in anatomy*, 1931; *clinical professor of otorhinolaryngology*, (1964)

Emmett, Edward, M.D., *clinical assistant in medicine*, 1942

Emmott, Ralph Cameron, M.D., *visiting lecturer in urology*, 1962–(64)

Epps, Curtis Howard, M.D., *instructor in clinical pathology*, 1940–42

Erdos, Ervin George, M.D., *professor of pharmacology*, 1963–(64)

Erwin, Paul D., M.D., *clinical assistant in surgery*, 1954; *assistant professor*, (1964)

Eskridge, James Burnett, Jr., M.D., *instructor in medicine and in obstetrics*, 1924; *clinical professor of obstetrics*, (1964)

Eskridge, James Burnett, III, M.D., *clinical assistant in obstetrics*, 1951; *assistant clinical professor*, (1964)

Essenburg, Jacob Martin, Ph.D., *associate professor of anatomy*, 1923–29

Estes, Hillard D., M.D., M.P.H., *consultant professor of research preventive medicine and public health*, 1960–61

Evans, Winfield W., M.S., *instructor in radiology*, 1952–(64)

Everett, Mark Allen, M.D., *instructor in dermatology*, 1958; *associate professor*, (1964)

Everett, Mark Reuben, Ph.D., *professor of physiological chemistry and pharmacology*, 1924; *regents professor of medical sciences and consulting professor of biochemistry and dean emeritus*, (1964); *dean and director of the University of Oklahoma Medical Center and superintendent of University Hospitals*, 1947–(64)

Ewing, William Finis, Jr., M.D., *clinical assistant in medicine*, 1957–58

Eyerer, Rudolf Emil, M.D., *assistant professor of pathology*, 1957–61

Fagin, Herman, M.D., *instructor in medicine*, 1932; *associate professor*, 1964

Fair, Ellis Edwin, M.D., *clinical assistant in surgery*, 1947; *visiting lecturer in psychiatry and neurology*, (1964)

Falks, John LeRoy, Ph.D., *consultant associate professor of preventive medicine and public health*, 1962–(64)

Faris, Brunel DeBost, M.D., *instructor in obstetrics*, 1937; *associate professor*, 1956

Farley, Nancy Bess, Ed.D., *research associate in pediatrics*, 1963–(64)

Farnam, Lorenzo Matthew, M.D., *assistant in surgery*, 1941; *instructor*, 1945

Farris, Edward Merhige, M.D., *clinical assistant in surgery*, 1948; *associate professor*, (1964)

Farris, Emil P., M.D., *clinical assistant in ophthalmology*, 1954; *assistant professor*, (1964)

Faulkner, Kenneth Keith, M.S., *instructor in anatomy*, 1954; *associate professor*, (1964)

Felton, Frances G., Ph.D., *assistant professor of research microbiology*, 1958; *associate professor*, (1964)

Felton, Jean Spencer, M.D., *associate professor of medicine and of preventive medicine and public health*, 1953; *professor of preventive medicine and public health and consultant in medicine*, 1957

Felton, Warren L., M.D., *clinical assistant in surgery*, 1958; *assistant professor*, (1964)

Felts, George R., M.D., *instructor in medicine*, 1936; *associate in pediatrics*, 1944

Ferber, Leon, M.D., *clinical assistant in psychiatry and neurology*, 1946–49

Ferguson, Charles Duncan, M.D., *instructor in ophthalmology, otology, rhinology, and laryngology*, 1912; *assistant professor of ophthalmology*, 1916

Ferguson, Edmund Gordon, M.D., *instructor in ophthalmology*, 1931; *professor*, (1964)

Ferguson, Edmund Sheppard, M.D., *professor of clinical ophthalmology, otology, rhinology, and laryngology*, 1910; *professor emeritus of ophthalmology*, 1941

Fesler, Paul H., *acting superintendent of University Hospital*, 1916–18; *superintendent of University Hospital*, 1918–20; *fiscal superintendent of University Hospital*, 1920–27; *administrator of University Hospitals*, 1946–47

Field, Clarence Henry, M.D., *instructor in gynecology*, 1912–13

Finch, James William, M.D., *visiting lecturer in medicine*, 1942–(64)

Finn, Thomas C., M.D., *clinical assistant in pediatrics*, 1957–59

Finney, Joseph Melville, M.D., *assistant in osteology*, 1905–1906

Fisher, Pearl D., Ph.D., *research associate in preventive medicine and public health*, 1959; *assistant professor*, (1964)

Fishman, Casriel J., M.D., *instructor in medicine and lecturer in clinical microscopy*,1911; *professor emeritus of medicine*, 1959

Fite, William Patton, M.D., *visiting lecturer in surgery*, 1941–61

Flanigan, Herman Floyd, M.D., *consulting professor of communication disorders*, (1964)

Fleming, Elizabeth P., M.D., *visiting lecturer in preventive medicine and public health*, 1958–(64)

Flesher, Marion A., D.D.S., *clinical assistant in dental surgery*, 1940; *clinical professor*, (1964)

Flesher, William Nason, D.D.S., *clinical assistant in dental surgery*, 1951; *associate professor (orthodontics)*, (1964)

Flock, Eugene Richard, M.D., *instructor in preventive medicine and public health*, 1954–58

Florence, John, M.D., *clinical assistant in orthopedic surgery*, 1951; *assistant professor of orthopedic and fracture surgery*, (1964)

Flux, Marinus, M.D., *clinical assistant in pediatrics*, (1964)

Foerster, Hervey Adolph, M.D., *instructor in dermatology and syphilology*, 1937; *clinical professor*, (1964)

Ford, Harry Cummings, M.D., *assistant in otorhinolaryngology*, 1938; *professor*, 1949

Forester, Virgil Ray, M.D., *clinical assistant in medicine*, 1952; *assistant professor*, (1964)

Forrest, William J., M.D., *clinical assistant in surgery*, (1964)

Foster, Albert Douglas, M.D., *professor of anesthesiology*, 1945–46

Foster, John Allan, M.S., *visiting lecturer in engineering in psychiatry, neurology, and behavioral sciences*, 1962–(64)

Foster, Richard Leland, M.D., *instructor in medicine and hygiene, sanitary science, and state medicine*, 1910; *assistant professor of medicine*, 1914

Fowler, William Alonzo, M.D., *instructor in obstetrics*, 1912; *professor of hygiene and public health*, 1942

Frank, Gael Raymond, M.D., *assistant professor of orthopedic and fracture surgery*, 1962–(64)

Frank, Louis S., M.D., *instructor in pediatrics*, 1948; *associate clinical professor*, (1964)

Freed, Leon C., M.D., *instructor in medicine*, 1954; *assistant professor*, (1964)

Freede, Charles Louis, M.D., *clinical assistant in pediatrics*, 1950; *associate clinical professor*, (1964)

Freeman, Charles W., M.D., *instructor in pediatrics*, 1941; *associate clinical professor*, (1964)

Frew, Athol Lee, Jr., D.D.S., M.D., *clinical assistant in dental surgery*, 1948; *associate professor of oral surgery*, (1964)

Friedberg, Wallace, Ph.D., *assistant professor of research biochemistry*, 1961–(64)

Friou, George J., M.D., *associate professor of medicine and research* microbiology, 1960–(64)

Fuller, Guy Wesley, M.D., *clinical assistant in medicine*, 1956; *instructor*, 1959

Fulton, Clifford Cannon, M.D., *assistant in surgery*, 1936; *associate professor*, 1956

Funnell, James Dean, M.D., *clinical instructor in gynecology-obstetrics*, (1964)

Funnell, Joseph W., M.D., *instructor in gynecology*, 1954; *assistant clinical professor of gynecology-obstetrics*, (1964)

Furman, Robert Howard, M.D., *associate professor of research medicine*, 1952–(64)

Gable, James Jackson, M.D., *instructor of mental diseases and medical jurisprudence*, 1920; *associate professor of mental diseases*, 1940

Gable, James Jackson, Jr., M.D., *clinical assistant in medicine*, 1948; *associate professor*, (1964)

Gafford, Tom Sid, Jr., M.D., *fellow in pathology*, 1948; *instructor*, (1964)

Galbraith, Hugh Malcolm, M.D., *instructor in neurology*, 1940; *assistant professor of psychiatry and neurology*, 1952

Galegar, William Clark, M.S., *instructor in preventive medicine and public health*, 1954–60

Gamble, Alice Frances, M.D., *instructor in anesthesiology*, 1963–(64)

Gamble, Shelby G., M.D., *professor of physical medicine*, 1954–59

Garnier, William Hampton, M.D., *clinical assistant in ophthalmology*, 1954; *assistant professor*, (1964)

Garrison, George Harry, M.D., *instructor in pediatrics*, 1930; *clinical professor*, (1964)

Gastineau, Felix Thomas, M.D., *instructor in pathology and clinical microscopy*, 1918–19

Gaston, John Zell, B.S., *assistant professor of anatomy*, 1920–22

Gatchell, Frank G., M.D., *clinical assistant in surgery*, 1959; *instructor*, (1964)

Geigerman, David Jackson, M.D., *instructor in anesthesiology*, 1951; *assistant professor*, (1964)

Gentry, Wanda, M.S.W., *clinical assistant in psychiatry, neurology, and behavioral sciences*, 1962–(64)

George, Ella Mary, M.D., *assistant professor of physical medicine*, 1949; *clinical professor*, (1964)

Geyer, James Robert, M.D., *clinical instructor in urology*, 1963–(64)

Geyer, Robert W., M.D., *instructor in radiology*, 1961–(64)

Green, Delmar L., Jr., M.D., *clinical assistant in pediatrics*, (1964)

Gibbs, Allen Gilbert, M.D., *assistant in medicine*, 1938; *assistant professor*, 1954

Gideon, Alma C., M.S.W., *clinical assistant in psychiatry, neurology, and behavioral sciences*, 1962–(64)

Gill, William Thomas, M.D., *visiting lecturer in pathology*, 1948–51

Gillaspy, Carrie S., B.A., *graduate assistant in anatomy*, 1938–41

Gilliland, Donald Carroll, M.D., *clinical instructor in ophthalmology*, (1964)

Ginn, Earl H., M.D., *assistant professor of medicine*, 1962–(64)

Glass, Albert Julius, M.D., *clinical professor of psychiatry, neurology, and behavioral sciences*, 1963–(64)

Glass, Howard George, Ph.D., *instructor in pharmacology*, 1944–46

Glasser, Samuel M., M.D., *instructor in radiology*, 1950; *associate professor*, (1964)

Glaze, Max A., M.D., *clinical assistant in psychiatry, neurology, and behavioral sciences*, 1958–59

Glismann, Marvin Brown, M.D., *assistant in medicine*, 1943; *assistant clinical professor*, (1964)

Goaz, Paul William, D.D.S., *instructor in research dental surgery*, 1953; *assistant professor of dental surgery and instructor in research microbiology*, (1964)

Goetzinger, Billy Richard, M.D., *instructor in anesthesiology*, 1962; *assistant clinical professor*, (1964)

Goff, Catherine, *dietitian*, 1919–20

Gogerty, John Harry, Ph.D., *assistant professor of pharmacology*, 1958–63

Gold, David, M.D., *clinical assistant in medicine*, 1955–57

Goldberg, Ira, Ph.D., *instructor in medical psychology in the department of psychiatry, neurology, and behavioral sciences*, 1960–61

Goldfain, Ephraim, M.D., *instructor in neurology*, 1929; *associate professor of medicine*, (1964)

Goldsmith, Joseph Benjamin, Ph.D., *assistant professor of histology and embryology*, 1931; *professor of preventive medicine and public health*, (1964)

Goodwin, Rufus Quitman, M.D., *instructor in medicine*, 1929; *professor*, (1964)

Googe, Mary, M.D., *assistant professor of anesthesiology*, 1954–55

Gordon, Douglas Meharg, M.D., *visiting lecturer in medicine*, 1941–51

Graham, Stephen Harry, M.D., *assistant in anatomy*, 1915–16

Gravelle, Harold Roy, D.D.S., *clinical assistant in oral surgery*, 1957; *instructor*, (1964)

Gray, Floyd, M.D., *instructor in obstetrics*, 1931; *associate professor*, 1946

Gray, Jacques Pierce, M.D., *professor of public health medicine*, 1946–47; *dean of the School of Medicine and superintendent of University Hospitals*, 1946–47

Gray, James K., M.D., *fellow in pathology*, 1938–39

Gray, Opal Willard, *instructor in massage (physical medicine)*, 1937; *lecturer*, 1943

Graybill, Charles Shelly, M.D., *fellow in orthopedic surgery*, 1949;

visiting lecturer, (1964)

Greaves, Donald C., M.D., *associate professor of psychiatry, neurology, and behavioral sciences*, 1955–58

Green, Charles Eugene, M.D., *visiting lecturer in pediatrics*, 1949–(64)

Green, James Albert, Ph.D., *associate professor of research biochemistry*, 1960–62

Green, Wilma Jeanne, Ph.D., *instructor in pathology*, 1931; *assistant professor*, (1964)

Greer, Allen E., M.D., *clinical assistant in surgery*, 1952; *associate professor*, (1964)

Gregg, Orion Russell, M.D., *visiting lecturer in preventive medicine and public health*, 1954–59

Griffin, David Wilson, M.D., *associate professor of mental diseases and medical jurisprudence*, 1916; *professor emeritus of psychiatry and neurology*, 1953

Groover, Marshall E., Jr., M.D., *associate professor of medicine*, 1961–(64)

Gruss, Sarah, B.A., *instructor in physical therapy*, 1955

Guin, Jere D., M.D., *visiting lecturer in dermatology*, 1960–63

Gumbreck, Laurence Gable, Ph.D., *assistant professor of anatomy*, 1957–(64)

Gunn, Chesterfield Garvin, Jr., M.D., *assistant professor of preventive medicine and public health*, 1956; *associate professor of physiology and medicine and assistant professor of preventive medicine and public health*, (1964)

Gussen, John, M.D., *assistant professor of psychiatry, neurology, and behavioral sciences*, 1955–57

Gussen, Ruth R., M.D., *instructor in pathology*, 1955–57

Guthrey, George Henry, M.D., *clinical assistant in psychiatry and neurology*, 1948; *clinical professor*, (1964)

Guthrie, Austin Lee, M.D., *instructor in otology, rhinology, and laryngology*, 1917; *associate professor*, 1936

Guthrie, Thomas Joseph, D.D.S., *clinical assistant in dental surgery*, 1961; *instructor*, (1964)

Gwinn, Margaret E., M.S., *instructor in preventive medicine and public health*, 1954; *assistant professor of administrative medicine in preventive medicine and public health*, 1961

Haase, Gunter R., M.D., *associate professor of neurology in medicine and associate professor of psychiatry, neurology, and behavioral sciences*, 1960–(64)

Hackler, Harold Waton, M.D., *clinical assistant in psychiatry and neurology*, 1947; *assistant professor of psychiatry, neurology, and behavioral sciences*, 1963

Hackler, John Fielden, M.D., *professor of preventive medicine and public health*, 1943; *visiting lecturer*, 1958

Haddy, Francis J., Ph.D., M.D., *professor of physiology and associate professor of medicine*, 1961–(64)

Haddy, Theresa Brey, M.D., *instructor in pediatrics*, 1961; *assistant professor*, (1964)

Hagans, James A., M.D., Ph.D., *assistant professor of medicine*, 1955; *associate professor of medical biostatistics*, 1962

Hahn, Richard G., M.D., M.P.H., *assistant professor of medicine and assistant professor of preventive medicine and public health*, 1953; *associate professor of preventive medicine and public health*, (1964)

Haig, Karl James, M.D., *assistant professor of anatomy*, 1931; *associate professor*, 1933

Haight, Thomas Hulen, M.D., *assistant professor of medicine and of preventive medicine and public health*, 1954; *assistant professor of medicine and of preventive medicine and public health and consultant assistant professor of pediatrics*, 1958

Hain, Raymond F., M.D., *associate professor of pathology*, 1960–(64)

Hale, John Milton, Ph.D., *associate professor of bacteriology*, 1952; *professor*, (1964)

Hall, Clark Homer, M.D., *instructor in pediatrics*, 1922; professor emeritus, (1964)

Hall, David Connolly, M.S., *instructor in pharmacology*, 1903–1908

Hall, Elizabeth Rose, M.S., *instructor in bacteriology*, 1941–44

Hallum, Glen Dale, M.D., *clinical assistant in radiology*, (1964)

Halpert, Béla, M.D., *professor of clinical pathology*, 1942–49

Hamburger, Irvin Glenn, M.D., *assistant professor of anesthesiology*, 1957; *associate professor*, (1964)

Hamby, Wallace Bernard, B.S., *assistant in histology*, 1924–26

Hammarsten, James F., M.D., *assistant professor of medicine*, 1953; *professor*, 1962

Hamner, Charles Earnest, M.D., *assistant professor of bacteriology*, 1913–14

Hampton, Hollis E., M.D., *clinical assistant in gynecology*, 1958; *instructor*, (1964)

Hampton, James W., M.D., *clinical assistant in medicine*, 1960; *assistant professor*, (1964)

Haney, Taswell Paul, Jr., M.D., D.P.H., *visiting lecturer in preventive medicine and public health*, 1954–62

Hannas, Ralston Raymond, Jr., M.D., *clinical assistant in medicine*, 1958; *assistant clinical professor*, (1964)

Hargrove, Reuben Morgan, M.D., *professor of anatomy*, 1918–19

Harris, Henry Washington, M.D., *assistant in obstetrics*, 1937; *instructor*, 1954

Harris, Jan Owen, M.S.W., *clinical assistant in psychiatry, neurology, and behavioral sciences*, 1962–(64)

Harris, Richard Lowell, M.D., *clinical assistant in obstetrics*, 1948; *instructor*, 1954

Harris, Russell D., M.D., *clinical assistant in orthopedic surgery*, 1951;

associate professor, (1964)

Harrison, Stearley Pike, M.D., *graduate assistant in physiology*, 1935; *instructor in medicine*, 1951

Harrison, William S., M.D., *clinical assistant in medicine*, 1959; *instructor*, (1964)

Harroz, Joseph, M.D., *clinical assistant in gynecology-obstetrics*, 1963–(64)

Harsha, William Norris, M.D., *clinical assistant in orthopedic and fracture surgery*, 1956; *instructor*, (1964)

Hart, J. P., M.S., *research fellow in biochemistry*, 1937–39

Hart, Maynard Sterling, M.D., *instructor in clinical pathology*, 1940–42

Hartford, John Smith, M.D., *instructor in gynecology*, 1910; *professor*, 1924; *chief of dispensary staff*, 1912–16

Hartford, Walter Kenneth, M.D., *clinical assistant in gynecology*, 1948; *clinical professor of gynecology and obstetrics and consultant associate professor of pathology*, (1964)

Harvey, Charles M., M.D., *clinical assistant in medicine*, 1954; *assistant professor*, (1964)

Harvey, Rosemary Boles, M.D., *visiting lecturer in preventive medicine and public health*, 1954–56

Hassler, Ferdinand Rudolph, M.D., M.P.H., *instructor in hygiene and public health*, 1936; *visiting lecturer in preventive medicine and public health*, (1964)

Hassler, Grace Ellen Clause, M.D., *instructor in anesthesiology*, 1937; *clinical professor*, (1964)

Hatchett, John Archer, M.D., *professor of obstetrics and gynecology*, 1911; *professor emeritus of obstetrics*, 1940

Hathaway, Euel Park, M.D., *instructor in genitourinary diseases*, 1932–33

Hauty, George Thomas, Ph.D., *professor of research physiology and of psychiatry, neurology, and behavioral sciences*, 1960–(64)

Hayes, Basil Augustus, M.D., *instructor in surgery and genitourinary diseases*, 1922; *professor emeritus of urology*, (1964)

Hays, Marvin Bryant, M.D., *clinical assistant in orthopedic and fracture surgery*, 1953; *instructor*, 1955

Hazel, Onis George, M.D., *instructor in epidemiology and public health*, 1933; *clinical professor of dermatology and syphilology*, 1957

Head, John Francis, M.D., *research fellow in medicine*, 1950; *instructor*, 1952

Heaney, Robert Proulx, M.S., *instructor in medicine*, 1954–56

Heatley, John Evans, M.D., *instructor in dermatology, electrotherapy, and radiography*, 1920; *professor emeritus of radiology*, 1961

Heck, Lilah Bell, M.D., *librarian*, 1942; *assistant professor of medical library science*, (1964)

Hefley, Harold Martin, Ph.D., *fellow in bacteriology*, 1936–37

Helander, Dick Herbert F., M.D., *assistant professor of research medicine*, (1964)

Hellams, Alfred Allen, M.D., *instructor in psychiatry and neurology*, 1950; *assistant professor of psychiatry, neurology, and behavioral sciences*, (1964)

Hellbaum, Arthur Alfred, Ph.D., M.D., *assistant professor of physiology*, 1936; *research professor of pharmacology*, (1964)

Heller, Ben I., M.D., *professor of laboratory medicine*, 1963–(64)

Henderson, Jesse Lester, M.D., *instructor in neurology*, 1936–43

Hendren, Walter Scott, M.D., *clinical assistant in medicine*, 1949; *associate professor*, (1964)

Hendrix, Sam W., M.D., *clinical assistant in obstetrics*, 1958; *clinical instructor in obstetrics and gynecology*, (1964)

Henke, Joseph Reid, M.D., *clinical assistant in ophthalmology*, 1957; *assistant professor*, (1964)

Henley, Thomas Hunter, M.D., *clinical assistant in surgery*, 1962–(64)

Hennes, Allen R., M.D., *assistant professor of medicine*, 1958–62

Hensley, Jess N., M.D., *assistant professor of pathology*, 1963; *assistant clinical professor*, (1964)

Herbelin, Joseph Ted, M.D., *clinical instructor in anesthesiology*, 1962–(64)

Herndon, Robert Eugene, M.D., *clinical assistant in pediatrics*, 1956; *clinical instructor*, (1964)

Herrmann, Jess Duval, M.D., *assistant in surgery*, 1936; *clinical professor*, (1964)

Hicks, Melvin Clause, M.D., *instructor in radiology*, 1958; *assistant professor*, (1964)

Hightower, Harry G., M.D., *clinical assistant in psychiatry, neurology, and behavioral sciences*, 1955; *assistant professor*, (1964)

Hill, Joseph MacGlashan, M.D., *assistant professor of pathology*, 1932; *assistant professor of anatomy*, 1934

Hill, Virgil Thomas, Ph.D., *visiting lecturer in psychiatry, neurology, and behavioral sciences*, 1959–(64)

Hinman, Edgar Harold, M.D., Ph.D., *professor of preventive medicine and public health*, 1949–51

Hinshaw, Lerner B., Ph.D., *associate professor of research physiology*, 1961–(64)

Hirner, Sister Mary Bonaventure, M.S., *instructor in nutrition*, 1951; *assistant professor*, 1962

Hirschi, Robert Graham, D.D.S., *clinical assistant in dental surgery*, 1949; *associate professor of dental surgery and visiting lecturer in preventive medicine and public health*, (1964)

Hirshfield, Albert Clifford, M.D., *instructor in materia medica*, 1910; *professor of obstetrics*, 1926

Hiser, Ernest Freeman, B.A., *medical artist*, 1930; *assistant professor of medical illustration*, (1964)

Hitchcock, Waldo Philip, B.A., *assistant in physiology*, 1936–39

Hladky, Frank, Jr., B.S., *research fellow in biochemistry*, 1943–44

Hodges, Thomas Oran, M.D., *clinical assistant in surgery*, 1955; *assistant professor*, 1958

Hohl, James F., M.D., *clinical assistant in medicine*, 1955–58

Hoke, Lillian M., M.D., *clinical assistant in pediatrics*, 1955; *clinical instructor*, (1964)

Holden, Everett Neal, M.D., *clinical assistant in preventive medicine and public health*, 1959–62

Hollis, Lynn E., M.D., *visiting lecturer in preventive medicine and public health*, 1954–57

Holt, Robert Perry, M.D., *clinical assistant in orthopedic surgery*, 1949; *associate professor of orthopedic and fracture surgery*, (1964)

Honick, Gerald L., M.D., *clinical assistant in medicine*, 1960; *instructor*, (1964)

Honick, Mary Duffy, M.D., *clinical assistant in medicine*, 1955; *instructor*, (1964)

Honska, Walter, M.D., *instructor in medicine and in preventive medicine and public health*, 1959; *instructor in medicine*, (1964)

Hood, Frederick Redding, M.D., *instructor in biochemistry and pharmacology*, 1928; *associate professor of medicine*, (1964)

Hood, Frederick Redding, Jr., M.D., *instructor in surgery* 1963–(64)

Hood, Phillip N., M.D., *reserch associate in pediatrics*, 1961–(64)

Hood, William E., M.D., *clinical assistant in obstetrics*, 1959; *assistant clinical professor*, 1962

Hooper, Henry Wade, M.S., *instructor in histology and embryology*, 1945–46

Hoot, Melvin Philip, M.D., *assistant in otorhinolaryngology*, 1938–42

Hoppock, Ruth Evelyn, B.A., *instructor in elementary dietetics*, 1928–30

Hopps, Howard Carl, M.D., *professor of pathology*, 1944–56

Horn, Bernard, M.D., *instructor in anesthesiology*, 1960–62

Horowitz, Leon, M.D., *visiting lecturer in pediatrics*, 1959–(64)

Houchin, Ollie Boyd, Ph.D., *instructor in pharmacology*, 1942; *assistant professor of research biochemistry and of psychiatry, neurology, and behavioral sciences*, (1964)

Hough, Jack Van Doren, M.D., *clinical assistant in otorhinolaryngology*, 1948; *associate professor*, (1964)

Houk, Paul Cullison, M.D., *clinical assistant in medicine*, 1963–(64)

Howard, Merle Quest, M.D., *instructor in neurology*, 1923

Howard, Robert Bruce, M.D., *assistant in surgery*, 1938; *clinical professor*, (1964)

Howard, Robert Mayburn, M.D., *professor of clinical surgery*, 1910; *professor emeritus*, 1963

Howard, R. Palmer, M.D., *associate professor of research medicine*, 1951–(64)

Howard, Walter Alonzo, M.D., *visiting lecturer in medicine*, 1941–51

Hoyt, Arthur W., M.D., *visiting lecturer in pediatrics*, 1948–53

Huber, Wolfgang Karl, M.D., *instructor in psychiatry, neurology, and behavioral sciences*, 1963–(64)

Hudnut, Herbert B., Jr., M.D., *clinical assistant in preventive medicine and public health*, 1959; *clinical assistant in medicine*, 1961

Hudson, Fred G., M.D., *clinical assistant in medicine*, 1955; *instructor*, 1961

Hudson, Katherine Kaufman, M.S., *assistant in psychosomatic teaching*, 1951; *instructor in social work and in psychiatry, neurology, and behavioral sciences*, (1964)

Huff, Dick Howard, M.D., *clinical assistant in medicine*, 1948; *assistant professor*, (1964)

Huff, Thomas Jefferson, Jr., M.D., *clinical assistant in surgery*, 1952; *instructor*, 1954

Huffman, Max Niel, Ph.D., *research professor of biochemistry*, 1950; *professor of research biochemistry*, 1963

Huggins, James Richard, M.D., *assistant in medicine*, 1938; *instructor*, 1954

Hughes, William Lyon, M.D., *clinical assistant in medicine*, 1962–(64)

Hull, Robert Lord, M.D., *lecturer in orthopedic surgery*, 1911; *associate professor*, 1919

Hull, Wayne McKinley, M.D., *instructor in clinical pathology*, 1937; *instructor in medicine*, 1945; *director of outpatient department*, 1935–37

Hunt, Davis T., M.D., *clinical assistant in obstetrics*, 1956; *clinical instructor*, 1963

Hunter, DeWitt T., M.D., *associate professor of pathology*, 1958–63

Hunter, George, M.D., *instructor in obstetrics*, 1914; *instructor in genitourinary diseases*, 1926

Hunter, L. Virginia, M.D., *instructor in pediatrics*, 1958; *clinical instructor*, 1963

Hyroop, Gilbert Louis, M.D., *clinical assistant in surgery*, 1953; *assistant professor*, (1964)

Hyroop, Muriel Hall, M.D., *instructor in psychiatry and neurology*, 1952; *assistant professor*, 1958

Ice, Clark Hawkins, M.S., *research fellow in pharmacology*, 1941–42

Ingle, John Daniel, M.D., *clinical assistant in surgery*, 1951; *associate professor*, (1964)

Ingram, Charles Dean, M.A., *instructor in medical library science*, 1963–(64)

Ishmael, William Knowlton, M.D., *assistant in medicine*, 1936; *associate professor*, (1964)

Ivey, Michael H., Ph.D., *associate professor of preventive medicine and public health*, (1964)

Jabbour, J.T., M.D., *assistant professor of neurology in psychiatry, neurology, and behavioral sciences and assistant professor of pediatrics*, 1961–(64)

Jacobs, John Theodore, Jr., M.D., *research fellow in orthopedic surgery*, 1942–46

Jacobs, Minard Friedberg, M.D., *instructor in medicine*, 1933; *clinical professor*, (1964)

Jansky, Cyril Methodius, B.S., *professor of physics and of electrical engineering*, 1905–1908

Janszen, Herbert H., M.D., *associate professor of psychiatry, neurology, and behavioral sciences*, 1958–61

Jaques, William E., M.D., *professor of pathology*, 1957–(64)

Jenkins, Joseph Basil, D.D.S., *instructor in dental surgery*, 1923–29

Jennings, George Harry, M.D., *clinical assistant in gynecology*, 1956; *assistant clinical professor of gynecology and obstetrics*, (1964)

Jeter, Hugh Gilbert, M.D., *assistant professor of clinical pathology*, 1927; *consultant associate professor of pathology*, (1964)

Jobe, Virgil R., M.D., *instructor in hygiene and public health*, 1936; *instructor in surgery*, 1947

Joel, Walter, M.D., *assistant professor of pathology*, 1949; *professor*, (1964)

Johnson, David Byars Ray, M.A., *dean and professor of pharmacy*, 1919–26

Johnson, Fred Schroeder, B.S., *instructor in diet therapy*, 1937–44

Johnson, Mark Royal, M.D., *instructor in medicine*, 1952–(64)

Johnson, Philip Carl, M.D., *assistant professor of medicine*, 1955; *associate professor*, 1958

Johnson, Porteous Elmore, M.D., *associate in orthopedic surgery*, 1946–47

Johnson, Tom Lamar, M.D., *instructor in ophthalmology*, 1962–(64)

Johnston, Richard E., M.S., *instructor in physics in radiology*, 1959–62

Jolly, William James, M.D., *professor of principles and practice of surgery*, 1910; *professor of surgery*, 1914; *acting dean of the School of Medicine*, 1913–14

Jones, Hugh Clifford, M.D., *instructor in gynecology*, 1931–34

Jones, Jake, Jr., M.D., *visiting lecturer in pediatrics*, 1961–(64)

Jones, Margie C., M.S., *instructor in nutrition*, 1958–(64)

Jones, Phyllis Emmaline, M.D., *clinical assistant in dermatology and syphilology*, 1946; *clinical professor of dermatology*, (1964)

Kalbfleisch, John M., M.D., *clinical assistant in medicine*, 1961; *instructor*, (1964)

Kahn, Robert W., M.D., *clinical assistant in medicine*, 1949; *associate professor*, (1964)

Kalmanson, George M., B.S., *fellow in bacteriology* 1936–37

Kalmon, Edmond H., Jr., M.D., *clinical assistant in radiology*, 1950; *associate professor*, (1964)

Katzberg, Allan Alfred, Ph.D., *instructor in histology*, 1949; *assistant professor of anatomy*, 1958

Kauth, John E., M.D., *visiting lecturer in radiology*, (1964)

Kavan, Lucien C., M.D., *instructor in urology*, 1959; *assistant professor*, (1964)

Kay, Jacob L., M.D., *instructor in pediatrics*, 1960; *assistant professor*, (1964)

Kearns, Harry James, Jr., M.D., *clinical assistant in radiology*, (1964)

Keaty, Ellen Corine, Ph.D., *research fellow in pharmacology*, 1946; *associate in research in the department of pharmacology and consulting research associate in dermatology and syphilology*, 1957

Keele, Doman K., M.D., *assistant professor of pediatrics*, 1958; *associate professor*, 1962

Keele, Marjorie S., M.D., *instructor in pediatrics*, 1959–62

Keeping, Eleanor S., Ph.D., *research associate in microbiology*, 1962–63

Keeping, Ernest Sydney, A.R.C.S., D.I.C., *consultant professor of preventive medicine and public health*, 1962–63

Keith, Howard Barton, M.D., *clinical assistant in surgery*, 1962–(64)

Keller, Wilbur Floyd, M.D., *instructor in medicine*, 1933; *clinical professor of pathology*, (1964)

Kelley, James W., M.D., *instructor in surgery*, 1957–(64)

Kelling, Jordan Albert, M.D., *clinical assistant in psychiatry and neurology*, 1946

Kelly, Florene Cora, Ph.D., *assistant professor of bacteriology*, 1944; *professor*, (1964)

Kelly, John W., Ph.D., *associate professor of pathology*, 1961–(64)

Kelso, Joseph Willard, M.D., *instructor in gynecology*, 1929; *professor*, (1964)

Keltz, Bert Fletcher, M.D., *instructor in medicine*, 1930; *clinical professor*, (1964); *director of outpatient department*, 1933–35

Kemler, Stanley M., M.D., *instructor in psychiatry, neurology, and behavioral sciences*, 1958; *assistant professor*, (1964)

Kemp, David Edward, Ph.D., *instructor in psychiatry, neurology, and behavioral sciences*, 1963–(64)

Kent, Herbert L., L.R.C.P., *associate professor of physical medicine*, 1955; *associate professor of physical medicine and of preventive medicine and public health*, (1964)

Kenyon, Rex E., M.D., *instructor in pathology*, 1955; *assistant professor*, (1964)

Kerekes, Ernest S., M.D., *visiting lecturer in radiology*, (1964)

Kersey, Barbara June, M.L.S., *instructor in medical library science*, 1963–(64)

Keso, Larson Russell, D.D.S., *clinical assistant in dental surgery*, 1960; *instructor*, (1964)

Keyl, M. Jack, Ph.D., *assistant professor of physiology*, 1957; *associate professor*, (1964)

Keys, John Walter, Ph.D., *professor of speech and director of Speech and*

Hearing Clinic, 1945; *consulting audiologist in otorhinolaryngology and professor of communication disorders*, (1964)

Kimball, George Henry, M.D., *assistant in surgery*, 1936; *clinical professor*, (1964)

Kimerer, Neil B., M.D., *clinical assistant in psychiatry and neurology*, 1950; *associate professor of psychiatry, neurology, and behavioral sciences*, (1964)

King, Robert Wallace, M.D., *clinical assistant in ophthalmology*, 1954; *assistant professor*, (1964)

Kirkman, Henry N., M.D., *assistant professor of pediatrics*, 1959; *professor of biochemistry and associate professor of pediatrics*, (1964)

Klinges, Karl Guy, M.D., *clinical instructor in gynecology-obstetrics*, 1963–(64)

Klopfenstein, Keith A., M.D., *instructor in medicine*, 1962–(64)

Knight, Laurence Lyle, M.D., *instructor in pathology*, 1962–(64)

Knowles, Frank Elwood, Ph.D., *instructor in physics*, 1904–1905

Knox, Frank C., Jr., M.D., *instructor in psychiatry, neurology, and behavioral sciences*, 1960–(64)

Knox, Gaylord Shearer, M.D., *associate professor of radiology*, 1961–(64)

Kochakian, Charles D., Ph.D., *professor of research biochemistry*, 1951–56

Kraft, David I., M.D., *clinical assistant in medicine*, 1956; *instructor*, (1964)

Kramer, Robert Lewis, M.D., *instructor in ophthalmology*, 1960–(64)

Krieger, Carl, Jr., M.D., *instructor in anesthesiology*, 1952; *associate professor*, (1964)

Kuchar, Vaclav, M.D., *professor of physical therapy*, 1928–36

Kuhn, John Frederick, M.D., *lecturer in clinical surgery*, 1912; *professor emeritus of gynecology*, 1942

Kuhn, John Frederick, Jr., M.D., *instructor in anatomy and gynecology*, 1935; *clinical professor of gynecology*, (1964)

Kuritz, Albert B., M.D., *clinical assistant in surgery*, (1964)

Kurtz, Alton Clair, Ph.D., *assistant professor of biochemistry*, 1942; *professor*, (1964)

Kurzner, Meyer, M.D., *assistant in pediatrics*, 1940; *instructor*, 1947

Kusakari, Takashi, M.D., *reserach associate in pharmacology*, (1964)

Kutkam, Ahmet L., M.D., *research associate in pathology*, 1961–(64)

Kutkam, Yildiz, M.D., *instructor in anesthesiology*, 1962–(64)

Kyriacopoulos, Adrian A., M.D., *clinical assistant in medicine*, 1960; *instructor*, (1964)

Kyriacopoulos, John D., M.D., *instructor in medicine*, 1961–(64)

Lachman, Ernest, M.D., *assistant professor of anatomy*, 1934; *professor of anatomy and radiology*, (1964)

Lain, Everett Samuel, M.D., *professor of dermatology, electrotherapy, and radiography*, 1910; *professor emeritus of dermatology*, (1964)

Lamb, John Henderson, M.D., *instructor in dermatology and syphilology*, 1936; *clinical professor of dermatology*, 1961

LaMotte, George Althouse, M.D., *professor of clinical medicine*, 1910; *professor emeritus*, 1959

Landy, Jerome J., M.D., *assistant professor of surgery*, 1955--56

Langston, Wann, M.D., *instructor in histology and bacteriology and in pathology and clinical microscopy*, 1916; *professor emeritus of medicine*, (1964); *medical superintendent of University Hospital*, 1920–29; *administrative officer of University Hospitals*, 1929–31; *director of outpatient department*, 1931–33; *dean and superintendent of University Hospitals*, 1945–46

Lane, Henry Higgins, M.A., Ph.D., *instructor in zoology and embryology*, 1906; *professor*, 1918

Larsen, Earl G., Ph.D., *assistant professor of biochemistry*, 1955; *associate professor*, (1964)

Lategola, Michael T., Ph.D., *assistant professor of physiology*, 1956; *associate professor of research physiology*, (1964)

LaTorre, Phillip, M.S., *instructor in preventive medicine and public health*, 1956–57

Lawler, Francis Cornelius, D.Sc., *assistant professor of bacteriology*, 1937; *assistant professor of bacteriology and of hygiene and public health*, 1941

Lawrence, Charles Hillman, Ph.D., *instructor in preventive medicine and public health and clinical instructor in radiology*, 1964

Lawson, Patrick Henry, M.D., *instructor in genitourinary diseases and syphilology*, 1933–39

Lawson, Robert C., M.D., *clinical assistant in medicine*, 1947; *associate professor*, (1964)

Lee, Clarence Edward, M.D., *instructor in clinical microscopy*, 1910–11

Lee, Norman K., M.D., *instructor in pathology*, 1959; *assistant professor*, 1962

Lehman, Arnold John, M.D., Ph.D., *assistant professor of pharmacology*, 1937–39

Leidigh, Mary, *assistant administrative dietitian*, 1944–45

Lemmon, William B., Ph.D., *consultant professor of psychology in psychiatry, neurology, and behavioral sciences*, 1959–(64)

Lemmon, William Gladstone, B.S., *assistant in pathology and bacteriology*, 1906; *assistant in pathology and bacteriology and in anatomy*, 1908

Lemon, Cecil Willard, M.D., *instructor in physiology*, 1928; *instructor in anesthesiology*, 1952

Leney, Fannie Lou Brittain, M.D., *instructor in pediatrics*, 1930–36

Leonard, Charles Edward, M.D., *assistant in medicine*, 1941; *clinical professor of psychiatry, neurology, and behavioral sciences*, (1964)

Leslie, Samuel B., M.D., *clinical assistant in ophthalmology*, 1959;

instructor, (1964)

Lester, Boyd K., M.D., *assistant professor of psychiatry, neurology, and behavioral sciences*, 1958; *associate professor*, (1964)

Levitt, Seymour H., M.D., *associate professor of radiology*, 1963–(64)

Levy, Bertha Marion, M.D., *instructor in pediatrics*, 1943; *associate clinical professor*, (1964)

Lewis, Arthur Rimmer, M.D., *special lecturer on applied therapeutics*, 1918–20

Lewis, John Emmett, D.D.S., *clinical assistant in dental surgery*, 1954; *instructor*, (1964)

Lhevine, Dave Bernard, M.D., *visiting lecturer in radiology*, 1952; *assistant professor*, (1964)

Lhotka, John Francis, Jr., M.D., Ph.D., *assistant professor of anatomy and histology*, 1951; *associate professor of anatomy*, (1964)

Li, Yu-Teh, Ph.D., *assistant professor of research biochemistry*, (1964)

Liebrand, Clair, M.D., *clinical assistant in medicine*, 1954–57

Limes, Barney Joe, M.D., *instructor in urology*, 1962–(64)

Lincoln, Richard B., M.D., *clinical assistant in medicine and consulting clinical assistant in psychiatry and neurology*, 1953; *assistant professor of psychiatry, neurology, and behavioral sciences*, (1964)

Lindeman, Robert D., M.D., *clinical assistant in medicine*, 1960–63

Lindner, Anton, M.D., *associate professor of pathology*, 1960–(64)

Lindsay, Ray Harvey, M.D., *visiting lecturer in surgery*, 1941–(64)

Lindsey, David C., M.D., *clinical instructor in medicine*, 1962–(64)

Lindstrom, William Carl, M.D., *assistant in obstetrics*, 1938; *instructor*, 1948

Lingenfelter, Forrest Merle, M.D., *instructor in medicine, surgery, and obstetrics*, 1925; *professor of surgery*, (1964)

Lisle, Achilles Courtney, M.D., *clinical assistant in surgery*, 1949; *associate professor*, (1964)

Little, Jesse Samuel, M.D., *clinical instructor in radiology*, (1964)

Lockwood, Wayne B., M.D., *clinical assistant in orthopedic and fracture surgery*, 1963–(64)

Long, LeRoy, M.D., *professor of surgery*, 1915–31; *dean of the School of Medicine and superintendent of University Hospitals*, 1915–31

Long, LeRoy, M.D., *clinical assistant in surgery*, 1963–(64)

Long, LeRoy Downing, M.D., *instructor in surgery*, 1924; *clinical professor*, (1964)

Long, Wendell McLean, M.D., *instructor in gynecology*, 1929–31

Loney, William Robert, M.D., *visiting lecturer in dermatology*, (1964)

Looney, Robert Elmore, M.D., *professor of obstetrics*, 1910; *associate professor*, 1929

Loucks, James E., M.D., *clinical assistant in gynecology*, 1952; *instructor*, 1955

Loughmiller, Robert Farris, M.D., *clinical assistant in otorhinolaryngology*, 1946; *assistant professor*, 1959

Lowbeer, Leo, M.D., *visiting lecturer in pathology*, 1948–(64)

Lowe, Robert Chester, M.D., *assistant professor of medicine*, 1946; *associate professor of preventive medicine and public health and of medicine and research consultant in hospital organization and administration*, (1964); *director of outpatient department*, 1946–49; *medical director of University Hospitals*, 1949–56; *superintendent of University Hospitals*, 1957–58

Lowell, James R., M.D., *clinical assistant in medicine*, 1957; *instructor*, (1964)

Lowry, David Charles, M.D., *instructor in radiology*, 1951; *associate professor*, (1964)

Lowry, Dick Moss, M.D., *clinical assistant in otorhinolaryngology*, 1950; *associate professor*, (1964)

Lowry, Richard Clyde, M.D., *instructor in obstetrics*, 1921; *professor*, 1941

Lowry, Thomas Claude, M.D., *instructor in medicine*, 1920; *dean of the School of Medicine and superintendent of University Hospitals*, 1942–45

Loy, Robert Lowe, Jr., M.D., *clinical assistant in obstetrics*, 1949; *instructor*, 1956

Loy, William Arlin, M.D., *associate professor of preventive medicine and public health*, 1945; *instructor in medicine*, (1964)

Lubin, Emanuel Nathan, M.D., *visiting lecturer in urology*, 1953–(64)

Luton, James Polk, M.D., *assistant in ophthalmology*, 1938; *professor*, (1964)

Lybrand, Walter Archibald, J.D., *lecturer in medical jurisprudence*, 1930; *associate professor emeritus*, (1964)

Lynch, Luiese Husen, B.S., *instructor in physical therapy*, 1959; *assistant professor of physical therapy*, (1964)

Lynn, Thomas Neil, Jr., M.D., *clinical assistant in medicine*, 1959; *associate professor of preventive medicine and public health and assistant professor of medicine*, (1964)

Lysaught, James Neill, M.D., *clinical assistant in pediatrics*, 1949; *associate clinical professor*, (1964)

Lythcott, George Ignatius, M.D., *clinical assistant in pediatrics*, 1956; *assistant clinical professor*, (1964)

Lytle, Roy Cobb, LL.B., *assistant professor of medical jurisprudence*, 1950; *associate professor emeritus*, (1964)

Mabry, Elba Kenneth, D.D.S., *dentist in outpatient department*, 1920; *instructor in dentistry in outpatient department*, 1921

McBride, Earl Duwain, M.D., *instructor in orthopedic surgery*, 1926; *clinical professor of orthopedic and fracture surgery*, (1964)

McCampbell, Stanley R., M.D., *clinical assistant in medicine*, 1957; *instructor in medicine and in preventive medicine and public health*, 1962

McCarley, Tracey Holland, M.D., *visiting lecturer in medicine*, 1941–51

McCarley, Tracey H., Jr., M.D., *assistant professor of psychiatry*, *neurology, and behavioral sciences*, 1955

McCarty, Catherine M., M.S., *instructor in nutrition and in preventive medicine and public health*, 1963–(64)

McCay, Paul Baker, Ph.D., *instructor in physiology*, 1955; *assistant professor of research biochemistry*, (1964)

McClellen, Betty Jane, M.D., *associate professor of pathology*, (1964)

McClure, Coye Willard, M.D., *clinical assistant in ophthalmology*, 1946; *associate professor*, (1964)

McClure, Lawrence E., Ph.D., *assistant professor of research biochemistry*, 1957–58

McClure, William Charles, M.D., *assistant in medicine*, 1943; *assistant professor*, 1954

McCollum, Wiley Thomas, M.D., *fellow in pathology*, 1945; *assistant professor*, (1964)

McCreight, William George, M.D., *clinical assistant in dermatology and syphilology*, 1949; *associate professor*, (1964)

McCullough, Gerald W., M.D., *clinical assistant in surgery*, 1963–(64)

McDonald, George Fred, M.D., *clinical assistant in surgery*, 1959; *instructor*, (1964)

McDonald, Georgia Helen, *dietitian*, 1919

McDonald, John Edwin, M.D., *visiting lecturer in orthopedic surgery*, 1948–59

MacDonald, Joseph C., M.D., *instructor in otology, rhinology, and laryngology*, 1924; *professor emeritus of otorhinolaryngology*, 1961

MacDonald, Thomas Mark, M.D., *assistant professor of pathology*, 1925; *associate professor*, 1947

McDuffie, Norton Graham, Ph.D., *assistant professor of research biochemistry*, (1964)

McGaffey, Hazel I., M.D., *assistant professor of pathology*, 1960–(64)

McGee, James Patton, M.D., *instructor in ophthalmology*, 1928; *professor emeritus*, 1956

McGoldrick, Elizabeth, M.A., *instructor in psychiatric social work*, 1930–31

McGregor, Frank Harrison, M.D., *clinical assistant in surgery*, 1954; *assistant professor*, (1964)

McHenry, Dolph D., M.D., *instructor in otorhinolaryngology and in ophthalmology*, 1912–13

McHenry, Lawrence Chester, M.D., *instructor in otology, rhinology, and laryngology*, 1928; *professor of otorhinolaryngology*, (1964)

MacKay, Robert Carroll, M.D., *assistant professor of pathology*, (1964)

McKee, Robert Doreck, M.D., *clinical assistant in obstetrics*, 1949; *associate clinical professor of gynecology and obstetrics*, (1964)

McKenzie, Jess Mack, Ph.D., *assistant professor of research physiology*, 1960–(64)

McKinney, Milam Felix, M.D., *instructor in medicine*, 1936; *assistant professor*, 1955

McKinney, Ruth Alden, Ph.D., *instructor in clinical pathology*, 1943–44

Maclaren, John Dice, M.D., *professor of physiology and therapeutics*, 1908; *professor of physiology and therapeutics and of experimental medicine*, 1911

McLaughlin, Robert A., M.D., *clinical assistant in surgery*, 1957; *instructor*, (1964)

McLean, Andrew Parks, M.S., *instructor in pharmacology*, 1937–39

McLean, George Davidson, M.D., *instructor in surgery*, 1916–20

McMullen, Donald Bard, D.Sc., *assistant professor of bacteriology*, 1938; *professor of preventive medicine and public health*, 1952

McNeill, Philip Marsden, M.D., *instructor in medicine*, 1926; *professor*, (1964)

Macomber, Charles W., M.D., *clinical assistant in gynecology-obstetrics*, (1964)

Maguire, Hugh Francis, D.D.S., *clinical assistant in oral surgery*, 1959; *instructor*, (1964)

Maier, Edwin R., M.D., *clinical assistant in orthopedic surgery*, 1958; *assistant professor*, (1964)

Mankin, Haven Winslow, M.D., *clinical assistant in radiology*, 1956; *assistant professor*, (1964)

Mannerberg, Frederick D., M.D., *clinical assistant in medicine*, 1962–(64)

Margo, Elias, M.D., *clinical assistant in orthopedic surgery*, 1946–48

Margo, Marvin K., M.D., *clinical assistant in orthopedic and fracture surgery*, 1955; *assistant professor*, (1964)

Marianos, Joanne, M.S., *instructor in nutrition*, 1960–61

Marsh, Donald W., M.D., *clinical assistant in ophthalmology*, 1963–(64

Marsh, Homer Floyd, Ph.D., *assistant professor of bacteriology*, 1941; *associate professor*, 1952

Marshall, Carl E., M.D., *consultant professor of biostatistics and of preventive medicine and public health*, 1958–(64)

Marshall, Richard A., M.D., *assistant professor of preventive medicine and public health and instructor in medicine*, 1962–(64)

Martel, Serge Bourgault, M.D., *clinical assistant in pediatrics*, (1964)

Martin, Frank John, M.D., *clinical assistant in medicine*, 1955–58

Martin, Harry, Ph.D., *instructor in psychiatry, neurology, and behavioral sciences*, 1959; *assistant professor*, (1964)

Martin, Joseph Louis, M.D., *clinical assistant in anesthesiology*, 1959; *assistant clinical professor*, (1964)

Martin, Joseph Thomas, M.D., *instructor in obstetrics*, 1910; *professor emeritus of medicine*, 1962

Mason, Edward Charles, M.D., Ph.D., *professor of physiology*, 1928–57

Massey, John Barry, M.D., *instructor in psychiatry, neurology, and behavioral sciences*, 1961–(64)

Massion, Walter H., M.D., *research associate in anesthesiology*, 1957; *associate professor*, (1964)

Masterson, Maude Merle, M.D., *clinical assistant in medicine*, 1946;

assistant professor, (1964)

Mathews, Newman Sanford, M.D., *assistant in medicine*, 1943; *associate professor*, (1964)

Matthews, Grady Fred, M.D., *lecturer in hygiene and public health*, 1939; *professor of preventive medicine and public health*, 1963

Mauritson, Donald Forsyth, M.D., *visiting lecturer in radiology*, (1964)

Mayberry, Ruben Hilton, M.D., *instructor in anesthesiology*, 1953; *visiting lecturer in preventive medicine and public health*, (1964)

Mayes, Robert Harold, M.D., *visiting lecturer in preventive medicine and public health*, 1954–(64)

Mayfield, Meredith, B.A., *instructor in elementary dietetics*, 1927–28

Mayfield, Robert Charles, M.D., *clinical assistant in surgery*, 1955; *instructor*, (1964)

Mayfield, Warren Troutman, M.D., *instructor in physical diagnosis*, 1926–29

Mays, James Ernest, Jr., M.D., *clinical instructor in pediatrics*, 1960–(64)

Meador, Eric B., Jr., M.D., *clinical assistant in pediatrics*, 1955; *clinical instructor*, (1964)

Mcchling, George Seanor, M.D., *instructor in anesthesiology*, 1936; *assistant professor*, 1952

Mee, Mary, B.S., *instructor in diet therapy*, 1927–28

Melgaard, J. Marie, M.S., *instructor in dietetics*, 1937–45

Melton, Carlton E., Jr., M.S., *associate professor of research physiology*, 1961–(64)

Melvin, Walter W., Jr., M.D., D.Sc., *associate professor of preventive medicine and public health*, 1958–60

Mencke, Eugene Oliver, Ph.D., *assistant professor of communication disorders*, 1963–(64)

Menguy, Rene, M.D., Ph.D., *assistant professor of surgery*, 1957–60

Mercer, Robert D., M.D., *clinical assistant in anesthesiology*, 1956; *assistant clinical professor*, (1964)

Merrill, James A., M.D., *professor of gynecology and obstetrics*, 1961–(64)

Messenbaugh, Joseph Fife, M.D., *instructor in medicine and pediatrics*, 1910; *assistant professor of medicine*, 1924

Messenbaugh, Joseph Fife, M.D., *assistant in surgery*, 1936; *clinical professor*, (1964)

Messinger, Robert P., M.D., *clinical assistant in medicine*, 1952; *assistant professor*, (1964)

Meyer, John, M.D., *consultant clinical assistant in psychiatry and neurology*, 1954–55

Meyers, Samuel M., M.A., *research associate in psychiatry, neurology, and behavioral sciences*, 1957; *instructor in research psychiatry, neurology, and behavioral sciences*, (1964)

Meyers, William Arthur, M.D., *assistant professor of biochemistry and pharmacology*, 1927; *assistant professor of pathology*, 1932

Middleton, William S., M.D., *visiting professor of medicine*, 1963–(64)

Milburn, Braxton, M.A., *instructor in communication disorders*, 1960–61

Miles, Walter Howard, M.D., *instructor in medicine and in epidemiology and public health*, 1920; *assistant professor of preventive medicine and public health*, 1954

Miley, Thomas Harvey, D.D.S., *clinical assistant in dental surgery*, 1952; *associate professor*, (1964)

Miller, Charles Henderson, M.D., *visiting lecturer in preventive medicine and public health*, 1955–58

Miller, Clinton M., III, Ph.D., *assistant professor of preventive medicine and public health*, 1962–(64)

Miller, James R., D.D.S., *clinical assistant in dental surgery*, 1946; *associate professor*, 1963

Miller, Jess E., M.D., *fellow in pathology*, 1948; *assistant professor of urology*, (1964)

Miller, Nesbitt Ludson, M.D., *instructor in medicine*, 1931; *assistant professor*, 1954

Miller, Robert Joseph, M.D., *clinical assistant in orthopedic and fracture surgery*, 1955–56

Miller, William Arthur, M.D., *graduate fellow in anatomy*, 1948; *assistant professor of orthopedic and fracture surgery*, (1964)

Mills, James Berry, M.D., *instructor in ophthalmology*, 1963–(64)

Mills, Richard C., M.D., *assistant in obstetrics*, 1940; *instructor*, 1948

Milowsky, Jack, M.D., *assistant professor of anesthesiology*, 1946

Minor, Dwane B., M.D., *visiting lecturer in dermatology*, 1960–(64)

Mishler, Donald L., M.D., *clinical assistant professor of otorhinolaryngology*, 1962–(64)

Mitchell, Dan, Jr., M.D., *clinical instructor in radiology*, (1964)

Mock, David Clinton, M.D., *clinical assistant in medicine*, 1956; *associate professor*, (1964)

Moffett, John Alfred, M.D., *instructor in anesthesiology*, 1930; *associate professor of medicine*, 1943

Mohler, Stanley R., M.D., *associate professor of research preventive medicine and public health*, 1961–(64)

Monnet, Julian Charles, M.D., *clinical assistant in orthopedic and fracture surgery*, (1964)

Montroy, John Fay, M.D., *clinical assistant in anesthesiology*, 1956; *instructor*, (1964)

Moody, Herman C., M.D., *clinical assistant in surgery*, 1957–60

Moor, Hiram Dunlap, M.D., *assistant professor of bacteriology*, 1920; *professor*, 1952

Moore, Clifford W., M.D., *visiting lecturer in preventive medicine and public health*, 1954–(64)

Moore, Ellis Nathaniel, M.D., *instructor in medicine and in genitourinary diseases and syphilology*, 1925; *instructor in urology*, 1947

Moore, Joanne I., Ph.D., *assistant professor of pharmacology*, 1961–(64)

Moore, Samuel Turner, M.D., *clinical assistant in orthopedic surgery,* 1948; *associate professor of orthopedic and fracture surgery,* (1964)

Moorman, James Floyd, M.D., *instructor in medicine,* 1928; *associate professor,* (1964)

Moorman, Lewis Jefferson, M.D., *professor of physical diagnosis,* 1910; *professor emeritus of medicine,* 1954; *dean of the School of Medicine and superintendent of University Hospitals,* 1933–35

Mordkoff, Arnold M., Ph.D., *assistant professor of psychiatry, neurology, and behavioral sciences,* (1964)

Morey, John Barnhart, M.D., *visiting lecturer in medicine,* 1946–(64)

Morgan, Philip E., M.D., *instructor in preventive medicine and public health,* 1954–55

Morgan, Robert Jesse, M.D., *graduate fellow in dermatology and syphilology,* 1948; *associate professor,* (1964)

Morledge, John Walker, M.D., *instructor in medicine,* 1930; *clinical professor emeritus,* (1964)

Morrison, Henry Clinton, M.D., *clinical assistant in obstetrics,* 1946–47

Morrison, Robert Dean, Ph.D., *consultant assistant professor of biostatistics in preventive medicine and public health,* 1958–(64)

Mosley, Kirk Thornton, M.D., D.P.H., *professor of epidemiology and consulting professor of preventive medicine and public health,* 1951; *professor of preventive medicine and public health,* (1964)

Moseley, Russell LeRoy, Ph.D., *assistant professor of anatomy,* 1940–43

Moth, Michael Victor, M.D., *instructor in medicine,* 1943–48

Muchmore, Harold G., M.D., *graduate fellow in pharmacology,* 1946; *assistant professor of medicine and of preventive medicine and public health and of microbiology,* 1962; *acting director of outpatient department,* 1949–52

Muenzler, William Stanley, M.D., *instructor in ophthalmology* (1964)

Mulvey, Bert Ernest, M.D., *instructor in medicine,* 1936; *clinical professor of radiology,* (1964)

Mummer, Lloyd M., M.D., *clinical assistant in medicine,* (1964)

Munnell, Edward Robert, M.D., *instructor in surgery,* 1956; *assistant professor,* (1964)

Murdoch, Raymond Lester, M.D., *instructor in surgery,* 1920; *professor,* (1964); *chief of outpatient staff,* 1925–31

Murphy, Ralph William, M.D., *visiting lecturer in pediatrics,* 1954–59

Murray, E. Cotter, M.D., *visiting lecturer in preventive medicine and public health,* 1954; *clinical assistant in medicine,* (1964)

Musallam, Sam N., M.D., *clinical assistant in medicine,* 1953; *assistant professor,* (1964)

Musick, Elmer Ray, M.D., *instructor in medicine,* 1930; *clinical professor,* (1964)

Musick, Vern Herschel, M.D., *assistant in medicine,* 1936; *assistant professor,* 1950

Mussill, William Marcus, M.D., *instructor in otology, rhinology, and laryngology*, 1930; *assistant professor of otorhinolaryngology*, 1959
Myers, Leroy Lynn, M.D., *clinical assistant in medicine*, 1962–(64)
Myers, Robert Emmett, M.D., *instructor in pediatrics*, 1960–63
Myers, William Sylvester, M.D., *clinical assistant in medicine*, 1962–(64)
Nagel, Carl Behr, M.D., *instructor in surgery*, (1964)
Nagle, Patrick Sarsfield, M.D., *instructor in surgery*, 1931; *associate professor*, 1957
Nakano, Jiro, M.D., *assistant professor of pharmacology*, 1961–(64)
Namiki, Hideo, M.D., *instructor in pathology*, 1959–61
Nations, Frankie Nell, M.D., *assistant professor of anesthesiology*, 1959–(64)
Nau, Carl August, M.D., *assistant professor of physiology*, 1930; *professor of preventive medicine and public health*, (1964)
Naughton, John Patrick, M.D., *clinical assistant in medicine*, 1961; *instructor*, (1964)
Navin, Kenneth W., M.D., M.P.H., *visiting lecturer in preventive medicine and public health*, 1954–(64)
Neal, Loraine, M.S., *instructor in medical library science*, 1959
Neel, Roy Laurence, M.D., *clinical assistant in radiology*, 1956; *assistant professor*, (1964)
Neel, Roy Lawrence, M.D., *clinical assistant in otorhinolaryngology*, 1946–47
Neff, Everett Baker, M.D., *assistant in surgery*, 1938; *clinical professor*, 1960
Neill, Alma Jessie, Ph.D., *assistant professor of physiology*, 1920; *associate professor*, 1928
Nelson, Franklin, Ph.D., *instructor in medical psychology in psychiatry, neurology, and behavioral sciences*, 1960; *assistant professor*, 1962
Nelson, Ivo Amazon, M.D., *visiting lecturer in clinical pathology*, 1943; *associate professor*, 1946
Nettleship, Anderson, M.D., *associate professor of pathology*, 1944
Newsom, William Taylor, M.D., *assistant professor of pediatrics*, 1951–54
Nice, Leonard Blain, Ph.D., *professor of physiology*, 1913–27
Nicholson, Ben Hamilton, M.D., *instructor in pediatrics*, 1932; *clinical professor*, (1964)
Nicholson, James Leonidis, M.D., *visiting lecturer in preventive medicine and public health*, 1946–51
Nix, Thomas E., Jr., M.D., *instructor in dermatology*, 1962; *assistant professor*, (1964)
Noble, James D., *research associate in radiology*, 1962–63
Noell, Robert Leonard, M.D., *instructor in orthopedic surgery*, 1936; *clinical professor of orthopedic and fracture surgery*, 1957
Norcia, Leonard N., Ph.D., *instructor in research biochemistry*, 1955;

associate professor, 1960

Northrip, Ray Ulman, M.D., *visiting lecturer in pathology*, 1951–(64)

Norwood, O'Tar, M.D., *clinical instructor in dermatology*, (1964)

Nozik, Robert Alan, M.D., *clinical instructor in ophthalmology*, (1964)

Nuhfer, Patrick Armour, B.A., *research associate in pharmacology*, 1937–38

Nunnemacher, Rudolph Fink, Ph.D., *instructor in histology and embryology*, 1938–39

Obermann, Charles Frederick, M.D., *assistant professor of psychiatry and neurology*, 1948; *clinical professor of psychiatry, neurology, and behavioral sciences*, (1964)

Obert, Paul Michael, M.D., *instructor in pathology*, 1951; *assistant professor*, 1955

O'Brien, Larry J., Ph.D., *associate professor of research physiology*, 1961–63

O'Donoghue, Don Horatio, M.D., *instructor in orthopedic surgery*, 1928; *professor of orthopedic and fracture surgery*, (1964)

Oesterreicher, Don L., M.D., *clinical assistant in surgery*, 1954; *assistant professor*, 1959

Ogle, Emogene, M.S., *assistant professor of nutrition*, 1961; *assistant professor of nutrition and of preventive medicine and public health*, (1964)

Olds, Virginia Newton, R.N., M.S.W., *instructor in preventive medicine and public health*, 1963–(64)

O'Leary, Charles Marion, M.D., *instructor in surgery*, 1939; *clinical professor*, (1964)

Olsen, Egil Thorbjorn, M.D., *lecturer on hygiene and public health*, 1935–40; *medical director of University Hospitals*, 1935–40

Olson, Robert L., M.D., *clinical assistant in dermatology* (1964)

Omundson, Dorothy, B.A., *research fellow in bacteriology*, 1940–41

O'Neil, Hugh Barrett, M.D., *assistant professor of medicine and of psychiatry, neurology, and behavioral sciences*, 1957; *clinical assistant professor of medicine and assistant professor of psychiatry, neurology, and behavioral sciences*, 1959

Outlaw, Robert J., M.D., *instructor in psychiatry, neurology, and behavioral sciences*, 1962–(64)

Overbeck, Henry West, M.D., *instructor in medicine*, 1963–(64)

Owen, Cannon Armstrong, M.D., *assistant in surgery*, 1938–39

Owens, James Newton, Jr., M.D., *visiting lecturer in pathology*, 1948; *assistant professor* (1964)

Owens, Lloyd A., M.D., *instructor in dermatology*, 1957; *assistant professor*, (1964)

Palik, Emil E., M.D., *visiting lecturer in pathology*, 1948–51

Paredes, Alfonso, M.D., *research associate in psychiatry, neurology, and behavioral sciences*, 1958; *assistant professor*, (1964)

Park, Riley W., M.D., *clinical assistant in anesthesiology*, 1960–61

Parker, Ira Tom, M.D., *clinical assistant in medicine*, 1961–(64)

Parker, Joe Marion, M.D., *clinical assistant in surgery*, 1946; *clinical professor*, (1964)

Parrish, John Martin, M.D., *assistant in obstetrics*, 1942; *clinical assistant professor of gynecology and obstetrics*, (1964)

Parrish, Pamela Prentice, M.D., *clinical assistant in medicine*, 1956; *instructor in clinical medicine*, (1964)

Parrish, R. Gibson, M.D., *instructor in anesthesiology*, 1950; *clinical assistant professor*, (1964)

Parry, William L., M.D., *professor of urology*, 1962–(64)

Parsons, Oscar Albert, Ph.D., *professor of medical psychology in psychiatry, neurology, and behavioral sciences*, 1959–(64)

Paschal, William R., M.D., *clinical assistant in medicine*, 1952; *assistant professor*, (1964)

Pascucci, Lucien Michele, M.D., *visiting lecturer in radiology*, (1964)

Patel, Natoo C., M.D., *instructor in medicine*, 1959–63

Patnode, Robert Arthur, Ph.D., *associate professor of microbiology*, 1960–(64)

Patterson, C. Dowell, M.D., *clinical assistant in medicine*, (1964)

Patterson, Robert Urie, M.D., C.M., LL.D., *dean of the School of Medicine and superintendent of the University Hospitals*, 1935–42

Patzer, Reynold, M.D., *assistant professor of surgery*, 1945; *associate professor*, 1947

Paulson, Alvin W., M.D., *clinical assistant in medicine*, 1958–59

Paulus, David Dare, M.D., *associate in medicine*, 1937; *associate professor*, (1964)

Payne, Ralph E., M.D., *clinical assistant in orthopedic and fracture surgery*, 1962; *instructor*, (1964)

Payne, Richard Weston, M.D., *graduate fellow in pharmacology*, 1946; *assistant professor of medicine*, (1964)

Payte, James Ira, M.D., *clinical assistant in medicine*, 1946

Pearce, Charles Merrett, M.D., *lecturer in hygiene and public health*, 1936–39

Pearson, Orrin Walter, D.D.S., *instructor in dental surgery*, 1961–(64)

Pedersen, Thelma, M.A., *assistant professor of physical therapy*, 1954; *professor*, (1964)

Penick, Grider, M.D., *instructor in surgery and in gynecology*, 1926; *professor of gynecology*, 1950

Penrod, John Norman, M.D., *visiting lecturer in dermatology*, (1964)

Perlmutt, Joseph H., Ph.D., *assistant professor of physiology*, 1949–50

Peter, Maurice L., M.P.H., M.D., *visiting lecturer in preventive medicine and public health*, 1954; *associate professor*, (1964)

Peters, Dale W., M.D., *assistant professor of psychiatry, neurology, and behavioral sciences*, 1956; *associate professor*, (1964)

Peters, Vera Iva Parman, M.S., *instructor in dietetics*, 1948; *assistant professor of nutrition*, (1964)

Petway, Aileen, M.D., *assistant in anesthesiology*, 1940–41

Pfundt, Theodore Robert, M.D., *assistant professor of pediatrics*, 1955; *assistant professor of preventive medicine and public health*, 1958

Phillips, James Gartrelle, M.D., *instructor in urology*, 1947–52

Phillips, Robert R., M.D., *visiting lecturer in psychiatry*, 1960–(64)

Pickard, John Copeland, M.D., *instructor in otorhinolaryngology*, 1932; *clinical professor*, (1964)

Pierce, Alexander W., Jr., M.D., *assistant professor of pediatrics*, 1962–(64)

Pierce, Bruce R., M.A., *instructor in communication disorders*, 1961; *assistant professor*, (1964)

Pierce, Chester M., M.D., *assistant professor of psychiatry, neurology, and behavioral sciences*, 1960; *associate professor*, (1964)

Pigford, Russell Clarke, M.D., *visiting lecturer in medicine*, 1941–51

Pilkingon, Lou Ann, Ph.D., *instructor in physiology*, 1961–63

Pippin, Bascum C., D.D.S., *clinical assistant in dental surgery*, 1957; *instructor*, (1964)

Pishkin, Vladimir, Ph.D., *associate professor of medical psychology in psychiatry, neurology, and behavioral sciences*, 1962–(64)

Pitts, James Burton, Jr., M.D., *instructor in gynecology*, 1954; *assistant clinical professor*, (1964)

Plowman, Paul E., D.D.S., *clinical assistant in dental surgery*, 1958; *assistant professor*, (1964)

Points, Thomas Craig, M.D., *assistant in obstetrics*, 1943; *associate clinical professor of obstetrics and assistant professor of preventive medicine and public health*, (1964)

Pollock, Harold R., D.D.S., *clinical assistant in oral surgery*, 1955; *assistant professor*, (1964)

Pollock, Ira O., M.D., *clinical assistant in surgery*, 1952; *associate professor*, (1964)

Porter, Earle Sellers, M.A., *instructor in chemistry*, 1912–13

Porter, Marilyn, M.D., *instructor in pediatrics*, 1961–(64)

Pounders, Carroll Monroe, M.D., *instructor in pediatrics*, 1922; *professor emeritus*, (1964)

Pratt, Tony Willard, M.S., *instructor in physiology*, 1931–32

Price, George Townley, D.V.M., *instructor in pathology*, 1952; *assistant professor*, (1964)

Price, Richard B., M.D., *clinical assistant in radiology*, 1959; *instructor*, (1964)

Price, William E., M.D., *clinical assistant in surgery*, 1962; *assistant professor*, (1964)

Prier, William Milton, M.D., *fellow in pathology*, 1946–47

Proctor, James T., M.D., *clinical professor of child psychology in psychiatry, neurology, and behavioral sciences*, 1962–(64)

Prosser, Moorman Paul, M.D., *instructor in psychiatry*, 1939; *clinical professor of psychiatry, neurology, and behavioral sciences*, (1964)

Pruitt, Francis Willard, M.D., *instructor in medicine*, (1964)

Puckett, Carl, M.D., *special lecturer in public health and sanitation*, 1925; *visiting lecturer in medicine*, 1951

Pugsley, William S., M.D., *instructor in medicine*, 1953; *assistant professor*, (1964)

Puls, Jerry Lee, M.D., *clinical assistant in medicine*, (1964)

Pumpian-Mindlin, Eugene, M.D., *professor of psychiatry, neurology, and behavioral sciences*, 1963–(64)

Puntenney, Mary E., M.D., *clinical assistant in medicine*, (1964)

Pyeatte, Jesse Eugene, M.D., *instructor in ophthalmology*, 1963–(64)

Quenzer, Fred August, M.D., *instructor in surgery*, 1948; *associate professor*, 1958

Rahhal, Lindberg J., M.D., *clinical assistant in radiology*, 1960; *instructor*, (1964)

Ramana, C. B., Diplomate, *research associate in psychology in psychiatry, neurology, and behavioral sciences*, 1957–(64)

Ramsey, Hal Harrison, III, Ph.D., *assistant professor of bacteriology*, 1952; *associate professor of microbiology*, 1958

Ramsey, John Earl, Jr., M.D., *instructor in gynecology and obstetrics*, 1961–(64)

Randel, Harvey Ollis, M.D., *assistant in ophthalmology*, 1940; *professor*, 1950

Ray, Thomas S., Ph.D., *research associate in psychiatry, neurology, and behavioral sciences*, 1957; *assistant professor*, (1964)

Rayburn, Charles Ralph, M.D., *instructor in neurology*, 1929; *professor of psychiatry and neurology*, 1948

Rebell, Gebert, B.S., *associate in research bacteriology and dermatology*, 1953; *associate in research microbiology and dermatology*, 1958

Reck, John Arthur, M.D., *instructor in gynecology*, 1914; *assistant professor*, 1930

Records, John William, M.D., *assistant in obstetrics*, 1939; *clinical professor*, (1964)

Redmond, Robert Franklin, M.D., *graduate fellow in pharmacology*, 1948; *assistant professor*, (1964)

Reece, C. Herman, D.D.S., *clinical assistant in dental surgery*, 1958; *assistant professor*, (1964)

Reed, Emil Patrick, M.D., *assistant in surgery*, 1936–37

Reed, Horace, M.D., *professor of surgical pathology and diagnosis*, 1910; *professor of clinical surgery*, 1935

Reed, James Robert, M.D., *assistant in anatomy*, 1925; *professor of ophthalmology*, (1964)

Reese, Lewis Laban, M.D., *lecturer in medicine*, 1940–41; *medical director of University Hospitals*, 1940–41

Reichert, Rudolph Joe, M.D., *assistant in medicine*, 1943; *instructor*, 1951

Reichmann, Francis J., D.D.S., *instructor in dental surgery*, 1927; *clinical professor emeritus*, (1964)

Reid, George Willard, D.Eng., *consultant professor of preventive medicine and public health*, 1962–(64)

Reifenstein, Edward C., Jr., M.D., *professor of research medicine*, 1950–54

Reiff, William H., M.D., *clinical assistant in medicine*, 1948; *assistant professor*, (1964)

Reinhardt, Herbert P., Jr., M.D., *visiting lecturer in preventive medicine and public health and clinical assistant in medicine*, 1962; *clinical assistant in medicine*, (1964)

Reisenberg, Herman Andrew, R.N., B.S.N., *clinical assistant in psychiatric nursing in psychiatry, neurology, and behavioral sciences*, 1963–(64)

Renfrow, William Branch, M.D., *instructor in anesthesiology*, 1955–(64)

Revsin, Alvin Morton, Ph.D., *assistant professor of research pharmacology*, (1964)

Reynolds, Charles Lee, Jr., M.D., *clinical assistant in urology*, 1960; *instructor*, (1964)

Reynolds, George Edward, Jr., D.D.S., *clinical assistant in dental surgery*, 1951; *associate professor*, (1964)

Rhinehart, Don Forrest, M.D., *clinical assistant in surgery*, 1963–(64)

Rice, Edgar Elmer, M.D., *instructor in gynecology*, 1911; *assistant professor*, 1915

Rice, Guy Vivian, M.D., *assistant professor of preventive medicine and public health*, (1964)

Rice, Paul Brewer, M.D., *clinical assistant in medicine*, 1946–52

Richardson, Sylvia O., M.D., *assistant professor of pediatrics*, 1958–(64)

Richardson, William R., M.D., *professor of pediatric surgery*, 1957–(64)

Richey, Harvey Mac, M.D., *instructor in surgery*, 1945–46

Richter, Kenneth Murrell, Ph.D., *research fellow in pathology*, 1939; *professor of histology and embryology in anatomy*, (1964)

Ricks, James Ralph, Jr., M.D., *clinical assistant in medicine*, 1946; *instructor*, (1964)

Ridgeway, Elmer, Jr., M.D., *clinical assistant in medicine*, 1946; *clinical assistant in obstetrics*, 1949

Ridings, Gus Ray, M.D., professor of radiology, 1957–62

Rieger, Joseph Anton, M.D., *instructor in mental diseases*, 1939; *clinical professor of psychiatry, neurology, and behavioral sciences*, (1964)

Riely, Leander Armistead, M.D., *associate professor of clinical medicine*, 1910; *professor emeritus of medicine*, 1959

Riggall, Jack Lee, M.D., *clinical assistant in medicine*, 1955; *instructor*, (1964)

Riggall, James R., M.D., *clinical assistant in surgery*, 1955; *assistant professor*, (1964)

Rigual, Jose Rafael, M.D., *assistant professor of otorhinolaryngology*, 1958; *associate professor*, (1964)

Riley, Harris D., Jr., M.D., *professor of pediatrics*, 1958–(64)

Riley, John William, M.D., *professor of fractures, dislocations, and minor surgery*, 1910; *professor of genitourinary surgery*, 1919
Riley, Robert Hickman, *assistant in pathology and bacteriology*, 1908–1909
Rinkel, Herbert John, M.D., *instructor in medicine*, 1932–33
Risser, Arthur Strohm, M.D., *visiting lecturer in surgery*, 1941–57
Rix, Robert Alvin, Jr., M.D., *clinical assistant in surgery*, 1948; *associate professor*, (1964)
Robbins, Galen Patchell, M.D., *clinical assistant in medicine*, 1959; *instructor*, (1964)
Robertson, Dean, D.D.S., *clinical assistant in dental surgery*, 1950; *assistant professor (pedodontics)*, (1964)
Robertson, Edwin Norris, Jr., M.D., *clinical assistant in ophthalmology*, 1947; *associate professor*, (1964)
Robertson, John Millard, D.D.S., *clinical assistant in surgery*, 1935; *associate professor of dental surgery*, 1963
Robinson, Charles W., Jr., M.D., *instructor in medicine*, (1964)
Robinson, John Harrison, M.D., *instructor in obstetrics and in surgery*, 1931; *clinical professor emeritus of surgery*, (1964)
Robinson, Norman J., M.D., *assistant professor of pediatrics*, 1950–51
Robinson, Ralph R., M.D., *clinical assistant in obstetrics and gynecology*, 1954; *assistant professor*, 1955
Robison, Clarence, Jr., M.D., *graduate fellow in pathology*, 1949; *assistant professor of surgery*, (1964)
Rock, John Lestrange, *laboratory assistant in physiology*, 1912–13
Roddy, John Augustus, M.D., *instructor in medicine*, 1943–45
Rogers, Joe O., M.D., *instructor in preventive medicine and public health*, 1956; *assistant professor of administrative medicine in preventive medicine and public health*, (1964)
Rogers, William Gerald, M.D., *instructor in gynecology*, 1935; *clinical professor*, (1964)
Rohrer, George Victor, M.D., *clinical assistant in medicine*, 1961; *instructor*, (1964)
Roland, Marion Mansfield, M.D., *instructor in dermatology, electrotherapy, and radiography*, 1916; *associate professor of dermatology and radiography*, 1935
Rolater, Joseph Brown, M.D., *lecturer in clinical surgery*, 1911–12
Romanell, Patrick, Ph.D., *professor of medical philosophy in medicine*, 1962–(64)
Rosenbaum, Paul Joseph, M.S., *research associate in radiology*, 1949–50
Rosenstein, Robert, Ph.D., *instructor in research pharmacology*, 1962–(64)
Roth, Raymond Edward, M.S., *visiting professor of preventive medicine and public health*, 1962–63
Rountree, Charles Ross, M.D., *instructor in orthopedic surgery*, 1929; *clinical professor of orthopedic and fracture surgery*, (1964)

Royce, Owen, Jr., M.D., *instructor in medicine and director of outpatient department*, 1940–41

Royer, Charles Abraham, M.D., *clinical assistant in ophthalmology*, 1946; *associate professor*, (1964)

Rubenstein, Alfred Ian, M.D., *graduate assistant in anatomy*, 1947–48

Rubio, Thomas, M.D., *clinical assistant in pediatrics*, (1964)

Rucks, William Ward, Sr., M.D., *associate in medicine*, 1937–39

Rucks, William Ward, Jr., M.D., *instructor in medicine*, 1932; *clinical professor*, (1964)

Rue, John Davison, Jr., M.A., *associate professor of chemistry*, 1911–13

Ruhm, Howard B., Ph.D., *assistant professor of audiology in communication disorders*, 1960–(64)

Russell, George T., M.D., *visiting lecturer in pediatrics*, 1958–(64)

Russell, Glen Alexander, M.D., *instructor in anatomy*, 1930–31

Russell, Henry Thomas, M.D., *visiting lecturer in pathology*, 1954; *assistant professor*, (1964)

Russman, Sumner, D.D.S., *clinical assistant in dental surgery*, 1950; *assistant professor*, (1964)

Russo, Peter Ernest, M.D., *assistant in roentgenology*, 1943; *professor of radiology*, 1963

Rutledge, Bob Jack, M.D., *clinical assistant in surgery*, 1954; *assistant professor*, (1964)

Sackett, Lloyd Melville, M.D., *instructor in gynecology*, 1916; *associate professor*, 1934

Sadler, LeRoy Huskins, M.D., *instructor in gynecology*, 1935; *associate professor*, 1951

Salsbury, Carmen Russell, M.D., *assistant professor of anatomy*, 1929; *professor*, 1933

Sands, Able Jay, M.D., *clinical assistant in medicine*, 1956–59

Sanger, Fenton Almer, M.D., *instructor in surgery*, 1931; *assistant professor*, (1964)

Sanger, Fenton Mercer, M.D., *instructor in gynecology*, 1916–39

Sanger, Welborn Ward, M.D., *clinical assistant in ophthalmology*, 1946; *associate professor*, (1964)

Sapper, Herbert Victor Louis, B.S., B.A., *laboratory assistant in bacteriology and histology*, 1912; *instructor in bacteriology*, 1915

Sapper, Herbert Victor Louis, M.D., *clinical assistant in pediatrics*, 1949; *associate clinical professor*, (1964)

Savage, William L., M.D., *clinical assistant in psychiatry, neurology, and behavioral sciences, 1962; instructor*, (1964)

Schechter, Marshall D., M.D., *professor of child psychiatry in psychiatry, neurology, and behavioral sciences and consultant professor of pediatrics*, (1964)

Schilling, John Albert, M.D., *professor of surgery*, 1956–(64)

Schmidt, Arthur, M.D., *instructor in medicine*, 1954; *assistant clinical professor*, (1964)

Schmidt, Edna, M.Ed., *instructor in physical therapy*, 1957; *assistant professor*, (1964)

Schmidt, Helen Hughes, M.D., *clinical assistant in radiology*, 1959; *instructor*, (1964)

Schmidt, Henry Louis, Jr., M.D., *assistant professor of medicine*, 1951–54

Schmidt, Loraine, M.D., *visiting lecturer in preventive medicine and public health*, 1954–56

Schneider, Edward Martin, M.D., *instructor in medicine*, 1953; *assistant professor*, 1956

Schneider, Robert A., M.D., *assistant professor of medicine*, 1952; *associate professor of medicine and of psychiatry, neurology, and behavioral sciences*, (1964)

Schnitz, Sidney E., M.D., *clinical assistant in pediatrics*, 1957; *clinical instructor*, (1964)

Schottstaedt, Mary Frances, M.D., *clinical assistant in medicine*, 1954; *assistant professor*, (1964)

Schottstaedt, William W., M.D., *assistant professor of preventive medicine and public health*, 1953; *professor of preventive medicine and public health, associate professor of medicine, and consultant professor of psychiatry, neurology, and behavioral sciences*, (1964)

Schow, Carl Emil, D.D.S., *clinical assistant in dental surgery*, 1953; *associate professor of oral surgery*, (1964)

Schultz, Wayne H., M.D., *clinical assistant in radiology*, 1958; *instructor*, (1964)

Scott, Jerry Benjamin, Ph.D., *research associate in physiology*, 1961; *assistant professor*, (1964)

Scott, John Robert, M.D., *visiting lecturer in preventive medicine and public health*, 1963–(64)

Scott, Lawrence Vernon, D.Sc., *assistant professor of bacteriology*, 1950; *professor of microbiology*, (1964)

Scruggs, Anna T., *research associate in pediatrics*, 1958–62

Scruton, Wilbert James, D.D.S., *assistant professor and consultant in dental surgery*, 1922–36

Seeley, J. Rodman, M.D., *associate professor of pediatrics*, 1963–(64)

Seeman, William, Ph.D., *associate professor of medical psychology in psychiatry, neurology, and behavioral sciences*, 1955–58

Seifter, Joseph Johann, M.D., *instructor in pharmacology*, 1935–37

Sell, Lawrence Stanley, M.D., *assistant in orthopedic surgery*, 1941; *assistant professor*, 1949

Sepkowitz, Samuel, M.D., *instructor in pediatrics*, 1953; *associate clinical professor*, (1964)

Serwer, Milton John, M.D., *instructor in obstetrics*, 1937; *professor of clinical gynecology and obstetrics*, (1964)

Sevelius, Gunnar George, M.D., *instructor in medicine*, 1962; *research associate*, (1964)

Sevelius, Hilli, M.D., *clinical assistant in medicine*, 1961; *instructor*, (1964)

Sewell, Dan Roy, M.D., *instructor in anatomy*, 1934; *instructor in surgery*, 1948

Sewell, Margery Ardrey, B.S., *instructor in dietotherapy*, 1928–37

Seymour, James, Ph.C., *instructor in pharmacy*, 1904

Shackelford, Paul D., M.D., *visiting lecturer in dermatology*, 1959–(64)

Shackleford, John William, M.D., *assistant professor of preventive medicine and public health*, 1946; *associate professor*, (1964)

Shackleford, Margaret F., M.S., *instructor in preventive medicine and public health*, 1948; *associate professor of statistics in preventive medicine and public health*, (1964)

Shadid, Ernest George, M.D., *clinical assistant in psychiatry, neurology, and behavioral sciences*, 1961; *instructor*, (1964)

Shaffer, Jerome Daniels, M.D., *clinical assistant in pediatrics*, 1949; *assistant clinical professor*, (1964)

Shaffer, Ward Loren, D.D.S., *instructor in dentistry*, 1930; *associate professor of dental surgery*, 1963

Shanholtz, Mack Irvin, M.D., *assistant professor of preventive medicine and public health*, 1948–51

Shanklin, Kitty, B.A. (Mrs. Rountree), *instructor in social services and dietetics*, 1927; *assistant professor of medical social work*, 1933; *social service director*, 1925–34

Shaver, Sylvester Robert, M.D., *assistant in otorhinolaryngology*, 1942; *clinical professor*, (1964)

Shaw, Russell Franklin, M.D., *clinical assistant in pediatrics*, 1963–(64)

Shelby, Hudson Swain, M.D., *instructor in anesthesiology*, 1936–47

Sheldon, Albert John, D.Sc., *assistant professor of bacteriology*, 1937–42

Sheppard, Fay, M.S., *assistant in biochemistry and pharmacology*, 1926; *instructor in biochemistry*, (1964)

Sheppard, Mary Virginia Sawyer, M.D., *assistant in bacteriology*, 1918; *assistant professor of medicine*, (1964)

Sherif, Carolyn W., Ph.D., *consultant assistant of social psychology in psychiatry, neurology, and behavioral sciences*, 1963–(64)

Sherif, Muzafer, Ph.D., *consultant professor of social psychology in psychiatry, neurology, and behavioral sciences*, 1956–(64)

Shetlar, Marvin Ray, Ph.D., *research associate in biochemistry*, 1946; *research professor*, (1964)

Shewmaker, Kenneth Lee, Ph.D., *instructor in medical psychology in psychiatry, neurology, and behavioral sciences*, 1962–(64)

Shideler, Alfred Max, M.D., *assistant professor of pathology*, 1954–57

Shifrin, Richard G., M.D., *clinical assistant in anesthesiology*, 1955; *assistant clinical professor*, (1964)

Shircliff, Edward Emmett, Jr., M.D., *clinical assistant in medicine*, 1942, *instructor*, (1964)

Shissler, George Edward, M.D., *clinical assistant in pediatrics*, 1962–(64)

Shoemaker, Harold Adam, Ph.C., Ph.D., *assistant professor of biochemistry and pharmacology*, 1925; *professor of pharmacology and toxicology*, 1960; *acting dean of the School of Medicine and superintendent of University Hospitals*, 1942–43

Shons, Kenneth W., D.D.S., M.S.D., *instructor in dental surgery*, 1959; *assistant professor*, (1964)

Shopfner, Charles E., M.D., *associate professor of radiology*, 1962–(64)

Shorbe, Howard Bruce, M.D., *instructor in orthopedic surgery and anatomy*, 1936; *clinical professor of orthopedic and fracture surgery*, (1964)

Shurley, Jay Talmadge, M.D., *professor of psychiatry, neurology, and behavioral sciences*, 1957; *reserach professor*, (1964)

Siebert, Frank Thomas, Jr., M.D., *instructor in clinical pathology*, 1940–41

Siegal, Peter Vincent, M.D., *assistant professor of research preventive medicine and public health*, 1963–(64)

Simcoe, Charles William, M.D., *clinical instructor in ophthalmology*, (1964)

Simon, Jimmy L., M.D., *instructor in pediatrics*, 1960; *assistant professor*, (1964)

Simon, William Hale, M.D., *visiting lecturer in pediatrics*, 1960–(64)

Singleton, Harry Fields, M.D., *clinical assistant in medicine*, 1954; *assistant professor*, (1964)

Sisney, Vernon V., Ph.D., *instructor in medical psychology in psychiatry, neurology, and behavioral sciences*, 1958; *assistant professor*, (1964)

Skouge, Oren T., M.D., *assistant professor of medicine*, 1957; *associate professor*, (1964)

Slagle, William F., Jr., D.D.S., *clinical assistant in dental surgery*, 1961; *instructor*, (1964)

Slatkin, Harry, *laboratory assistant in anatomy*, 1912–13

Sleeper, Harold G., M.D., *clinical assistant in psychiatry, neurology, and behavioral sciences*, 1948; *assistant professor*, 1961

Sloan, Mary N., M.S.S. (Mrs. Hall), *instructor in psychiatry, neurology, and behavioral sciences*, 1959–(64)

Smiley, Robert H., M.D., *clinical assistant in surgery*, (1964)

Smith, Bobby Gene, M.D., *assistant professor of urology*, (1964)

Smith, Byran Freemont, M.D., *clinical assistant in medicine*, 1948; *assistant clinical professor*, (1964)

Smith, Carl Ray, M.D., *instructor in ophthalmology*, (1964)

Smith, Carl W., M.D., *assistant professor of medicine*, 1958–(64); *director of outpatient department*, 1961–(64)

Smith, Charles Andrew, M.D., *assistant in medicine and clinical assistant in psychiatry and neurology*, 1936; *clinical professor of psychiatry, neurology, behavioral sciences*, (1964)

Smith, Charles E., Jr., M.D., *instructor in psychiatry, neurology, and behavioral sciences*, 1958; *assistant professor*, (1964)

Smith, Delbert Gilmore, M.D., *assistant in obstetrics*, 1940; *clinical professor of gynecology and obstetrics*, (1964)

Smith, Edward Needham, M.D., D.Sc., *associate professor of obste* trics, 1940; *clinical professor*, 1951

Smith, Ella, B.S., *instructor in physical education (physical medicine)*, 1936; *lecturer in physical education*, 1945

Smith, J.B., M.D., *superintendent of University Hospitals*, 1931–33

Smith, James William Hickman, M.D., *assistant professor of physiology*, 1951; *professor of physiology and consultant in medicine*, 1961

Smith, John Darrel, M.D., *associate professor of pediatrics*, (1964)

Smith, Millington, M.D., *professor of surgery*, 1910; *professor emeritus of gynecology*, 1936

Smith, Paul Winston, Ph.D., *assistant professor of pharmacology*, 1941; *professor of research pharmacology*, (1964)

Smith, Philip Edward, D.Sc., *assistant professor of preventive medicine and public health*, 1952; *professor of parasitology in preventive medicine and public health*, (1964)

Smith, Phillip B., M.D., *clinical assistant in psychiatry, neurology, and behavioral sciences*, 1957–58

Smith, Ralph Argyle, M.D., *assistant in medicine*, 1936; *associate clinical professor*, (1964)

Smith, Ralph Vernon, M.D., *instructor in surgery*, 1911; *assistant professor*, 1915

Smith, Sam Corry, Ph.D., *assistant professor of biochemistry*, 1951; *associate professor*, 1955

Smith, Vivian Sweibel, Ph.D., *consultant assistant professor of preventive medicine and public health*, 1953; *consultant associate professor of parasitology in preventive medicine and public health*, (1964)

Smith, Wendal Doop, M.D., *assistant professor of histology and embryology*, 1926–28

Smith, Wendell Logan, M.D., *instructor in medicine*, 1935; *clinical assistant in surgery*, 1948

Smith, William O., M.D., *clinical assistant in medicine*, 1955; *associate professor*, (1964)

Smotherman, Howard, M.D., *clinical instructor in gynecology-obstetrics*, (1964)

Smythe, Olivia M., M.A., *assistant professor of public health nursing in preventive medicine and public health*, 1960–62

Snoddy, William Thomas, M.D., *instructor in pathology*, 1953; *assistant professor*, (1964)

Snow, Clyde Collins, Ph.D., *research associate in medicine*, (1964)

Snow, James Byron, M.D., *instructor in medicine*, 1928; *professor of clinical pediatrics*, (1964)

Snow, James Byron, Jr., M.D., *assistant professor of otorhinolaryngology*, 1962; *professor*, (1964)

Snyder, David Deal, M.D., *clinical assistant in surgery*, 1962–(64)

Snyder, James Howard, M.D., *clinical assistant in psychiatry and neurology*, 1949; *instructor*, 1953

Snyder, Laurence Hasbrouck, D.Sc., *professor of medical genetics*, 1947–58

Sokatch, John R., M.D., *assistant professor of microbiology*, 1958; *associate professor*, (1964)

Sorgatz, Frank Bruner, M.D., *instructor in medicine*, 1911; *associate professor of clinical pathology research*, 1918

Soule, Edward Easton, LL.B., *assistant professor of medical jurisprudence in the Department of Medicine*, 1960–(64)

Soutar, Richard Gray, B.S., *professor of physical education*, 1914–17

Sowell, Harlan Keith, M.D., *instructor in anesthesiology*, 1947; *assistant professor*, (1964)

Spangler, Arthur Stephenson, B.S., *research fellow in pharmacology*, 1938–39

Speed, Louis Elliott, M.D., *clinical assistant in surgery*, 1956–(64)

Spencer, Jack D., M.D., *instructor in orthopedic and fracture surgery*, 1962–(64)

Spencer, Robert W., M.D., M.Sc., *clinical assistant in ophthalmology*, 1955; *assistant professor*, 1962

Spengos, Michael N., D.D.S., *clinical assistant in dental surgery*, 1962–(64)

Springall, Arthur N., M.D., *assistant professor of preventive medicine and public health*, 1958–(64)

Spuehler, Henry Ernest, M.D., *consultant in otorhinolaryngology*, 1958–60

Stacy, John Raymond, M.D., *clinical assistant in orthopedic surgery*, 1949; *associate professor of orthopedic and fracture surgery*, (1964)

Stanbro, Gregory Everett, M.D., *assistant in surgery*, 1936; *clinical professor*, 1962

Stanley, Allan John, Ph.D., *assistant professor of physiology*, 1943; *professor*, (1964)

Starry, Leo Joseph, M.D., *instructor in surgery*, 1924; *professor emeritus*, (1964)

Start, Armond H., M.D., *clinical instructor in pediatrics*, 1963–(64)

Stavinoha, William B., Ph.D., *assistant professor of research pharmacology*, 1960–(64)

Steele, Elizabeth Julia, B.S. (Mrs. Eley), *assistant in histology and pathology*, 1919; *instructor in pathology*, 1925

Steen, Carl T., M.D., *instructor in psychiatry*, 1935; *assistant professor of psychiatry, neurology, and behavioral sciences*, (1964)

Steen, Wilson David, Ph.D., *research associate in preventive medicine and public health*, 1958; *assistant professor*, (1964)

Steinmann, Leroy William, M.D., *assistant professor of preventive medicine and public health*, 1952–54

Stephenson, Joseph Clark, Ph.D., M.D., *professor of anatomy*, 1919–31

Sternlog, Richard Edward, Ph.D., *research associate in preventive medicine and public health and instructor in medical psychology in psychiatry, neurology, and behavioral sciences*, (1964)

Stewart, Frank William, D.M.D., *clinical assistant in dental surgery*, 1952; *associate professor*, (1964)

Stocking, Charles Howard, Ph.C., *dean of the School of Pharmacy and professor of pharmacy*, 1912–13

Stone, Herman Hull, M.D., *clinical assistant in medicine*, 1949; *instructor*, 1951

Stone, Merlin Jones, M.D., *assistant professor of anatomy*, 1920; *associate professor*, 1923

Stone, Samuel Newton, M.D., *clinical assistant in surgery*, 1946; *clinical professor*, (1964)

Stoops, Roy Philson, M.D., *instructor in physiology*, 1903; *professor of anatomy*, 1908; *acting dean of the School of Medicine*, 1904–1908

Stout, Hugh Albert, M.S., M.D., *clinical assistant in medicine and instructor in pathology*, 1948; *assistant professor of pathology*, (1964)

Stout, Landon Clarke, Jr., M.D., *assistant professor of medicine*, 1963–(64)

Stout, Marvin Elroy, M.D., *instructor in surgery*, 1916–21

Stream, Lawrence, M.D., *assistant professor of anesthesiology*, 1954; *associate professor*, (1964)

Strecher, William Edgar, M.D., *assistant in gynecology*, 1939; *instructor in surgery*, 1963

Strenge, Henry Bonheyo, M.D., *assistant professor of pediatrics*, 1947; *professor*, 1957

Studebaker, Gerald Arthur, Ph.D., *assistant professor of communication disorders*, 1962; *assistant professor of communication disorders and consultant in audiology in otorhinolaryngology*, (1964)

Sturm, Robert Theodore, M.D., *clinical assistant in surgery*, 1946; *assistant professor*, (1964)

Sugg, Alfred R., M.D., *visiting lecturer in urology*, 1953–60

Sukman, Robert, M.D., *instructor in radiology*, 1954; *associate clinical professor*, (1964)

Swenson, Alvin L., M.D., *assistant in orthopedics*, 1942–43

Tackwell, Elizabeth M., M.A., *clinical assistant (psychiatric social worker) in psychiatry, neurology, and behavioral science*, 1963–(64)

Talaat, Samir, M.B., D.S., M.Ch., *visiting lecturer in surgery*, 1962–63

Tampietro, P. F., Ph.D., *associate professor of research physiology*, 1961–(64)

Tang, Jordan J. N., Ph.D., *research associate in research biochemistry*, 1962; *assistant professor*, (1964)

Tang, Pei Chin, Ph.D., *associate irofessor of research physiology*, 1960–(64)

Tapp, Ernest Martin, M.D., *clinical assistant in medicine*, 1948–49

Tapuz, Jaime Tobias, M.D., *clinical assistant in anesthesiology*, (1964)

Taybi, Hooshang, M.D., *assistant professor of radiology*, 1960–62
Taylor, Ardell Nichold, Ph.D., *assistant professor of physiology*, 1946; *professor*, 1961
Taylor, Charles Benjamin, M.D., *instructor in genitourinary diseases and syphilology*, 1916; *professor emeritus of urology*, 1959
Taylor, Coleman, M.D., *associate professor of ophthalmology*, 1962–(64)
Taylor, Gladys, B.S. (Mrs. Stuard), *instructor in dietotherapy*, 1932–37
Taylor, James Mabury, M.D., *instructor in urology*, 1941; *clinical professor*, (1964)
Taylor, Lewis Carroll, M.D., *instructor in anesthesiology*, 1945; *associate professor*, (1964)
Taylor, Pleasant Addison, *laboratory assistant in anatomy and physiology*, 1911–13
Taylor, William Merritt, M.D., *lecturer in children's diseases*, 1911; *professor emeritus of pediatrics*, 1957
Teed, Roy W., M.D., *instructor in ophthalmology*, 1957; *associate professor*, 1963
Thompson, James Barrett, M.D., *visiting lecturer in surgery*, 1954–(64)
Thompson, John B., M.D., *instructor in medicine*, 1962–(64)
Thompson, Steven Wright, M.D., *instructor in medicine*, 1959; *assistant professor of medicine and instructor in psychiatry, neurology, and behavioral sciences*, (1964)
Thompson, Willard Van Voorhis, M.D., *instructor in medical jurisprudence*, 1946; *teaching fellow in oncology*, 1949
Thompson, William Best, M.D., *clinical assistant in medicine*, 1952; *assistant professor*, (1964)
Thornton, Lowell F., M.D., *visiting lecturer in pathology*, 1957–(64)
Threlkeld, Lal Duncan, M.D., *clinical assistant in obstetrics*, 1948; *associate clinical professor*, (1964)
Thuringer, Joseph Mario, M.D., *professor of histology and embryology*, 1920–51
Thurston, Thomas Watson, M.D., *clinical assistant in pediatrics*, 1962–(64)
Tilton, Edith Ruth, B.S. (Mrs. Aitken), *instructor in dietetics*, 1926–32
Tipton, Albert C., D.D.S., *clinical assistant in dental surgery*, 1955; *assistant professor*, (1964)
Todd, Harry Coulter, M.D., *professor of otology, rhinology, and laryngology*, 1910–36
Tollett, Charles Albert, M.D., *clinical assistant in surgery 1957; instructor*, (1964)
Tompkins, Jack E., M.S., *research associate in medicine*, 1962–(64)
Tompkins, S. Fulton, M.D., *clinical assistant in orthopedic surgery*, 1951; *associate professor of orthopedic and fracture surgery*, (1964)
Tool, Donovan, M.D., *assistant in medicine*, 1943; *assistant professor of pathology*, 1963
Torrey, John Paine, M.D., *instructor in physical diagnosis*, 1915; *acting*

professor of anatomy, 1920

Townsend, Myron Thomas, Ph.D., *associate professor of histology and embryology*, 1928–30

Tracewell, George L., M.D., *instructor in otorhinolaryngology*, 1962–(64)

Traub, Sidney P., M.D., *professor of radiology*, 1963–(64)

Trent, Robert Irvine, M.D., *assistant in ophthalmology*, 1939; *clinical professor*, (1964)

Trites, David K., Ph.D., *associate professor of medical psychology in psychiatry, neurology, and behavioral sciences*, 1960–(64)

Troop, Robert Cecil, Ph.D., *instructor in physiology*, 1954; *assistant professor*, 1955

Trucco, Raul Esteban, Ph.D., *assistant professor of research biochemistry*, 1957; *professor*, 1963

Tucker, Kenneth Merlin, D.D.S., *instructor in dental surgery*, (1964)

Turley, Louis Alvin, Ph.D., *instructor in pathology and neurology*, 1908; *professor emeritus of pathology*, 1953; *acting dean of the School of Medicine and superintendent of the University Hospitals*, 1935

Turner, Henry Hubert, M.D., *instructor in medicine*, 1925; *clinical professor* (1964); *acting medical superintendent of University Hospitals*, 1924–25

Turner, Maxine, M.S., *instructor in preventive medicine and public health*, 1946–48

Ullestad, Rolf J., D.D.S., *clinical assistant in dental surgery*, 1955; *assistant professor*, (1964)

Upjohn, Lawrence Northcote, M.D., *instructor in anatomy and physical culture*, 1900; *professor of anatomy and pathology*, 1904; *administrator of the School of Medicine*, 1900–1904

Valin, Jack Louis, M.D., *assistant professor of anesthesiology*, 1943–45

Vandever, Harry Wallace, M.D., *instructor in pediatrics*, 1957; *clinical instructor*, (1964)

Van Duyne, Charles Michael, M.D., *assistant professor of gynecology-obstetrics*, 1963–(64)

Van Matre, Reber, M.D., *clinical assistant in psychiatry and neurology*, 1948; *instructor*, 1953

Van Vleet, Albert Heald, Ph.D., *professor of biology*, 1900–1909

Vega, Arthur, Jr., M.A., *research associate in psychiatry, neurology, and behavioral sciences*, 1963–(64)

Viavant, William, Ph.D., *consultant associate professor of computer science in preventive medicine and public health*, 1960–63

Vickers, Paul Merton, M.D., *instructor in surgery*, 1945; *clinical professor*, (1964)

Villet, Lieonnir Janeal, B.S., *graduate assistant in biochemistry*, 1944–45

Von Saal, Frederick H., M.D., *fellow in orthopedic surgery*, 1938–39

Von Wedel, Curt Otto, Jr., M.D., *lecturer in minor surgery and bandaging and superintendent of dispensary*, 1912; *acting professor of* anatomy and assistant professor of surgery, 1916; superintendent of dispensary, 1911–12

Wade, Albert B., M.A., *instructor in psychiatry, neurology, and behavioral sciences*, 1958–59

Wagner, Milton Lee, M.D., *clinical instructor in radiology*, (1964)

Wails, Theodore Grant, M.D., *instructor in ophthalmology*, 1922; *professor emeritus of otorhinolaryngology*, (1964)

Wainwright, Tom Lyon, M.D., *assistant in surgery*, 1938; *assistant professor*, 1949

Waites, Lucius, M.D., *assistant professor of pediatrics and assistant professor of psychiatry, neurology, and behavioral sciences*, 1958–61

Walcher, Helen Ross, M.A., *assistant professor of communication disorders*, 1960; *associate professor*, (1964)

Waldrop, William L., M.D., *clinical assistant in orthopedic surgery*, 1949; *associate professor of orthopedic and fracture surgery*, (1964)

Walker, Ethan Allen, Jr., M.D., *clinical assistant in otorhinolaryngology*, 1952; *associate professor*, (1964)

Walker, James Robert, M.D., *instructor in anesthesiology*, 1947; *associate professor*, (1964)

Wallace, William Jones, M.D., *assistant professor of genitourinary diseases*, 1914; *professor of genitourinary diseases and syphilology*, 1934

Ward, Audray Delbert, M.D., *assistant professor of orthopedic surgery*, 1947–48

Ward, Vernon G., M.D., *clinical assistant in medicine*, 1960

Warner, Francis James, M.D., *associate professor of anatomy*, 1924–25

Warren, McWilson, Ph.D., *assistant professor of preventive medicine and public health*, 1957; *associate professor*, 1962

Washburn, Homer Charles, Ph.C., *instructor in pharmacy*, 1904; *professor of pharmacy and materia medica and dean of the School of Pharmacy*, 1911

Watson, Leigh Festus, M.D., *lecturer in operative surgery*, 1911; *assistant professor*, 1917

Watson, O. Alton, M.D., *instructor in otology, rhinology, and laryngology*, 1936; *professor of otorhinolaryngology*, (1964)

Watson, Raymond Delbert, M.D., *assistant in surgery*, 1938–46

Webb, Paul Paine, M.D., *assistant professor of physiology* 1951–54

Weber, Henry Clarence, M.D., *visiting lecturer in surgery*, 1941–51

Weber, Marion, B.S., *instructor in dietetics*, 1932–37

Wehrs, Roger E., M.D., *instructor in otorhinolaryngology*, 1963–(64)

Weiss, Kurt A., Ph.D., *associate professor of research physiology*, 1961–(64)

Weitzenhoffer, Andre Muller, Ph.D., *associate professor of psychiatry, neurology, and behavioral sciences*, 1962–(64)

Wells, Barbara, M.S., *instructor in bacteriology and in preventive medicine and public health*, 1948; *instructor in preventive medicine and public health*, 1951

Wells, Lois Lyon, M.D., *associate in anesthesiology*, 1938; *professor emeritus*, (1964)

Wells, Shirley L., M.S., *associate research professor of nutrition*, 1951–(64)

Wells, Walter William, M.D., *instructor in obstetrics*, 1916; *professor emeritus*, 1950

Welsh, Jack Daryl, M.D., *instructor in medicine*, 1959; *assistant professor*, (1964)

Welt, Peter J. L., M.D., *assistant professor of anesthesiology*, 1958–(64)

Werthessen, Nicholas T., Ph.D., *associate research professor of gynecology-obstetrics and associate professor of physiology*, 1962–(64)

West, Archa Kelly, M.D., *professor of principles and practice of medicine*, 1910; *professor of medicine*, 1925

West, Kathryn L., B.A., *research associate in psychiatry, neurology, and behavioral sciences*, 1958–(64)

West, Kelly McGuffin, M.D., *clinical assistant in medicine*, 1952; *associate professor of medicine and professor of continuing education*, (1964)

West, Louis Jolyon, M.D., *professor of psychiatry and neurology*, 1954; *professor of psychiatry, neurology, and behavioral sciences*, (1964)

West, Willis Kelly, M.D., *instructor in surgery*, 1919; *professor of orthopedic and fracture surgery*, 1962

Westfall, Leslie Marshall, M.D., *instructor in ophthalmology*, 1917; *professor emeritus*, 1956

Wettstein, Margaret Doepfner, Ph.D., M.D., *assistant professor of psychiatry, neurology, and behavioral sciences*, 1957–61

Wheeler, Preston, D.D.S., *clinical assistant in dental surgery*, 1960; *instructor in dental surgery*, (1964)

Whelan, Mary, M.S., *instructor in biochemistry and pharmacology*, 1930; *instructor in pharmacology*, 1936

Whitcomb, Walter H., M.D., *clinical assistant in medicine*, 1956; *assistant professor of medicine and of radiology*, (1964)

White, Arthur Weaver, M.D., *instructor in gastrointestinal diseases*, 1910; *professor emeritus of clinical medicine*, 1945

White, Charles Lincoln, D.D.S., *clinical consultant in dental surgery*, 1917; *associate professor*, 1941

White, Joseph M., M.D., *professor of anesthesiology*, 1955–(64); *acting dean of the School of Medicina and superintendent of University Hospitals*, 1964

White, Oscar Rogers, M.D., *instructor in surgery*, 1932; *clinical professor emeritus*, (1964)

Wickham, Mallalieu McCullagh, M.A., *instructor in histology, embryology, and zoology*, 1922; *instructor in histology and pathology*, 1924

Wienecke, Robert M., M.D., *assistant professor of psychiatry, neurology, and behavioral sciences*, (1964)

Wiggins, Carryle W., M.D., *clinical assistant in medicine*, 1955; *instructor*, (1964)

Wigler, Paul W., Ph.D., *assistant professor of research biochemistry*, 1960; *associate professor*, (1964)

Wilbanks, George Dewey, Jr., M.D., *clinical instructor in gynecology-obstetrics*, 1963–(64)

Wilber, Gertrude Helen, M.S., *assistant professor of histology and embryology*, 1930–31

Wildman, Stanley Francis, M.D., *instructor in genitourinary diseases and syphilology*, 1933; *assistant professor of urology*, 1947

Wiley, A. Ray, M.D., *visiting lecturer in surgery*, 1951–59

Wiley, George A., M.D., *clinical assistant in ophthalmology*, 1948; *associate professor*, 1959

Wilkins, Harry, M.D., *assistant in anatomy*, 1925; *professor of surgery*, (1964)

Wilkinson, Mary, B.A., *instructor in foods and nutrition*, 1937–40

Will, Arthur Anderson, M.D., *instructor in rectal surgery*, 1910; *associate professor*, 1926

Williams, Edward Marsh, B.S., *instructor in pathology and histology*, 1905; *instructor in pathology and bacteriology*, 1908

Williams, George Rainey, M.D., *assistant professor of surgery*, 1958; *professor*, (1964)

Williams, Guy Yandell, Ph.D., *instructor in chemistry*, 1907; *associate professor*, 1912

Williams, Harold L., Ph.D., *research professor of psychology in psychiatry, neurology, and behavioral sciences*, (1964)

Williams, Onie Owen, M.D., *assistant professor of pathology*, 1937–39

Williams, Robert Findlater, M.D., *professor of clinical medicine*, 1911–13; *dean of the School of Medicine*, 1911–13

Williams, T. Glyne, M.D., *associate professor of preventive medicine and public health and of psychiatry, neurology, and behavioral sciences*, 1961–63

Williamson, Frances, *assistant in histology and embryology*, 1944–45

Williamson, Lawrence McCoy, M.D., *clinical assistant in otorhinolaryngology*, 1946–47

Willie, James Asa, M.D., *instructor in neurology*, 1941; *instructor in psychiatry and neurology*, 1946

Wilner, Sal, M.D., *visiting lecturer in radiology*, (1964)

Wilson, Charles Hugh, M.D., *clinical assistant in surgery*, 1946; *associate professor*, (1964)

Wilson, James Ward, M.D., *clinical assistant in medicine*, (1964)

Wilson, Thomas Edward, Ph.D., *assistant professor of research microbiology*, 1957–59

Winkleman, George William, M.D., *clinical assistant in psychiatry and* neurology, 1947; *instructor in medicine*, 1956

Winn, George Louis, M.D., *clinical assistant in medicine*, 1949; *assistant professor*, (1964)

Winter, Charles Allen, Ph.D., *assistant professor of physiology*, 1944; *associate professor*, 1946

Winter, Irwin Clinton, Ph.D., *assistant professor of pharmacology*, 1939–1942

Wisdom, Norvell Edwin, B.S., *research associate in pharmacology*, 1936–37

Witcher, Jones E., M.D., *instructor in otorhinolaryngology*, 1963–(64)

Witten, Harold Brian, M.D., *clinical assistant in psychiatry and neurology*, 1947; *visiting lecturer in psychiatry, neurology, and behavioral sciences*, (1964)

Wolf, Stewart George, M.D., *professor of medicine*, 1952; *professor of medicine and consultant professor of psychiatry, neurology, and behavioral sciences*, (1964)

Wolff, John Powers, M.D., *assistant in surgery*, 1936; *clinical professor*, (1964)

Woods, Alexander H., M.D., *instructor in medicine*, 1958; *assistant professor of medicine and assistant professor of research immunology in microbiology*, (1964)

Woodward, Neil Whitney, M.D., *assistant in surgery*, 1936; *clinical professor*, 1962

Wooldridge, Wilfred Erwin, M.D., *visiting lecturer in dermatology*, 1959–(64)

Worsham, Bertrand Ray, M.D., *clinical assistant in psychiatry, neurology, and behavioral sciences*, 1959; *instructor*, (1964)

Wortham, Ruby Allen, M.A., *instructor in histology*, 1939–44

Wright, Leroy David, D.M.D., *clinical assistant in dental surgery*, 1948; *associate professor*, (1964)

Wulff, Johan Adolf, M.D., *clinical assistant in medicine*, 1960; *instructor*, (1964)

Wynn, Noble Franklin, M.D., *instructor in pharmacology*, 1943–44

Wyrick, Richard, M.D., *clinical assistant in ophthalmology*, 1952; *associate professor*, (1964)

Yamamoto, Joe, M.D., *assistant professor of psychiatry, neurology, and behavioral sciences*, 1955–58

Yang, Hsiu-Ying, Ph.D., *research associate in pharmacology*, (1964)

Yeager, Douglas A., D.D.S., *clinical assistant in dental surgery*, 1950; *assistant professor*, (1964)

Yeakel, Earl LeRoy, M.D., *instructor in bacteriology*, 1917–18

Young, Andrew Merriman, M.D., *instructor in obstetrics*, 1912–17

Young, Andrew Merriman, III, M.D., *clinical assistant in urology*, 1946; *instructor*, 1957

Young, Antonio DeBord, M.D., *professor of nervous and mental diseases*,

1910; *professor of neurology*, 1930

Young, C. Jack, M.D., *instructor in dermatology and syphilology*, 1954; *associate professor*, (1964)

Young, Edgar W., Jr., M.D., *graduate fellow in pharmacology*, 1948; *instructor*, 1955

Zahasky, Mary C., B.S., *associate professor nutrition*, 1948; *associate professor of nutrition and of preventive medicine and public health*, (1964)

Zaricznyj, Basilus, M.D., *assistant professor of orthopedic and fracture surgery*, 1957–60

Appendix V.
Preceptors of the School
of Medicine, 1949–65

Atkins, Charles N., M.D., Oklahoma City, 1958–59
Bailey, Carl H., M.D., Stroud, 1950–60
Barnes, Lynn C., M.D., Nowata, 1955–65
Barnes, S. D., M.D., Hollis, 1963–64
Bell, Eugene S., M.D., Tishomingo, 1963–65
Benjegerdes, T. D., M.D., Beaver, 1950–51
Blender, John X., M.D., Cherokee, 1955–56
Buell, A. L., M.D., Okmulgee, 1950–52
Burleson, Ned, M.D., Prague, 1950–54
Byrd, Wallace, M.D., Coalgate, 1952–53
Carson, John M., M.D., Shawnee, 1952–59
Conley, R. A., M.D., Watonga, 1964–65
Connell, M. A., M.D., Picher, 1952–59
Cook, Edward T., Jr., M.D., Anadarko, 1956–64
Cunningham, C. S., M.D., Poteau, 1964–65
Dersch, Walter H., Jr., M.D., Shattuck, 1953–65
Devanney, P. J., M.D., Sayre, 1962–63
Duer, Joe L., M.D., Woodward, 1949–65
Emmott, Ralph C., M.D., Stilwell, 1957–58
Finch, J. William, M.D., Hobart, 1949–56, 1961–65
Freed, Leon C., M.D., Perkins, 1951–54
Fried, David, M.D., Mangum, 1954–57
Fry, E. P., M.D., Stillwater, 1963–65
Gathers, George B., M.D., Stillwater, 1954–63
Gibson, Robert B., M.D., Ponca City, 1954–62
Godfrey, Kenneth E., M.D., Okeene, 1955–60
Graham, J. A., M.D., Pauls Valley, 1960–65
Green, Burdge F., M.D., Stilwell, 1956–65
Holland, C. K., M.D., McAlester, 1958–65
Johnson, C. L., Jr., M.D., Bartlesville, 1954–57
Johnston, L. A. S., M.D., Holdenville, 1959–63
Kinsinger, R. R., M.D., Blackwell, 1954–55
Kirby, Lester R., M.D., Cherokee, 1953–55
Lindley, E. C., M.D., Duncan, 1960–65

Lindsay, Ray H., M.D., Pauls Valley, 1949–56
Little, A. C., M.D., Minco, 1949–52
Lowrey, Robert W., M.D., Poteau, 1960–63
Masters, Herbert A., M.D., Tahlequah, 1949–52
Mollison, Malcolm, M.D., Altus, 1959–65
McCurdy, W. C., Jr., M.D., Purcell, 1949–65
McDonald, Glen W., M.D., Pawhuska, 1953–56
McDougal, R. C., M.D., Holdenville, 1963–65
McGrew, E. A., M.D., Beaver, 1949–63
McIntyre, John A., M.D., Enid, 1952–57
McMillan, J. M., M.D., Vinita, 1949–50
McMurray, James F., M.D., Sentinel, 1949–52
Newman, O. C., M.D., Shattuck, 1950–53
Parmley, Van S., M.D., Mangum, 1951–54
Patterson, O. H., M.D., Sapulpa, 1963–65
Petty, James S., M.D., Guthrie, 1949–58
Pryor, V. W., M.D., Holdenville, 1949–50
Ray, C. Cody, M.D., Pawhuska, 1956–65
Rhea, Thomas E., M.D., Idabel, 1953–56
Rose, Daton M., M.D., Okemah, 1958–60
Schaff, H. V., M.D., Holdenville, 1954–59
Shirley, Edward T., M.D., Wynnewood, 1954–65
Smith, Carlton E., M.D., Henryetta, 1955–65
Spence, Ray E., M.D., Pauls Valley, 1956–60
Srigley, Robert S., M.D., Hollis, 1950–55
Stowers, Aubrey E., M.D., Sentinel, 1952–58
Tallant, George A., M.D., Frederick, 1959–65
Taylor, John R., M.D., Kingfisher, 1949–55
Traverse, C. A., M.D., Alva, 1949–59
Wainwright, Tom L., M.D., Mangum, 1957–64
Walker, Roscoe, M.D., Pawhuska, 1949–52
Weedn, A. J., M.D., Duncan, 1949–50
Whinery, K. E., M.D., Sayre, 1963–65
Wilhite, L. R., M.D., Perkins, 1949–52
Williams, C. H., M.D., Okeene, 1963–65
Winters, R. L., M.D., Poteau, 1963–64
Wolfe, Henry D., M.D., Hugo, 1949–56
Woodson, Earl M., M.D., Poteau, 1949–50
York, J. F., M.D., Madill, 1949–56

Appendix VI.
Superintendents and Medical Directors of the University Hospitals, 1911–64

Cowles, Annette B., R.N., *superintendent*, 1911–15
Hill, Lucy Renette, R.N., *superintendent*, 1915–16
Workman, H. Mary, R.N., *superintendent*, 1916
Long, LeRoy, M.D., *dean and superintendent*, 1915–31
Fesler, Paul H., *acting superintendent*, 1916–18
Fesler, Paul H., *superintendent*, 1918–20
Fesler, Paul H., *fiscal superintendent*, 1920–27
Langston, Wann, M.D., *medical superintendent*, 1920–29
Turner, Henry H., M.D., *acting medical superintendent*, 1924–25
Langston, Wann, M.D., *administrative officer*, 1929–31
Smith, J. B., M.D., *superintendent*, 1931–35
Moorman, Lewis J., M.D., *dean and superintendent*, 1933–35
Turley, Louis Alvin, Ph.D., *acting dean and superintendent*, 1935
Jeter, Hugh G., M.D., *medical director*, 1935
Patterson, Robert Urie, M.D., *dean and superintendent*, 1935–42
Olsen, Egil Thorbjorn, M.D., *Medical Director*, 1935–40
Reese, Lewis Labon, M.D., *medical director*, 1940–41
Barry, George Newton, M.D., *medical director*, 1941–44
Shoemaker, Harold A., Ph.D., *acting dean and superintendent*, 1942–43
Lowry, Thomas Claude, M.D., *dean and superintendent*, 1942–45
Barry, George Newton, M.D., *medical director*, 1944–45
Langston, Wann, M.D., *dean and superintendent*, 1945–46
Fesler, Paul H., *administrator*, 1946–47
Gray, Jacques Pierce, M.D., *dean and superintendent*, 1946–47
Everett, Mark R., Ph.D., *dean and superintendent*, 1947–(64)*
Cushing, Vernon D., M.D., *acting medical director*, 1948
Cushing, Vernon D., M.D., *medical director*, 1949
Lowe, Robert Chester, M.D., *medical director*, 1949–56
Lowe, Robert Chester, M.D., *superintendent*, 1957–58
Crews, Raymond Drake, LL.B., *superintendent*, 1959–(64)
White, Joseph M., M.D., *acting dean and superintendent*, 1964
Dennis, James L., M.D., *dean and superintendent*, 1964

* When 1964 appears in parentheses, it indicates that this was not the final year of appointment.

Appendix VII.
Directors of the
Outpatient Department, 1911–64

Von Wedel, Curt Otto, Jr., M.D., *superintendent of the dispensary*,
 1911–12
Hartford, John Smith, M.D., *chief of dispensary staff*, 1912–16
Clymer, Cyril Ebert, M.D., *chief of dispensary staff*, 1917–24
Murdoch, Raymond Lester, M.D., *chief of outpatient department staff*,
 1925–31
Langston, Wann, M.D., *director*, 1931–33
Keltz, Bert F., M.D., *director*, 1933–35
Hull, Wayne McKinley, M.D., *director*, 1935–37
Barry, George N., M.D., *director*, 1937–40
Royce, Owen, Jr., M.D., *director*, 1940–41
Barry, George N., M.D., *reappointed director*, 1941–42
Avey, Harry Thompson, Jr., M.D., *director*, 1942–46
Lowe, Robert Chester, M.D., *director*, 1946–49
Muchmore, Harold G., M.D., *acting director*, 1949–52
Colmore, John P., M.D., *director*, 1952–61
Smith, Carl W., M.D., *director*, 1961–(64)*

* When 1964 appears in parentheses, it indicates that this was not the final year of
appointment.

Appendix VIII.
Social Service Directors,
1921–64

Tolbert, Virginia, 1921–25
Shanklin, Kitty, B.A., (Mrs. Rountree),* 1925–34
Carr, Helen, B.A., * 1934–41
Foulks, Ketourah, M.S., 1941–45
Lowery, Ruth, M.S., 1945–51
Walton, Elizabeth, M.S.W., 1951–55
Schroeder, Edith, M.S.W., *acting director*, 1955–56
Barnes, George, M.S.,* 1956 58
Smith, Ether, M.S.W., *acting director*, 1958–59
Connery, Jennie, M.S.W.,* 1959–61
Hornor, Katherine E., M.S.S.W., *acting director*, 1961–62
Hornor, Katherine E., M.S.S.W., 1962–(64)**

* Members of the faculty of the School of Medicine.
** When 1964 appears in parentheses, it indicates that this was not the final year of appointment.

Appendix IX.
Dietetic Internship Directors,
1928–64

Aitken, Edith Ruth Tilton, B.S., 1928–32
Sewell, Margery Ardrey, B.S., 1932–36
Melgaard, J. Marie, M.S., 1936–45
Peters, Vera Parman, M.S., 1945–48
Zahasky, Mary C., B.S., 1948–(64)*

* When 1964 appears in parentheses, it indicates that this was not the final year of appointment.

Appendix X.
Dietetic Interns, 1928–64

1928
Winifred R. Daily

1929
Mary C. Barnes
Marian Hanson

1930
Cleo Lambrecht
Anna B. Griffith

1931
Ida Osborn
Eva Galt

1933
Vivian T. Pobar
Esther Dinwiddle Phillips

1934
Roberta Cole
Opal Bradley Shinn
Lesey B. Kinsel

1935
Mary E. Leidigh

1936
Ruby Lambert Harp
Marjorie Frich
Pauline Griffin Kearns

1938
Muriel Tice Nelson

1939
Mary S. Hiatt
S. Novelle Tucker Eppler
Helen Inverso

1940
Helen Pachak
Maurine Lovell

1941
Wilma Hayter, R.D.
Ethel Lienhardt Gould
Jean Hondrum Graham

1942
Alcy W. Goldsmith
Juanita Hope

1943
Bernice Duncan
Carol Swain Huggins
Joyce P. Jemison
Opal Jane Austin
Ellen Brasted
Catherine Bardsley Eisenburg

1944
Jeanne House Hutchinson
Rosemary Holm

1945
Mary Lankford, Jr.
Bonnie Sewick

1946
Marian Meyers
Catherine Cullen
Nancy Jameson Herrin
Mary Collins

1947
Emilie R. Oldfield
Shirley Wallace Hearn

1948
Eunice Wilson
Anne C. Logan

1949
Mary Norris
Nancy Johnson Tidmore
Sara Walter

1950
Betty Voorheis
Gloria Spradley
Patsy Drucker Lee

1951
Mary Lou McDonald
Maudell Baxley Doner
Beverly Collier Hilleary

1952
Sharon Orrick Belindo
Eloise C. Runolfson
June Kettering
Dorothalee Hayes

1953
Olga Cartwright
Charlotte Slemp
Onah K. Bayless

1954
Nell Jane McCormack
Lucille Perez
Felicitas F. Piedad Pascual
Catherine Forest
Mary F. Collins

1955
Patricia Merritt
Shirley Smith

1956
Nancy Davis Robertson
Phyllis Lee Duckworth
Meredith J. Bell
Dorothy Siemann

1957
Joanne Yeager
Maxine S. Summers

1958
Norma L. Jones
Bente Morch
Lanora Barnes

1959
Clara McCord Day
Jean Akerley Gray
Rosalie Hughey
Mary Louise Cole, III
Janice Black, Jr.
Barbara Martin
Marlene Easter

1960
Glenda Pullin Ray
Dorothy Dowling
Margaret Smith

1961
Linda Lacefield

1962
Lorna Moya Crum
Janis Peak
Mary Melia, Jr.
Madeline J. Jennings

1963
Kathlyn Smithson
Judy Gardner Dunlap

1964
Margaret Wall
Barbara Mayo Deal
Colleen Wilson
Marilyn Reilly
Janet Wenzel

Appendix XI.
Librarians, 1924–64

Jameson, Agnes, 1924–27
Cassidy, Grace Swain, 1927–31
Hughes, Ruth Thompson, 1931–38
Sigerfoos, Grace Robeson, A.B., 1938–42
Heck, Lilah Bell, M.S., 1942–62
Eddy, Leonard, M.L.S., 1962–(64)*

* When 1964 appears in parentheses, it indicates that this was not the final year of appointment.

Appendix XII.
Doctor of Medicine Degrees Conferred on Graduates of the University of Oklahoma School of Medicine, 1911–64

Abbott, Mary Ida Irby, 1957
Abelarde, Jose Francisco, 1930
Abernethy, Alton Coy, 1930
Abernethy, James Harold, 1939
Abshere, Lynn Wallace, 1956
Acers, Thomas Edward, 1959
Adair, John Ralph, 1954
Adams, George Mullins, 1943
Adams, Henry Grady, 1915
Adams, James Elston, 1917
Adams, Jerome M., 1953
Adams, Marcus Webb, Jr., 1959
Adams, Sylva, 1924
Adams, Walter B., 1911
Adelman, Frank Leo, 1943
Afinowicz, John Robert, 1964
Akin, Robert Howe, 1928
Albright, John D., 1962
Aldredge, William Max, 1941
Alexander, Bronson Raye, 1954
Alexander, Everett Tweed, 1920
Alexander, James Leon, 1943
Alexander, John Robert, 1961
Alexander, Richard Kent, 1959
Alexander, Robert Lin, Jr., 1961
Alexander, Samuel Howard, 1928
Alexander, Thomas Crawford, 1963
Allen, Clifford Ward, 1944
Allen, George T., 1932
Allen, Ray F., 1960
Allen, Rollie Edward, 1953
Allen, Russell Floyd, 1963

Allensworth, Edward Wayne, 1961
Allgood, Edward Allphin, 1945
Allgood, Elvus Jene, 1930
Allgood, John Milton, 1928
Allgood, Richard Jene, 1964
Alling, Emery Ernest, 1925
Allison, Robert Lee, 1953
Allred, Robert Louis, 1963
Alston, William Corder, Jr., 1937
Ambrister, Jerome Warner, 1943
Amdall, Robert Owen, 1953
Amspacher, Jimmie Charles, 1943
Amspacher, William, 1936
Anderson, Haskell Reynolds, 1934
Anderson, Hubert Manley, 1942
Anderson, Irene Freda, 1939
Anderson, Lanny Gordon, 1961
Anderson, Paul Sanford, 1935
Anderson, Ralph Doyle, 1942
Anderson, Roy W., 1939
Anderson, Thomas Page, 1943
Anderson, William Douglas, 1931
Andreskowski, W. Theodore, 1919
Angerer, Alden Lee, 1946
Angus, Donald Adelbert, 1933
Angus, Howard, 1938
Annadown, Ruth Vivian, 1946
Appleton, Meredith Marcus, 1934
Archer, Homer Vincent, 1943
Arky, Albert Milton, 1955
Armstrong, W. O., 1924
Arndt, Jerome Harrison, 1958

Arnold, James Kerley, 1956
Arrendell, Cad Walder, Jr., 1945
Arrendell, Eugene Hamlin, 1943
Arrington, Carl Thomas, 1930
Arthurs, Donald Duane, 1958
Arthurs, Melvin Ross, 1954
Asher, James Ottley, 1941
Ashley, Robert E., 1955
Askins, John Robert, Jr., 1950
Atherton, Charles V., 1932
Athey, Clanton Ray, 1953
Atkin, John Drew, 1961
Auriemma, Pasquale Richard, 1928
Austin, Frank Herbert, Jr., 1946
Austin, George Nicolo, 1950
Austin, John David, 1947
Aycock, Byron Wolverton, 1940
Baggett, Rex T., 1962
Bagwell, Kenneth Hugh, 1957
Bahr, Walter Julien, 1955
Bailey, Albert Stanley, Jr., 1955
Bailey, Byron James, 1959
Bailey, Byron Louis, 1947
Bailey, Carl Horatio, 1933
Bailey, Harry Kenneth, 1953
Baines, Roy Dixie, Jr., 1959
Baird, Cecil Dryden, 1927
Baird, Wilson Davis, 1926
Baker, Cecil Camak, Jr., 1956
Baker, Charles Ernest, 1951
Baker, Loren V., 1925
Baker, Loren V., Jr., 1955
Baker, Marguerite Madigan, 1927
Baker, Petey Hughey, 1964
Baker, Wilbur K., II, 1960
Baker, William L., 1960
Bakken, Richard Lowell, 1949
Ballard, Jack Duane, 1943
Ballard, Noble Lee, 1964
Ballard, Ray Halcomb, 1939
Ballinger, Thomas Irwin, 1953
Baltazar, Alejandro Christi, 1927
Baltazar, Bertha Mueller, 1927
Balyeat, Ray Morton, 1918
Barb, Kirk Bentley, 1915
Barb, T. J., 1921

Barb, Thomas John, Jr., 1933
Barbee, Richard Franklin, 1957
Barber, Forest Chester, 1950
Bare, Lawrence E., 1962
Barger, John Blanchard, 1931
Barker, Clyde James, Jr., 1935
Barker, Marcus Spero, 1948
Barker, Robert Duane, 1943
Barkett, N. F. Vander, 1939
Barlow, Ronald S., 1962
Barnes, Harry Edward, 1935
Barnes, Lynn Carl, Jr., 1952
Barnes, Robert Nelson, 1934
Barnes, Shelby Dee, 1954
Barnett, Duane Alfred, 1952
Barney, Donald Charles, 1958
Barney, Jack Alroy, 1956
Barnhill, John Willis, 1959
Barno, Alex, 1944
Barrett, Paul Arthur, 1963
Barrow, Llewellyn Lancelot, 1931
Bartel, Jack Orvis, 1930
Barton, Clyde Wheeler, 1958
Bash, Vincent Clarence, Jr., 1951
Bassett, Clifford Monroe, 1930
Bast, Lowell E., 1960
Bates, Clarence Edgar, 1920
Baton, Bobby G., 1960
Battenfield, John Young, 1937
Baugh, Harold Timberlake, 1930
Baum, Ernest Eldon, 1928
Baxter, Earl Dale, 1964
Baxter, Virgil Clifford, 1939
Bayless, James Mason, 1947
Baylor, Richard A., Jr., 1962
Baze, Roy, 1936
Bealmear, Kent Drake, 1963
Beasley, Gerald LeRoy, Jr., 1953
Beaty, C. Sam, 1935
Beaty, George Lewis, 1929
Beavers, James Clyde, 1955
Beck, Charles Edward, 1952
Beck, L.D., 1935
Becker, Fred William, 1946
Beckloff, George N., 1962
Beckloff, Gerald Lee, 1961

Bedner, Gerald, 1940
Beeler, Thomas Taylor, 1937
Beiderwell, Paul Leo, 1938
Bell, Ben, 1942
Bell, Bruce Gene, 1963
Bell, Eugene Steven, 1952
Bell, Howard Bryant, 1951
Bell, James Preston, 1952
Bell, James Thomas, 1935
Bell, Joseph Price, 1943
Bell, Orville E., 1936
Bell, Robert Frank, 1961
Beller, Cleve, 1943
Belter, Lester Francis, 1946
Belter, Louis Clayton, 1956
Bender, Herman Robert, 1941
Bennett, Wayne Eugene, 1953
Benward, John H., 1939
Berger, Elmer Stanley, 1944
Berger, Martin, 1947
Bergman, Donald R., 1962
Berkenbile, Glen Lee, 1946
Bernamonti, Don, Jr., 1955
Bernard, Clarence Rolla, 1925
Bernell, William, 1942
Bernhardt, Keith I., 1962
Bernhardt, Samuel C., 1960
Bernhardt, William Gene, 1958
Bernstein, Samuel S., 1916
Berrey, Leo Alonzo, 1916
Berry, James Eason, 1959
Berry, John Curtis, 1937
Berry, Spencer Edgar, 1950
Betson, Johnnie Richard, Jr., 1955
Beumer, Oliver Chester, 1943
Bickford, Colon Underwood, 1948
Bida, John Frank, 1948
Biehler, Larry L., 1962
Billingsley, James Glazebrook,
   1955
Bilsky, Nathan, 1924
Binkley, Frank Carlton, 1939
Binkley, James G., 1917
Bird, Billy Joe, 1957
Birge, Jack Paul, 1931

Bishop, Calmes P., 1937
Bishop, David William, 1958
Bissell, Robert Gene, 1959
Blackburn, Robert Neil, 1961
Blackert, Dorothy Frances, 1943
Blackketter, Donald Ewing, 1952
Blackwelder, Stephen Elliott, 1964
Blair, Clifford Jennings, 1939
Blair, J. V., 1921
Blair, Wilma Jeanne, 1955
Blanchard, William Grant, 1955
Blankenship, Jerry B., 1962
Blaschke, John Ahrens, 1950
Bledsoe, Joe Thomas, 1959
Blender, John Xavier, 1946
Blevins, Billy E., 1960
Blevins, James W., III, 1955
Blevins, Walter Eugene, 1951
Blinde, Oscar J., 1935
Bliss, Bryce Owen, 1957
Bloom, Nathan Nehemia, 1916
Bloss, Claude M., Jr., 1937
Blue, Johnny A., 1934
Boatman, Karl Kenneth, 1952
Boatright, Lloyd C., 1931
Boaz, John T., III, 1960
Bobek, Donald W., 1955
Bodine, Charles David, 1943
Boggs, Harold Earl, 1964
Boggs, James Thomas, 1946
Bohlman, Wilbur Frederick, 1937
Bolene, John Frederick, 1955
Bolene, Robert Victor, 1948
Bolene, William Dean, 1958
Boles, Gerald William, 1957
Boles, Robert Dale, 1953
Bolton, Houck Ernst, 1943
Bond, Eugene Cralle, 1948
Bond, Ira Tarlton, Jr., 1927
Bond, William Lawrence, 1947
Bondurant, Charles P., 1924
Bonham, Russell Farber, 1926
Boone, Clifton U., 1932
Booth, George Randolph, 1944
Boothby, Paul Revere, 1943

Borecky, George L., 1923
Boren, Paul G., 1962
Borron, Robert Kenneth, 1959
Boswell, William Eugene, 1933
Bosworth, William C., 1960
Bottomley, Richard Harold, 1958
Bottomley, Robert G., 1962
Bowers, Neville, 1939
Bowers, Robert Carl, 1950
Bowers, William Edward, Jr., 1955
Bowie, Carl Walton, 1946
Bowlan, Walter Lewis, 1961
Boyd, Tom Madison, 1917
Boyd, Wayne Johnson, 1950
Boyer, Harold Lester, 1941
Boyle, James Stanton, 1948
Bozalis, George Sam, 1935
Braden, Barbara Foster, 1957
Braden, Donald Kent, 1957
Bradfield, Eldon O., 1936
Bradfield, Samuel Jackson, 1915
Bradford, Arthur Calvin, 1955
Bradford, Reagan Howard, 1961
Bradford, Vance Arthur, 1938
Bradley, Frank, 1936
Bradley, Harold C., 1917
Brady, Jack Harry, 1936
Brake, Charles Arthur, 1917
Brake, Charles Murray, 1951
Braly, Berton Edward, 1951
Braly, Murlin Knight, 1947
Brandes, Herman G., 1911
Brandt, Edward N., Jr., 1960
Branham, Donald W., 1925
Brashear, Eddie Alvin, 1958
Brauchi, John Tony, 1955
Brauer, Siegfried Herman, 1926
Braun, Jacob Peter, 1930
Brawner, Donald Leon, 1947
Brawner, Luther Clifton, 1939
Breco, Davis, 1933
Bressie, Jerry Lee, 1958
Brett, Dale Edward, 1958
Brewer, August Malone, 1927
Brewer, Lt. Kenneth Arthur, 1930

Bricker, Earl M., Jr., 1953
Bridal, Loy D., 1960
Bridges, Delta Walker, Jr., 1963
Bridges, Robert Goltra, 1958
Bridwell, Malcolm Edward, 1964
Brightwell, Gaines Levy, 1931
Brightwell, Richard Justice, 1941
Brill, Melvyn Leon, 1961
Brittain, Fanny Lou, 1927
Britton, Bloyce Hill, 1928
Britton, Bloyce H., Jr., 1960
Brixey, Albin Monroe, Jr., 1943
Broadrick, Broadway, 1945
Brock, Bill L., 1954
Brockman, Hiram Leroy, 1920
Brooks, Harold Lloyd, 1963
Brooks, J.T., 1945
Brooks, Quentin Thomas, 1953
Broome, Robert Ogie, 1958
Browder, Sue Elizabeth, 1945
Brown, Arthur Merton, Jr., 1945
Brown, Benjamin Henton, 1949
Brown, Bruce H., 1947
Brown, Byron Brandon, 1925
Brown, Charles Leonard, 1921
Brown, Charles Reiff, 1957
Brown, Claude H.B., 1953
Brown, Clifford Alton, 1943
Brown, David Randolph, 1949
Brown, David William, 1964
Brown, DeLon Nello, 1945
Brown, Forest R., 1936
Brown, George MacMillan, Jr.,
   1943
Brown, Gerster William, 1930
Brown, Horace Jacquelin, 1959
Brown, Irwin Hubert, 1945
Brown, Isadore, 1932
Brown, James Winter, 1914
Brown, John Harrold, 1954
Brown, Leonard Harold, 1945
Brown, Mary Louise Mathews,
   1964
Brown, Olin Edwin, 1928
Brown, Spencer Henton, 1940

Brown, Thomas Guy, 1929
Brownlee, Leslie G.A., 1912
Brownson, Richmond Jay, 1964
Brundage, Bert, 1936
Brundage, Carl L., 1920
Bryon, Richard Stephen, 1950
Buchanan, F. Randall, 1942
Buckholts, Col. Walter H., 1929
Buell, Arthur Louis, 1939
Buffington, Fred Courtney, 1935
Buffington, Gordon Warren, 1950
Buford, Elvin Lee, 1941
Bugg, Robert Nelson, 1943
Buice, William Alfred, 1930
Bulla, Gordon G., 1930
Bullard, Ray Elva, 1924
Buller, Ralph Leland, 1956
Bunch, Allen Henry, 1950
Bungardt, Alfred Hiller, Jr., 1939
Burg, Fred Allen, 1939
Burgert, E. Omar, Jr., 1947
Burgess, Eugene Pierce, 1955
Burgett, Robert Ernest, 1958
Burgtorf, Richard Herbert, 1945
Burke, Martha Jene, 1945,
Burks, Arthur Lynn, 1939
Burleson, Hopson Ned, 1930
Burleson, Michael Ned, 1961
Burnett, Hal Arthur, 1943
Burnett, Jack F., 1939
Burr, Donald C., 1962
Burr, John Clarence, 1957
Burris, Otis Franklin, 1955
Burtis, Buffington Bonheur, 1964
Burton, Leonard Eugene, 1954
Busboom, Robert Gray, 1946
Bush, John D., 1960
Bush, Jordan Morgan, 1939
Buswell, Arthur Wilcox, 1952
Butcher, John M., 1936
Butcher, Orby L., Jr., 1955
Buttram, Clarence Abram, 1938
Buttram, Harold Eugene, 1958
Butts, Donald Terry, 1963
Butts, Imogene,. 1933

Buxton, Merwin Thomas, Jr., 1947
Bynum, Chester Lee, 1957
Bynum, Turner Edward, 1964
Bynum, William Robert, 1951
Cagle, Ronald Edward, 1958
Cailey, Leo F., 1925
Cain, James Henry, 1942
Caldwell, Avalo Vergne, 1950
Caldwell, Delmar Ray, 1961
Cales, John Othal, 1942
Calhoon, Ed Latta, 1950
Calhoon, Harold Wayne, 1958
Calhoon, James Hal, 1956
Calkin, Alan Charles, 1956
Calkins, Robert S., 1947
Callahan, J. Stanley, 1924
Cameron, Alan S., Jr., 1950
Camp, Carl D., 1962
Campbell, James A., 1915
Campbell, James Franklin, 1928
Campbell, John Roy, 1935
Campbell, Philip J., 1960
Campbell, Robert Emerson, 1954
Campbell, William J., 1939
Canada, J. Clayton, 1929
Cantrell, David Emerson, Jr., 1934
Cantrell, Emma Jean, 1933
Cantrell, Capt. Roy Foster, 1928
Cantrell, William Howard, 1940
Capehart, John Daniel, 1946
Capehart, Maurice Phillip, 1944
Capehart, Samuel Alfred, 1948
Carey, Philip O., 1953
Carl, Roy Barton, 1955
Carleton, Lawrence H., 1917
Carlile, William Finley, 1961
Carlton, Theodore, 1946
Carmack, Charles Allen, 1955
Carney, John Harvey, 1956
Carr, William Austin, 1918
Carroll, James Robert, 1959
Carson, Harold Bryan, 1949
Carson, John, 1936
Carter, Claude E., 1932
Carter, Donald R., 1960

Carter, Herschel Gray, 1943
Carter, Merle Dean, 1959
Cartmell, Larry Wayne, 1964
Casey, Earle Addison, 1935
Casey, James G., 1954
Casey, Robert Elsworth, 1945
Casey, Robert Louis, 1963
Cash, Gerolis Shelton, 1940
Cason, Peter L., 1960
Casper, Pete D., 1946
Casper, Stark Michael, 1923
Cassidy, John McCarty, 1931
Cassidy, Robert J., 1955
Casteel, Charles Kempe, 1959
Castle, Eugene Allen, 1953
Castronova, Joseph, 1929
Cathey, Charles Wesley, 1953
Caughron, John R., 1960
Cavanaugh, William Johnson, 1920
Cavener, Jessie Lee, 1939
Cawley, Francis Patrick, 1944
Cawley, John J., Jr., 1938
Cawley, Leo Patrick, 1952
Chaffin, Zale, 1936
Chamberlin, Cecil Rhodes, Jr.,
   1955
Chambers, Clint Edwin, 1959
Chambers, Evander Evans, 1940
Chambers, Jean Frances, 1949
Chambless, William Stephen, 1959
Chandler, Harold M., 1960
Chandler, Herbert Norman, 1946
Chapman, Frank Deuel, 1961
Chapman, Paul Benton, 1946
Charney, Louis H., 1928
Chatfield, Robert B., 1962
Chatterjee, Surendra N., 1919
Chaves, Enrique, 1963
Cheatwood, William Randolph,
   1937
Chesher, Earl Clifford, 1928
Chesnut, Dan Edwin, 1963
Chesnut, John Kent, 1959
Childers, Stanley Gray, 1945
Childress, Marvin Allen, 1945

Choice, Robert William, 1938
Christensen, Marion D., 1952
Christian, Paul Christopher, 1914
Chumley, Channer P., 1916
Clabaugh, West Addis, 1964
Clanin, James Olin, 1931
Clark, Ben Prestridge, 1934
Clark, Frank Wilson, 1951
Clark, John Vincent, 1939
Clark, Ralph Otis, 1936
Clark, Ronald David, 1961
Clarkson, Alvin Marshall, 1926
Classen, Jeannine Archer, 1954
Classen, Kenneth Leon, 1954
Clay, Richard Allen, 1943
Cleaver, William Raymond, 1958
Clemans, David Clifton, 1952
Clemens, Ted, Jr., 1952
Clements, Donald Gene, 1947
Clevenger, Alva Ben, 1964
Click, William Claude, 1949
Clift, Merl Cecil, 1923
Clifton, Curtis Neil, 1955
Clifton, Jerry Taylor, 1956
Clingan, Frank Add, 1956
Clinger, John Milton, Jr., 1949
Clopton, James William, 1945
Close, John H., 1962
Cloud, Robert Sidney, 1959
Clough, Charles Atherton, 1959
Clymer, John Hatchett, 1944
Coates, John Albert, 1955
Coates, Rugie Reynold, 1937
Coats, Jack L., 1957
Cochran, Bryce Holmes, 1951
Cochran, Roy L., 1919
Cochrane, Charles Riley, 1947
Coe, William Henry, 1949
Coen, James Randolph, 1927
Coffey, Clinton Maurice, 1958
Coggins, Farris Webb, 1947
Cohen, Eugene Saul, 1946
Cohen, Samuel Lewis, 1943
Coil, Jenner George, 1946
Coin, Carl Gene, 1951

Coin, James Walter, Jr., 1951
Cokey, John Kenner, Jr., 1934
Coldwell, James George, 1955
Cole, Orville Wilbur, 1930
Cole, Rosser Ryan, 1963
Cole, Royce Murray, 1963
Cole, William Charles, 1941
Coleman, Billy O., 1947
Collins, Donald Dee, 1959
Collins, Glenn Jessie, 1935
Collins, Glenn Samuel, Jr., 1948
Collins, Herbert Dale, 1926
Collins, Joe Ed, 1948
Collins, William Robert, 1953
Colvert, James Robert, 1941
Colwick, James Thomas, Jr., 1952
Colyer, Ardell Benton, 1941
Combs, Leon Doyle, 1944
Compton, Avery Paul, 1957
Cone, Jesse Donald, 1947
Cone, John Allen, 1964
Conley, Richard Albert, 1959
Conn, Julian Harold, 1943
Connell, Matt A., 1932
Conner, Hugh McDonald, Jr., 1952
Conners, Thomas Patrick, 1937
Connor, Edwin Earl, 1926
Conrad, Betty Louise, 1944
Conrad, Loyal Lee, 1943
Cook, Charles Edgar, Jr., 1942
Cook, Edward Tiffin, 1938
Cook, Odis A., 1931
Cook, William Zachariah, Jr., 1955
Cooke, Everette Ellis, 1943
Cooley, Ben Hunter, 1921
Cooley, Percy Paul, 1923
Cooper, Alice Cora, 1938
Cooper, Frank Harry, 1958
Cooper, Kenneth Hardy, 1956
Copeland, Edwin King, 1930
Copeland, Evan Leonard, 1944
Coppedge, Orville Newelle, 1933
Corbett, Lewis B., 1924
Corbin, Damon Elliott, 1929
Cordonnier, Byron, 1932

Cordum, Myron A., 1962
Corley, Bert N., 1962
Cornelius, George Robert, 1957
Cornelsen, Ernest Edwin, 1943
Cosby, Glenn Wendelle, 1943
Coston, Rolls McKinney, 1929
Cotner, Jerry Bob, 1959
Cotner, Norman Andrew, 1958
Cotteral, John Robert, 1929
Cotton, Bert Hollis, 1937
Cotton, William Walker, 1935
Couch, Jim C., 1962
Courtright, Ann, 1951
Courtright, Claiborne Lee, 1951
Coussons, Richard Timothy, 1963
Covey, James Henry, 1964
Cowling, Robert Emmett, 1935
Cox, Arlo, 1932
Cox, Walter Mason, 1953
Coyle, John Jerome, 1943
Coyner, Wallace Roosevelt, 1947
Coyner, Wallace Ware, 1963
Crabtree, James Alan, 1957
Craft, Wilma E., 1933
Craig, Kenneth Burton, 1958
Craig, Nancy Ryan, 1949
Craig, William Joseph, 1951
Cramer, Ralph, Jr., 1964
Crane, Francis S., 1933
Cravens, Clem, 1950
Crawford, James Wallace, 1963
Crawford, Perry F., 1953
Crawford, Sterling Thomas, 1942
Crick, Lloyd Earp, 1934
Crittendon, William Floyd, 1954
Crockett, Herbert Gillis, 1934
Crockett, William Anders, 1961
Croom, William Sterling, 1948
Crosthwait, Marion Joe, 1955
Crowell, Bill Bruce, 1964
Crump, James Leonard, 1955
Cullen, Marvin LeRoy, 1943
Culmer, Ausmon Edgar, Jr., 1940
Culwell, Don W., 1962
Culwell, William Burk, 1938

Cunningham, Charles Donald, 1938
Cunningham, Charles Stewart, 1945
Cunningham, Curtis B., 1935
Cunningham, Hugh Alexander, 1934
Cunningham, John, 1936
Cunningham, John Henry, 1950
Cunningham, William Alfred, 1958
Curb, Delos Griffith, 1933
Currie, John Morgan, 1963
Curry, Roy Lee, 1931
Curtess, Ross Lee, Jr., 1949
Curtis, Lt.Col., Selvie Jewell, 1928
Curtiss, William Phelps, 1946
Cushman, Harry Rutledge, 1935
Daffer, Ernest R., 1962
Daily, Raymond E., 1932
Dakil, Louis, 1936
Dakil, Samuel Edward, 1950
Danel, Joe Randolph, 1961
Daniel, Thomas Gerald, 1958
Danielson, Arthur D., 1932
Darden, Paul Martin, 1942
Dardis, Walter Traynor, 1911
Dardis, Walter Traynor, Jr., 1945
Darnell, Elmer E., 1911
Darrough, Forrest M., Jr., 1963
Darrough, James Breese, 1933
Darrough, John Walton, 1930
Darrow, Robert Stewart, 1939
Daugherty, Rex Wilson, 1954
Davenport, Charles D., 1953
Davenport, Howard Sample, 1952
Davidson, Harold D., 1962
Davidson, Wallace Norman, 1919
Davidson, Wallace Norman, Jr., 1951
Davie, Eugene Newton, 1940
Davie, Victor Vance, 1943
Davis, Charles Fletcher, 1914
Davis, Emmer Palmore, 1912
Davis, George Fred, 1916
Davis, George Henry, 1951
Davis, George Munroe, Jr., 1939
Davis, Guy Clark, 1946

Davis, John Benjamin, 1935
Davis, Joseph Paul, Jr., 1942
Davis, Randell Eugene, 1951
Davis, Robert Gaylord, 1959
Davis, Robert Sears, Jr., 1954
Davis, Samuel M., 1956
Davis, Wesley Warren, 1941
Davis, William Orville, 1943
Davison, Chester Oliver, 1915
Dawson, Clarence Benton, 1943
Dawson, Ora O., 1912
Day, Ben Hill, 1912
Day, John Charles, 1959
Dean, Charles Edward, 1961
Dean, Robert E., 1947
Dean, Robert William, 1955
Dean, William Forest, 1926
Deardorff, Max Allard, 1959
DeArman, Thomas Milton, 1928
Deaton, David Grady, 1927
Dehart, Ollie Wayne, 1961
DeJarnette, John Franklin, Jr., 1948
Delhotal, Charles Earl, 1947
Demand, Francis Asbury, 1917
Demas, Ross Pete, 1946
DeMeules, Edgar A., Jr., 1938
Dennehy, Timothy H., 1960
Denney, Laurence Albert, 1946
Dennis, James Lowden, 1940
Dennis, Robert Pinkerton, 1945
Denny, Ralph Carol, 1952
Denny, William F., 1953
Denyer, Hillard Earl, 1941
DePorte, Seymour, 1919
Deputy, Ross, 1935
Dersch, Walter Henry, 1917
Dersch, Walter Henry, Jr., 1945
DeShan, Preston Warren, Jr., 1961
Desmuke, Lamar Donald, 1961
Deupree, Harry, 1936
Devanney, Phil J., 1931
Devine, J. C., 1953
Devore, James Kilgore, 1947
Devore, John Woodrow, 1945
Diacon, James Lewis, 1952

Diaz, Carlos J. H., 1929
Dickerson, Jay L., 1954
Dickerson, William Joseph, 1955
Dickinson, Wylie Paul, 1948
Dickson, James Richard, 1955
Dietrich, Bailey L., 1953
Dillingham, Cecil Homer, Jr., 1945
Dillman, Robert Eldon, 1946
Dillman, Theodore Erman, 1946
Diment, Dean H., 1960
Dinkler, Fred, 1947
Disiere, John Eldred, 1963
Dixon, Gerald Rugh, 1958
Dixon, James Lowell, 1940
Dixon, Robert Wendell, 1944
Dodson, George Edward, 1940
Dodson, Harrell Chandler, 1941
Dolenz, Bernard Joseph, 1957
Dolph, Chancey H., 1926
Donaghe, Roy Wallace, 1947
Donald, E. Wendell, 1942
Donald, Jack William, 1954
Donaldson, Ronald Jack, 1963
Donat, Paul E., 1962
Doner, Richard Earl, 1963
Donica, Thomas Marion, 1964
Donnell, John, 1943
Dooley, Robert Thomas, 1958
Doran, Charles Kendrick, 1963
Dorr, Clyde Hudson, II, 1961
Dorrough, John Levi, 1915
Dorsey, Elizabeth, 1936
Dotter, Billy Dale, 1959
Dotter, Richard Gene, 1959
Doty, Roy Joseph, 1958
Dougan, Archie F., 1936
Dougherty, Raymond Joseph, Jr., 1947
Dougherty, Virgil F., 1924
Dougherty, William Henry, Jr., 1954
Douglas, Herschel L., 1960
Douthit, Thomas Eugene, Jr., 1954
Dowdell, Roy Wesley, 1963
Dowdy, Gerald S., Jr., 1953

Dowdy, Kemp Holman, 1940
Dowell, Carr Thomas, Jr., 1929
Dowling, William Jackson, 1946
Downing, Joseph Jackson, 1946
Dozier, Barcley Evans, 1923
Drake, Dale Wilfred, 1948
Drake, John Shahan, 1942
Draughon, Clyde William, 1954
Dreher, Henry Samuel, 1915
Drennan, Stanlay Lewis, 1941
Drew, May Adah Twyford LaTorra, 1913
Drewry, Robert Hill, 1959
Drummond, N. Robert, 1936
Duckett, Jim G., 1955
Dudley, Alberta Pasch Webb, 1942
Dudley, Patrick William, 1958
Duer, Joe L., 1932
Duewall, Rudolph Henry, 1938
Duff, Fratis L., 1939
Duffy, Joseph, 1964
Duffy, Mary Loretta, 1953
Dugan, Victor Henry, 1956
Dugger, James Atwood, 1946
Dulaney, Richard B., 1960
Dunbar, Milton J., 1919
Duncan, Cloyce Louis, 1946
Duncan, Darrell Gordon, 1928
Duncan, Kenneth Craig, 1955
Duncan, Robert W., 1936
Dunlap, Harold Earl, 1955
Dunn, John Siever, 1949
Dunnington, William Glenn, 1934
Dunton, Loren Alonzo, 1945
Duran, Robert Jackson, 1947
Durham, Wilson Ervin, 1957
Dutton, Adena C., 1926
Dycus, David Sprouse, 1961
Dycus, Don Lee, 1957
Dyer, James William, 1959
Eades, Dee William, 1930
Eads, Charles Henry, 1933
Eager, Ella Leota, 1949
Earls, Jim H., 1962
Earnest, Earl R., 1960

Earnheart, Harold E., 1929
Earp, Ancel, Jr., 1947
East, John, 1937
East, William Robert, 1961
Eastland, William Edgar, 1923
Eberhart, Marjorie Graham, 1930
Echols, Raymond Samuel, 1943
Eddington, Allen Boyce, 1953
Edmonds, Paul Bryan, 1961
Eley, Julia Steele, 1944
Eley, Norphlette Price, 1922
Edge, Jodie L., 1955
Edwards, Martin Dale, 1945
Edwards, Stan Lee, 1956
Edwards, William Louis, 1964
Egan, James William, 1956
Egelston, James Russell, 1955
Eggenberg, David M., Jr., 1955
Elkin, William Paul, 1935
Elkins, Marvin Galloway, 1938
Elkins, Ronald C., 1962
Elkouri, Harvey Don, 1954
Ellifrit, William Oron, 1959
Elliott, Arthur Furman, 1945
Elliott, Charles C., 1962
Elliott, James Howard, 1952
Ellis, Leonard James, Jr., 1942
Ellis, Richard Allison, 1945
Ellis, Robert Keith, 1957
Ellison, Gayfree, Jr., 1940
Ellzey, Robert Franklin, 1954
Emanuel, Roy Edgar, 1926
Emenhiser, Lee Kenneth, 1931
Endres, Robert Kendall, 1948
England, Myron, 1936
Engles, Charles Franklin, 1951
Engles, Estelle Smith, 1954
Engles, Leroy Lawson, 1948
Engles, Loretta Graham, 1951
Engles, Raymond Leslie, 1953
Engles, Robert Everett, 1954
Ennis, John Hine, 1954
Enos, Jack Paul, 1950
Ensey, James Elbert, 1928
Epley, Verne C., 1942

Erwin, Chesley Para, 1951
Erwin, Constance Rabb, 1951
Erwin, Paul Dair, 1946
Eskridge, James B., Jr., 1921
Eskridge, James Burnette, III, 1945
Esparza, Edward, 1959
Estes, Jesse Franklin, 1926
Evans, Alfred M., 1930
Evans, Arthur George, 1958
Evans, Gary Gene, 1963
Evans, John Patrick, 1963
Evans, Leo R., 1927
Evans, Logan I., 1916
Evans, Robert Erle, 1934
Evatt, Bruce Lee, 1964
Everett, Elwood Dale, 1963
Everett, Mark Allen, 1951
Ewing, William Finis, Jr., 1953
Fagin, Herman, 1923
Fair, Ellis Edwin, 1941
Fair, Thomas Hackler, 1947
Faris, Brunel DeBost, 1927
Farnam, Larry Matthew, Jr., 1939
Farr, Charles Henry, 1961
Farr, Louise Kinkead, 1943
Farris, Edward Merhige, 1941
Farris, Emil P., 1950
Faulkner, Mortimer Sharpe, 1942
Faust, Hugh Harvard, 1940
Feigley, Charles Anderson, 1950
Felactu, James, 1962
Felts, George R., 1932
Ferguson, Edmund Gordon, 1929
Ferguson, Emmett Bonlore, Jr.,
   1959
Ferguson, Lawrence Wynn, 1928
Ferrell, Donald Patrick, 1963
Fife, Phillips Raymond, 1943
Finch, James William, 1931
Findlay, John Robert, 1952
Finley, H. Webb, 1912
Finn, Thomas Charles, 1953
First, Safety Reual, 1943
Fisher, Harry E., Jr., 1952
Fisher, Robert Darryl, 1964

Fitch, Eldon E., 1960
Fitz, Rudolph Guilford, 1920
Fitzgerald, Dean Turner, Jr., 1961
Flanigin, Herman Floyd, Jr., 1943
Fleetwood, Doyle Homer, 1941
Flesher, David A., 1962
Flock, Eugene Richard, 1951
Flood, William Robert, 1941
Florence, John, 1943
Florence, Robert William, 1941
Floyd, John H., 1953
Fluhr, William Forrest, 1943
Flynn, Samuel Fulton, 1955
Foerster, David William, 1958
Foerster, Hervey Adolph, 1927
Ford, Frederick Roscoe, 1944
Ford, Harry Cummings, 1933
Ford, Joseph Wesley, 1931
Ford, Richard Bland, 1928
Forester, Virgil Ray, 1944
Forrest, William J., 1955
Forsythe, Thomas Gordon, 1926
Foster, Claude Franklin, Jr., 1948
Foster, Lloyd Galloway, 1934
Foster, Riley Payton, 1947
Fox, Fred Thomas, 1930
Fox, William Wade, 1926
Fraley, Thomas Haskell, Jr., 1959
Francis, John Wesley, 1911
Francisco, F. Glenn, 1916
Frankel, Jerome Jerry, 1954
Franken, Edmond Anthony, Jr.,
    1961
Franklin, Mildred Ann, 1961
Franz, Robert George, 1959
Franz, Roger Abie, 1961
Frederickson, John Wardell, 1947
Freede, Charles Louis, 1945
Freede, Henry James, 1942
Freeman, Charles Winfred, 1941
Fried, David, 1940
Friedman, Daniel, 1947
Frieze, Harold William, 1954
Fry, Francis, 1936
Fry, Powell Everett, 1934

Fryer, Samuel Richard, 1933
Fugate, Edward Munroe, 1947
Fuhring, Shirley, 1932
Fuller, Alen Munson, 1961
Fuller, Guy Wesley, 1955
Fuller, Harlin Griffin, 1949
Fuller, William Banks, 1923
Fulton, Warren Carlton, 1955
Funk, Gustavus DeLana, 1933
Funnell, James D., 1960
Funnell, Joseph Willard, 1949
Fuquay, Maurice Coyle, 1952
Gable, James Jackson, 1915
Gable, James Jackson, Jr., 1942
Gable, Tom Powell, 1943
Gaddis, Herman W., 1936
Gafford, Tom Sid, Jr., 1947
Gaines, John F., 1947
Gallagher, Clarence Alfred, 1937
Galloway, Nova Linda, 1951
Gambill, Alice Frances, 1949
Gardiner, Howard Glenn, 1935
Gardner, Elsworth Louis, 1935
Gardner, John Edward, 1959
Garis, John Arthur, 1963
Garlin, Jack Birden, 1945
Garlington, Elmer Franklin, 1915
Garner, James H., Jr., 1962
Garnier, William Hampton, 1935
Garrison, Dale Allen, 1940
Garrison, George Bolar, 1956
Garside, G. Earl, 1923
Garst, Ronald Joseph, 1948
Gaspar, Harold Eugene, 1955
Gaspar, Harvey Lee, 1961
Gastineau, Clifford Felix, 1943
Gastineau, Felix T., 1918
Gastineau, Robert Milton, 1950
Gatchell, Frank Gaffney, 1948
Gathers, George Burley, Jr., 1950
Gatti, Robert R., 1955
Gayman, Byron Roosevelt, 1924
Gayman, Mark Willis, 1917
Gayman, Samuel Ellsworth, 1912
Gebetsberger, Charles Joseph, 1957

Gedosh, Edgar A., 1960
Geigerman, David Jackson, 1944
Gentry, E. Lee, 1950
Gentry, Raymond, 1932
George, Joseph Mathews, 1921
Gephardt, Maurice Carl, 1943
Gerard, Rene Gabriel, 1943
Geurkink, Nathan Alvin, 1959
Ghormley, James Grant, 1934
Gibbens, Murray Everett, 1938
Gibbs, Allen G., 1932
Gibson, Charles Roy, 1955
Gibson, Robert Berry, 1915
Gibson, Samuel Wallen, 1954
Giesen, Andrew Frederick, 1925
Gilbert, John Berry, 1943
Gilchrist, Ronald W., 1960
Gilliland, Donald C., 1960
Gilliland, James O., 1932
Gilliland, Lloyd Nance, Jr., 1940
Gingles, Charles Harold, 1936
Gingles, Robert Hal, 1936
Gist, Joel Keith, 1964
Glasgow, Jack Green, 1942
Glaze, Max A., 1951
Glenn, James Clarence, 1950
Glismann, John David, 1946
Glomset, John Larson, Jr., 1963
Goddard, Roy Keene, 1912
Godfrey, James Timothy, 1940
Godfrey, Kenneth Eugene, 1950
Godley, Milton Lloyd, 1952
Goerke, Lenor Stephen, 1936
Goetzinger, Billy Richard, 1956
Goggin, Chester William, 1941
Goldberg, Jed Edwin, 1948
Goldfeder, Jesse, 1924
Goldner, Abraham, 1916
Gonzales, I. Ernest, 1958
Gonzales, Juan Samson, 1927
Gooch, Lloyd Donald, 1963
Goodman, Abram Robert, 1917
Goodman, C. Leroy, 1964
Goodman, George LeRoy, 1927
Goodman, Hubert T., 1936

Goodman, Thomas Allen, 1957
Goodman, Thomas G., 1960
Gorby, Alvin Levi, 1925
Gordon, Glenn Warren, 1958
Gordon, James Maurice, 1927
Gordon, William T., Jr., 1958
Gorc, Dorothy Elizabeth, 1945
Gorena, Adan Luis, Jr., 1961
Gorrell, Benjamin Franklin, 1945
Grady, Charles W., 1918
Graham, Rex Myron, 1942
Graham, Robert Norvell, 1926
Graham, Stephen Harry, 1915
Grant, George Nolan, 1956
Gray, Billy Neil, 1950
Gray, Floyd, 1928
Graybill, Charles Shelly, 1943
Grayson, Arthur, 1956
Green, Gergory Albert, 1958
Green, James Douglas, 1957
Green, James L., Jr., 1947
Green, Paul Anderson, 1946
Green, Phillip Edward, 1956
Greer, Allen Eddy, 1942
Greer, Rex E., 1933
Gregg, Damon Donald, 1959
Gregston, Jack L., 1945
Griffin, John Edward, 1958
Grigsby, Orville Lee, 1945
Grimes Ira Ross, 1954
Grimes, Wilford Arden, 1950
Grisham, Philip L., 1962
Grisham, Richard Saint Clair, 1958
Gross, Francis Warren, 1937
Groves, Fred Bascom, 1956
Groves, Hassell Eugene, 1948
Guenther, Bernard Enloe, 1955
Guffy, Joseph Laymon, 1933
Guild, Carl Holmes, 1918
Guild, Carl Holmes, Jr., 1944
Gullatt, Ennis M., 1932
Gunn, Marvin Ray, 1954
Gunter, Caldeen D., 1948
Gunter, Jack Pershing, 1963
Guss, Louis, 1941

Guthrey, George Henry, 1944
Guthrie, John Alexander, 1917
Gutsche, Paul William, Jr., 1935
Gwartney, Warren G., 1950
Gyles, William Taylor, 1948
Hackler, Harold Waton, 1933
Hackler, John Fielden, 1933
Hackney, John Louis, 1961
Haddad, George Norman, 1957
Haddock, James L., 1932
Hahn, Charles Ray, 1964
Hake, Orin Joseph, 1949
Haldeman, Jack Carroll, 1937
Hale, Arthur Edward, 1945
Hale, Arthur Eugene, 1950
Hale, Charles Harrison, 1961
Hale, Forrest Howard, 1925
Hale, William John, 1963
Hall, Jerry Daniel, 1956
Hall, Robert M., 1938
Hall, Ronald Ross, 1964
Hall, William Edward, 1955
Hallendorf, Leonard Charles, 1942
Hallford, Jasper Carl, 1952
Hallum, Glen D., 1960
Hamburger, Irvin Glenn, 1954
Hamby, Wallace Bernard, 1928
Hamilton, James, 1935
Hamilton, Mary Wiseman, 1927
Hamilton, Robert Luther, 1925
Hammond, James H., 1937
Hampton, Hollis Eugene, Jr., 1948
Hampton, James Barnett, 1944
Hampton, James Wilburn, 1956
Hamra, Henry M., 1937
Hamra, Sam T., 1963
Hancock, Allison R., 1919
Haney, Arthur Ceberry, 1914,
Haney, Arthur H., 1927
Hanks, Norman Ned, 1963
Hanna, William Ricks, 1964
Hansen, Arthur Franklin, 1925
Hansen, Daniel George, 1951
Hanson, Orcina Harry, 1928
Hanson, Paul J., 1936

Hanson, Victor Eugene, 1959
Haralson, Prescott Herndon, 1951
Hardegree, Harvey Columbus, Jr.,
    1950
Hardman, Thomas James, 1934
Hardy, Homer Dwight, Jr., 1949
Hardy, Samuel Isaac, 1944
Harff, John R., 1918
Hargrove, Fred Turner, 1934
Hargrove, Robert Donald, 1950
Harmon, Thomas Fredric, 1935
Harms, Edwin Martin, 1934
Harms, Frank Louis, 1939
Harms, Harold Harvey, 1941
Harper, Jack S., 1962
Harper, Richard Fred, 1956
Harrell, Don Grant, 1936
Harris, Clyde E., 1943
Harris, Frank M., 1931
Harris, George G., 1917
Harris, Henry Washington, 1927
Harris, Jack Allen, 1953
Harris, Richard Lowell, 1945
Harrison, Alexander Vayle, 1939
Harrison, Gene Howard, 1950
Harrison, Grover C., Jr., 1960
Harrison, Lynn Henry, 1940
Harrison, Richard Edward, 1956
Harrison, William Smith, 1953
Harroz, Joseph, 1956
Hart, Dillis Leroy, 1964
Hart, Mabel M. Eckstedt, 1928
Hart, Marshall Oscar, 1927
Hartford, Walter Kenneth, 1940
Hartzog, Joe Thomas, 1964
Harvey, Meldrum Johnston, 1964
Harvey, William Gipson, 1953
Haslam, Gilbert E., Jr., 1962
Hassler, Ferdinand Rudolph, 1937
Hassler, Ferdinand R., Jr., 1955
Hassler, Grace Clause, 1935
Hathaway, Euel Park, 1929
Hathaway, Helen Sue, 1954
Hathaway, Paul Walter, 1964
Hathaway, William Ellison, 1954

Haunchild, Charles Dennis, 1961
Hawes, Charles Richard, 1946
Hawkins, Larry Edward, 1963
Hawley, William Dean, 1964
Hayes, Harrison Frensley, 1961
Hayes, Robert H., 1960
Haygood, Charles Wendell, 1935
Haynes, Charles Elmer, 1915
Haynie, Weldon Keller, 1933
Hays, Carolyn Collins, 1947
Hays, Gary G., 1960
Hays, Marvin Bryant, 1945
Hays, Powell Lambert, 1914
Hazel, Onis George, 1931
Head, Philip Wayne, 1964
Head, Robert William, 1948
Hearin, James Thomas, 1945
Heath, William D., 1956
Heberlein, Charles Robert, 1941
Hefner, James Richard, 1963
Heiligman, Haskell, 1931
Heilman, Elwood Hess, 1941
Heinrichs, William L. 1958
Hellams, Alfred Allen, 1938
Helvie, Henry E., 1960
Hemphill, William Joseph, 1947
Henderson, Ernest Aubrey, 1938
Hendren, Walter Scott, 1941
Henke, Joseph Reid, 1937
Henley, Billie Gene, 1948
Henley, Marvin Dumas, 1922
Henley, Thomas H., 1950
Hennessey, Howard Lawrence,
 1954
Henry, Colvern Dewey, 1926
Henry, Mary Azalea Mitchell, 1926
Henry, Russell Cole, 1940
Hensley, Jess, 1959
Henson, Minnie Marie, 1944
Henton, Rossler Hampton, 1951
Herbelin, Joseph Ted, 1954
Herndon, Noel Elwood, 1955
Herndon, Robert Eugene, 1948
Herrick, Robert S., 1960
Herrin, Bob J., 1955

Herrington, David John, 1917
Herrington, Van Dolph, 1925
Herrmann, Jess Duval, 1931
Hesser, James Matthew, 1941
Hewett, Horace E., 1957
Hewitt, Perry E., Jr., 1937
Hicks, Melvin Claude, Jr., 1949
Hicks, Paul Johnson, 1956
Highland, John Eugene, 1939
Hightower, Harry Gray, 1948
Hilbig, Albert Lionel, 1930
Hilderbrand, Harold Eugene, 1943
Hill, James Avon, 1963
Hill, Jesse King, 1950
Hill, John Morrie, Jr., 1958
Hill, Larry Wayne, 1964
Hill, Riley A., 1954
Hillis, Robert Ray, 1959
Hinkle, Alfred Burke, 1951
Hinkle, Royce Albert, 1963
Hinshaw, J. Raymond, 1946
Hinshaw, Joseph Raymond, 1921
Hirose, Frank Mitsuo, 1951
Hirschfield, Herman, 1935
Hladky, Frank, Jr., 1946
Hobgood, Richard Guy, 1945
Hodge, James Carlton, 1948
Hodge, Tommy G., 1960
Hodges, Thomas O., 1950
Hodgson, Clella Monroe, 1927
Hoffer, Maxine Ruth, 1941
Hoffmeister, William Edward, 1958
Hogue, Robert James, Jr., 1961
Hohl, James Fitton, 1944
Hoke, Bob, 1958
Hoke, Lillian Marie, 1949
Holcomb, William Maynard, 1956
Holland, Charles Dale, 1954
Holley, Paul Sullivan, 1957
Hollingsworth, Francis Willis, 1944
Hollingsworth, Robert, 1937
Holloway, Harry Charles, Jr., 1958
Holman, Douglas Campbell, 1949
Holman, James Horace, 1951
Holt, Orville U., 1952

Ison, Lee A., 1962
Jack, Samuel Corwin, 1955
Jackson, Alvin Ross, 1930
Jackson, Paul Pierce, 1942
Jacob, John Benton, 1948
Jacobs, Luster I., Jr., 1953
James, Frank Marshall, 1947
Janco, Leon, 1918
Jarman, Joe Bob, 1961
Jarrett, Thirl, 1936
Jay, George R., 1962
Jayne, Elta Howard, 1957
Jeffress, Vinnie Hale, 1930
Jelsma, P. Franklin, 1925
Jenkins, Henry B., 1929
Jenkins, Paul Alexander, 1934
Jennings, Col. Aubrey L., 1929
Jennings, George Harry, 1952
Jennings John Douglas, 1954
Jennings, Kenneth D., 1924
Jeter, Grady L., 1962
Jeter, Perry Raleigh, 1928
Jeter, Wiley Price, Jr., 1953
Jimerson, Gordon Kent, 1964
Jobe, Charles Louis, Jr., 1961
Jobe, James Philip, 1951
Jobe, Virgil R., 1933
Jobe, Virgil R., Jr., 1960
Jobe, William Louis, 1964
Johnson, Alpha Louis, 1926
Johnson, Charles Leon, 1943
Johnson, Donald Edwin, 1954
Johnson, Doyle Eugene, 1959
Johnson, Egbert Guy, 1918
Johnson, Erma Ossip, 1934
Johnson, Henry Lee, 1917
Johnson, Henry Myles, 1940
Johnson, Howard Raymond, 1964
Johnson, John Walker, Jr., 1954
Johnson, L. A., 1936
Johnson, L. G., 1935
Johnson, Mark Royal, 1946
Johnson, Max Edwards, 1939
Johnson, Raymond Leroy, 1931
Johnson, Richard Bard, 1957

Johnson, Robert Adair, 1956
Johnson, Robert Ray, 1944
Johnson, Roger Gene, 1954
Johnson, William M., 1960
Johnson, William Thomas, Jr.,
   1954
Jones, Benjamin G., 1917
Jones, Edward F., 1956
Jones, Ester Lee, 1915
Jones, Harry B., 1955
Jones, Jake, Jr., 1954
Jones, James Stewart, 1964
Jones, Jerry Clark, 1963
Jones, Laurence Lewis, 1943
Jones, Oliver William, Jr., 1957
Jones, Phyllis Emmaline, 1940
Jones, Robert Austen, 1942
Jones, Robert Buckner, 1951
Jones, Ruth Belcher, 1936
Jones, Stephen Tisdal, 1952
Jones, William I., 1960
Jones, Wilton Noah, 1951
Jordon, Michael Lee, 1964
Joseph, Philip George, 1940
Josephson, Aaron M., 1949
Joyce, Frank T., 1936
Judd, Loyd Wesley, Jr., 1950
Kahn, Bernard I., 1934
Kahn, Robert W., 1939
Kalbfleisch, Frank David, 1956
Kalbfleisch, John M., 1957
Kaldahl, Paul E., 1960
Kantor, Norman, 1955
Kaplan, Sidney, 1944
Karnes, William Ernest, 1955
Karns, Donald C., 1960
Kasha, Herman Leon, 1925
Katz, Morris Elliott, 1941
Kay, Felix Ross, 1959
Kay, James Robert, 1959
Kearns, Harry James, Jr., 1957
Keen, Frank M., 1932
Keeran, Michael Garnett, 1963
Keith, Howard Barton, 1957
Keller, Grape Frank, 1934

Lane, Camille Cecelia, 1943
Lane, Kenneth Stephen, 1950
Lane, Lloyd C., 1929
Lane, Marie Thaxton, 1949
Lang, Frederick L., 1957
Lang, Silas A., 1932
Langford, Orville LeRoy, 1956
Langston, Wann, 1916
Lanning, John A., 1960
Larkin, Henry Watson, 1920
Lashley, Floyd J., Jr., 1960
Latta, Jo Ellen, 1959
Lattimore, Frank C., 1932
Lauderdale, Thomas LeRoy, 1913
Laughlin, Lycurgus Orrin, 1959
LaVon, Rosalie Anderson, 1964
Lawson, Patrick Henry, 1929
Lawton, Lawrence Michael, 1949
Layton, Donald Dewey, Jr., 1954
Layton, Otto Earl, 1937
Layton, Rex Gordon, 1939
Leap, Paul A., 1960
Leatherman, Douglas Dione, 1958
Leathers, Hollis Kirkpatrick, III, 1964
Ledbetter, Edgar Otis, 1956
Ledbetter, Marion Kenneth, 1946
Ledbetter, William Harry, 1939
Lee, Daniel Webster, 1955
Lee, Judah K., 1923
Lee, Robert Ray, 1933
Lee, Robert Rex, 1955
LeFevre, Sam Frank, 1911
Lehew, Elton Wilmot, 1930
Lehew, John Leslie, Jr., 1927
Lehew, John Leslie, III, 1955
Lehmann, Harold Theron, 1940
Lehmer, Elizabeth E., 1920
LeMaster, Dean W., 1924
Lembke, Robert Leon, 1950
Lemon, Cecil Willard, 1931
Lenaburg, Herbert H., 1960
LeNeve, Robert Thomas, 1946
Leonard, Charles E., 1932
Leonard, Edward LeRoy, 1952

Lerblance, William Penn, Jr., 1945
Leslie Samuel Brewster, Jr., 1942
Lester, Boyd Kenneth, 1954
Lester, Eugene Fay, 1941
Lester, Joseph Karl, 1952
LeValley, Steve Allen, 1963
Leverett, Cary L., 1963
Lewis, Billie, 1959
Lewis, Russell W., 1932
Lewis, Vivian Moon, 1959
Lewis, Wilbur Curtis, 1955
Lewis, Wilburt Fielding, 1939
Ley, Eugene B., 1938
Lhevine, Dave Bernard, 1945
Lhevine, Morris Boise, 1917
Limes, Barney Joe, 1955
Lincoln, Richard Benjamin, 1946
Lindberg, Charles O., 1924
Linde, Leonard Melvin, 1956
Lindeman, George Munro, 1950
Lindsay, Wren Allie, 1928
Lindsey, Joseph Henry, 1950
Lindstrom, W. Carl, 1934
Lingenfelter, Forrest Merle, 1923
Lingenfelter, Paul Brann, 1933
Lisle, Achilles Courtney, Jr., 1943
Little, Aaron Chalfant, 1931
Little, James H., 1962
Little, Jesse Samuel, 1959
Little, John Rudolph, 1929
Lively, Claude E., 1934
Lively, Gerald Andrew, 1953
Livingston, David Eugene, 1957
Llewellyn, Thomas Sylvester, III, 1961
Lockwood, Gerald Warren, 1948
Logan, Clifford K., 1920
Long, Fred Mac, 1951
Long, James Downing, 1959
Long, Larry Lee, 1963
Long, Leonard, 1932
Long, Loyd Lee, Jr., 1946
Long, Lyda Louise, 1964
Long, Ray Hubert, 1930
Long, Warren David, Jr., 1963

Long, Willie George, 1952
Lorenz, Max P., 1962
Loucks, James Erickson, 1947
Loughbridge, Billy Paul, 1961
Loughmiller, Robert F., 1937
Love, Albert Joseph, 1941
Lowe, Alvin Louis, 1951
Lowe, Kenneth Gilbert, 1955
Lowell, James R., 1953
Lowenthal, Philip J., 1938
Lowery, Larry Lee, 1956
Lowry, David Charles, 1946
Lowry, Dick, 1916
Lowry, Dick Moss, 1945
Lowry, Robert W., 1936
Lowry, Tom, 1916
Loy, Richard Warren, 1949
Loy, Robert Lowe, Jr., 1947
Loy, William A., 1937
Lucas, Vance, 1942
Lumpkin, Lee Roy, 1953
Lung, John Alvin, 1964
Lunsford, William Frederick, 1923
Luton, James Polk, 1933
Lykins, Robert Willis, 1946
Lynch, Russell Hugh, 1926
Lynn, Bernard Anthony, 1956
Lynn, Clyde Arthur, 1958
Lynn, Doss Owen, 1937
Lynn, Thomas Neil, Jr., 1955
Lyon, James Benton, Jr., 1956
Lyons, Mason Russell, 1940
McAdams, Alpha Mal, 1921
McAlister, John Edwards, 1961
McArthur, Charles Ernest, 1938
McArthur, Lloyd Glenn, 1957
McBride, David LeMarr, 1956
McBride, Ollie, 1937
McCabe, Jack Merrill, 1953
McCabe, William Robert, 1953
McCann, Beryl Royce, 1956
McCann, William Edward Francis, 1948
McCants, Ralph Samuel, 1950
McCartney, Vivian Mae, 1928

McCarver, Charles L., 1962
McCarver, Robert Roy, Jr., 1954
McCauley, Donald W., 1943
McCauley, Joe Wheeler, 1955
Mackey, Abner, 1939
Mackey, Dan Michael, 1963
Mackler, David Lee, 1957
McClain, Mack I., 1962
McCleery, James M., 1952
McClellan, James Thomas, 1942
McClelland, Charles William, 1941
McClure, Coye Willard, 1940
McClure, Hubert L., 1960
McClure, Joy Lancelot, 1929
McClure, William, 1936
McCollough, Billy Lee, 1958
McCollum, Estel B., 1932
McCollum, Wiley Thomas, 1940
McConnell, Archie Bernice, 1915
McCormick, Jay Earl, 1939
McCoy, Donald, 1947
McCreight, William George, 1940
McCrimmon, Herman Patrick, 1925
Macrory, Paul David, 1943
McCullough, Gerald William, 1954
McCune, Edward Allison, 1955
McCurdy, Robert Edwin, 1946
McCurdy, William Claude, II, 1964
McDonald, Glen Webster, 1934
McDoniel, James William, 1956
McDonnold, George Fred, 1952
McDougal, Royce Carmack, 1955
McElwee, Mary Louise, 1950
McFadden, Candour A., 1929
McFarland, James Riley, 1953
McFarling, John M., 1935
McGeary, William Clyde, Jr., 1949
McGee, Harry, 1944
McGehee, Charles Leo, 1931
McGill, Ralph Albert, 1922
McGinnis, Delbert H., 1957
McGovern, James L., 1952
McGovern, Joseph D., Jr., 1953
McGrath, Thomas James, 1927
McGraw, Willard Lyal, 1944

McGregor, Frank Harrison, 1950
McGregor, Robert Aubrey, 1952
McGuire, Ivan Alonzo, 1939
McHale, Thomas Cecil, 1928
McHenry, Lawrence Chester, Jr.,
  1955
McInnis, Dalton Blue, 1945
McInnis, James Thermon, 1937
McIntosch, Robert Keer, Jr., 1937
McIntyre, John Aubrey, 1943
McIntyre, Ray Vern, 1951
McKay, Edward Danson, 1935
McKee, Patrick A., 1962
McKeehan, Guy Oliver, 1926
McKerracher, Robert Daniel, 1955
McKinne, Richard Alan, 1964
McKinney Milam Felix, 1930
McKinnon, Jeanne Elise, 1941
McLauchlin, James Rayburn, Jr.,
  1943
McLauchlin, James R. Grave, 1911
McLauchlin, Robert Allen, 1948
MacLeod, Sherburne, 1933
McMaster, Audrey Jeanne, 1964
McMillan, Charles B., 1917
McMillan, James Moughan, 1933
McMullen, Thomas, 1943
McNeill, Philip Marsden, 1923
McPheron, William Graves, 1942
McPike, Lloyd Henry, 1935
McQuown, Albert Louis, 1941
Macrory, Paul David, 1943
McSpadden, Floyd Fuller, 1944
McWhirter, Wallace Warren, 1951
Madeley, Howard Randall, 1934
Maguire, Philip J., 1960
Mahan, Frank Lewis, 1953
Mahone, Marion Wilson, 1939
Maimbourg, Charles Louis, 1958
Maldonado, Wilfred E., 1958
Mann, Lawrence Earl, 1954
Mannerberg, Frederick Donald,
  1959
Manning, Wesley Thacker, 1950
Mansfield, Richard Elwood, 1961

Mansur, Harl D., Jr., 1939
Marder, Leon, 1949
Margo, Marvin Kenneth, 1948
Mariel, Joe J., 1936
Maril, William David, 1940
Market, George C., 1960
Markland, Ralph Richard, 1956
Marks, John William, 1954
Marks, Mark M., 1928
Marsh, Charles Edward, 1954
Marsh, Donald Wayne, 1958
Marsh, John Henry, 1963
Marshall, Albert Henry, 1914
Marshall, Charles E., 1960
Marshall, Richard Allen, 1955
Martin, Charles Edward, 1948
Martin, Chesley Marion, 1915
Martin, Clarence Adolph, Jr., 1963
Martin, Emmett Otis, 1921
Martin, Fred Richard, 1957
Martin, Howard Choice, 1929
Martin, James Daugherty, 1939
Martin, John William, 1930
Martin, Thomas Reynolds, 1928
Martin, William Allen, 1915
Marx, Ralph L., 1932
Mason, William Sterling, 1920
Massad, Paul Eugene, 1964
Massad, Woodrow W., 1950
Massey, John Barry, 1954
Masters, Harold Arnold, 1956
Masters, Herbert Alfred, 1934
Masters, Paul Leroy, 1953
Masterson, Maude, 1936
Mathews, Charles Robert, 1945
Mathews, Grady Frederick, 1925
Mathias, Charles M., 1929
Matter, Billy Joe, 1959
Matthews, Newman Sanford, 1937
Matthey, William Alan Alfred,
  1950
Mauldin, Howard Paul, 1953
Maupin, Clinton S., 1934
Mavity, Ralph Page, 1915
May, June Carolynn, 1961

Mayes, Robert Harold, 1940
Mayfield, Robert Charles, 1950
Mayfield, Warren T., 1920
Mead, William Wesley, 1937
Meador, George Emery, 1940
Means, Melvin Thistle, 1923
Means, Royce Bryan, 1947
Meares, Cecil Haynes, Jr., 1952
Medcalf, Winfred Louis, 1957
Mechling, George S., 1932
Medley, Seth Raymond, 1921
Meece, Leo, 1960
Meinhardt, Kenneth Dean, 1957
Meinhardt, Ralph Eugene, 1951
Meis, Armon M., 1943
Meis, Donna Lea Hammer, 1943
Mench, Robert Montgomery, 1940
Mengel, Chester Kenzer, 1939
Mercer, Herman A., 1922
Mercer, J. Wendall, 1925
Mercer, Robert D., 1951
Merkley, George Elmer, Jr., 1952
Merrell, Webber Warren, 1942
Merrifield, Vernon Conrad, 1945
Merritt, Lawrence Stevens, 1962
Mershon, Helen Ruth, 1949
Messenbaugh, Joseph Fife, 1933
Messenbaugh, Joseph F., III, 1958
Messinger, Robert Phillip, 1938
Metcalf, Robert Paul, 1964
Meyer, Retta Ruth, 1949
Meyer, William Donald, 1955
Meyers, William Arthur, 1927
Michael, Harvey R., 1962
Michaelson, Leon Jack, 1928
Michener, Frank R., 1960
Miears, Claude H., 1925
Mileham, Jack Cecil, 1946
Miles, John B., 1927
Miles, Walter H., 1918
Miller, Bonnie Gibson, 1959
Miller, Cecil Ewing, 1938
Miller, Duane C., 1960
Miller, Elnora Gertrude, 1946
Miller, Floyd Freeman, 1956

Miller, George Lance, 1964
Miller, Griffith Champion, 1961
Miller, Jack Eaton, 1939
Miller, James V., 1962
Miller, Jess E., 1947
Miller, Nesbitt Ludson, 1927
Miller, Noel Eugene, 1959
Miller, Raymond Delbert Niles, 1945
Miller, Robert Joseph, 1947
Miller, Ross Hayes, 1946
Miller, William Arthur, 1947
Miller, William Richey, 1942
Mills, Richard C., 1928
Mills, Victor David, 1938
Milton, Leroy Marvin, 1959
Mings, Harold Harvey, 1957
Minnig, Donald Irwin, 1938
Minor, Dwane Blake, 1954
Mitchell, Bob Gunter, 1956
Mitchell, Clarence, 1931
Mitchell, Dan, Jr., 1958
Mitchell, Ernest Dale, 1954
Mogab, John Haikal, 1943
Mohr, John Anthony, 1964
Moline, Lester Lee, 1954
Mollison, Malcolm, 1946
Monfort, John J., 1932
Monfort, Mariam Felicia, 1950
Monnet, Julien Charles, 1956
Montgomery, Hazel Irene, 1941
Montgomery, William Ewel, 1911
Moody, Herman Carter, 1952
Moore, Benjamin Harrison, Jr., 1953
Moore, Clifford Wesley, 1927
Moore, Ellis Nathaniel, 1921
Moore, George C., 1962
Moore, James Davis, 1961
Moore, John Morgan, 1952
Moore, Larue, 1923
Moore, Robert, 1953
Moore, Samuel Turner, 1938
Moore, Tom Dickson, 1954
Moore, Walter Mason, 1945

Moore, William Manning, 1955
Moore, William Richard, 1953
Moose, Robert Ronald, 1961
Moran, Willard Brown, Jr., 1961
Morehead, Jackson Frank, 1937
Morgan, Carl Clifton, 1946
Morgan, Charles Thomas, 1956
Morgan, Chesley Andrew, 1929
Morgan, Edward Alexander, 1917
Morgan, Francis M., 1943
Morgan, James Dale, 1961
Morgan, Johnny Jack, 1954
Morgan, Louis Starner, Jr., 1948
Morgan, Nova Lemoine, 1950
Morgan, Omar J., 1962
Morgan, Philip Edward, 1951
Morgan, Robert F., 1953
Morgan, Robert Jesse, 1944
Morgan, Royce Harvey, 1953
Morgan, Thomas Richard, 1928
Morgan, Troy Olen, Jr., 1956
Morgan, Vance Frederick, 1934
Morgan, William L., 1953
Morgan, William Richard, Jr., 1958
Morkin, Eugene, Jr., 1959
Morris, David Gordon, 1934
Morris, Jessie Lee, 1949
Morris, Richard Earl, 1963
Morris, William A., 1937
Morris, William T., 1960
Morrison, John Wildey, 1944
Morrison, J. Scott, 1962
Morrow, Jerry Fleming, 1963
Morse, James Otto, 1953
Morter, Roy Alton, 1913
Morton, Donald Gene, 1953
Morton, Ralph Warren, 1940
Moseley, Jack Ellis, 1953
Mosely, Ray Ruel, 1918
Mosher, Donovan Dillon, 1926
Mosley, Wiley Henry, 1959
Moss, Charles Basil, 1949
Mote, Paul, 1924
Mote, Wesley Robert, 1958
Mote, Wesley Russell, 1927

Motley, Ray Franklin, 1959
Mount, Houston Faust, 1946
Moyer, Herman John, 1955
Mrez, Gerald Lincoln, 1941
Muchmore, Harold Gordon, 1946
Muenzler, William S., 1960
Mulholland, James Andrew, Jr., 1964
Mullins, J. Arthur, 1911
Mullins, William B., 1937
Mulmed, Earl I., 1937
Mulvey, Bert E., 1930
Murphree, James Wallace, 1947
Murphy, Charles Percy, 1912
Murphy, Elmer Grant, 1945
Murphy, Ralph William, 1949
Murphy, Weldon Odell, 1935
Murray, Edward Cotter, 1930
Murray, Ella Hasemeier, 1949
Murray, Forney Long, 1937
Myers, Jack Wendell, 1943
Myers, Leonard Albert, 1922
Myers, Lynn Leroy, 1959
Nagle, Patrick Sarsfield, 1928
Nash, Howard Lavern, 1957
Naughton, John Patrick, Jr., 1958
Nave, Richard Randall, 1958
Naylor, Bruce Addis, 1964
Neal, Billy James, 1963
Neal, John Robert, 1914
Neal, Laile Gould, 1925
Neal, Victor Ray, 1957
Needham, Clarence Fred, 1924
Neel, James Hal, 1943
Neel, Roy Lawrence, 1938
Neely, Samuel Eugene, 1948
Neely, Shade Durrett, 1920
Neff, Everett B., 1936
Neill, Elaine M., 1962
Nelson, Arnold Gordon, 1952
Nelson, Henry John, 1930
Nelson, Iron Hawthorne, 1940
Nelson, Ivo Amazon, 1925
Nelson, James Mack, 1934
Neugebauer, M. Kenith, 1956

Neugebauer, Victor Wayne, 1963
Neumann, Milton A., 1930
New, William Nell, 1934
Newlin, William H., 1932
Newport, Norsuda Monteville, 1935
Newton, Norris Lynn, Sr., 1956
Nicholas, Hugh B., 1948
Nichols, Ray Ernest, 1930
Nicholson, James Leonidas, 1931
Nicklas, Thomas O., 1962
Nickolls, Charles Leslie, 1955
Nida, Jerry R., 1960
Nisbet, Alfred A., 1938
Noell, Robert Leonard, 1928
Norman, E. Wade, 1963
Norris, Claud Bazil, 1921
Norris, Frances L., 1936
Northrip, Ray Ulman, 1938
Northrup, Robert Alan, 1948
Nuernberger, Louis G., 1955
Nugent, Goldwin I., 1914
Nunnery, Arthur W., 1916
Nunnery, Arthur W., 1953
Oakes, John Robert, 1942
O'Bar, Paul Rupert, 1957
Obermiller, Ralph G., 1932
Obert, Paul M., 1947
Oesterreicher, Donald Lawson,
    1949
Ogg, Kenneth Gale, 1948
Oglesbee, Carson Leroy, 1937
O'Leary, Charles Marion, 1934
Olson, Donald Henry, 1943
Olson, Forrest William, 1948
Olson, Virginia, 1936
O'Neal, John Talmage, 1964
Opper, Marshall, 1944
Orbin, John Andrew, 1957
Orr, Herbert Stokes, Jr., 1942
Orr, Ronald, 1962
O'Shea, James George, Jr., 1948
Otis, Paul Joseph, 1945
Overbey, Charles Brown, 1941
Overstreet, Robert John, 1953
Owen, Cannon Armstrong, 1934

Owen, Herbert Leo, 1950
Owen, John Roy, 1958
Ownby, Ralph, Jr., 1949
Oxley, William Nathan, 1944
Ozias, Charles Ralph, 1914
Padberg, Elder Dunham, 1940
Page, Crockett Henry, 1961
Palmer, Clara Frances, 1940
Paramore, Charles Francis, 1924
Paris, David, 1941
Park, Riley W., Jr., 1957
Parker, Ira Tom, Jr., 1958
Parker, James William, 1946
Parker, William Lee, 1956
Parkhurst, Yale Eugene, 1948
Parks, Jeff Thompson, 1943
Parks, Kirtland Garvin, 1923
Parks, Stephen, 1952
Parrish, Jack Walker, 1953
Parrish, Roy Gibson, 1944
Parrish, Stuart Leland, 1943
Parrish, Wilmer Eugene, 1943
Parsley, Frank E., 1927
Parsons, Bernie, 1961
Parsons, Orval Loewen, 1933
Paschal, William Raymond, 1945
Patrick, Alvin W., 1960
Patten, William Robert, 1952
Patterson, Andrew Mack, 1929
Patterson, Frank Baumgardner,
    1927
Patterson, James Lindley, Jr., 1947
Patterson, Leon L., 1911
Patterson, Oliver Hamilton, 1955
Patton, Michael J., 1963
Patzkowsky, Lawrence Willis, 1950
Patzkowsky, Paul D., 1960
Paul, Press Mansfield, Jr., 1949
Paul, Roger Ray, 1957
Paul, Thomas Otis, 1939
Paul, William Gordon, 1939
Paulus, David Dare, Jr., 1955
Payne, Charles Leon, 1963
Payne, Donald E., 1952
Payne, Douglas Wilton, 1942

Payne, Ralph Edward, 1948
Payne, Ralph Edward, Jr., 1956
Payne, Richard Weston, 1943
Payte, James Ira, 1930
Payte, James Thomas, 1957
Payton, Hugh William, 1945
Peacher, Kenneth Lee, 1948
Pearce, Elizabeth K. Youngman,
 1911
Pearce, Henry Johnson, 1964
Pearlstine, Maurice, 1923
Pearson, Daniel Bester, 1941
Pearson, Murble Henry, 1938
Peck, Thelma Gwendolyne, 1948
Peffly, Elmer Dale, 1953
Pendergraft, Leonard Olen, Jr.,
 1964
Pendergrass, Clayton Ina, 1930
Pendleton, Alice Antoinette, 1937
Penico, Peter E., 1947
Penrod, John Norman, 1956
Percefull, Sabin Crawford, 1945
Perry, Daniel Lafayette, 1926
Perry, Fred, 1936
Perry, Fred Thomas, 1933
Perry, Hugh, 1926
Perry, Hugh, Jr., 1958
Perry, James Sidney, 1925
Perry, John Claud, 1923
Perry, John Milton, Jr., 1946
Perryman, Robert Gentry, 1946
Peter, Maurice Lyle, 1933
Peter, Maurice Lyle, Jr., 1957
Peters, James Coldren, 1944
Peterson, Robert Francis, 1957
Petrie, Robert Bryce, 1953
Petty, James Sturgis, 1935
Petway, Aileen, 1937
Pfeifer, Donald Richard, 1959
Pfundt, Robert Theodore, 1944
Pfundt, Theodore Robert, 1944
Phelan, Ralph Stewart, 1939
Phelps, Joseph T., 1919
Phelps, Willis Franklin, 1963
Phillips, Donald Morris, 1957

Phipps, John, 1944
Phipps, Tilden Hendricks, Jr., 1937
Pickard, John Copeland, 1926
Pickhardt, Woodson Louis, 1937
Pierce, Gerald G., 1956
Pierson, Dwight D., 1932
Pinkerton, C. B., 1953
Piper, Arthur Sylvester, 1911
Piper, Charles Leslie, 1915
Pitts, Herman C., 1962
Pitts, James Burton, 1946
Plummer, Kenneth Garolyn, 1961
Plummer, Thomas Orlando, 1935
Poarch, John Ellis, 1964
Pogoloff, Samuel Hirsch, 1923
Pointer, Edwin Lowell, 1956
Points, Blair, 1911
Points, Thomas Craig, 1941
Poling, Fowler Border, 1940
Pollard, James Eugene, 1943
Poole, Sam Lee, 1963
Popkess, Fred G., 1943
Poplin, Lenard, A., 1962
Porte, Daniel, 1926
Porter, Marilyn Gregory, 1956
Porter, Warren Harvey, 1951
Powell, Jack Dean, 1961
Powell, Jay A., 1918
Powell, Paul Thurston, 1941
Powell, Tracy O., 1931
Power, Robert Earl, 1953
Prather, Charles Edward, 1964
Pratt, Tony Willard, 1938
Prentice, Pamela Richardson, 1944
Prentiss, Harley M., 1918
Presson, Virgil Guy, 1923
Preston, Russell M., 1955
Preston, William Jack, 1963
Price, Charles Hugh, 1955
Price, Harris Pierce, 1913
Price, Joe Holmes, 1928
Price, Joel Scott, 1928
Price, King Graham, 1957
Price, Neel Jack, 1942
Price, Richard Brooke, 1951

Price, Richard Dean, 1946
Price, Terrill Eyre, Jr., 1961
Price, William Edmund, Jr., 1946
Prier, William Milton, 1943
Priest, James Robert, 1964
Prosser, Moorman Percy, 1935
Puckett, Tony G., 1962
Pugh, Robert E., 1936
Pugsley, William Silvey, 1945
Puls, Jerry Lee, 1961
Punsalang, Jose Vitug, 1923
Purviance, Carlton C., 1930
Pyeatte, Jesse Eugene, 1955
Pyeatte, Joella Campbell, 1954
Pyle, Oscar Snow, 1926
Quillen, Pauline Barker, 1912
Rabon, Nancy Ann, 1959
Rader, Lloyd Edwin, Jr., 1959
Ragan, Tillman A., 1932
Rahhal, George Metray, 1945
Rahhal, Lindbergh John, 1953
Raines, James Richard, 1935
Raines, Morris M., 1937
Raisen, Kenneth Herman, 1948
Ramey, Dayne W., 1960
Randall, Donald Lee, 1959
Randels, George Robert, 1952
Ranson, Robert Fike, 1947
Ratliff, Hansel L., 1962
Raub, Roy Raymond, 1946
Ray, C. Cody, 1950
Ray, Raymond Gerald, 1933
Ray, Robert Hartley, 1949
Rayburn, Charles R., 1925
Razook, Jerry D., 1962
Read, Theodore Porter, Jr., 1954
Rector, William Lee, Jr., 1943
Reddin, Robert L., 1955
Reding, Anthony Charles, 1935
Redmond, Robert F., 1947
Reed, Bert Thomas, 1963
Reed, Charles W., 1933
Reed, Emil Patrick, 1931
Reed, Howard Leonard, 1916
Reed, James Robert, 1927

Reed, James S., 1962
Reed, Karl Asbury, 1933
Reeves, Claude L., 1931
Reeves, Walter Paul, 1948
Reichelt, Edward G., 1964
Reichenberger, Jerome Anthony, 1963
Reid, Donald A., 1962
Reid, Frank Isaac, 1927
Reid, John Robert, 1921
Reid, John Robert, Jr., 1956
Reid, Oren Creighton, 1945
Reid, William Richard, 1955
Reiff, William Henry, 1941
Reigel, David George, 1961
Reimer, Gerald Ray, 1963
Reimer, Jacob Paul, Jr., 1957
Reinschmiedt, Edwin Ruben, 1956
Reiss, Merrell Dee, 1955
Reiter, Arthur William, Jr., 1949
Rempel, John H., 1962
Rempel, Paul Harvey, 1934
Renfrow, William Branch, 1950
Renfrow, William Frank, 1926
Rentfrow, James William, Jr., 1950
Resler, Donald R., 1960
Reynolds, Bill J., 1949
Reynolds, Ernest West, Jr., 1946
Reynolds, Freddie A., 1962
Reynolds, Joe B., 1962
Reynolds, Stephen Woodson, 1914
Rhine, John Richard, 1953
Rhinehart, Don Forrest, 1958
Rhoades, Everett Ronald, 1956
Rhodes, Ivan Eugene, 1949
Ricchetti, Warren F., 1960
Rice, Paul Brewer, 1938
Richard, Robert Max, 1961
Richard, Warren Edward, 1940
Richardson, Darwin Lloyd, 1947
Richardson, Jessie Floyd, 1958
Richardson, Samuel M., Jr., 1956
Rickey, Orville Lee, Jr., 1958
Ricks, James Ralph, Jr., 1938
Ridgeway, Elmer, 1940

Rieger, Joseph A., 1932
Rigual, Rafael, Jr., 1950
Riley, Lee Hunter, Jr., 1957
Riley, Robert Hickman, 1913
Ringrose, Robert Edward, 1963
Rinn, Odville Alton, 1957
Rippy, Orville Main, 1939
Ritan, John Leif, 1957
Ritchey, Charles Leroy, Jr., 1959
Rivers, William Miley, 1915
Robards, Victor Lycurgus, Jr., 1961
Robberson, Morton Early, 1934
Roberson, Arvin Craig, 1954
Roberts, Buford Benjamin, 1927
Roberts, Clarence Rochelle, Jr., 1956
Roberts, David A., 1932
Roberts, Elisha H., 1916
Roberts, Kenneth Nott, 1940
Roberts, Marvin Talmadge, 1954
Roberts, Paul E., 1960
Roberts, Robert Eugene, 1926
Robertson, Charles Walter, 1928
Robinson, Charles Watson, Jr., 1957
Robinson, Earl Moore, 1943
Robinson, Franklin Pierce, 1914
Robinson, John H., 1925
Robinson, Mildred Irene, 1937
Robinson, Roscoe Ross, 1954
Robison, Clarence, Jr., 1948
Rocco, Albert Francis, 1948
Rock, Robert Lee, 1958
Rockett, Louis Stong, 1943
Rockwell, Don Arthur, 1963
Rockwood, Charles Adelbert, Jr., 1956
Rodriquez, Mamiliano Juan, 1931
Rogers, David G., 1962
Rogers, Galen Alonzo, 1933
Rogers, Gloria Denezie Akin, 1961
Rogers, Kenneth Alfred, Jr., 1961
Rogers, William Gerald, 1930
Rohrer, George Victor, 1958

Rolle, Paul Nesson, 1930
Rollins, James Hugh, 1944
Rollins, John Gordon, 1950
Rollo, James Wilson, 1913
Rollow, John Arch, III, 1943
Rorie, Jean Early, 1945
Rosales, Godofredo Dilay, 1926
Rose, David Dean, 1959
Rose, Dayton Morrison, 1948
Rose, Ernest, 1936
Ross, George Thompson, 1935
Ross, Hope Annette, 1935
Roth, Herman W., 1932
Rothenberger, Monty Leray, 1961
Rowland, Herbert, 1964
Rowland, Robert Hazel, 1941
Roys, Harvey Curtis, Jr., 1943
Roys, Richard Dennis, 1939
Royse, Robert Dayton, 1958
Royster, Ralph L., 1930
Ruble, George Clyde, 1922
Rucker, Ralph, 1936
Rude, Evelyn Mae, 1935
Rude, Joe C., 1930
Runser, Richard Henry, 1959
Rupp, Robert Ray, 1956
Russell, David Stanton, 1963
Russell, Lum Elbert, 1933
Russell, Richard Lee, 1949
Ruth, Weldon Kenneth, 1933
Rutherford, Vester M., 1932
Rutledge, Art Henry, 1944
Rutledge, Ben Allen, 1944
Rutledge, Bob Jack, 1948
Ryan, Henry Grady, II, 1947
Ryan, Robert O., 1937
Ryan, Warren Albert, 1931
Ryder, Judith Harcourt, 1958
Sablan, Ralph Guerrero, 1959
Saddoris, Marvin LeRoy, 1927
Sadler, LeRoy Huskins, 1929
Sadler, Paul Eugene, 1952
Salamy, Joseph, 1944
Salkeld, Phil Lloyd, 1941
Salman, Phineas, 1918

Sanden, Austin Oliver, 1922
Sanders, Harold Ray, 1943
Sanders, Ron R., 1960
Sanders, Wallace Robert, 1956
Sandford, John Lee, 1960
Sandlin, Dean Clifford, 1941
Sandlin, Robert Edward, 1943
Sands, Abel Jay, 1946
Sanford, Herbert Marvin, 1938
Sanford, Roy Keith, 1941
Sanger, Fenton Almer, 1926
Sanger, Paul Griffith, 1931
Sanger, Walter Bailey, 1935
Sanger, Welborn Ward, 1931
Sapinoso, Pastor Ramirez, 1922
Sapper, Herbert Victor Louis, Jr., 1944
Sargent, John Frank, 1921
Satterfield, J. B. Lowery, 1954
Savage, William Lee, 1957
Saviers, Boyd Miller, 1947
Sawyer, William Claude, Jr., 1951
Sayers, Capt. James Rolland, 1929
Saylor, Charles Richard, 1963
Saylor, Robert Martin, 1929
Scates, Julius L., 1960
Schaff, Hartzell Vernon, 1942
Schlicht, Mabelle Blanche, 1946
Schloesser, Harvey Leopold, 1951
Schloesser, Patricia Turk, 1949
Schmidt, Helen Hughes, 1948
Schnoebelen, Rene, 1940
Schoolar, Earl Jerome, Jr., 1964
Schultz, Norman Jerry, 1955
Schurter, Lonis Leon, 1946
Scivally, Kenneth R., 1962
Scoggin, Eddie B., 1962
Scott, Don Engle, 1964
Scott, Nathan Earl, 1954
Scott, Richard D., 1962
Seba, Chester Randall, 1938
Sebastion, J. J. B., 1936
Sebring, Milton Harvey, 1940
Seelig, Darrell Arnold, 1953
Seeman, Roy Dean, 1958

Sehested, Herman Charles, 1931
Seibold, George Joseph, Jr., 1934
Selby, David Moore, 1961
Selders, Raymond Everett, 1927
Self, Jane, 1961
Senter, Jerald Raydell, 1952
Sexton, Jack M., 1955
Shackelford, Paul Olden, 1944
Shadid, Edward A., 1960
Shadid, Ernest George, 1955
Shadid, Frederick Victor, 1940
Shane, Ramon A., 1962
Shanks, Edwin Patrick, 1946
Sharpe, Joseph H., 1947
Shaver, Robert Paul, 1961
Shaver, Sylvester Robert, 1937
Shaw, Charles Joseph, 1961
Shaw, Clinton McKinley, Jr., 1945
Shaw, Dwight Beach, 1926
Shearer, Joseph Michael, 1942
Sheets, Marion Edrington, 1928
Sheets, Ronald Rex, 1964
Sheffel, Donald James, 1953
Shelby, Hudson Swain, 1933
Shellenberger, Charles Gibson, 1945
Shelton, Joel A., 1934
Shepherd, Phillip Leighton, 1959
Shepherd, Virgil Jerry, 1958
Sherrod, Dale Byars, 1961
Shibley, George John, 1957
Shidelar, Alfred Max, 1950
Shields, Clarence, Jr., 1963
Shields, Herbert B., Jr., 1937
Shiflet, Albert Woods, 1933
Shipp, Jesse Day, 1933
Shippey, William Laton, 1927
Shirley, Edward Thornton, 1934
Shirley, Jack David, 1956
Shofstall, William Howard, 1941
Shore, Robert Lee, 1949
Short, Laurence Oliver, 1951
Shriner, Richard Floyd, Jr., 1944
Shupe, Henry Wren, 1949
Shuttee, Robert David, 1944

Shwen, Ralph Otto, 1943
Shyrock, Leland Franklin, 1940
Siddons, Ivan Doyle, 1957
Siebs, John A., 1947
Siegel, Arthur, 1943
Silverthorn, Louis Edward, 1934
Simmering, James Virgil, 1955
Simcoe, Charles William, 1959
Simmons, Charles E., 1954
Simon, Bill J., 1947
Simon, Floyd, 1943
Simon, Ralph, 1944
Simon, Robert Bowman, 1957
Simon, William Hale, 1954
Singleton, Harry Fields, 1946
Sisler, Frank Herbert, 1940
Skeehan, Raymond Aloysius, Jr., 1949
Slagle, Gene Watts, 1947
Sledge, Claire Blount, 1948
Slight, John Rigby, 1961
Smalley, Tim Kent, 1964
Smiley, Robert Hoyland, 1956
Smith, Addison B., 1932
Smith, Bobby Gene, 1955
Smith, Bradley Edgerton, 1957
Smith, Byron Freemont, 1945
Smith, Carl Roy, 1959
Smith, Carl Walter, Jr., 1953
Smith, Carlton Earl, 1934
Smith, Charles Edward, Jr., 1954
Smith, David A., 1962
Smith, Delbert Gilmore, 1929
Smith, Earl E., Jr., 1954
Smith, Edward Eugene, 1959
Smith, Francis Elmo, 1950
Smith, Gene Richard, 1957
Smith, Gladys Christine, 1947
Smith, Haskell, 1934
Smith, Henry Clinton, 1945
Smith, Henry Percy, 1961
Smith, Jackson Algernon, 1943
Smith, James Ronald, 1944
Smith, Jarroud Benonia, Jr., 1938
Smith, John Darrell, 1951

Smith, John Herbert, Jr., 1956
Smith, John Irving, 1961
Smith, John Richard, 1957
Smith, Lester Pennington, 1925
Smith, Morris William, 1928
Smith, Neldagae, 1955
Smith, Newton Converse, 1945
Smith, Paul Frederick, 1941
Smith, Paul Greer, 1951
Smith, Philip B., 1951
Smith, Phillip J., 1937
Smith, Raymond O., 1932
Smith, Raymond Orval, Jr., 1963
Smith, R. Earle, 1913
Smith, Richard Wendall Doop, 1932
Smith, Robert Cecil, 1956
Smith, Robert Marchand, 1961
Smith, Ronald Carl, 1956
Smith, Rupard Glenn, 1938
Smith, Thomas Joseph, 1959
Smith, Virgil Dan, 1934
Smith, Wendell Logan, 1933
Smith, Willard Haynes, 1940
Smith, William Howard, 1947
Smith, William Orlando, 1925
Smith, William Orlando, Jr., 1957
Smith, William Robert, 1956
Smithpeter, Roger Lee, 1963
Smithson, Carl Bryan, 1933
Smithson, John Richard, 1955
Smotherman, Howard, 1958
Sneed, Norma L., 1960
Snider, James Rhodes, 1956
Snoddy, William Thomas, 1944
Snow, Otis E., 1949
Snyder, James Howard, 1943
Sockler, David Lee, 1956
Soma, Yonekichi, 1920
Sorenson, Eric John, 1964
Souda, Robert M., 1960
Soutar, Richard Gray, 1922
Souter, John Ellis, 1919
Southworth, James Larry, 1938
Sowell, Harlan K., 1943

Spann, Joe Louis, 1948
Spann, Logan A., 1934
Speakman, Walter Fred, 1945
Speed, Henry Kirven, Jr., 1933
Speed, Henry K., III, 1962
Spence, Ray Elmo, 1946
Spence, Wayman R., 1960
Spencer, David Alan, 1964
Spencer, Jack David, 1954
Sprehe, Daniel Joseph, 1957
Springer, Homer Clarence, 1931
Stacey, Norman R., Jr., 1962
Stafford, Joseph William, 1954
Stakle, Sylvia, 1958
Stamps, Phil, 1963
Standifer, John James, 1953
Standifer, Orion Cecil, 1924
Stanley, Thomas Moore, 1963
Stansberry, Cecil Ray, Jr., 1957
Stark, Jodie Adams, 1958
Starkey, Wayne Anthony, 1934
Stauber, Robert Andrew, 1956
Steelman, Gerald Matthew, 1945
Steen, Carl T., 1914
Steffen, Harlow Leland, 1954
Stehr, Danny L., 1962
Steinig, Harry William, 1925
Stephens, Audy Bryan, 1928
Stephens, Frank Gordon E., 1934
Stephenson, Ishmael F., 1929
Stephenson, Jack McKinley, 1957
Stephenson, Philip Logan, 1958
Steward, Rodney Dwight, 1957
Stewart, Joe Allen, 1949
Stewart, Oscar Wilhelm, 1934
Stewart, Walter Edgar, 1912
Stickle, Arthur Waldo, 1943
Stillwell, Robert J., 1929
Stites, Hugh Dinsmore, 1924
Stobaugh, Robert E., 1960
Stockton, Robert Louis, 1959
Stockton, William James, 1956
Stokes, Lowell, 1936
Stone, Burl Eugene, 1952
Stone, William Tex, 1954

Stonecipher, Harlan Keith, 1963
Stoner, Raymond Ward, 1930
Storts, Daniel Ray, 1956
Storts, Richard Alvin, 1959
Story, Thomas McNeil, 1959
Stough, Daniel Freeman, Jr., 1927
Stough, Daniel Ross, 1964
Stout, Billy Herman, 1964
Stout, Harold, 1960
Stout, Hugh Albert, 1937
Stover, Robert Mahl, 1953
Stover, William Harrison, 1945
Strader, Simon Ernest, 1917
Strahan, Ronald Wayne, 1963
Strange, Jimmy Ray, 1959
Stratton, Forrest Leroy, 1926
Stream, Lawrence, 1949
Stream, Millicent Marrs, 1950
Strecker, William, 1936
Strickland, Luther Jearl, 1961
Strode, Jack William, 1944
Strong, Clinton Riley, 1943
Strong, Joseph Pershing, 1946
Stroup, Clayton King, 1926
Stuard, Charles Goodson, Jr., 1937
Stullman, Walter Seymour, 1964
Sturgell, Joseph Carroll, 1938
Sturgeon, H. Violet, 1933
Sturm, Robert Theodore, 1938
Sudduth, Herschel Cochran, 1942
Sullivan, Clarence Bennett, 1922
Sullivan, Dan T., 1962
Sullivan, Don Duane, 1964
Sullivan, Jerry Wayne, 1957
Sullivan, Robert Raymond, 1955
Sullivan, Sullins Grenfell, 1935
Sundquist, Glenn Vernon, 1945
Svoboda, Catherine Anna, 1953
Swan, Josetph J., 1939
Swanda, David Eugene, 1948
Swanson, Homer S., 1936
Switzer, Fred D., 1936
Swyden, Robert Gene, 1956
Sykes, Walter Peter, 1949
Tackett, Orville H., 1939

Tallant, George, 1936
Talley, Charles N., 1923
Talley, Evans E., 1934
Talley, John Edward, 1957
Talley, Thomas Evans, 1964
Tate, Harry Brackenridge, 1963
Tate, Robert Victor, 1964
Tatlow, Byron Webster, Jr., 1945
Tatom, John Henry, 1958
Taylor, Billy B., 1952
Taylor, Clarence Pierce, 1947
Taylor, Fred Wilbur, 1943
Taylor, Harold Wilford, Jr., 1951
Taylor, James R., 1962
Taylor, John Robert, 1934
Taylor, Larry R., 1962
Taylor, Lewis Carroll, 1938
Taylor, Lloyd Wilson, 1941
Taylor, Robert Anthony, 1964
Taylor, Robert Leroy, 1942
Taylor, Thomas Warren, 1953
Tefertiller, Charles Lester, 1942
Templer, Lowell Nelson, 1961
Tenney, Richard Frank, 1959
Terrell, Marvin Silas, 1942
Theimer, Louis Michael, Jr., 1951
Thiessen, Harold Dean, 1961
Thomas, Denton Barney, 1950
Thomas, Edwin Crawford, 1914
Thomas, Leo Dexter, 1956
Thomason, Frank, 1917
Thompson, Benjamin D., 1926
Thompson, Lawrence E., Jr., 1952
Thompson, Marylyn Ann, 1950
Thompson, Wayman J., 1929
Thompson, Wayman J., Jr., 1960
Thompson, Willard Van Voorhis, 1944
Thompson, William Best, 1943
Thornton, Lowell Francis, 1948
Thorp, Edward McLain, 1942
Threlkeld, Lal Duncan, 1940
Throne, Bert Ennis, 1950
Thuringer, Carl Bernard, 1946
Thurston, Thomas Watson, 1957

Tichenor, Ernest LaPoint, 1933
Tidwell, Robert Austin, 1937
Tipps, Bill, 1956
Tisdal, James Harold, 1945
Tisdal, William Charles, 1933
Todd, John Broadus, 1929
Tolbert, Jack Burgess, 1943
Toma, Helen J., 1960
Tomlin, Clyde Edward, 1945
Tool, C. Donovan, 1931
Townsend, Horace Dean, 1959
Townsend, John Lionel, 1959
Townsley, Humphrey C., 1962
Tozer, Howard Grafflin, 1945
Tracy, Gilbert W., 1938
Trammell, John Raymond, 1959
Trapp, Irvin B., 1929
Traverse, Clifford Austin, 1933
Traweek, Albert Carroll, Jr., 1930
Trent, David Lee, 1964
Trotter, Lanny F., 1962
Trow, Thomas Archie, Jr., 1942
Trzaska, Henry Constantine, 1943
Tullius, Philip G., 1942
Tupper, Walter R., 1936
Turnbow, William Ray, 1935
Turner, Edwin Charles, 1943
Turner, James Sterling, 1963
Tuttle, Howard Dale, 1951
Tutwiler, Elizabeth Irby, 1943
Tyler, John Myron, 1955
Ungerman, Arnold Harold, 1934
Ungerman, Milford Shael, 1945
Vahlberg, Ernest Raginald, 1923
Valder, David Clarence, 1951
Valderas, Sylvino Luna, 1924
Vallion, Robert Dean, 1964
Vammen, Adolph Nathaniel, 1944
Van Buren, William Edward, 1961
Van Deventer, Loyd Roy, Jr., 1947
Van Hoesen, Daisy Gertrude, 1937
Vanlandingham, Homer Walter, 1934
Vann, Paul Neeley, 1957

Van Valkenburgh, Glennwood
  Milford, 1931
Vaughn, Daniel L., 1955
Vaughn, Thomas Neil, 1957
Veatch, Everett Parker, 1926
Veirs, Charles Robert, 1952
Vesley, Don Ray, 1959
Viers, Wayne Allen, 1956
Vincent, Duke William, 1917
Vinson, Harold Augustus, 1935
Vint, William Allison, 1952
Vinyard, V. Lee, 1954
Violett, Theodore Willis, 1956
Vogt, Milton Wayne, 1956
Vogt, William, 1936
Waddell, Bill D., 1956
Wade, Donald F., 1960
Wade, Glen Franklin, 1944
Wade, Lisby Lucius, 1917
Wadsworth, Ray Maxwell, 1942
Wagner, John Clifford, 1919
Wagner, Taylor Dan, 1963
Wagnon, Marion C., 1960
Wails, Theo. G., 1921
Wainwright, Tom Lyon, 1933
Waldrop, William Loving, 1942
Walker, Agnew Astley, 1924
Walker, Ethan Allen, Jr., 1943
Walker, James Robert, 1943
Walker, Joseph D., 1922
Walker, Price Mars, 1922
Walker, Russell H., 1932
Walker, Thomas A. W., 1956
Walker, William Archibald, 1927
Wall, Henry Leo, 1953
Wall, Leonard Allen, 1951
Wallace, Deloss Arnold, 1934
Wallace, Helen Irene Travia, 1950
Wallace, Jimmy Byron, 1964
Wallace, Virgil May, 1911
Wallace, Virgle Wesley, 1942
Walters, Philip Greenwood, 1957
Wamack, William Scott, 1954
Ward, Delbert Audray, 1931
Ward, John Wayne, 1951

Ward, John William, 1956
Warren, Darrell R., 1960
Warren, Earle W., 1938
Warren, Roy C., 1928
Waterbury, Cecil Ray, 1945
Waters, Claude Bryan, 1934
Waters, Floyd Leo, 1934
Waters, Philip Cook, 1944
Waters, William Alfred, 1947
Watkins, Wanda Lorraine, 1957
Watson, I. Newton, 1935
Watson, O. Alton, 1929
Watson, Price Thorne, 1933
Watson, Raymond Delbert, 1929
Webb, Dale Isaac, 1964
Webb, Floyd Edmond, Jr., 1957
Webb, James Albert, 1953
Webb, Joan Liebenheim, 1959
Webb, Roy Abner, 1916
Weber, Fred Warner, 1951
Weedn, Alton James, 1935
Weedn, Henry John, 1916
Weedn, Joseph Dwight, 1954
Weeks, Bertram Allen, 1941
Weidner, Larry Wayne, 1963
Weigand, Dennis Allen, 1963
Weisiger, Ross Wilson, 1930
Welborn, Orange Miller, 1946
Wenger, Theodore R., 1949
Werner, Dean Franklin, 1948
West, Harriet Katherine, 1942
West, Kelly McGuffin, 1948
West, Willis Kelly, 1915
Westbrook, Brock Rogers, Jr., 1946
Whalen, Michael H., 1962
Wheaton, William, 1950
Wheeler, Homer Clark, 1938
Wheeler, J. Lawrence, Jr., 1952
Wheeler, Pinckney Raymond, 1956
Whinery, Kenneth E., 1955
Whitcomb, Walter Henry, 1953
White, Arthur E., 1932
White, Eric, 1936
White, James Edwin, 1954
White, James Halley, 1934

White, John Vernon, 1958
White, Lorance Mitchell, 1948
White, Nelson Paschal Hamlin, 1963
White, Nelson Stuart, 1920
White, Robert Glenn, Jr., 1956
White, Ronald Hugh, 1963
White, Travis E., 1962
White, Wayne Franklin, 1957
Whitely, Seals Leftwich, Jr., 1949
Whiteneck, Rhonald Alven, 1943
Whitener, Betty Lou, 1959
Whitlock, Boyd O., 1962
Whitsett, Thomas L., 1962
Whittlesey, Wes A., 1963
Wickham, Mallalieu Maccullagh, 1926
Wienecke, Robert Miller, 1956
Wiggins, Everett L., 1954
Wiggins, Frances Polaski, 1921
Wiggins, Howell, 1936
Wilbanks, Charles E., Jr., 1950
Wilber, Gertrude Helen, 1937
Wild, William Bronnie, 1925
Wildman, Dora Ellen, 1926
Wildman, Stanley F., 1924
Wiley, Alvin Ray, 1913
Wilhite, Lee Roy, 1916
Wilkerson, Bernie Jewel, 1930
Wilkerson, Douglas Clifton, Jr., 1959
Wilkerson, John M., 1932
Wilkins, Afton Norvell, 1935
Wilkins, Harold Dean, 1959
Wilkins, Harry, 1927
Willard, Delbert C., 1929
Willhoite, David Roy, 1963
Williams, Benjamin T., Jr., 1955
Williams, Claude, 1940
Williams, Claude Harold, 1950
Williams, Gordon Darnall, 1927
Williams, Guy Herson, 1934
Williams, James Garth, 1964
Williams, James Sanford, 1958
Williams, Jon Thomas, 1950

Williams, Judy Dyan, 1964
Williams, Leonard Charles, 1920
Williams, Levona Sarah, 1951
Williams, Raymond A., 1938
Williams, Raymond McKinley, 1930
Williams, Richard Goree, 1953
Williams, Theodore Sherman, 1938
Williamson, Paul Shan, 1946
Williamson, Walter Scott, 1950
Wilson, Charles Hugh, 1937
Wilson, Douglas Earl, 1947
Wilson, James Ward, 1958
Wilson, Jay Deane, 1944
Wilson Kenneth Johnson, 1916
Wilson, Larkin Monroe, Jr., 1958
Wilson, Robert Edwin, 1950
Wilson, Russell Howard, 1940
Winkelman, George William, 1940
Winn, Donald Allen, 1957
Winn, George Louis, 1943
Winningham, Elbert Vance, 1949
Winston, Hamilton M., 1960
Winston, John R., 1933
Winterringer, James Riley, 1945
Winters, Richard Lee, 1953
Wisdom, Cranfill Karl, 1955
Witcher, Jones E., 1943
Witt, Richard Earl, 1941
Witten, Harold, 1936
Witter, Stanton Lee, 1961
Wolever, LeRoy Allen, 1950
Wolfe, Ted Wallace, 1961
Wolff, Eugene G., 1934
Wolff, John Powers, 1936
Woll, James C., Jr., 1917
Womack, Granville Jean, 1952
Wood, Dorothy Antonia, 1963
Wood, Harold A., 1930
Woodruff, Bill Eugene, 1958
Woods, Frank Mosely, 1935
Woods, Leon Perry, Jr., 1956
Woods, Louis Edgar, 1926
Woodson, Fred Edward, 1931
Woodson, Orville McClure, 1933

Woodward, Neill W., 1929
Woodward, Neil Whitney, Jr., 1956
Wootan, George Allen, 1963
Word, Emery France, 1941
Word, Harlan L., 1936
Workman, Milton Rice, 1961
Worley, James W., 1960
Worthen, French LaZelle, 1958
Wright, Asa, 1913
Wright, Flora A., 1925
Wright, Phillip Jay, 1961
Wright, William Thomas, 1950
Wuerflein, Robert Dean, 1964
Wyand, Hesler Hiram, 1922
Wynn, Noble F., 1942
Wyrick, Richard, 1949
Yarbro, Jesse Lee, 1948
Yates, Donald Leslie, 1958
Yates, Loren Kent, 1957
Yeakel, Earl Leroy, Jr., 1943

Yeakel, Samuel Victor, 1951
Yeakley, Robert A., 1960
Yeary, Edwin Curtis, 1939
Yeary, Glenn Hillis, 1929
Young, Andrew Merriman, 1937
Young, Banff Ogden, 1947
Young, Charles J., Jr., 1947
Young, Charles W., 1922
Young, Clarence Calhoun, III, 1963
Young, Edgar Wade, Jr., 1947
Young, James Walker, 1964
Young, Larry Ivan, 1963
Young, Millington Oswald, 1944
Youngblood, Billy J., 1954
Zeiders, James W., 1960
Zeigler, Joel, 1934
Zeigler, Paul, 1934
Zimmerman, Kenneth Dale, 1955
Zumwalt, Gerald, 1956
Zumwalt, Robert Burton, 1953

Appendix XIII.
Directors of the
School of Nursing,
1911–64

Cowles, Annette Bourbon, R.N., 1911–15
Hill, Lucy Rennette, R.N., 1915–16
Workman, H. Mary, R.N., 1916
Holland, Edna, 1916–19
Mackenzie, Mary Ard, 1919
Monfort, Candice, 1919–24
Crocker, Ada Reitz, 1924–27
Smith, Mable E., M.A., 1928–29
Lee, Candice Monfort, R.N., 1929–37
Triplett, Edythe Stith, 1937–41
Wangen, Clare Marie Jackson, M.A., 1941–43
Krammes, Kathlyn A., M.N., 1943–47
Jones, Clara Wolfe, R.N., *acting director*, 1944–45
Crocker, Ada Reitz, *acting director*, 1947–48
Caron, Mary Rosch, R.N., M.A., 1948–51
Hawkins, Ada, R.N., M.S., 1951–60
Patterson, Helen, R.N., M.A., *dean*, 1960–(64)*

*When 1964 appears in parentheses, it indicates that this was not the final year of appointment.

Appendix XIV.
Faculty of the
School of Nursing,
1911–64

Armstrong, Thelma Louise, R.N., *teaching assistant in nursing*, 1953–54
Bain, Joyce, *teaching assistant in nursing (operating room)*, 1953–54
Barlow, Donna, R.N., B.S., *instructor in nursing (public health)*, 1954–57
Bartlett, Elissa Isaacson, R.N., B.S.N., *instructor in nursing (maternal and child health)*, 1961; *instructor in nursing (public health)*, 1963
Bastion, Ethel Maxine, G.N., *assistant in nursing*, 1943; *assistant instructor in nursing*, 1944
Battles, Barbara Amdell, R.N., B.S., *instructor in communicable disease nursing*, 1946–47
Baudendistel, Rosalie Dresner, R.N., *instructor in nursing*, 1955–56
Beuchler, C. Jane, R.N., *public health coordinator*, 1947–48
Bickford, J. Ruth Cotton, R.N., B.S., *instructor in nursing*, 1950–53
Bierbauer, F. Elaine Brady, R.N., *instructor in nursing (obstetrics)*, 1950; *instructor in nursing (surgery)*, 1952
Blakley, Ruby, R.N., *instructor in operating room technique,* 1946–47
Bolton, Margaret, *instructor in nursing education,* 1941
Borella, Mary Elizabeth, G.N., *instructor in principles and practice of nursing*, 1933–35
Brewer, Edith, G.N., *instructor in obstetrical nursing*, 1927–29
Brock, Edith L., R.N., *instructor in nursing arts*, 1950–51
Burnet, Caroline, T., G.N., *instructor in practical nursing*, 1928–29
Caron, Mary Rosch, R.N., M.A., *professor of nursing and director of the School of Nursing*, 1948–51
Chapman, Jessie Laverne, R.N., *instructor in operating room technique*, 1947–51
Clark, Francile, R.N., *instructor in nursing (pediatrics)*, 1955–56
Clark, Joe Ann Keeley, R.N., B.S.N., *teaching assistant in nursing*, 1955; *instructor in nursing*, 1958
Conae, Ivy White, R.N., *instructor in nursing and educational director,*

---

* When 1964 appears in parentheses, it indicates that this was not the final year of appointment.

1949

Cowles, Annette Bourbon, R.N., *superintendent of University Hospital, with rank of instructor*, 1911–15

Crocker, Ada Reitz, G.N., *associate professor of nursing education and director of the School of Nursing*, 1924–27; *acting director of the School of Nursing*, 1947–48

Crowell, Evelyn Roberta, R.N., *clinical instructor in medical nursing*, 1948–49

Daniel, Josephine L. (Mrs. Andes), R.N., M.A., *associate in public health nursing*, 1955–63

Deborra, Elaine L., R.N., B.S., *instructor in nursing education*, 1941; *instructor in nursing arts*, 1947

Denton, Ruth Irlene, *teaching assistant in nursing*, 1957

Dewar, Margaret, R.N., *teaching supervisor in operating room technique*, 1946–47

Dittig, Olga Broks, A.M., *assistant director of the School of Nursing*, 1941–42

Dorffeld, Mildred E., R.N., M.A., *assistant professor of nursing*, 1952; *associate professor of nursing*, 1957

Duff, Ruby, R.N., *instructor in operating room technique*, 1940–41

Fair, Elizabeth, G.N., B.A., *instructor in nursing education*, 1940; *educational director of the School of Nursing*, 1943

Farmer, Nellie Jensen, R.N., *teaching assistant (pediatrics)*, 1954; *assistant professor of nursing (pediatrics)*, 1961

Fassett, Edna, R.N., *teaching assistant (operating room)*, 1955–57

Fitzgerald, Margaret, G.N., *instructor in surgical technique*, 1929

Fleming, Katherine, G.N., *instructor in nursing education*, 1929; *superintendent of Crippled Children's Hospital and assistant director of the School of Nursing*, 1937

Flinner, Emma Kay, R.N., B.S., M. Litt., *assistant professor of nursing*, 1956–62

Flood, Josephine O., R.N., B.S., *associate in industrial nursing*, 1955–60

Follansbee, Bernice, R.N., *instructor in pediatric nursing*, 1925–26

Foster, Verna, G.N., *instructor in theoretical nursing*, 1928–29

Fuchs, Ora (Mrs. Ryan), G.N., *instructor in nursing education*, 1937

Gallaspy, Mary Jane (Mrs. Simpson), R.N., *teaching assistant (operating room)*, 1956–58

Garrett, Marie, R.N., B.S., *instructor in nursing education*, 1939; *instructor in practical nursing sciences*, 1941

Gillis, Eugene A., M.P.H., M.D., *lecturer on contagious diseases*, 1940–41

Grandin, Carmen, R.N., *clinical instructor in pediatric nursing*, 1949

Granger, Juanita, *instructor in nursing arts (part-time)*, 1943–44

Grant, Dorothy C., R.N., B.S., *supervisor of clinical instruction and instructor in pediatrics*, 1950; *assistant professor of nursing and supervisor of clinical instruction*, 1955

Gray, Jane Dorothy, R.N., B.S., *instructor in nursing (public health)*, 1953–54

Gray, Opal Willard, *instructor in massage and physiotherapist*, 1937; *lecturer on massage*, 1943

Gunther, Hulda, B.S., *instructor in nursing arts*, 1942–43

Halsell, Marilyn Anne, B.S.N., M.S., *instructor in nursing*, 1961; *assistant professor of nursing*, 1963

Hamburger, Margaret S. (Mrs. Scott), R.N., B.S., *instructor in pediatrics*, 1946; *supervisor of clinical instruction*, 1948

Hamil, Evelyn Marie, B.S., M.N., *instructor in pediatrics and supervisor of clinical instruction at Children's Hospital*, 1949; *assistant professor of nursing*, 1953

Hart, Frances, R.N., M.A., *assistant professor of nursing*, 1960–(64)*

Hawkins, Ada, R.N., M.S., *instructor in practical nursing*, 1925–28; *director of the School of Nursing*, 1951–60; *professor of nursing*, 1951–(64)

Hawkins, Maria Berry, R.N., *educational director*, 1949–50

Henke, Ella Marie, B.S., *assistant superintendent of nurses in University Hospitals*, 1942–43

Henry, Frances Victoria (Mrs. Powell), R.N., B.A., *instructor in nursing education*, 1937; *ward teaching supervisor*, 1946

Hermanstoffer, Goldia (Mrs. Shaeffer), G.N., *instructor in principles and practice of nursing*, 1935; *instructor in orthopedic nursing*, 1937

Hewett, Bonnie, G.N., *instructor in nursing arts*, 1944–45

Highfill, Lela (Mrs. Brock), R.N., B.S., *teaching assistant in nursing (surgical)*, 1956; *assistant professor of nursing*, 1958

Hill, Lucy Rennette, R.N., *superintendent of University Hospital*, 1915–16

Hinnenkamp, Wilhelmina, G.N., *instructor in operating room technique*, 1929–31

Holland, Edna, G.N., *superintendent of nurses*, 1916–19

Hollis, Dorothy, R.N., B.S., *teaching assistant in nursing*, 1956–58

Hubbard, Jenell Dykstra, R.N., B.S.N., *assistant instructor in nursing arts*, 1948; *instructor in nursing arts*, 1950

Hubbard, Sybil, R.N., *instructor in practical nursing education*, 1937–38

Hughes, Effie, R.N., *instructor in medical nursing*, 1946–47

Ingram, Florence, R.N., *instructor in obstetrical nursing*, 1929–36

Inzer, Frances L., R.N., B.S.N., *instructor in nursing*, 1960–65

James, Minnie Elsie, R.N., M.A., *assistant professor of nursing*, 1961–64

Jetziniak, Zofia L., *instructor in nursing*, 1961–62

Jones, Clara Wolfe, R.N., *acting director of the School of Nursing and acting superintendent of nurses*, 1944–45

Jones, Lillian Whitaker, R.N., B.S.N., M.A., *assistant professor of nursing (maternal and child health)*, 1960–(64)

Jones, Mary Ella, G.N., *instructor in principles and practices of nursing*, 1929–37

Jordon, Edward Raymond, *instructor in psychology*, 1955–56
Krammes, Kathlyn Allison, M.N., *director of the School of Nursing and superintendent of nurses*, 1943–47
Lacy, Ruth, R.N., *instructor in operating room technique*, 1935–44
Lansky, Ida Gertrude, R.N., *instructor in public health nursing*, 1949–1951
Lee, Candice Monfort, R.N., *superintendent of nurses*, 1919–24; *associate professor of nursing education; director of the School of Nursing and superintendent of nurses*, 1929–37
Loo, Fe Villafloras, B.S.N., *instructor in nursing (maternal and child health)*, 1961–62
Lord, Gloria Lee (Mrs. Webb), R.N., B.S.N., *instructor in nursing (pediatrics)*, 1956–57
Lower, Alvida (Mrs. Moore), R.N., B.S., M.P.H., *assistant professor of nursing (public health)*, 1958–62
Macaulay, S. Marian, R.N., *research associate in nursing*, 1951–61
McComas, Caroline Stephanie, R.N., B.S.N., *clinical instructor in surgical nursing*, 1948–49
McCullough, Helen, B.S.N., M.A., *assistant professor of nursing*, 1958–60
McElvogue, Edna, G.N., *instructor in pediatrics*, 1939–41
Mackenzie, Mary Ard, *superintendent of nurses*, 1919
McMinn, Elaine, R.N., M.S., *assistant director of the School of Nursing*, 1957; *associate professor and director of the School of Nursing*, 1960
Marshall, Janet Kathryn, *instructor in nursing*, 1961
Martin, Julia, G.N., *instructor in theoretical nursing*, 1929–30
Martin, Mary Jane (Mrs. Deardorff), R.N., *instructor in operating room technique*, 1933–35
Matter, Lois June, *teaching assistant in nursing*, 1960
Matthews, Patricia Ann, *teaching assistant in nursing*, 1956
Mayes, Fayrene Bennett, R.N., B.A., *assistant clinical instructor*, 1949; *instructor in orthopedic nursing*, 1953
Mesley, Josephine, R.N., *instructor in pediatric nursing*, 1930–37
Messi, Carolee Ann, B.S.N., *instructor in nursing*, 1961–64
Mink, Marie Cecelia McKnight, R.N., M.S., *teaching assistant in nursing*, 1953; *assistant professor of nurses*, (1964)
Moody, Maureen Janet (Mrs. Morgan), *instructor in nursing*, 1958–61
Moore, Odessa R., R.N., *teaching assistant in nursing (public health)*, 1959–60
Muelhauser, Florence H., R.N., B.S., *educational director*, 1945–46
Mueller, Floriene Ann, G.N., *instructor in pediatric nursing*, 1929–30
Murdock, Betty, R.N., B.S., *instructor in nursing (surgery)*, 1953; *assistant professor of nursing (surgery)*, 1955
Nigh, Pansy, R.N., B.S., *instructor in nursing*, 1951–53
Olmstead, Betty Joy (Mrs. Simmons), R.N., *teaching assistant in nursing*

(surgery), 1954–55

Pamintuan, Helen, R.N., M.S.N., *assistant professor of nursing (psychiatry)*, 1960–63

Patterson, Georgia Elizabeth, R.N., A.B., *clinical instructor in medical nursing*, 1949; *supervisor of clinical instruction in medical and surgical nursing*, 1950

Patterson, Helen Evelyn, R.N., M.A., *instructor in nursing and director of nursing services*, 1948; *professor of nursing and dean of the School of Nursing*, 1960–(64)

Peace, Julia, R.N., *instructor in nursing education*, 1929; *assistant director of the School of Nursing*, 1941

Peters, Vera Parman, M.S., *instructor in dietetics*, 1948; *assistant professor of nutrition*, (1964)

Phelps, Frances Jergen, R.N., *instructor in orthopedic nursing*, 1949–50

Phillips, Margaret Lilliam (Mrs. Anderson), R.N., *instructor in pediatrics*, 1948–50

Poindexter, Ruth Wadsworth, R.N., *instructor in nursing education*, 1924–28

Powell, Thirza Ann, R.N., *instructor in nursing*, 1926; *instructor in nursing (obstetrics)*, 1955

Priebe, Jean (Mrs. Holt), R.N., *instructor in nursing (surgery)*, 1955–57

Richbourg, Mavis, B.S., *instructor in nursing education*, 1930–33

Roepe, Ruby L., R.N., *supervisor of clinical instruction at Children's Hospital*, 1943–48

Russell, Monica Medill, R.N., B.S., *assistant instructor in nursing (pediatrics)*, 1951; *instructor in nursing*, 1954

Ruth, Elaine, R.N., M.S., *instructor in nursing arts*, 1948; *assistant professor of nursing in medicine*, 1955

Schmelzenbach, Mary Kate, B.A., *assistant in nursing arts*, 1943

Schreiner, Freda S. (Mrs. Inda), R.N., B.S.N., *teaching assistant in nursing (pediatrics)*, 1958; *instructor in nursing (pediatrics)*, 1961

Slief, Golda B., R.N., M.A., *administrative assistant in the School of Nursing*, 1950–51

Smith, Effie Katherine (Mrs. Root), G.N., *instructor in pediatrics*, 1937–39

Smith, Ella, B.S., *instructor in physical education and physiotherapist*, 1936; *lecturer in physical education*, 1945

Smith, Glennita, R.N., B.S.N., *teaching assistant in nursing*, 1958–60

Smith, Mabel E., M.A., *associate professor of nursing education and director of the School of Nursing*, 1928–29

Smythe, Olivia, R.N., M.A., *assistant professor of nursing (public health)*, 1960–62

Souders, Bessie, R.N., *instructor in surgical nursing*, 1943; *clinical instructor in surgical nursing*, 1948

Stacy, Teresa, R.N., *teaching assistant (pediatrics)*, 1956; *teaching assistant in nursing*, 1959

Standish, Dorothy, R.N., *teaching assistant in nursing (pediatrics)*, 1956–58

Stephens, Evelyn, R.N., B.A., *instructor in practical nursing*, 1938–39

Stranathan, Doris Jane, R.N., *instructor in orthopedic nursing*, 1945–46

Stuve, Phyllis M., R.N., *instructor in nursing (obstetrics)*, 1953–54

Swenson, Alice Olson, B.S., *instructor in nursing education*, 1941–42

Takacs, Margaret Marion, R.N., B.S., *clinical instructor in surgical nursing*, 1949

Tayrien, Dorothy, R.N., *instructor in nursing arts*, 1949–50

Terrell, Lucile (Mrs. Holland), R.N., B.S., *assistant professor of public health nursing*, 1958; *assistant professor of nursing*, 1961

Trinque, Bonnie L. (Mrs. Fulton), R.N., *instructor in communicable diseases*, 1946–48

Triplett, Edythe Stith, G.N., *instructor in nursing education*, 1929; *director of the School of Nursing and superintendent of nurses; associate professor of nursing education*, 1937–41

Troyer, Loretta Lee Edwards, R.N., B.S.N., *teaching assistant in nursing (operating room technique)*, 1960; *instructor in nursing (operating room technique)*, 1963

Turner, Anna Bowling, *teaching assistant in medical research and surgical nursing*, 1956

Vrooman, Vivian Lucille (Mrs. Bramley), R.N., B.S.N., *instructor in nursing (pediatrics)*, 1953; *assistant professor of nursing (pediatrics)*, 1956

Waddell, Margaret (Mrs. Lamb), G.N., *instructor in operating room technique*, 1931–33

Wangen, Clare Marie Jackson, M.A., *director of the School of Nursing and superintendent of nurses*, 1941–43

Watson, Beverlyn (Mrs. Allen), R.N., B.S.N., *teaching assistant in nursing (operating room)*, 1958; *instructor in nursing*, 1960

Weber, Flora, R.N., *instructor in nursing education and assistant director of the School of Nursing*, 1925–29

White, Commorah H. E., R.N., B.S.N., M.N., *assistant professor of nursing*, 1958–61

Wilson, Jesscelia Abram, R.N., B.S.N., *instructor in nursing (medicine)*, 1956–(64)

Wirick, Edith Clarkson, R.N., B.S., *instructor in public health nursing*, 1958–60

Wolfe, Marjorie Louise, R.N., B.S., *instructor in nursing*, 1951–53

Wolfe, Mary Jane Campbell, R.N., B.S.N., *assistant in nursing (general)*, 1950; *assistant professor of nursing*, 1956

Woods, A. Martyne, R.N., *acting instructor in nursing arts*, 1946–47

Workman, H. Mary, R.N., *superintendent of University Hospital*, 1916

Zimmerman, Martha Eggleston, R.N., *assistant superintendent of University Hospital, with rank of instructor*, 1912–14

Appendix XV.
Graduates of the
University of Oklahoma
School of Nursing,
1913–1964

Abshire, Claire, 1932
Adams, Anna Jean, 1932
Adams, Burnace, 1922
Adams, Fern, 1945
Adams, Lucille, 1925
Adams, Virginia Mae, 1935
Adkins, Barbara Bross, 1961
Adwan, Emileen, 1947
Adwan, Kathleen, 1947
Akors, Patricia, 1947
Aldridge, Maureen Townsend, 1951
Alexander, Norene, 1930
Allen, Beverlyn, R.N., B.S.N.,
    1957
Allred, Carol Sue Owens, 1963
Alpers, Eva Lou, 1932
Amdall, Barbara, 1943
Amos, Ruby Ellen, 1941
Anderson, Jenna Vee, 1937
Anderson, Louise, 1930
Anderson, Noreen, 1944
Andrews, Vernita Carolyn Helms,
    1960
Androskowski, Irene, 1920
Anthony, Lois Irene, 1941
Archer, Katherine, 1948
Arman, Emma Bode, 1944
Arnold, Marilyn, 1956
Ashley, Una, 1921
Atkins, Jeanette, 1927

Atteberry, Mary A., 1946
Atwood, Marion, 1924
Avery, Joyce Brown, 1955
Ayers, Carole Pitzer, 1964
Babb, Helen, 1926
Bacon, Anna Marie, 1951
Baguhm, Dorothea Jean Burchardt,
    1953
Bailey, Frances, 1946
Bailey, Jeannette, 1942
Bain, Joyce Carter Burnett, 1953
Baird, Marion Rice, 1935
Baird, Marjorie, 1932
Baker, Alyce, 1924
Baker, Clara, 1918
Baker, Delphine, 1948
Baker, Eloise, 1944
Baldwin, Elizabeth, 1959
Ballard, Wanda Fay Mason, 1952
Banks, Norma Sue Ford, 1951
Barker, Reba Nell Turner, 1951
Barlow, Dorothy, 1941
Barlow, Margaret, 1944
Barnes, Ethel, 1925
Barnes, Jo Ann Wikle, 1955
Barnes, Virginia, 1956
Barnett, Norma Jean, 1951
Barton, Shirley, 1959
Bassham, Dorothy, 1957
Bastion, Ethel Maxine, 1943

Bates, Hazel Allene, 1937
Beam, Oleta, 1959
Beard, Frieda Cletha, 1942
Beaubien, Laura, 1918
Beaver, Lennie, 1933
Becker, Ella, 1926
Beckett, Hazel Lee, 1919
Beggs, Katherine, 1934
Bell, Juanita Manans, 1938
Bell, Lucy, 1924
Bennedum, Lucille, 1934
Bennett, LyVonne, 1957
Bentley, Julia, 1932
Bergsten, Mary Casteel, 1961
Bernard, Vera, 1945
Berndt, Gertrude Lucy, 1940
Berry, Alice Esta, 1940
Bettes, Joyce Florene, 1962
Bevers, Lazette, 1960
Bickel, Violet, 1921
Biddler, Thelma, 1928
Biddy, Frances Ellonor, 1942
Bieberle, Anna, 1943
Biggs, Freeda Floe, 1940
Biggs, Joann Young, 1957
Bigham, Maxine, 1936
Bigham, Mescal, 1947
Bigham, Ramona Bernandine, 1936
Blacks, Lillian, 1932
Blackwood, Ann, 1950
Blair, Florence, 1918
Blair, Jean, 1956
Blakley, Marie Elaine, 1944
Blakley, Ruby Ivalee, 1944
Bland, Aileen Louise Gunniz, 1953
Block, Alma, 1950
Bloont, Alberta, 1945
Boa, Jean Elizabeth Hill Ferguson,
    1955
Boarman, Elizabeth, 1927
Boatman, Kathleen Cassady, 1964
Boatright, Leota, 1931
Boaz, Susie Evelyn, 1935
Boczkiewicz, Helen, 1942
Boden, Bertha Ann Wilson, 1953

Bomar, Birdie, 1925
Bonham, Gyn, 1931
Bonham, Jonita, 1943
Borella, Emma Jean, 1933
Borella, Mary Elizabeth, 1932
Borror, Hester Louise, 1942
Boss, Marianlee Wilson, 1951
Bourlier, Alma, 1941
Bowen, Martha, 1928
Bowlin, Nancy, 1961
Boyd, Gerturde, 1939
Boyles, Patricia, 1955
Bradford, Thelma James, 1953
Bradley, Mary Nell, 1945
Bradley, Sarah, 1963
Bradshaw, Evelyn Jo Morrison,
    1952
Brand, Dolores Sharleen S. L.,
    1953
Brandley, Ann Clark, 1948
Branham, Florence Nadine, 1940
Branscome, Emma Jewel, 1937
Brasseur, Marie Irene, 1940
Bray, Pauline, 1936
Brewer, Clara, 1933
Brewer, Edith, 1926
Bridge, Mary, 1948
Bridges, Floriene, 1937
Bridwell, Roberta Lee Smith, 1954
Brittain, Cleo, 1921
Broady, A., 1950
Brock, Leona, 1948
Brooks, Josephine, 1934
Brooks, Velma May, 1940
Brower, Janice Lynn Spradling,
    1958
Brown, Alice, 1913
Brown, Betty Lou Kapka, 1951
Brown, Isabel, 1928
Brown, Jewel Janet, 1930
Brown, Marjorie, 1948
Brown, Mary Helen, 1947
Brown, Ruby Jean, 1959
Brown, Shirley, 1956
Brownson, Sondra Cooper, 1963

Bruns, Blanche Beatrice, 1939
Bryan, Estelle, 1921
Bryan, Rosa Lee, 1939
Bryant, Alice H., 1947
Bucknum, Dorothy, 1930
Bucknum, Ora, 1930
Bumgarner, Helen, 1948
Bump, Beula, 1943
Burch, Winnie, 1927
Burger, Jo Dcc Hurdcn, 1952
Burgess, Geneva Mae, 1949
Burgess, Loretta Muriel Church, 1951
Burris, Marjean Ford, 1963
Burrus, Nina, 1947
Burton, Karol Alyne, 1954
Burton, Mary F., 1959
Burton, Wilma Rose, 1946
Busby, Jonnie Lucille, 1938
Buswell, Jo Ann Sherrill, 1951
Bynum, Doris Ward, 1956
Bynum, Jessie Winifred, 1944
Bynum, Margaret, 1932
Byron, Blanche, 1929
Caesar, Alberta, 1922
Cahil, Marjory Leila, 1937
Campbell, Margaret, 1933
Canary, Alma, 1922
Cant, Nellie, 1933
Cantrell, Ethel, 1938
Carlton, Pauline, 1933
Carman, Yukola, 1935
Carpenter, Elizabeth E., 1947
Carrett, Ethel, 1933
Carrington, Mae, 1931
Carter, Altha, 1932
Carter, Claudia Joan, 1941
Carter, Elois, 1943
Carter, Marilyn Roberta Every, 1955
Carter, Naomi, 1956
Caskey, Flore Kirby, 1942
Castelburry, Mary E., 1943
Chadwick, Deloris, 1956
Chambers, Genevia, 1948

Chance, Sue, 1938
Chandler, Jonnie Pauline, 1942
Chaney, Lwana Sue, 1961
Chapman, Jessie LaVerne, 1946
Chapman, Valta, 1929
Chappell, Ada Ruth, 1933
Charvoz, Patsy Mayo, 1951
Chase, Sondra Sue Snyder, 1961
Chausse, Donna Bond, 1955
Chavcs, Vilma Peralta, 1963
Chilton, Gertie Lou, 1932
Chitwood, Maxine, 1935
Cisper, Helen, 1963
Clark, Joe Ann, B.S.N., 1955
Clark, Mary Frances, 1937
Clark, Patricia, 1959
Clark, Patricia Ann Meeks, 1960
Clement, Dorotha Olene, 1951
Cline, Marlene, 1958
Clum, Alice, 1940
Coble, Lorraine Louise, 1944
Cochran, Jo Mildred, 1937
Cochran, Ruby Mae, 1939
Cocks, Stella Louise, 1925
Codgill, Iris, 1933
Coleman, Paula, 1958
Collier, Linda, 1950
Compton, Carol Shaffer, 1963
Conerly, Cora Eugenia, 1934
Connoway, Marilyn Ann Harper, 1962
Conway, Kathleen, 1946
Cook, Jessie Marie, 1928
Cooke, Blanche, 1921
Cooke, Doris Jean, 1938
Cooley, Charlotte, 1947
Cooper, Beulah Bond, 1918
Copely, Naomi Catherine, 1934
Coppock, Mary Kathleen, 1940
Cosgrove, Doris Mae, 1946
Cousins, Tom, 1917
Coussins, Carole Handley, 1960
Covey, Pauline, 1947
Covington, Nell, 1931
Cox, Barbara, 1959

Cox, Olive, 1924
Coyner, Shirley Carolyn Stevens, 1951
Crabtree, Alberta Regina, 1938
Crawford, Deanna, 1961
Crawford, Jeanne, 1945
Crawford, Norma Jean Smith, 1952
Crews, Betty Eakins, 1951
Crimmett, Geraldine Lou, 1944
Crispins, Irene, 1933
Croan, Edith, 1917
Crook, Grace, 1922
Crook, Minnie, 1926
Crooks, Dora Ellen, 1936
Crouch, Geraldine, 1941
Crum, Irene, 1932
Crum, Mary Catherine, 1932
Crumrine, Norma Wiley, 1954
Culver, Ruth Hawkins, 1951
Culwell, Doris Evelyn, 1937
Culwell, Paula Janice, 1939
Cuppy, Mary Katherine, 1935
Curtis, Elizabeth Berky, 1951
Curtis, Ruth, 1943
Custer, Josephine Eloise, 1940
Cutler, Grace Ledbetter, 1944
Data, Josephine, 1931
Daugherty, Narcissa, 1932
Davidson, Margaret, 1931
Dawkins, Hattie, 1925
Dawson, Ruth Cleo, 1942
Dennis, Nancy Jane, 1961
Dersch, Dorothey, 1946
Dess, Virginia, 1945
Dewar, Margaret, 1945
DeWees, Frances, 1925
Dick, Eva Dean, 1945
Dickerson, Eugenia Hopkins Brand, 1953
Dickson, Grova Nelle, 1940
Diffle, Mary, 1931
Dillingham Sara, 1934
Dillman, Mary Joan Moore, 1955
Dittemore, Irene, 1950
Dodson, Elizabeth, 1928

Dolezal, Alice, 1956
Donat, Martha Gafford, 1962
Dooley, Anne Frances Murray, 1955
Doosing, Edith, 1929
Doosing, Naomi, 1930
D'Orsay, Joan Cravey, 1942
Dorsett, Dorothy, 1947
Dougherty, Lena, 1935
Douglas, Eugenia, 1928
Downen, Nina Ruth, 1947
Drye, Nellie, 1947
Duff, Alma, 1930
Duff, Ruby, 1930
Duffy, Sara Elden Ristell, 1960
Dugan, Nancy Jean Von Stetten, 1955
Duncan, Neva Juanita, 1935
Duncanson, June, 1943
Dunlap, Hazel, 1920
Dunn, Bernice Mae, 1938
Dunning, Eva, 1930
Dunscomb, Pearl, 1921
Dykes, Mary, 1947
Dys, Lillie B., 1919
East, Margaret, 1950
Easterling, Ruth, 1930
Ebarb, Clyo Ann Heck, 1960
Edgar, Kay, 1956
Edgar, Rachel, 1932
Edgerton, Amy Lois, 1939
Edmonds, Arlys Victorine Hodgson, 1960
Edmundson, Margaret, 1929
Edwards, Anna May Rickerd, 1954
Edwards, Betty, 1948
Edwards, Cleo, 1947
Edwards, Helen, 1936
Edwards, Ramona Keen, 1950
Eker, Martha Lynette Foster, 1957
Ellis, Josephine, 1939
Elwell, Mary, 1930
Enos, Mary Lou, 1942
Epperson, Nadine, 1947
Essary, Hazel, 1939

Estes, Fern, 1929
Evans, Nannette, 1931
Evans, Natalie, 1945
Evans, Rosie, 1950
Every, Margaret Mary, 1935
Eyler, Ruth Aryliene, 1941
Fair, Elizabeth, 1936
Fairless, Lucile Loretta, 1953
Fannin, Patt, 1925
Fanning, Willie, 1920
Farr, Goldie, 1933
Faulk, Irene, 1931
Faulkner, Isabel, 1924
Fellows, Beulah, 1925
Ferguson, Priscilla Whalen, 1964
Ferguson, Mildred Madeline, 1940
Ferguson, Sarah, 1945
Fields, Carolyn Ledbetter, 1957
Fimple, Joyce, 1950
Fimple, Thelma, 1943
Finnell, Imogene Adamson, 1959
Fiolle, Betty L., 1948
Fisher, Flossye, 1929
Fisher, Lois Williams, 1958
Fitch, Jo Crinklaw, 1960
Flanagan, Hazel, 1933
Flatt, Vivian Jewell, 1938
Fleming, Katherine, 1924
Fleming, Pauline, 1949
Flippin, Mary Elizabeth Marx, 1960
Flood, Eva Marie, 1919
Foale, Georgia Mae Holland, 1946
Forbes, Thelma Belle, 1937
Force, Rose Cellan, 1955
Ford, Joanne, 1957
Foster, Lula Ruth, 1920
Fox, Gladys, 1921
Francis, Edith Wilson, 1954
Freeny, June Merrick, 1955
Frost, Virginia Baldwin, 1962
Frye, Lela, 1933
Fuchs, Ora, 1934
Fuller, Ima Mae, 1948
Fulton, Bonnie Lorene, 1936
Fulton, Janice Brown, 1961
Gadberry, Minnie, 1932

Gadbow, Bethelyn Sue Jennings, 1961
Gallaspy, Mary Jane Simpson, 1953
Ganoung, Joy, 1948
Gardner, Dorothy Anna, 1955
Gardner, Yvonne Dorothy Bergner, 1954
Garner, Bonnie Jean, 1938
Garrett, Doris Ellen, 1942
Garrett, Ethel, 1924
Garrett, Eunice Kathlyn, 1939
Gastineau, Ellen Corinne Oliver, 1953
Geary, Francis Nutter, 1951
Gehrt, Irene Karr, 1955
Geiss, Edna, 1925
Gelsomino, C. Herberger, 1950
Gentner, Carolyn, 1959
George, Henryetta Frances, 1940
George, Thelma Geraldine Doty, 1954
Geter, Jacqueline Miller, 1962
Ghahremani, Dorothy Louise Smith, 1955
Gifford, Bonnie Belle Hughes, 1955
Gifford, Edglea Marie Mason, 1954
Gilbert, Ione, 1948
Gilbert, Jennie, 1930
Gist, Eloise, 1943
Gist, Martha Hazel, 1942
Gladden, Sarah Lee, 1952
Glenn, Fern, 1930
Glenn, Vera Hoe, 1925
Glennon, Loretta Weber, 1955
Glidewell, Cleo, 1925
Goldsmith, Helen, 1956
Goodson, Naomi Ruth, 1939
Goodwin, Virginia, 1943
Gookin, Wilma, 1933
Goose, Ima Jeanne, 1942
Gotcher, Jeanne McElroy, 1961
Gould, Margaret, 1918
Gowin, Mildred Roberts, 1937
Grandin, Carman, 1946
Graves, Drucilla L. Griggs, 1962
Graygo, Stella, 1933

Green, Evelyn Mae, 1944
Green, Frances, 1930
Green, Margaret Elsie, 1942
Green, Ruth, 1931
Griffin, Mae Etta, 1956
Griffith, Naomi, 1932
Griffy, Carolyn Dee, 1960
Grimes, Ara Naomi, 1940
Grover, Mary, 1929
Grubbs, Roxie Lillian, 1931
Gruenbaum, Anna, 1943
Gulich, Yvonne, 1934
Guthrie, Merry Mignon Thornton,
  1954
Halbrook, Helaine Kathleen, 1939
Hale, Helen Irene, 1941
Hall, Jerry, 1950
Hall, Joyce, 1956
Hall, Pauline, 1933
Hamburger, Margaret Sue, 1944
Hamil, Grace Ruth, 1946
Hammer, Joan, 1950
Hansard, Margaret, 1948
Hanson, Mary Ann, 1930
Harden, Ruth Erline Denton, 1955
Harder, Vesta, 1935
Hardin, Doris, 1957
Hardway, Beverly Jean Atkins,
  1954
Hardy, Florence, 1933
Hardy, Rosemary Antoinette
  Piering, 1944
Hargis, Linda Lou, 1954
Hargrove, Pauline, 1946
Harman, Bernice, 1925
Harmon, Margaret Ellen, 1944
Harms, Ruth Maydell James, 1941
Harper, Clarice, 1932
Harper, Esther, 1929
Harris, Billie Jo, 1948
Harris, Blanche, 1922
Harris, Mary Inez, 1940
Harris, Patsy Jo Ann Farris, 1952
Harris, Theda Jan Allen, 1957
Harrison, Claire Marie, 1939
Harrison, Georgia, 1920

Harvey, Betty Lois Barton, 1954
Hass, Clara, 1934
Hastings, Lois, 1929
Haug, Ruth, 1939
Hawkins, Ada, 1928
Hawley, Bessie, 1930
Hawthorne, Florence, 1932
Hayward, Mildred, 1938
Hazelton, Marie, 1931
Head, Mary Kathryn Gimlin, 1954
Heard, Charlotte Faye Tracy, 1954
Heaton, Edna, 1956
Henderson, Cordie, 1918
Henderson, Ethel, 1932
Hendricks, Jonnie, 1933
Hendrix, Billie Mae Cook, 1955
Henry, Francis Victoria, 1934
Hensley, Lela Florence, 1938
Henson, Elyse Smith, 1952
Herbelin, Wilma June Richardson,
  1953
Hermanstoffer, Goldia, 1921
Herrick, Grace Ann Ritchie, 1952
Hesser, Linda, 1956
Hester, Mildred, 1947
Hester, Virginia Charlene, 1944
Hewett, Bonnie Patterson, 1940
Hickman, Charlotte, 1938
Hicks, Coralie, 1955
Hicks, Elaine, 1956
Higginbotham, Opal, 1932
Hightower, Mary, 1946
Hilderbrandt, Agnes, 1924
Hill, Opal Viola, 1932
Hine, Dorothy, 1932
Hite, Lou, 1920
Hocket, Dolores Jean, 1955
Hofeld, Dottie, 1930
Hofley, Stella, 1927
Hogan, Dora, 1928
Hogue, Anna, 1945
Holcomb, Barbara Ann
  Montgomery, 1955
Holcomb, Lora, 1936
Holcomb, Vivian Sarah, 1936
Holt, Lessie, 1939

Holt, Lois Bland, 1939
Holt, Nina Lou, 1939
Holtzen, Verna Lee, 1955
Homes, Helen M. Bush, 1946
Hopkins, Bernice Triplett, 1946
Hornby, Viola Hicks, 1954
Hort, Marilyn Ann, 1952
Hostler, Margaret Link, 1946
Housh, Eula, 1948
Houston, Mildred, 1938
Houts, Marian, 1938
Howell, Vivian, 1934
Hubbard, Jenell Dykstra, 1946
Hudack, Emily, 1930
Huff, Frances Alice, 1938
Huff, Kathryn, 1947
Huffman, Rosa, 1926
Hughes, Effie Agnes, 1944
Hughcs, Janc, 1941
Hulet, Jerrie, 1964
Humphrey, Virginia, 1955
Hunnicut, Virginia, 1932
Hunt, Christine, 1943
Huntington, Edna Mae Snow, 1953
Hurlburt, Rosemary Carolin, 1940
Hussey, Helen Margaret, 1942
Hutchinson, Pattie, 1928
Hutchison, Billie Louise, 1944
Hutchison, Zoline, 1936
Hyde, Elsie Mae Brady, 1952
Hyde, Frances, 1945
Ice, Wanda Howell, 1950
Ickes, Louise Wildman, 1952
Inman, Ruth Walker, 1952
Irwin, Bessie Elizabeth, 1937
Irwin, Hazel Christina, 1941
Irwin, Ruth, 1920
Ivey, Zane, 1946
Jackson, Hester Mae, 1937
Jackson, Idella, 1958
Jackson, Julia Eithel, 1939
Jackson, Mabel Marie, 1937
James, Pauline, 1932
James, Stella Francis, 1940

James, Wilma, 1956
Jameson, Eunice, 1956
Jamison, Charlene W., 1946
Jantz, Lena, 1945
Jay, Doris, 1945
Jeffries, Lou Ann Pope, 1958
Jennings, Marilee Margaret, 1944
Jenry, Billie Jean, 1948
Jeter, Joan Keylon Hill, 1954
Johnson, Alma Mae, 1951
Johnson, Erma, 1933
Johnson, Jacqueline, 1946
Johnson, Jessie, 1918
Johnson, Joye Ann Wolfe, 1954
Johnson, June Lucille, 1938
Johnson, Lillian Mozelle, 1934
Johnson, Linda Arfstrom, 1962
Johnson, Lucille, 1929
Johnson, Mary Elizabeth Black,
   1954
Johnson, Vera Pauline, 1934
Johnston, E., 1943
Jolly, June, 1956
Jones, Betty Jo, 1948
Jones, Catherine (Kay) Warren,
   1954
Jones, Jennie, 1940
Jones, Lillian W., B.S.N., 1929
Jones, Margaret, 1913
Jones, Minnie Lou, 1952
Jones, Naomi, 1939
Jones, Naomi, 1947
Jones, Norma, 1959
Jones, Vesta, 1931
Jorgensen, Bobbie Jeanne Miller,
   1954
Kammerlocher, Ilene LaRae
   Widener, 1954
Kearney, Virginia, 1932
Kelly, Mary Jo, 1935
Kendrick, Kathy, 1959
Kennedy, Mary Jane, 1944
Kennedy, Mildred, 1952
Kensey, Betty, 1959

Kerley, Bobbie Patterson, 1951
Kerneck, Eula, 1925
Kernek, Della, 1926
Kerns, Lola, 1933
Killough, B., 1943
Killough, Bessie, 1925
Killough, Mary Maude, 1934
Kincaid, Mary F., 1947
Kincaid, Susan Wright, 1964
Kinchen, Madelaine, 1948
King, Billie R., 1946
King, Kathryn, 1933
King, Mattie, 1922
King, Rebecca, 1921
Kirby, Mabelle, 1934
Kissinger, Joan, 1943
Kissleburg, Thelma Blanche, 1938
Klein, LaVerne Faye, 1935
Kluck, Louise, 1933
Knight, Cora Sue, 1951
Koehn, Nettie, 1923
Kopacka, Marilyn, 1957
Kraybill, Sarah Louise, 1953
Kroaker, Edna Aleen, 1942
Kruger, Frieda, 1922
Kuhn, Edna, 1926
Kuhn, Minnie, 1927
Kurtz, Jean, 1964
Lacy, Carrie, 1924
Lacy, Rita Lou Dickson, 1953
Lacy, Ruth, 1924
Lamb, DeAnn, 1961
Lamb, Mildred, 1943
Lambert, Madie E., 1959
Lamons, Ruth, 1932
Lana, Sibyl, 1945
Lancaster, Florence Ethel, 1917
Landers, Jacqueline, 1947
Landreneau, June Marie Hewitt, 1964
Lane, Lotty Anna, 1941
Lane, Louise, 1946
Langley, Billie S., 1948
Lasiter, Temple Oleta, 1938

Latimer, Velma, 1930
Laubach, Charlene, 1957
Lauer, Mary, 1947
Laughlin, Harriet, 1923
Lawyer, Joanna, 1936
Layden, Etta Minnick, 1961
Lee, Bertha Margaret, 1933
Leeparm, Thelma, 1930
LeFavour, Jane, 1959
Legako, Irene Eva, 1941
Legg, Dorothy Armer, 1952
Leonard, Adnell, 1934
Leonox, Mildred, 1934
Lessley, Elizabeth, 1928
Leverich, Suzanne Sebring, 1962
Lewis, Cora Jean Green, 1954
Lewis, Evalyn, 1944
Lewis, Velma Belle, 1933
Lewis, Zenith, 1949
Likens, Wilbur Dan, 1962
Link, Laveta, 1950
Linn, Ann Loree, 1940
Linville, Clio, 1932
Linville, Neva Faye, 1934
Lister, Dardenella, 1943
Little, Elizabeth Janice, 1951
Little, Helen, 1926
Little, Ruth, 1948
Little, Wynona Lucille, 1938
Lloyd, Jane, 1940
Lloyd, Mary Patricia Markham, 1954
Logan, Altha, 1926
Long, Clara, 1945
Long, Marcella, 1935
Lord, Gloria Lee, B.S.N., 1955
Lorenson, Ruth Harris, 1955
Lorenz, Patricia, 1959
Lorrimer, Loretta, 1930
Loucks, Mattie, 1926
Lowder, Melba, 1956
Lowe, Nellie, 1946
Lowman, Edythe, 1930
Luddington, Bertha, 1929

Lukens, Helen Ruth, 1949
Lunsford, Mary Lou, 1959
Mabes, Ople Juanita, 1940
McAlister, Zelma Juanita, 1940
McCann, Vivian Eveline Cherry, 1955
McCartney, Judy, 1963
McCarver, Betty Louise McLendon, 1954
McCauley, Audrey Jackson, 1954
McClain, Jean Claire, 1951
McClain, Mariam Louisa, 1940
McClary, Fern Gilpen, 1955
McCleery, Dorothy Dixon Barrett, 1953
McClure, Della Lee, 1935
McCord, Dortha, 1948
McCormack, Leola, 1934
McCormack, Zora, 1950
McCoy, Wilma, 1930
McCracken, Betty Jean, 1952
McCracken, M., 1950
McDaniel, Betty Lou, 1943
McDonald, Waldrine, 1933
McElroy, Ruth, 1927
McEntire, Ruth Ann Moore, 1962
McGee, Anne, 1925
McGehee, Irene, 1934
McGilbrey, Vera Dick, 1947
McGill, Arlene, 1948
McGuire, Maude, 1927
McIlvoy, Jeannie Rose, 1938
McIntyre, Lillian, 1930
McKerracher, Ethel, 1944
McKinnon, M. Edna, 1917
Macklin, Barbara, 1945
McKool, Ruth Anne Hicks, 1961
McManus, Mildred Florence, 1939
McMillan, Patricia, 1943
McMurray, Helen, 1932
Madden, Judy Maxine, 1943
Magee, Marilyn, 1959
Mahan, Jean Gaedke, 1952
Maitlen, Florence, 1919
Maker, Elnora, 1948

Manitowa, Lorena, 1926
Manning, Anna Ruth Goad, 1951
Mansfield, Ernestine Farrell, 1961
Marianos, Louise Casey, 1952
Marlow, Polly, 1950
Marrs, Louise, 1933
Marrs, Shirley, 1947
Marsh, Patrika Jean, 1920
Martin, Carol S., 1947
Martin, Mae, 1927
Martin, Mary Jane, 1930
Martin, Nanetta, 1950
Martin, Thelma, 1933
Martin, Zela Fay, 1936
Mason, Rose Marie Hussman, 1954
Matheny, Ida, 1925
Mathews, Bonnie Ray, 1936
Matrin, Sandra Hale, 1961
Mattacks, Laura Alling Kibbe, 1955
Matthews, Patricia Ann Heinzig, 1954
Mealer, Leila, 1929
Meinhardt, Dolores Elayne Cole, 1952
Melton, Josephine, 1925
Menzer, Emma, 1934
Meriwether, Lena, 1933
Mervine, Beth, 1948
Mesley, Eloise, 1932
Mesley, Josephine, 1929
Meyers, Martha Maise, 1947
Michener, Jeanette Wood, 1960
Miles, Bernice, 1934
Milford, Mildred Louise, 1942
Miller, Annette Virginia, 1940
Miller, Barbara, 1956
Miller, Charla Kay Mills, 1960
Miller, Doris Aleen, 1935
Miller, Helen, 1931
Miller, Lottie, 1930
Miller, Lucretia, 1948
Miller, Mary Virginia, 1935
Miller, Nadine, 1936
Miller, Ruby, 1930
Miller, Shirley, 1958

Milligan, Melba Tucker, 1951
Mills, Lavena, 1959
Mills, Patsy Marilyn, 1951
Milner, Mary Rebecca Smith, 1952
Mingus, Ruby Jean, 1936
Minter, Willie Alma, 1934
Miracle, Mae, 1927
Mitch, Margaret, 1936
Mitchell, Harryette Margaret, 1951
Mitchell, Lula Grace, 1915
Moad, Lucille, 1943
Moad, Margaret, 1948
Moak, Katy Lee, 1926
Monday, Dolly Mae, 1934
Mondoza, Ruth, 1934
Moody, Maureen Janet, 1954
Mooneyham, Virginia Ione, 1940
Moore, Arzelia Sylvia, 1954
Moore, Harriett, 1927
Moore, LaVerne, 1933
Moore, Letha Johnson, 1953
Moore, May Belle, 1938
Moore, Patricia, 1959
Moore, Patti Jeanne Callihan, 1952
Morgan, Glenda Stevens, 1961
Morgan, Vera Adams, 1941
Moriarity, Vera, 1926
Moritz, Sue Ann, 1955
Moritzky, Fleeta, 1933
Morris, Tommie, 1956
Morris, Virginia, 1945
Morrison, Dorothy, 1931
Morrow, Hattie, 1933
Moss, Bennie, 1950
Mouck, Jewel Very, 1939
Mouschke, Volita Rehle, 1937
Muchmore, Donna Marie Stevens, 1954
Mueller, Reba Joy Kent, 1951
Murphy, Beryl Irene, 1938
Muse, Betty Jo Hewitt, 1951
Musick, Clarence Kathryn, 1937
Myers, Martha, 1947
Myers, Vinita, 1946
Nagel, Lillian, 1947

Nagel, Velma, 1956
Nance, Georgia Dee, 1933
Neinhuser, Hope Sprowls, 1963
Nesbit, Norman, 1929
Newman, Harriette, 1964
Nichols, Dianne, 1963
Nichols, Irene Simpson, 1935
Nichols, Sandra, 1961
Niles, Juanita, 1946
Nordstrom, Eva Emily, 1937
Norman, Evelyn, 1944
Norman, Maxine, 1944
Northcutt, Jennie Suzette Lalanne, 1960
Oberhouse, Peggy Virginia, 1942
Odell, Abbie, 1913
Ogan, Edith Sue, 1939
Ogilbee, Velma Jane Grubaugh, 1952
Oldham, Mae, 1925
Oliphant, Carmen, 1932
Oliver, Alzada, 1959
Omara, Betty Lou, 1947
O'Neil, Marguerita, 1945
O'Neill, Frances, 1945
Oneth, Helen Virginia, 1946
Orman, Emma Bode, 1945
Osborn, Mabel Lurene, 1946
Osteen, Amelia Correia, 1949
O'Toole, Joretta Nugent, 1953
Owen, Dora Alice, 1935
Owen, Guinn, 1948
Owens, Pattie, 1923
Page, Essie, 1920
Page, Lahoma, 1931
Pahcheka, Bernice, 1946
Palmer, Frances, 1935
Palmer, Marcella Evylin, 1942
Parks, May Belle, 1913
Parr, Blanche Elizabeth, 1957
Parr, Erma, 1930
Parrish, Colleen Lockhart, 1950
Parsons, Anna, 1959
Parsons, Ruth Imogene Scott, 1952
Patrick, Marilyn, 1957

Patterson, Geneva Audry, 1936
Patterson, Georgia Elizabeth, 1941
Patterson, Helen Evelyna, 1941
Patton, Doris, 1948
Payne, Betty Zink, 1952
Payne, Melva Vaughan, 1961
Peck, Nadine, 1945
Pendergraft, Carolyn Sue, 1964
Penrod, Lillian Brown, 1951
Perrin, Maple Malone, 1954
Phillips, Bobbye, 1948
Phillips, Margaret Lillian, 1944
Phipps, Cora Etta, 1913
Pickens, Pearl, 1943
Pinson, Lucille Bullard, 1952
Pitcock, Lucille, 1920
Platt, Elizabeth, 1924
Poindexter, Ruth, 1924
Polaski, Lena, 1920
Polson, Dortha, 1952
Pope, Ruth, 1949
Porter, Glenda Faye Potts, 1962
Porter, Susie, 1931
Portschy, Hilda, 1934
Poulter, Louise Van Horn, 1951
Pounds, Margaret Lorene, 1939
Powell, Judy Mae Smith, 1960
Prentice, Dorothea Beach, 1937
Presley, Lois, 1948
Preston, Mary Lou Baity, 1955
Price, Georgia Lorraine, 1944
Price, Victoria Lee, 1942
Priebe, Jean, 1945
Pritchard, Mary, 1943
Pritchett, Mary Annie Mae, 1935
Pritchett, Vera, 1940
Privette, Wilma, 1948
Proctor, Doris Oleta, 1946
Prollock, Betty, 1947
Pyatt, Shirley Eickhoff, 1951
Quillen, Mary Jean, 1941
Rader, Cynthia Reid Hayes, 1962
Railey, Julia Anne, 1939
Rainbolt, Flora, 1932
Ramsey, Anna Elizabeth, 1937

Rapp, Doris Laverne, 1940
Rapp, Helen Lorse, 1939
Rau, Faydelle Kuhlmann, 1952
Ray, Carol June, 1964
Reading, Ora Lee, 1918
Redpath, Pauline, 1927
Reed, Betty Beckett, 1952
Reed, Estelle Liles, 1940
Reed, Lois Nadine, 1940
Reed, Vida Tate, 1954
Reese, Henryette Jane, 1927
Reeves, J. Parr, 1950
Reevis, Etta Vee, 1947
Reggin, Mary Aleen Mabry, 1951
Regier, Lillie, 1959
Reimers, Doris Atteberry, 1951
Reinke, Dorothy Jane, 1941
Reynolds, Edith Melba, 1941
Reynolds, Ina Barton, 1933
Reynolds, Mamie, 1921
Reynolds, Olive Ruth, 1925
Rhodes, Edl Lee Foster, 1957
Rice, Nora, 1915
Rich, Helen, 1945
Richard, Freeda, 1946
Richard, Mary Katherine, 1930
Richardson, Jane, 1959
Richardson, Patricia, 1959
Richardson, S., 1943
Richburg, Predirta Lucille, 1946
Richerd, Helen Fay, 1954
Ricks, Trebreh, 1941
Riley, Beulah, 1922
Riley, Louise Robbins, 1949
Ritter, Jean, 1948
Rittersbacher, Opal Betty, 1941
Roark, Maydell, 1946
Roark, Maydell, 1946
Roark, Polly, 1950
Roberts, Edith, 1945
Roberts, Frances Morgan, 1955
Roberts, Hazel Maudine, 1940
Roberts, Helen, 1943
Roberts, Marie Steed, 1957
Roberts, Nina, 1933

Roberts, Rebecca, 1923
Roberts, Sally Frierson, 1946
Robertson, Clarice, 1921
Robey, Lenore, 1925
Robinson, Dixie, 1959
Robinson, Florence, 1930
Robinson, Jessie, 1948
Robinson, Lela, 1932
Robinson, Mona McGraw, 1953
Robinson, Wanda Mae, 1955
Robinson, Wayman, 1930
Roeber, Johnnie, 1946
Rogers, Ardath, 1941
Rogers, Sally Jo Eisenbeck, 1954
Roop, Mary Ellen, 1946
Ross, Jean Ann Ladwig, 1964
Ross, Mary Ellen, 1946
Ross, Ruth, 1949
Ross, Thelma Jean Beall, 1951
Roulet, Florence, 1935
Rowley, Hellen Emmaline, 1937
Roysden, Bobbie Marie, 1964
Rush, Mary Alice, 1945
Russell, Grace, 1919
Ryan, Rose Nell, 1942
Ryberg, Marie, 1934
St. Germain, Myrl, 1920
Sale, Mary Ann, 1935
Samson, Nelecta, 1946
Sanders, Billye Bob Hall, 1952
Sanders, Suzanne, 1945
Sarasin, Beverly, 1949
Savage, Alice Bernice, 1940
Sawyer, Geraldine Gallager, 1935
Sayre, Ethel, 1919
Scharnhorst, Loveda May, 1944
Schlecter, Ruth, 1930
Schmit, Zofia Irene Jedziniak, 1955
Schreiner, Freda, B.S.N., 1957
Schultz, Elouise Moore, 1957
Scott, Kathryn Marie, 1941
Scott, Nina Lynn, 1941
Scott, Ola Virginia, 1940
Scott, Sarah Jane Fortmann, 1957
Seamans, Mary Elizabeth, 1940

Seaton, Leon, 1964
Seaton, Roberta Wehrenberg, 1963
Seeger, Joy Lotspeich, 1957
Seelke, Martha, 1928
Sehested, Pernie, 1931
Shackelford, Avis, 1947
Shaefer, Catherine Martin, 1950
Shanks, Lottie Belle, 1933
Sharp, Connie Louise Atkins, 1951
Shaw, Velda, 1935
Shelton, Lometa Ozell, 1938
Sherril, Bette, 1946
Shields, Myrna, 1947
Shillington, Ellen, 1948
Shillington, Hellen, 1948
Shipley, Iva, 1946
Shire, Clara, 1934
Shire, Shirley Aileen, 1947
Shoemaker, Maurietta, 1930
Short, Cheryl Bernice Elerick, 1952
Shultz, Bernice May, 1940
Sieh, Marcia Kay Midkiff, 1963
Silvey, Billie June Hopkins, 1952
Simmerling, Velma, 1948
Simmons, Betty Joy Olmstead,
  1953
Simmons, Jean Marilyn McCreary,
  1951
Skinner, Alberta, 1924
Slama, Mary Jo, 1946
Slate, Virginia, 1959
Slemmer, Harriett, 1940
Slemmer, Mabel, 1923
Smalley, Jo Ann, 1948
Smedley, Helen, 1926
Smith, Agnes, 1935
Smith, Ann Dodd, 1955
Smith, Barbara, 1956
Smith, Clara Jane Johnson, 1954
Smith, Effie Katherine, 1923
Smith, Elaine Estelle Branson, 1954
Smith, Ethel Estelle, 1944
Smith, Glenita, 1957
Smith, Grace Cowdy, 1948
Smith, Hattie Belle, 1941

Smith, Hilda, 1936
Smith, Jo Moore, 1950
Smith, Lena, 1925
Smith, Lola, 1932
Smith, Loree, 1945
Smith, Mabel, 1921
Smith, Margaret Williams, 1951
Smith, Mary Ann Muskrat, 1951
Smith, Maxine, 1954
Smith, Miriam, 1935
Smith, Shirley, 1958
Smith, Shirley, 1959
Snider, Dulin Mae King, 1961
Snyder, Cora, 1934
Sommerville, Ruth Emmaline, 1935
Souders, Bessie, 1930
Southard, Laverda June High, 1952
Southwell, Blanche, 1947
Spencer, Geneva Winifred, 1941
Spencer, Mary Jane, 1939
Spengos, Patricia Carlisle, 1955
Spradling, Janice Brower, 1958
Spurgeon, Norma Ruth Walker,
    1952
Stafford, Gwendolyn Jean
    Boudreau, 1955
Stafford, Hermoine, 1935
Standish, Dorothy, 1956
Standley, Esther Elenora, 1941
Stapp, Mabel, 1930
Stark, Bessie, 1932
Stark, Dorothy Elaine, 1961
Stark, Frances, 1932
Stark, Lottie Irene, 1927
Stark, Medora Jane, 1940
Starkey, Winnie Mae, 1941
Starr, Barbara, 1958
Stauffer, Gladys, 1922
Steele, Julia Juanita, 1936
Stein, Patricia Anne Collum, 1953
Stephens, Barbara Ruth, 1943
Stephens, Sallie, 1916
Stephenson, Opal, 1943
Sterling, Dorothea, 1946
Sterling, Ida, 1956

Stevans, Etta Lee, 1930
Stiles, Ada, 1931
Stimson, Frances, 1946
Stolpe, Anna, 1927
Stone, Maribel, 1938
Stone, Nancy Lou Adcocok, 1953
Stone, Roberta, 1950
Storie, Betty, 1956
Story, Helen, 1946
Stovall, Barbara Frances Boles,
    1953
Stranathan, Doris Jana, 1943
Streck, Cleo Irene, 1941
Strong, Patricia, 1964
Stucker, Juanita, 1946
Studor, Betty, 1945
Sturgis, Flora Mae, 1949
Sullenberger, Lora Mae, 1938
Sullivan, Georgia Ann, 1934
Swain, Lillian, 1934
Swallow, Mildred, 1932
Swanson, Peggy, 1933
Sweatte, Ruth Elaine Wilson, 1954
Sykes, Michelle, 1963
Taber, Thelma, 1956
Tabor, Lucille, 1950
Tahkofper, Arlene Sue, 1954
Tanner, Lizzie James, 1933
Taylor, Alice, 1959
Taylor, Doris, 1927
Taylor, Gertrude, 1931
Taylor, Katherine, 1925
Taylor, Lillian, 1928
Taylor, Marilyn Jewart, 1946
Taylor, Pauline, 1931
Teders, Ella Louise Grove, 1954
Templeton, Mildred Edna, 1939
Terbush, Bonnie, 1932
Terbush, Edna, 1932
Terbush, Martha Genevieve, 1938
Thaxton, Helen E., 1940
Thickstun, Jo Esther Lewis, 1953
Thiessen, Thelma, 1945
Thompson, Anna, 1946
Thompson, Mabel, 1928

Thompson, Reba, 1946
Thompson, Virginia Dorlye, 1942
Tilley, Shirley, 1956
Tilton, Geraldine L., 1946
Tilton, Patricia, 1948
Timbers, Blanche, 1919
Tomasek, Ann Elizabeth Smyth,
   1954
Town, Tallie, 1959
Towne, Marilyn Carol, 1962
Townsend, R., 1943
Townsley, Rebecca, 1946
Triplett, Edythe Stith, 1923
Tuck, Hazel, 1927
Tucker, Dorene Eloise, 1939
Tucker, Sue, 1959
Tunnissen, Charlotte May, 1937
Turbeville, Donna, 1956
Turner, Barbara Ann, 1960
Turner, Bessie, 1928
Turner, Dolores Murphy, 1951
Turner, Grace Owens, 1938
Turrentine (Mrs. Harrison), 1930
Upp, Florence Marie, 1936
Utsey, Eileen Bandy, 1941
Utsey, Laura Smith, 1950
Van Leeuwen, Barbara Sawatsky,
   1958
Vammen, Alta, 1947
Vammen, Ardis R., 1946
Vanderhook, Penny, 1959
Van de Mark, Laura, 1927
Van Doren, Adelyn, 1929
Vaughan, Grace Elizabeth, 1941
Vickers, Una, 1934
Vincent, Mary Opal, 1931
Vinson, Tharyn Modine, 1941
Vogel, Maria, 1938
Waddell, Margaret, 1929
Wagnon, Essie, 1929
Waldby, Echo Geneva, 1946
Walker, Mary Jewell, 1941
Wallace, Janyth Morgan, 1957
Wallace, Martha Ann, 1951
Walters, Lela M. Walker, 1955

Walton, Winnie Estelle, 1936
Ward, Janice, 1936
Ward, Oleta, 1939
Ware, Betty Jean, 1955
Warhurst, Betty Madge, 1942
Washington, Clara, 1945
Washmon, Mina, 1948
Waterbury, Nina, 1932
Waters, Eva Annette Chambers,
   1954
Watkins, Marilyn Kay, 1962
Watkins, Nan, 1956
Watts, Winifred Fay, 1955
Weaver, Constance, 1961
Webb, June Barbara Marrow, 1952
Weber, Evelyn, 1934
Weber, Wilma, 1957
Webster, Zola Mae Hagin, 1953
Weems, Modine Velda, 1938
Weigand, Janet White, 1961
Wells, Lorene, 1943
West, Grace, 1925
Westmoreland, Susan Elizabeth,
   1913
Wettengel, Patricia, 1946
Wheeler, Alma Jean Helm, 1962
Wheeler, Beth, 1945
Wheeler, Fannie, 1932
Whisenant, Kathryn Sandlin, 1957
White, Margie, 1948
White, Nita, 1924
White, Tommy Jo, 1929
Whitis, Mary Jo, 1948
Whitlock, Myrna Tarkington, 1961
Whitlow, Katherine, 1927
Whitsell, Darlene Trosper, 1960
Whittaker, Alberta, 1929
Whittaker, Betty Bonneil, 1933
Wibking, Roberta, 1941
Wiebe, Matilda Elizabeth, 1939
Wiley, Joy, 1945
Wilhelm, Marjorie Turner, 1951
Wilkerson, Adelee June Hoffert,
   1955
Wilkens, Kathleen, 1945

Willey, Karen McElfish, 1963
Williams, Arnetta, 1948
Williams, Jamie Sue, 1957
Williams, Judith Dondelinger, 1952
Williams, Rosamund Cicely, 1964
Williams, Ruby, 1946
Wilson, Carol Bozarth, 1952
Wilson, Florence, 1948
Wilson, Madelyn L., 1946
Wilson, Margie, 1948
Wilson, Pauline, 1931
Wilson, Peggy Jo, 1944
Winburn, Billye Newton, 1951
Wishon, Dayse L., 1946
Wisler, Mabel Ruth, 1942
Wisner, Thurlene, 1964
Withiam, Phyllis, 1963
Witt, June Elizabeth, 1936
Witt, Mary Lee Reeves, 1946
Witwell, Alta, 1915
Wolfe, Opal, 1927

Wood, Dorothy Wertz, 1952
Wood, Muriel, 1945
Woodward, Dolores June Tingler, 1954
Wright, Lila, 1926
Wright, Verna, 1930
Wurman, Margaret Lininger, 1953
Wyatt, Billie, 1947
Yates, Madonna, 1959
Yeagley, Norma, 1947
Young, Gladys, 1928
Young, Jessie Jean, 1931
Young, Maxine, 1946
Young, Nora, 1921
Young, Ruth Evelyn Kramer, 1955
Youngblood, Emily Studdert, 1955
Yowell, Virginia, 1951
Zaleski, Martha Agnes, 1944
Zciders, Verna Lee Brammer, 1955
Ziegler, Charlene, 1945

Index of Persons

General Index

491